Staying Out of Trouble

in Pediatric Orthopaedics

Second Edition

David L. Skaggs, MD, MMM

Chief of Orthopaedic Surgery
Children's Hospital Los Angeles
Professor of Orthopaedic Surgery
University of Southern California Keck School of Medicine
Children's Hospital Endowed Chair of Pediatric Spinal
  Disorders
Los Angeles, California

John M. (Jack) Flynn, MD

Richard M. Armstrong, Jr, Endowed Chair
Chief of Orthopaedic Surgery
The Children's Hospital of Philadelphia
Professor of Orthopaedic Surgery
The University of Pennsylvania School of Medicine
Philadelphia, Pennsylvania

Mininder S. Kocher, MD, MPH

Chief, Division of Sports Medicine
Boston Children's Hospital
Professor of Orthopaedic Surgery
Harvard Medical School
Boston, Massachusetts

Kenneth J. Noonan, MD, MHCDS

Associate Professor
University of Wisconsin School of Medicine and Public
  Health
American Family Children's Hospital
Madison, Wisconsin

Michael G. Vitale, MD, MPH

Ana Lucia Professor of Pediatric Orthopaedic Surgery and
  Neurosurgery
Vice Chair, Quality and Strategy, Orthopedic Surgery
Columbia University Medical Center
Director, Division of Pediatric Orthopaedics
Chief, Pediatric Spine and Scoliosis Service
Morgan Stanley Childrens Hospital of
  New York – Presbyterian
New York, New York

Consulting Gurus

Lindsay Andras
Alexandre Arkader
Donald Bae
Jeffrey M. Bender
Laurel Claire Blakemore
Douglas L. Brockmeyer
Michael T. Busch
Elaine Butterworth
Michelle S. Caird
Henry G. Chambers
Haemish Crawford
Jon R. Davids
Alain Diméglio
John B. Emans

Mark A. Erickson
Nicholas D. Fletcher
Steven Frick
Theodore J. Ganley
Matthew A. Halanski
Martin J. Herman
Christopher Iobst
Lori A. Karol
Robert M. Kay
William Mackenzie
Todd A. Milbrandt
James O. Sanders
Wudbhav N. Sankar
Jeffrey R. Sawyer

Jonathan Schoenecker
Suken A. Shah
Kevin G. Shea
Benjamin J. Shore
Paul D. Sponseller
Daniel J. Sucato
Vernon T. Tolo
Paul S. Viviano
Kristy L. Weber
Ira Zaltz

Staying Out of Trouble
in Pediatric Orthopaedics

Second Edition

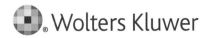. Wolters Kluwer

Philadelphia • Baltimore • New York • London
Buenos Aires • Hong Kong • Sydney • Tokyo

Director, Medical Practice: Brian Brown
Senior Development Editor: Stacey Sebring
Editorial Coordinator: Cody Adams
Production Project Manager: Sadie Buckallew
Design Coordinator: Joseph Clark
Manufacturing Coordinator: Beth Welsh
Prepress Vendor: TNQ Technologies

9 8 7 6 5 4 3 2 1

Printed in China

Library of Congress Cataloging-in-Publication Data

ISBN-13: 978-1-975103-95-8

Cataloging in Publication data available on request from publisher.

---

shop.lww.com

Dedications

This book is dedicated to my wife Val who supports me, makes me better, and is fun to share life with. I am grateful for my children Jamie and Clay who are my workout partners and friends who keep me humble. I am proud to report since the first edition my daughter Kira has entered medical school and tells me I no longer embarrass her (at least not too much). Finally, I am grateful to work with the team at Children's Hospital Los Angeles every day who joyfully share the high mission of caring for children.

—DLS

I dedicate this work to two groups of humans dear to me. First and foremost, my wife Mary, the love of my life, and our four children Erin, Colleen, John, and Kelly—poised to be a legacy that will bring us great pride and joy. Secondly, to all the great teachers and advisers I've had in pediatric orthopaedics who taught me how to stay out of trouble. If the wisdom in this book helps in the care of just one child, then the thousands of hours are surely time well spent.

—JMF

I dedicate this book to my family, my wife Mich and kids Sophia, Izzy, Calvin, Ava, and Henry, for their love, support, encouragement, and patience; my clinical mentors Drs. David Sabiston, John Feagin, John Hall, and Richard Steadman, who taught me not only how to stay out of trouble but also how to do the right thing when you find yourself in trouble; my colleagues at Boston Children's Hospital who bring out the best in each other and are the epitome of a high-functioning team; and finally to my patients who make it all worthwhile.

—MSK

This book is dedicated to my amazing wife Kristan, who is the most compassionate pediatric provider I know. I further recognize my five amazing children; Claudia, Samuel, Peter, Emma, and Claire, all who have a desire to serve others. It is the fact that I see my children in the eyes of my patients and the love in my patient's families that drives me to be the best I can be in service, research, and education. It is a privilege to do what I do.

—KJN

This book is dedicated to my wife (Andrea) and kids (Alexandra, Lucas, Nicholas, Marcus, and Michael) who keep me focused on what's right and important in this busy life. And to my father, the original Dr. Vitale, who continues to skillfully and compassionately serve his orthopaedic patients all these years later—and who modeled for me how to do the same. And finally to my patients and their families who constantly remind me what a solemn responsibility we have to do our best and stay out of trouble.

—MV

Consulting Gurus

Lindsay Andras, MD
Assistant Professor of Orthopedics
Department of Orthopedic Surgery
University of Southern California
Los Angeles, California

Alexandre Arkader, MD
Associate Professor of Orthopedic Surgery
Perelman School of Medicine at the
    University of Pennsylvania
Children's Hospital of Philadelphia
Philadelphia, Pennsylvania

Donald Bae, MD
Associate Professor
Department of Orthopedics
Harvard Medical School
Boston, Massachusetts

Jeffrey M. Bender, MD
Associate Professor
Department of Pediatrics
Keck School of Medicine at University of
    Southern California
Los Angeles, California

Laurel Claire Blakemore, MD
Professor and Chief, Pediatric
    Orthopaedics
Shriners Hospitals in Pediatric
    Orthopaedics
Orthopaedics and Rehabilitation
University of Florida
Gainesville, Florida

Douglas L. Brockmeyer, MD
Professor of Neurosurgery
Chief, Division of Pediatric Neurosurgery
Department of Neurosurgery
University of Utah
Salt Lake City, Utah

Michael T. Busch, MD
Consulting Associate
Department of Orthopaedic Surgery
Duke University
Durham, North Carolina

Elaine Butterworth, RN, BSN, CPN
Registered Nurse
Department of Orthopaedic Surgery
Children's Hospital Los Angeles
Los Angeles, California

Michelle S. Caird, MD
Associate Professor
Department of Orthopaedic Surgery
University of Michigan
Ann Arbor, Michigan

Henry G. Chambers, MD
Professor of Clinical Orthopedic Surgery
Department of Orthopedic Surgery
University of California
San Diego, California

Haemish Crawford, FRACS
Paediatric Orthopaedic Surgeon
Department of Paediatric Orthopaedic
    Surgery
Starship Children's Hospital
Auckland, New Zealand

Jon R. Davids, MD
Professor, Ben Ali Chair
Department of Orthopaedics
University of California Davis Medical
    Center
Sacramento, California

Alain Diméglio, MD
Professor
Department of Pediatric Orthopedic
Medical School University
Montpellier, France

John B. Emans, MD
Professor
Department of Orthopedic Surgery
Harvard Medical School
Boston, Massachusetts

Mark A. Erickson, MD, MMM
Professor
Department of Orthopedic Surgery
University of Colorado
Aurora, Colorado

Nicholas D. Fletcher, MD
Associate Professor of Orthopaedic
  Surgery
Department of Orthopaedic Surgery
Emory University
Children's Healthcare of Atlanta
Atlanta, Georgia

Steven Frick, MD
Professor and Vice Chair
Department of Orthopaedic Surgery
Stanford School of Medicine
Stanford, California

Theodore J. Ganley, MD
Professor
Department of Orthopaedic Surgery
The University of Pennsylvania School of
  Medicine
Philadelphia, Pennsylvania

Matthew A. Halanski, MD
Associate Professor
Department of Orthopaedic Surgery
University of Nebraska Medical Center
Omaha, Nebraska

Martin J. Herman, MD
Professor
Department of Orthopedic Surgery
Drexel University College of Medicine
Philadelphia, Pennsylvania

Christopher Iobst, MD
Director, Center for Limb Lengthening
  and Reconstruction
Department of Orthopedic Surgery
Nationwide Children's Hospital
Columbus, Ohio

Lori A. Karol, MD
Professor
Department of Orthopaedic Surgery
University of Texas Southwestern Medical
  Center
Dallas, Texas

Robert M. Kay, MD
Professor
Department of Orthopaedic Surgery
Keck School of Medicine at University of
  Southern California
Los Angeles, California

**William Mackenzie, MD, FRCSC,
FACS**
Professor
Department of Paediatric Orthopaedic
  Surgery
Sidney Kimmel Medical College
Thomas Jefferson University
Philadelphia, Pennsylvania

Todd A. Milbrandt, MD
Associate Professor
Department of Orthopedic Surgery
Mayo Clinic
Rochester, Minnesota

James O. Sanders, MD
Frank C. Wilson Distinguished Professor
Chair Department of Orthopaedics
University of North Carolina at Chapel
  Hill, North Carolina

Wudbhav N. Sankar, MD
Associate Professor
Division of Orthopaedic Surgery
The University of Pennsylvania
Philadelphia, Pennsylvania

Jeffrey R. Sawyer, MD
Professor
Department of Orthopaedic Surgery
University of Tennessee – Campbell Clinic
Memphis, Tennessee

Jonathan Schoenecker, MD, PhD
Associate Professor and Jeffrey Mast
  Chair of Orthopaedics
Departments of Orthopaedics,
  Pharmacology, Pathology and Pediatrics
Vanderbilt University Medical Center
Nashville, Tennessee

Suken A. Shah, MD
Associate Professor
Departments of Orthopaedic Surgery and
  Pediatrics
Sidney Kimmel Medical College
Thomas Jefferson University
Philadelphia, Pennsylvania

Kevin G. Shea, MD
Professor & Vice Chief
Department of Orthopaedic Surgery
Stanford School of Medicine
Stanford, California

Benjamin J. Shore, MD
Associate Professor
Department of Orthopedic Surgery
Harvard Medical School
Boston, Massachusetts

Paul D. Sponseller, MD
Professor of Orthopaedic Surgery
Department of Pediatric Orthopaedics
John Hopkins University
Baltimore, Maryland

Daniel J. Sucato, MD, MS
Professor
Department of Orthopaedic Surgery
University of Texas Southwestern Medical
    Center
Dallas, Texas

Vernon T. Tolo, MD
John C. Wilson, Jr., Professor of
    Orthopaedics
Department of Orthopaedic Surgery
Keck School of Medicine at University of
    Southern California
Los Angeles, California

Paul S. Viviano
President and CEO
Department of Administration
Children's Hospital Los Angeles
Los Angeles, California

Kristy L. Weber, MD
Professor
Department of Orthopaedic Surgery
University of Pennsylvania
Philadelphia, Pennsylvania

Ira Zaltz, MD
Professor
Department of Orthopaedic Surgery
Oakland University William Beaumont
    School of Medicine
Royal Oak, Michigan

Contributing Authors

Richard C. E. Anderson, MD
Associate Professor
Neurological Surgery
Columbia University
New York, New York

Alexandre Arkader, MD
Associate Professor of Orthopedic Surgery
Perelman School of Medicine at the
    University of Pennsylvania
Children's Hospital of Philadelphia
Philadelphia, Pennsylvania

John M. (Jack) Flynn, MD
Richard M. Armstrong, Jr., Endowed
    Chair
Chief of Orthopaedic Surgery
The Children's Hospital of Philadelphia
Professor of Orthopaedic Surgery
The University of Pennsylvania School of
    Medicine
Philadelphia, Pennsylvania

Robert M. Kay, MD
Professor
Department of Orthopaedic Surgery
University of Southern California Keck
    School of Medicine
Los Angeles, California

Mininder S. Kocher, MD, MPH
Chief, Division of Sports Medicine
Boston Children's Hospital
Professor of Orthopaedic Surgery
Harvard Medical School
Boston, Massachusetts

Vincent S. Mosca, MD
Professor
Department of Orthopedics and Sports
    Medicine
University of Washington School of
    Medicine
Seattle, Washington

Kenneth J. Noonan, MD, MHCDS
Associate Professor
University of Wisconsin School of
    Medicine and Public Health
American Family Children's Hospital
Madison, Wisconsin

Ernest L. Sink, MD
Associate Professor of Orthopaedic
    Surgery
Hospital for Special Surgery
Weill Cornell Medical College
New York, New York

David L. Skaggs, MD, MMM
Chief of Orthopaedic Surgery
Children's Hospital Los Angeles
Professor of Orthopaedic Surgery
University of Southern California Keck
    School of Medicine
Children's Hospital Endowed Chair of
    Pediatric Spinal Disorders
Los Angeles, California

Michael G. Vitale, MD, MPH
Ana Lucia Professor of Pediatric
    Orthopaedic Surgery and Neurosurgery
Vice Chair, Quality and Strategy,
    Orthopedic Surgery
Columbia University Medical Center
Director, Division of Pediatric
    Orthopaedics
Chief, Pediatric Spine and Scoliosis Service
Morgan Stanley Children's Hospital of
    New York–Presbyterian
New York, New York

Klane K. White, MD, MSc
Professor
Department of Orthopaedics and Sports
    Medicine
University of Washington
Seattle, Washington

Contributing Authors

Preface

Orthopaedic textbooks generally come in two varieties:

1. Encyclopedic syntheses of the research literature, with background information on disease etiology, surgical indications, and authors' preferred methods for treatment. These texts are unbeatable references.
2. Technique manuals. These texts are great to review the night before a procedure that the practicing surgeon does not do regularly or that the surgeon in training is learning to do.

Both of these textbook types are valuable, and many competing versions are published each year and purchased by orthopaedic trainees, surgeons, and libraries.

Staying Out of Trouble in Pediatric Orthopaedics is a completely different concept. This is a book of wisdom, not just synthesized facts. You cannot Google this stuff. The editors, authors, and gurus have over 1,000 years combined experience of caring for children with orthopaedic problems. They are thought-leaders in the field (no chapter was written by a trainee or editorial assistant), and they aim to share all that they have learned about delivering the best possible care for children. The essence of this book is promoting safe and high-quality care—yes, preventing complications, but also optimizing interactions with families.

Rather than a book that you dust off a couple times a year to peruse a few pages about a specific condition or technique, *Staying Out of Trouble in Pediatric Orthopaedics* should live on the bedside table or beside your favorite chair and be read like a novel or a nonfiction thought-provoker. It contains loads of advice for dealing with situations, patients, families, and staff, completely based on real-life experience. We all know that despite the surgeon's very best efforts, stuff happens. Leaders in the field share problems they have encountered and bad outcomes they have experienced to help you avoid such "stuff" in your own practice. The writing style is designed to remind you of your best mentors, teaching you in the clinic or operating room. The material is covered with humor, empathy, and heaps of insight. Plus, there are cartoons.

This second edition of *Staying Out of Trouble in Pediatric Orthopaedics* reflects the explosive growth and increasing subspecialization of the field since the first edition was published in 2006. We have added new chapters on sports medicine, early-onset scoliosis, and the adolescent hip, reflecting areas of tremendous growth in the 21st century, plus another on leadership, as we could all use help with that. In addition to a designated expert guru or two for each chapter (who chime in with additional personal insight and tips), *Staying Out of Trouble in Pediatric Orthopaedics* incorporates input from the book's editors, whose opinions and reminders are likewise added to the voice of the chapter authors. The "discussion" that results from the multiple voices in each chapter increases both the diversity of opinion and the sheer volume of profound wisdom being offered to you by thought-leaders. The new features "Newsflash!" and "Orthopaedics 101" emphasize critical principles in caring for patients. A summary box of key points for staying out of trouble ends every chapter to hammer home the essentials. (We are all so easily distracted these days—summaries are needed!)

The editors of *Staying Out of Trouble in Pediatric Orthopaedics* have written literally hundreds of book chapters ourselves over the years. We did this book not to add to our CVs or as a favor to a senior author making request, but as a mission. We sincerely hope that those who care for children with orthopaedic problems will enjoy this read, share it with their trainees and partners, and avoid the "trouble" described and illustrated.

David L. Skaggs, MD, MMM

John M. (Jack) Flynn, MD

Mininder S. Kocher, MD, MPH

Kenneth J. Noonan, MD, MHCDS

Michael G. Vitale, MD, MPH

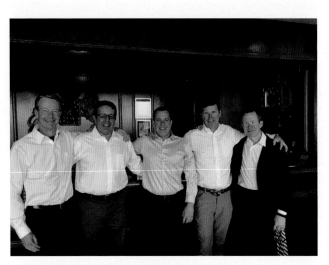

My best friend is the one who brings out the best in me.

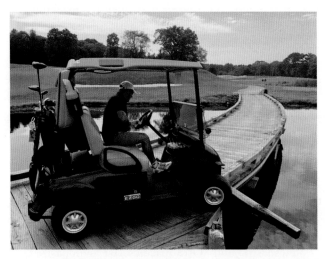

Studies show we are really not good at multitasking. Stay out of trouble by giving full attention to the task at hand.

Acknowledgments

The Editors would like to acknowledge Grace Caputo who we worked with often more than once each day. Grace saw the specialness of this text and took this on as her mission to help make this the best text possible.

Contents

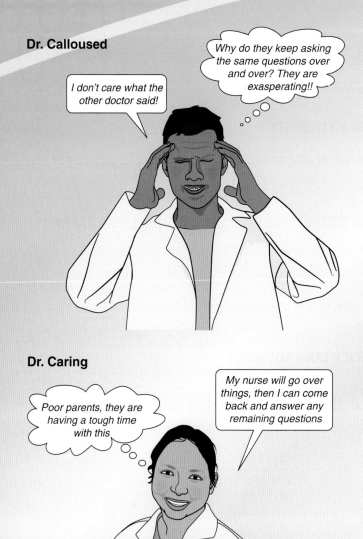

Chapter 1

Partnering With Families

DAVID L. SKAGGS, MD, MMM

Gurus: Elaine Butterworth, RN, BSN, CPN and Lori A. Karol, MD

There is no question that partnering with parents requires a significant amount of time and energy on the part of the doctor and entire health care team. At times, the demands may seem unreasonable. However, very few things in life compare to the sincere depth of gratitude we receive from parents, children, and others when caring for a sick or injured child. One of the wonderful things about caring for children's orthopaedic problems is that we can significantly improve, or cure, most of the children we care for, and we often become part of their lives for many years.

Psychologists tell us that the death of one's child is perhaps the most painful thing a human may experience; worse than divorce or loss of a spouse. By extension, when a child is in pain, sick, or at risk of harm, a parent may actually suffer more than the child. Anger or other irrational behavior on the parent's part is a common response to this stress. A child with health problems can be a severe stress to a marriage. Caregivers must have broad shoulders to carry the weight of the family's problems. Acknowledging a parent suffering and accepting responsibility to care for the parent as well as the child is an important aspect of a healthy doctor-family relationship.

Simply smiling and starting "from a place of yes" can set a positive tone. It is almost always possible to answer a demand with "Yes, we can do what you suggest, but must consider these consequences …" When a parent expresses anger toward you, monitor your emotions. It is natural to become defensive. Instead of being defensive, it may be better to say, "It was not my intent to make your child worried by discussing this complication."

If this seems a bit too touchy-feely, remember staying out of legal trouble in pediatric orthopaedic surgery may be more dependent on the family's feelings toward the doctor than technical skill or outcome.

Heightened Emotions Decrease Logical Understanding

Families are frequently so overcome with emotion after hearing their child may have a perceived serious medical condition, need surgery, or face risks and complications, that they are unable to process or remember much of what the doctor said. This can lead to confusion, anxiety, extra office visits, and multiple phone calls.

When family members repeat the same question multiple times, it is likely that the answer was not effectively communicated (given and/or received) the first couple of times, or they did not like the answer. Either way, this is a cry for help that more communication is needed. It may be tempting to ignore this during busy office hours when other families are waiting, but ignoring it will cause more problems in the long run and degrade your stature in the eyes of the family. Repeated questions are a time to lean in.

Busy physicians do not always physically have the time to answer every question, particularly repeated questions. We cannot stress how valuable it is when a nurse or physician assistant spends time with families after the doctor leaves the room to answer questions and make certain that the family "heard" what was said. Resources spent on patient education and relationship building are well worth it.

One technique for addressing repeated questions is to gently point out that the question was already asked and inquire if they understand the answer. This often elicits the parents' underlying concerns.

Dr. Flynn Adds

A concept to consider in dealing with a family is the profound difference between a family thrown into your lap by a serious injury that you meet moments before important surgery and that family you've been shepherding through bracing for 3 years and eight visits and that is now facing elective surgery. Those are very different dynamics.

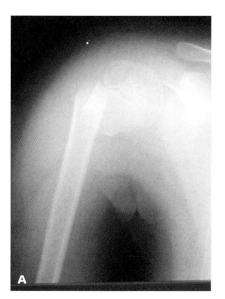 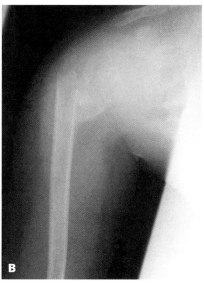 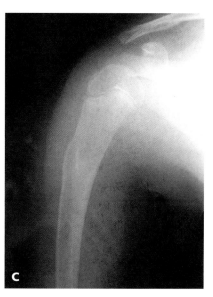

Figure 1-1 **A:** An 8-year-old boy with a proximal humerus fracture. The father was a medical malpractice plaintiff's attorney and was referred to me with a recommendation of surgery from the original orthopaedic surgeon. Treatment with a shoulder immobilizer was started. **B:** One month after injury, the patient's range of motion was poor and the father's concern was increased. Examples such as these X-rays that show remodeling of similar fractures were provided as teaching files to help relieve parents' and surgeon's anxiety. **C:** One year after injury, the patient had full range of motion with no sequelae.

Expectations

Understanding and managing parental expectations is a key step for staying out of trouble in pediatric orthopaedics. Parents' satisfaction with their child's care depends on their expectations almost as much as the outcome of surgery. Take the example of a 3-year-old girl with a midshaft femur fracture treated in a spica cast that healed in 5° of valgus with a minor limp persisting 3 months after injury. At this point many parents are concerned and even upset when they see that the bone has healed in a "crooked" position and that their daughter is not walking normally. In contrast, parents who have been adequately prepared may be thrilled that the femur healed in a nearly straight position that will continue to improve without their child needing surgery (which they learned carries risks and results in scars). Furthermore, they feel fortunate that her limp is almost gone already, as the doctor told them children often limp for 6 months following a femur fracture.

Sharing X-ray images of fracture remodeling (forearm, femur, and proximal humerus are good examples) with families is a highly efficient means of guiding parental expectations and preventing unwarranted anxiety before it occurs. Feel free to make copies of Figures 1-1 and 1-2 for your patients. A small amount of time spent at the beginning of treatment often saves large amounts of time later explaining "unexpected" progress and pays rich dividends toward the family's satisfaction and the doctor's reputation. A surgeon who warns a family ahead of time of loss of forearm rotation with a radial neck fracture looks like a prophet (Fig. 1-3). A surgeon who tries to explain it after the fact is more likely to be perceived as covering up bad results.

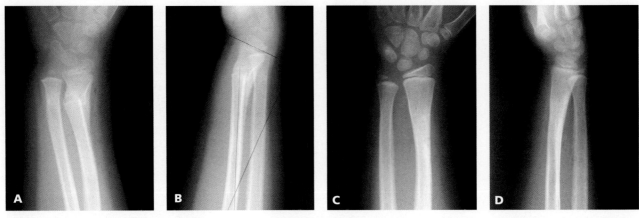

Figure 1-2 A, B: A 6-year-old girl with angulation on X-ray and a bump on her arm 1 month after injury. The mother, who is a doctor as well as my wife, was less than happy. X-ray examples of remodeling helped restore marital bliss. **C, D:** Six months later, the fracture had nearly fully remodeled.

All Kinds of Families

The care team should know the relationship of all the people in the room to the patient, such as parents, stepparents, uncle or aunt, friends, etc. Prior to treatment, clarify who is the legal guardian otherwise you may discover at the time of surgical consent, or worse on the day of surgery, that the child's legal guardian is unaware of the planned surgery. Often, extended family members or siblings may be useful, particularly in cases of language or comprehension challenges.

Beware that some parents going through a divorce consciously or unconsciously use their child's health care as a bargaining chip against each other. A surgeon may help diffuse this dynamic with an explicit reminder to both parents of the common goal of doing what is best for the child. Although it takes more time, it may be best to give each divorced parent a teaching handout and to meet with each parent separately or follow-up with a phone call to the absent parent at the end of the day. Document this, as I have seen these conversations brought up in divorce proceedings. It is important that neither parent senses you are taking sides or have secrets with the other parent; maintain neutrality. Make certain your responsibility to the child presides over any social discomfort on your part.

Who's in Charge Here Anyway?

Some interesting situations arise with the doctor-family relationship in terms of authority. A common scenario is that the parent wants you to pronounce what is "best" for the child and with the understanding that the parents will enforce the will of the adults. This is effective for a baby needing a vaccine, but can be emotionally devastating for the 13-year-old girl considering brace treatment for scoliosis. When a child transitions into a self-aware human participating in their own destiny, varies by family, social setting and child.

A common pitfall is to ignore the child and speak only to the parents. We recommend erring in the other direction. Early in the examination, talk to the child. Even if a young child may not grasp all you say, looking them in the eye, speaking gently, and showing them respect convinces the child you are on their side. The

Dr. Wise

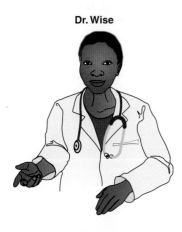

Dr. Defensive

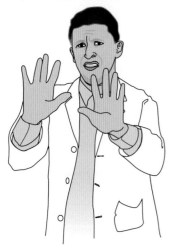

Figure 1-3 The difference between families thinking you are Dr. Wise or Dr. Defensive may be no more than how you initially set patient expectations.

parents will still hear your words, and just as importantly, they will recognize your caring approach to their child. I often turn to parents early in the visit and tell them I will answer all their questions before the visit is done, but I would like to chat with their child first.

Let us return to the scenario of the 13-year-old girl with newly diagnosed scoliosis who may be a candidate for brace treatment. Some parents state that the child will wear a brace at all times before the child has a chance to talk, which could increase the likelihood of bracing becoming an emotionally charged issue between family members.

A doctor with a high emotional intelligence will "read the room" and try to prevent family members to taking sides on issues until a balanced discussion of pros and cons has occurred. I have found it very helpful to tell the older child or adolescent that I work for them, that they own their body, and within reason I will not do anything to their body without their permission. Parents are usually quite appreciative of your genuine commitment to their child's well-being and of your respect for them as a person.

People Listen to You

When addressing a graduating class of medical students at Columbia University College of Physicians and Surgeons, television personality Larry King said, "The special thing about doctors is, people listen to their doctors more than any other profession." Be wary of how various treatment options are presented, because your prejudices will almost certainly come through. Providing a balanced view of various options and involving your nurse or physician assistant allows the family to participate in treatment decisions. If a child, and especially a teenager, feels they have chosen their course of treatment, everyone is happier, and compliance is more likely.

It is notable that for the past 17 consecutive years, the Gallup poll has found nursing to be the highest rated profession for honesty and ethics. We have found nurses and physician assistants with sufficient expertise, emotional intelligence, and dedication to be an invaluable resource for families throughout the course of their treatment. A great deal of a family's positive feelings about their medical care and their doctor results from their relationship with a nurse or physician assistant.

Nonaccidental Trauma

There is no easy way to tell a parent that nonaccidental trauma is suspected. The language used in this setting should be carefully chosen. The phrase "child abuse" is associated with parental blame or inadequacy and will most likely lead to defensiveness on the part of the parents. Saying "There is a possibility that someone may have injured the child" may be less likely to alienate the parents. This conversation should be held in a private setting, in an unrushed manner. If necessary, the physician may add that if there is any question of the possibility of nonaccidental trauma, the child must be evaluated or the physician could lose his or her license—this is the law. This may help the parents understand that the physician is not acting out of malevolence. Again, in keeping with the central themes of this chapter, if the parents feel that you genuinely care for the child, problems are uncommon. To stay out of trouble on the topic of nonaccidental trauma, if there is any suspicion, get the proper specialists involved. Be cognizant that some parents may react violently, particularly if alcohol or drugs are involved.

Dr. Flynn Adds

It's incredibly important to sit for conversations. Get the parents in chairs and the patient up on the examination table, higher than all. You sit on a low stool, so the child is looking down on you.

THE GURU SAYS...

I can't tell you how often families seek other opinions and allow the child to choose their doctor. Frequently, the moms tell me the kids chose the doctor who spoke to them, listened, and valued the child's opinion.

ELAINE BUTTERWORTH

THE GURU SAYS...

I find the best way to inform a family that I am calling in the child abuse team is to say, "It's my job to refer every single child like your baby that has (a femur fracture, multiple fractures, etc) for a formal child abuse evaluation. Nearly all families clear this evaluation without a problem, but I am required to identify the one in a hundred that has nonaccidental trauma."

LORI KAROL

Dealing With Challenges in the Relationship

Sometimes parents will be angry at doctors. They may not be having their best day. Good negotiators try to come back to common ground when things get heated. In this case, the common ground is easy to find, parents and the doctor wants what is best for the child. Simply telling parents, "My job is to give your child the very best care possible, we are on the same team" is generally all it takes. But remember, actions and body language speak louder than words.

If you don't feel that you are giving 100% for that child and family, or you feel that the family does not have faith in you or trust you, you should probably not be the child's doctor. One option is to state in a quiet and respectful fashion first verbally, then in the medical record, that you feel there is "not a good fit" between doctor and family and you recommend the family seek care elsewhere. Do not get into any details that can be argued; simply saying "not a good fit" is sufficient. In particular, do not proceed with elective surgery involving significant risks if it does not feel right in your gut. This will minimize trouble for you and your team. However, if this situation occurs more than a few times a year, it may be cause for concern about the doctor's professionalism.

"I Want Something Done About This."

"I have already been to two other doctors who won't do anything. I am not dumb, and I can see that Junior's (feet turn in/feet are flat/legs are bowed, etc.). I want something done about this" (Fig. 1-4). This is the time to take a Taoist approach,

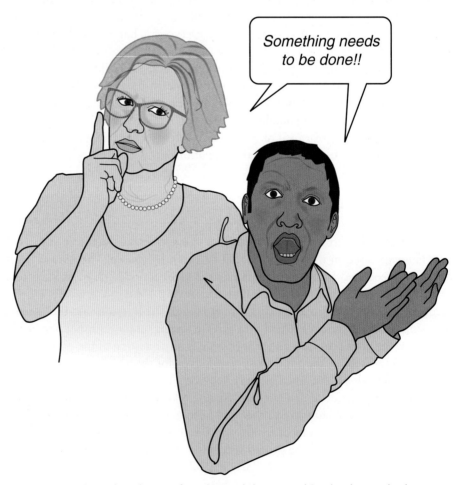

Figure 1-4 Patients' loved ones often demand that something be done, whether or not something *can* be done.

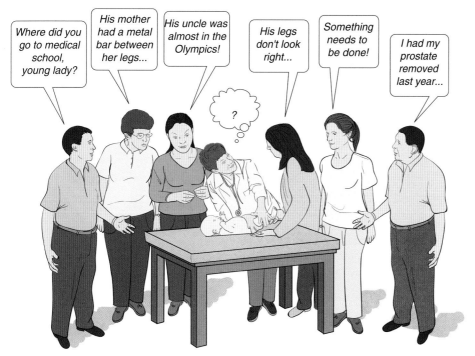

Figure 1-5 Nearly every orthopaedic chief resident has had the thought, "I really like pediatric orthopaedics; I'm just not certain I want to deal with parents."

avoid confrontation, and go with the parent's spirit of wanting what is best for the child. Your opinion that nothing needs to be done is based on knowledge that the parent does not have. Before stating your opinion, give parents the "data" on the condition without a recommendation, and they will hopefully conclude the same opinion that you have. Remember that parents generally want what is best for their children. If they are asking for something else, it is usually due to a lack of medical understanding, with education usually, but not always, being the cure. One must, however, ultimately do what is right for the patient and not just appease the parents (Fig. 1-5). It does not seem ethical to subject a child to a Dennis-Brown bar just to satisfy the parents.

When Things Go Wrong

Sometimes the most difficult aspect of having a complication is recognizing it and accepting it yourself. Confidence is necessary to be a good surgeon, but too much of it creates a blind spot. We have all seen overconfident surgeons; vow early in your career not to be that surgeon. The next challenge is explaining the complication to the family. It is best if parents hear it from you first. If they hear it from anyone else, particularly after they sought a second opinion or plaintiff attorney, it will erode your credibility in their eyes. It would be nice to be perfect, but most of us should simply aspire to recognize problems quickly and accept fault early. Any perception that a complication is being covered up or minimized could lead to anger and suspicion.

There is benefit both legally and clinically to sharing the case with trusted peers for advice and documenting this. Tell the family you did this, so they know you are taking the situation seriously and giving it extra attention. If handled correctly, families of children who have had complications often become your staunchest supporters.

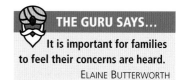
THE GURU SAYS...
It is important for families to feel their concerns are heard.
ELAINE BUTTERWORTH

Dr. Flynn Adds

If the same questions come from almost every family in a particular situation ("Your daughter needs an ACL reconstruction"), it's great to be able to offer clearly written and well-illustrated patient teaching handouts, answering FAQs. Don't make an electronic version—people will post it online. Hand them something to go home with. It feels like a tangible gift, and a great reference for when the mind and emotions settle. And, wow, a well-written and illustrated handout (such as shown in Fig. 1-6) can save a ton of phone calls to busy physician assistants and nurses.

Feet Turn In

Many children have feet that turn in. This is usually not a serious problem. It may be caused by the child's position while in the mother's uterus and usually corrects over time without treatment. These conditions generally do not cause any limitation in activity or delay normal growth and development.

A child's feet turning in is usually noticed in the first few years of life. It develops from one of three areas: the foot, the shin, or the thigh.

Foot: Metatarsus Adductus or Metatarsus Varus

This is most often recognized by parents during infancy and is very common. If the foot can be easily put in the correct position, no treatment is necessary, though your doctor may ask you to stretch the feet at home, and return to the office to make certain the feet are straightening with growth. In the unusual case that the foot cannot be easily straightened by gentle manipulation, your physician may recommend treatment, most frequently a cast. Scientific studies do not support using a brace or special shoes to help straighten the foot faster than normal growth.

Shin: Internal Tibial Torsion

The larger bone in the lower leg (tibia) may be slightly twisted or rotated inward and cause the foot to turn in. It is often first noticed when your child starts walking. Many parents believe the turned-in feet cause their children to trip more frequently. Fortunately, children usually grow out of this condition before age 10. If a child does not grow out of this condition, there is scientific evidence suggesting that internal tibial torsion is associated with being a faster sprinter. Many famous athletes have tibial torsion. There is no scientific evidence that bracing, special shoes, exercises or any other treatment short of surgery can correct the torsion. Surgery is very rarely needed in otherwise normal children.

Thigh: Femoral Anteversion or Torsion

This is caused by an inwards twisting of the thigh bone. When your child starts walking you may notice the feet and knee caps point inward. When the child runs, the feet may fly out sideways and make running appear clumsy. The turning in of the feet and knees may even appear to worsen in the first few years during the normal period of relaxation of the child's hips. Your child may be able to twist legs or sit in positions that would be uncomfortable for most adults. Fortunately, this condition will gradually improve over time (up till age 10) as your child grows and does not require treatment. Surgery is very rarely needed in otherwise normal children. There is no scientific evidence that braces, sitting position, exercises, or any treatment corrects or speeds up the natural improvement of this condition.

Special Shoes

In spite of a lack of scientific evidence, many parent and grandparents want something done, and feel that special shoes or braces couldn't hurt. Frequently, members of the family may have been treated with braces during childhood and their feet stopped turning in. It is important to remember that even if these people had not been treated with braces, their feet would have probably stopped turning in as a part of natural growth.

Researchers have found that adults who wore corrective shoes as children had lower self-esteem, a poorer self image, and recall being teased about their shoes. Corrective shoes or braces may hurt the child, and should not routinely be used to make the family feel that "something is being done."

Janet Jack, RN | John M. Flynn, MD | David L. Skaggs, MD

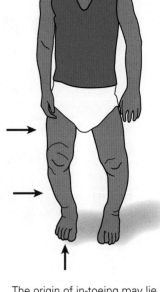

The origin of in-toeing may lie in the thigh, theshin, or the foot

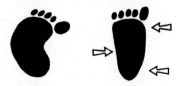

Three-point pressure straightens the foot

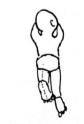

Thigh-foot angle

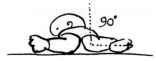

Hip rotation

Figure 1-6 Teaching handouts such as this can be a valuable resource for a patient's family. Include illustrations or photos to aid in understanding and put your name on it.

Complications cause surgeons mental anguish. It is a natural human tendency to avoid what causes us pain, but avoiding the family will harm your relationship. When things go wrong, make sure the family has your cell phone number and consider seeing the patient twice each day when they are in the hospital.

Dealing With Pain

When parents seem disproportionally anxious and worried about pain before surgery, it can affect the child's care. A study found that when parents tested one standard deviation high for generalized anxiety during a preoperative office visit, the children were more than twice as likely to be taking narcotics at the first follow-up visit after a spine fusion.[1] Quoting this study to parents seems to help. It also helps to share the downside of too much pain medicine (stop breathing). When a parent goes out of their way to state their child has a high pain tolerance, paradoxically this may be a red flag that the child actually has a low threshold for pain. Referring to multispecialty pain team with psychological capabilities is often best for families.

Handling Opinions of Other Caregivers

Other caregivers, such as physical or occupational therapists, chiropractors, and podiatrists, may spend more time with your patients than you do and develop a bond with the families. Their diagnoses and treatment recommendations may bear no semblance to anything you learned in medical school or can find in PubMed. In more than 20 years of practice, I have found that over 99% of children who see a podiatrist are told they need an orthosis. When seeing patients in my Beverly Hills office, I became worried that normal children no longer exist. Each child seemed to be a potential Olympic athlete with a private coach, or they were in therapy. I clearly remember one child who was seeing seven different therapists, but I was unable to discern any abnormalities with the child. The condition of excessive therapy seems limited to those with generous insurance policies or pocketbooks. With the advent of direct to consumer marketing and social media, many families will want the newest experimental treatment regardless of objective evidence. Unfortunately, surgeons jumping on the latest bandwagon can be effective marketing, particularly around large cities.

Avoid the pitfall of belittling other health care providers' opinions, as it erodes faith in the medical profession, makes the doctor look unprofessional, and can create conflicting loyalties in the family. Share objective data, give your recommendation, and perhaps even refer them to a trusted website or colleague for a tie-breaking opinion. A nurse or other member of your team speaking with the family without the doctor present may be of value (Fig. 1-6).

THE GURU SAYS...
Complications happen to all of us. The only way to avoid them is to never operate. Rather than running away from your problems, embrace them closely. What you do in the first 24 hours after a complication occurs has the greatest impact on your patient's recovery. Seek advice from your senior partners. We have all been there.
LORI KAROL

THE GURU SAYS...
Nurses are helpful in setting expectations of pain management, as well as providing emotional support and encouragement through treatment.
ELAINE BUTTERWORTH

THE GURU SAYS...
I am frequently asked what I would do if it were my child, and I give an honest answer. I think the cost of missed opportunity should be considered when weighing options, especially with treatments that have inadequate science or research behind them (such as scoliosis-specific exercises). The child's (and family's) time, money, and effort may be best spent playing sports, involved in afterschool activities, doing homework, or being with friends.
ELAINE BUTTERWORTH

Staying Out of Trouble When Partnering With Families

✳ The doctor and the parents want what is best for the child. Make sure the family feels you are on the same team.

✳ When a child suffers, the parent suffers. Care for the parent as well.

✳ Parent satisfaction is greatly influenced by pretreatment expectations: parents are happiest if expectations are restrained in the beginning and later surpassed.

✳ Nurses and other team members are highly valuable at family education and relationship building, as well as efficient use of surgeon's time.

✳ When a problem occurs: recognize it, accept it, and explain it to the family as soon as possible.

SOURCE OF WISDOM

1. Sarkisova N, Andras LM, Yang J, et al. High parental anxiety is associated with increased narcotic use in adolescent patients following spinal fusion. *J Ped Orthop*. 2020.

FOR FURTHER ENLIGHTENMENT

Bradberry T, Greaves J. *Emotional Intelligence 2.0*. San Diego, CA: TalentSmart; 2009.

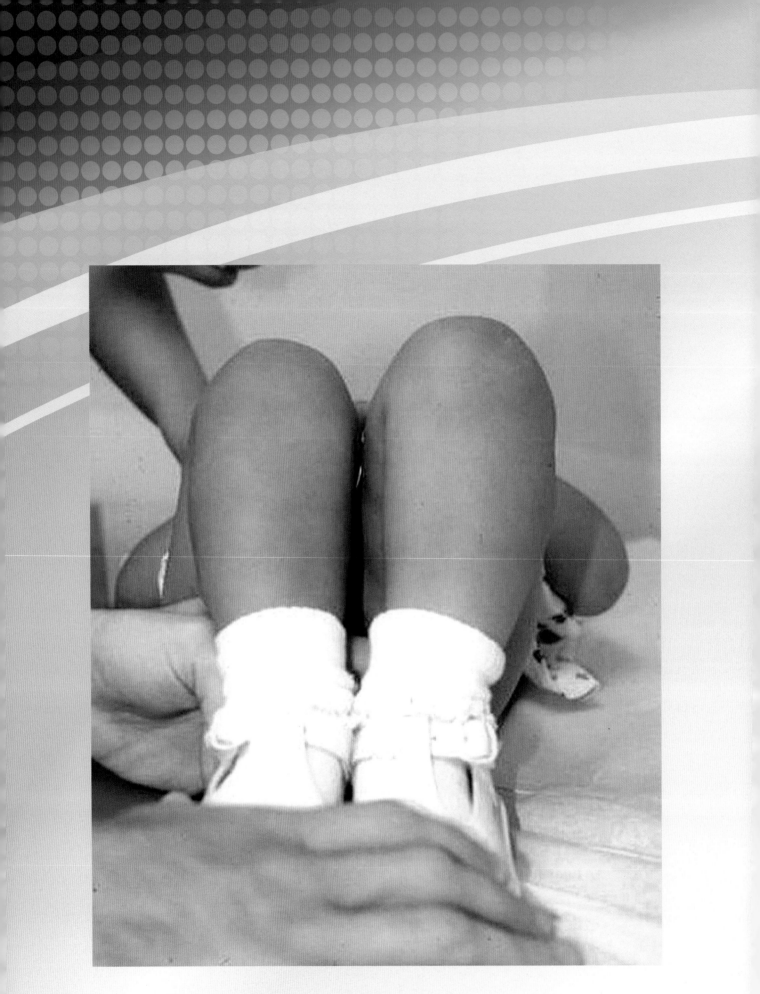

Chapter 2

The Pediatric Orthopaedic Physical Examination

MININDER S. KOCHER, MD, MPH

Guru: Henry G. Chambers, MD

General Approach

The musculoskeletal physical examination is why I went into orthopaedics. The ability to take a history and do a physical examination to diagnose an injured or dysfunctional structure, to correlate that to the patient's symptoms, to try to correct this through treatment, and then to re-examine the patient is miraculous. Although advanced imaging techniques such as MRI or ultrasound are useful in confirming the diagnosis or gaining additional information to guide treatment, everything is based on the history and physical examination. Young clinicians who rely too much on an MRI may get led astray by incidental or misleading findings. Master your exam, practice it, refine it, and treasure it!

The physical examination of children presents the orthopaedic surgeon with unique challenges and demands. Children between the ages of 14 months and 3 years often have an appropriately learned fear of doctors and needles and may be uncooperative. Nevertheless, the physician is expected to perform a reliable examination upon which the diagnosis and future decisions are based. This chapter focuses on those aspects of the physical examination, which are of special concern to pediatrics.

While this chapter focuses on aspects of the physical examination, elements of the history are unique to pediatrics. Birth history, such as prematurity, birth weight, perinatal complications, and number of days spent in the hospital may provide clues to an underlying disorder. The most useful developmental milestone is the age independent walking began. This may be considered normal if the child began walking by roughly 18 months of age, and frequently no further milestones are needed if this is the case. Grandparents may elucidate the family history, such as the patient's father walked on his toes till the age of 3 years. To stay out of trouble, proceed with the assumption that the parent or referring doctor is always right until proven otherwise by a thorough history and examination.

On entering the room, assess the child's level of apprehension and consider sitting as far away as possible from the child while chatting in a friendly manner with the parents and occasionally engaging the child in part of the conversation. Try to get low by sitting instead of towering over the child. A little effort in relationship building rapport with the child up front usually leads to a better examination (which may explain why pediatric orthopaedists wear such silly ties.) Treating even young children with genuine respect and not ignoring them while talking to parents goes a long way.

Carefully observe the child's movements and posture before touching them, because once the crying starts, the information that can be gained from observation will be quite limited. Some children, typically between 14 months and 3 years of age, will be completely uncooperative, and the only chance you will have to observe to their gait is when they walk into the room, so take advantage of that opportunity if possible. Distraction often works well with children. If they are tensing up or apprehensive, ask them questions about their pets, their favorite food, or the local sports team.

To help avoid missing serious underlying conditions, a good rule of thumb is to examine the hips and spine of every child younger than 5 years unless the patient has a fracture or other clearly localized complaint. This cursory examination may consist only of the Galeazzi test, abduction of the hips, and inspection and palpation of the spine under a child's shirt. It is quite easy to forget to examine parts of the body other than the chief complaint. To avoid this blunder, plan on examining the area of chief complaint last. For example, when an infant is brought to you for evaluation of a possible torticollis, examine the spine and upper and lower extremities first, before focusing in on the neck. The parents will not let you leave the room without examining the neck, but it is easy to forget to examine the hips.

Most areas of the body have more or less symmetrical sides; take advantage of this, by examining the "normal" side first for comparison. For example, you may think an injured knee is loose on examination; however, when you examine the contralateral knee, it is also loose indicating ligamentous laxity. Avoid loss of credibility in the parent's eyes by checking for muscle tone. Many children have already been evaluated by a therapist or other doctor and diagnosed (often overdiagnosed) with hypo- or hypertonia. Muscle tone of the upper and lower extremities may be tested by rapidly flexing elbows, knees, and ankles to assess the overall tone as well as a side-to-side comparison.

Increased tone on one side compared to the other may be indicative of cerebral palsy with spastic hemiplegia, while increased tone of the lower extremities compared to the upper extremities may be indicative of cerebral palsy with spastic diplegia. In order to avoid trouble with parents and referring doctors, consider referral to an appropriate specialist for evaluation of the child's increased muscle tone, rather than blurting out the emotionally laden diagnosis of cerebral palsy at the first visit.

Hypotonia is difficult to assess and may be more related to a child's state of wakefulness rather than an underlying disorder. When lifting a child of any age with the examiner's hands under the child's axilla, muscle tone about the shoulder girdle should be strong enough to support the child's weight. If a child slips through the examiner's hands, consider Duchenne muscular dystrophy or some other neuromuscular disorder.

Also, assess for laxity and stiffness. The Beighton score (Table 2-1) is useful in assessing generalized ligamentous laxity or suspicion of Ehlers-Danlos syndrome. Conversely, assess for tightness with inability to fully extend. Laxity and tightness often play a role in the development or manifestation of pediatric orthopaedic pathology.

Gait

If young children refuse to walk when asked, opening the door to the examination room and asking the parents if they would like to take their child for a walk in the hallway is often effective. If that doesn't work, taking the child away from the parents to observe the child walk back to the parents usually works. Toddlers can be expected to walk with a wide-based-waddling-gait pattern with the hands held wide for balance. While it is normal for children learning to walk to fall down frequently, a history of increasing falling should alert the physician to the possibility

TABLE 2-1 Beighton Score

There are 9 points, and a score of 4 or more is considered a sign of generalized joint hypermobility likely being present.
- One point if, while standing and bending forward, the patient can place their palms on the ground with the legs straight
- One point for each elbow that extends more than 10°
- One point for each knee that extends more than 5°
- One point for each thumb that, with the wrist flexed, can be manipulated to the forearm
- One point for each fifth finger that extends beyond 90°

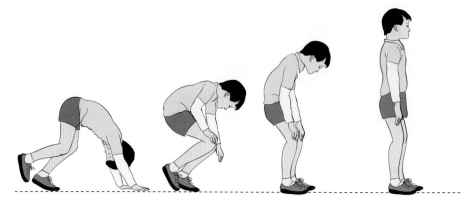

Figure 2-1 Weakness of proximal muscles that causes child to use arms to climb up legs on arising from sitting position is present in Duchenne muscular dystrophy and other conditions. The hardest part about this test is remembering to do it.

of a progressive neurologic condition, such as cerebral palsy, tumor, or other pathology. Where there is a history of progressive falling or weakness, a Gower test should be performed. To perform the Gower test, the child is asked to rise to a standing position from a sitting position on the floor. If the child uses their hands to climb up the legs and knees when arising, a muscular dystrophy should be suspected. A positive Gower test indicates proximal muscle weakness involving the gluteus maximus and the quadriceps muscles (Fig. 2-1). If a Gower test is positive, the calves should be inspected for pseudohypertrophy. If the patient has a positive Gower test with associated muscle weakness, a referral to a pediatric neurologist is recommended to evaluate for muscular dystrophy and a CPK blood test should be considered.

If you are having difficulty evaluating the child's gait pattern, it may be helpful to evaluate one aspect of gait at a time, moving from the feet, upward to ankles, knees, hips, torso, and arms. Walking up on one's toes should alert the physician to the possibility of cerebral palsy or other neuromuscular conditions. Running often helps amplify otherwise subtle gait disturbances such as a unilateral flexed elbow indicative of cerebral palsy with spastic hemiplegia (Fig. 2-2).

In the evaluation of intoeing, if the knees point straight ahead and the feet point inward during gait, this is consistent with internal tibial torsion. If both the feet and the knees point inward, this is consistent with internal femoral torsion. It is fairly easy to fall out of favor with the parents if they feel you have not spent sufficient time and attention analyzing their child's gait pattern. Bringing a parent into the hallway and having them point out their concerns about the child's gait pattern is usually time well spent. If you find some minor asymmetry in the gait and share this with parents it usually validates their concerns. If you are not certain whether a limp is present, closing your eyes and listening for an irregular cadence of foot strike often helps.

Hip

INFANTS

The examination of the infant's hips is fraught with trouble and deserves in-depth attention in this text, and your practice. Examination of an infant's hip should be performed first while the infant is calm and relaxed. Unlike many centers in Europe, with universal screening of infants' hips for developmental

THE GURU SAYS...

Taking a video (if your hospital allows it) and placing it in the electronic medical record is very helpful as one can take the time to watch the gait in slow motion and also compare to later examinations. As most of the pathology is in the sagittal plane, it is important to view the gait from the side of the patient (often difficult in small hallways). Of course, a three-dimensional computerized gait analysis should be considered if there is a complex gait abnormality.

Hank Chambers

dysplasia of the hip (DDH), the physical examination is usually the only chance of picking up a dislocated, subluxated, or dislocatable hip in most children in North America.

The newborn with DDH will typically have ligamentous laxity with hip instability which is elicited by performing the Ortolani and Barlow tests. Once the infant is 3 months of age, the ligamentous laxity decreases and the Ortolani and Barlow tests typically are normal. At this age, the clinician looks for asymmetric abduction or a limb length discrepancy (with the Galeazzi test) as a sign of DDH.

For simplicity, historical accuracy will be sacrificed, and provocative tests of hip stability will be referred to as Barlow and Ortolani tests, which attempt to dislocate and relocate the hip respectively. These tests are technically difficult, especially in light of how rarely the test is positive in most practitioner's hands. We recommend stabilizing the pelvis with one hand, with the thumb on the pubic symphysis and the fingers under the sacrum. While many physicians test both hips simultaneously, logic suggests that giving your full attention to one moving joint at a time is preferable in the setting of such an important examination.

In the Barlow maneuver (Fig. 2-3), while bringing the hip from abduction to adduction, the primary maneuver is pushing downward in line with the femoral shaft with your palm on the knee, while the secondary maneuver is pushing laterally on the medial proximal femur with your thumb. A positive finding is a palpable, and usually visible, posterior dislocation of the hip. It is not a high-pitch tissue click, but rather a deeper clunk, with significant motion such as going over a speed bump.

In the Ortolani maneuver (Fig. 2-4), while bringing the hip from an adducted to abducted position, the primary maneuver is gently lifting the hip into the socket with your long finger. As in the Barlow test, a positive finding is the palpable deep resonance of going over a speed bump. Usually a positive finding can be seen by others in the room. A high-pitched "click" is common and does not represent DDH, but probably a product of soft-tissue structures moving over bony prominences.

If a baby is crying, high quality provocative tests of the hip are impossible. This point cannot be overstated. Even a newborn's tight muscles may mask instability. Do whatever is necessary to obtain a hip examination in a calm baby, including pacifiers, reexamination after feeding, during feeding, or even rescheduling the examination for a different day. Unlike the Galeazzi test, the Barlow provocative test and the Ortolani tests may be performed on a parent's lap if this helps keep the infant calm. To stay out of trouble do not be afraid to consider an ultrasound

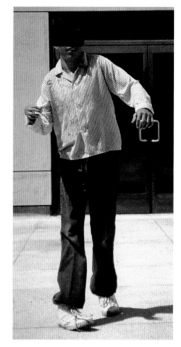

Figure 2-2 Child with hemiplegia demonstrates characteristic elbow flexion. Note that this child has posturing of both elbows, suggesting asymmetric. (Courtesy of Robert Kay, MD, Children's Orthopaedic Center, Los Angeles.)

THE GURU SAYS...

These are very gentle maneuvers using just mild rotations of your wrist and prodding with your fingers. These are not the same maneuvers used when examining a knee or shoulder.

HANK CHAMBERS

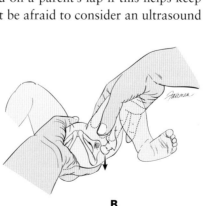

Figure 2-3 Barlow maneuver. **A:** Resting position. **B:** Provacative Position—palm pushes down on the knee in adduction to dislocate the hip posteriorly.

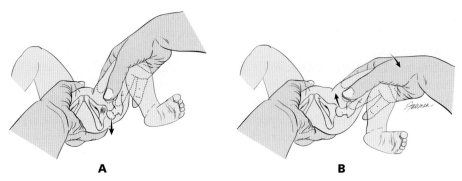

Figure 2-4 Ortolani maneuver. **A:** Resting Position. **B:** Provacative Position—fingers lift up on the greater trochanter in abduction to reduce the dislocated hip.

as an extension of the physical examination of a hip. There is no shame in sending the baby with an equivocal examination for an ultrasound with a repeat examination in 1 to 2 weeks. Decreased abduction is indicative of a dislocated or subluxated hip (Fig. 2-5). However, there are three pitfalls to avoid with this test. One, in the first few weeks of life an infant's hip joints may be hyperlax and abduct fully, even with a dislocated hip. Thus, testing hip abduction is of limited value in the evaluation of newborns. Once the infant is 3 months old, if the femoral head is still subluxated or dislocated, the adductor muscles become tight causing an adduction contracture of the hip. Two, in the case of bilaterally dislocated hips, abduction is symmetrical, though decreased. In most infants, one should be suspicious of DDH if the hips do not abduct more than 60° to 70°. And three, a child on a parents lap may be positioned with the pelvis slightly tilted, which may mask hip asymmetry. Thus, hip abduction should be better evaluated with the child supine on an examining table.

The appearance of asymmetrical skins folds is of questionable value. They are easily seen, but often are not always indicative of underlying DDH. The simplest test to perform is the Galeazzi test, in which the child lies supine, with the hips fully flexed, and the feet flat on the table and the ankles touching the buttocks (Fig. 2-6). If the knees are at different heights, this is indicative of a dislocated hip

Figure 2-5 Asymmetry of hip abduction is associated with a unilateral hip dislocation in the hip that abducts less. A potential pitfall is not leveling the pelvis on the examination table; subtle asymmetry may be missed in that event.

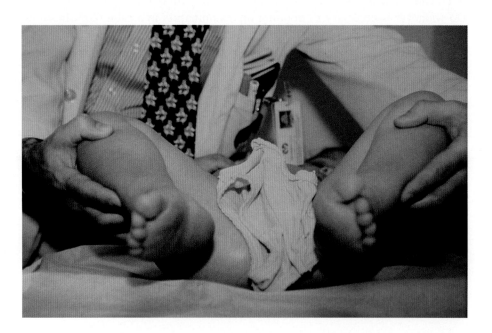

or other less common conditions such as proximal femoral focal deficiency, hemihypertrophy, etc. To stay out of trouble, this test is best performed on an examining table, not the mother's lap, with all diapers, blankets, and clothing out from under the baby, as even a 1 cm fold of clothing under the hemipelvis may mask a limb length discrepancy. Being peed on at times is just part of the job.

Be aware that the Galeazzi test may be negative in bilateral dislocated hips. In a newborn with bilateral dislocated hips, the only abnormality on physical examination may be a lack of the normal hip flexion contractures of infancy.

OLDER CHILDREN

The single most useful exam in the evaluation of an older child's hip is prone internal rotation. The child lies prone on the examining table, with the knees flexed 90° and the tibias pointing toward the ceiling. The ankles are then brought outwards as far as the child comfortably tolerates. Hip internal rotation is 0° if the tibia points toward the ceiling or 90° if they fall completely outward and become horizontal. Asymmetry of hip internal rotation usually defines intra-articular hip pathology in the hip with less rotation (Fig. 2-7). Common conditions causing limited internal rotation include transient synovitis, infection, and Legg-Calvé-Perthes disease. Uncommon causes of asymmetric internal rotation include a healed femur fracture with axial malalignment and asymmetric unilateral femoral torsion. This test should be performed in any child who is limping or complaining of leg pain without clear localization. Another pitfall with this test is not stabilizing the pelvis in neutral rotation, allowing pelvic tilt to mask the asymmetric internal rotation. The most common problem with this test is simply forgetting to do it. Remember that in children, hip pathology may cause referred pain to the thigh, or even the knee.

A related test to help determine the degree of hip irritation is the "log roll" test (Fig. 2-8). In this test, the child is supine, with the hip and knee fully extended. A child with an acute hip infection will often resist lying with the hip fully extended. Rolling the leg back and forth causes internal and external rotation of the hip. By pretending to examine the foot, an examiner often discovers much more motion than the nondistracted child would permit. This test is particularly useful in helping to distinguish between transient synovitis and septic arthritis. In septic arthritis, children are uncomfortable with nearly any internal rotation, while a child with transient synovitis will often allow up to 30° of internal rotation if the examiner is gentle and patient. This test will also uncover a slipped capital femoral epiphysis.

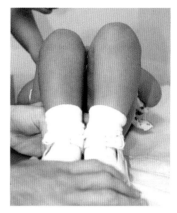

Figure 2-6 Galeazzi test is positive when knees are at different heights. When positive, there may be a unilateral dislocated hip or a leg length discrepancy.

THE GURU SAYS...

Sometimes, especially with a septic hip or femoral osteomyelitis, it is difficult to examine the child's hip when the child is supine as they want to hold it in flexion, abduction, and external rotation. Have the mother hold the child around her hip to help the child relax and allow you to gently rotate the hips to see if that elicits more pain. You can also palpate the limb when the child is more secure and comfortable.

HANK CHAMBERS

THE GURU SAYS...

Don't forget to examine hip extension. This can be done by flexing both hips up until the lumbar lordosis is corrected (assessed by placing one's hand under the lumbar spine) and the sequentially extending each hip. The Staheli method has you place the patient in a prone position with the ASIS on the edge of the table. Extend the hip until the pelvis rises. This is very accurate, but sometimes the children are apprehensive about hanging over the edge of the table.

HANK CHAMBERS

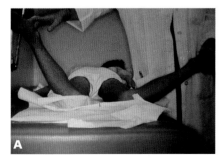
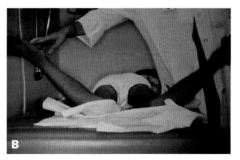

Figure 2-7 Asymmetry of internal hip rotation is best appreciated prone. Asymmetry localizes intra-articular pathology to the hip with less internal rotation. A potential pitfall occurs when the test is performed while the pelvis is not perfectly flat on the table, as noted by the seemingly different findings between **A** and **B**.

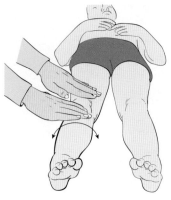

Figure 2-8 Log roll. Rolling the leg from side to side will help you distinguish between septic hip and transient synovitis.

THE GURU SAYS...

I find it easier to do this from behind the child and assess the posterior iliac crests. Look for knee flexion, equinus, or asymmetry of the foot (unilateral varus or valgus), which can also lead to a limb length discrepancy.

HANK CHAMBERS

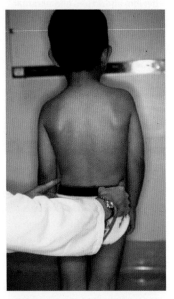

Figure 2-9 Limb lengths may be easily and accurately assessed, and demonstrated to parents, by placing your fingers on the iliac crests. A potential pitfall is the child with a significant limb length discrepancy who bends the short knee in an attempt to "stand up straight."

When testing for hip abduction or adduction in the supine position, place a hand across both anterior superior iliac spines in young children, or a forearm in larger children, to make certain you are not causing pelvic tilt and masking asymmetric hip abduction or adduction.

Hip flexion may be tested with the child supine, with one of the examiner's hands under the lumbar spine to feel when flexion of the lumbar spine begins to occur. It is surprisingly easy to join the club of doctors who have mistaken spine flexion for hip flexion in a patient with a hip fusion. If passive flexion of the hip is accompanied by obligate external rotation, a slipped capital femoral epiphysis may be present. Also, pain with hip flexion internal rotation should raise suspicion of SCFE. Remember, SCFE often presents as knee pain or distal thigh pain. Don't be that doc that diagnoses patellofemoral pain or scopes the knee instead of diagnosing SCFE!

Assessment of Limb Length

Assessing limb lengths from the anterior superior iliac spine to the medial malleolus is notoriously inaccurate, particularly in squirming and overweight children. A much simpler method is to place the examiner's fingers on the iliac crests when the child is standing (Fig. 2-9) and observing for asymmetric heights of the iliac crests. Blocks of various thicknesses can be used under the short leg to determine the leg length difference that equalizes the iliac crests. For nonambulators or uncooperative children, the Galeazzi test as described above is useful. The Galeazzi test is particularly useful in demonstrating to parents the presence or absence of a length discrepancy. A method to assess femoral and tibial lengths in a nonambulatory patient is to place the patient in the prone position with the hips in full extension and the knees flexed to 90°. In this position if the right knee is shorter than the left, it indicates a femoral length discrepancy. In this position if the right heel is lower than the left, it indicates a tibial length discrepancy.

A pitfall in the assessment of limb lengths is a unilateral hip abduction contracture, with the abducted leg giving the appearance of being longer in nearly all positions. To avoid this pitfall, make certain that pelvis is level during the Galeazzi test.

Legs

In children, the examination of the legs is often focused on angular and torsional deformities. A common pitfall is to mistake tibial torsion for genu varum, as discussed in Chapter 27 (Legs are bowed, Feet turn in, Who cares?). To avoid this pitfall, examine the child in the supine position, making certain the patellas point straight up with the legs fully extended. With internal tibial torsion, the feet will point inward. The thigh-foot angle is the angle between the axis of the thigh and the axis of the foot, with the knee bent to 90°.

If significant genu varum is present, the space between the knees may be measured when the ankles are together for future comparison. Similarly, in cases of genu valgum, with the knees lightly touching the space between the medial malleolus may be measured.

Knee

In a child presenting with knee or leg pain, the most important pitfall to avoid is to remember to examine the hips. Find the point of maximum tenderness about the knee and you can diagnose the majority of pediatric knee problems

(Fig. 2-10). In an acutely injured knee that hurts "all over," localizing the point of maximum tenderness may be impossible and best deferred to a return visit in 1 to 2 weeks. Patients that localize their knee pain by grabbing the front of the knee with their whole hand are demonstrating the "grab sign" characteristic of patellofemoral dysfunction. Traumatic knee effusions in children should be taken very seriously. Radiographs are always warranted, and if negative, then possibly an MRI. In a child with a traumatic effusion, everyone suspects an ACL injury, but a patellar dislocation or subluxation is commonly the cause of the effusion when the chief complaint is "my knee gave out." In the setting of trauma, remember a distal femoral Salter I fracture is possible in a child with open growth plates, while an MCL injury is more common in the adolescent. The two may be differentiated by point of maximal tenderness, radiographs (possibly with stress), or even an MRI.

For chronic knee pain, measuring the circumference of the leg 6 cm above and 10 cm below the patella provides objective evidence of the child's use of the limb. The first muscle in the quadriceps mechanism to atrophy is the vastus medialis obliquus (VMO), so do not measure too high on the thigh. Depending on the size of the child, 1 to 2 cm of increased circumference of the dominant thigh may be considered within normal limits. While most asymptomatic "clicking" about the knee is not of concern, children may have unstable discoid lateral menisci. The squat test—crouching like a catcher—will almost always produce pain in a patient with a meniscus tear.

Osteochondritis dissecans develops when part of the subchondral bone of the distal femur or patella loses its blood supply. Wilson sign is often sited as a key test to diagnose osteochondritis dissecans involving the distal femur, but it is often falsely negative. A positive Wilson sign occurs when the patient's knee is passively extended with the tibia internally rotated; at 30° of flexion, the patient experiences pain that is immediately relieved by externally rotating the tibia. In cases of chronic knee pain, radiographs including a notch view (beam directed 20° cephalad from a true AP) help evaluate for osteochondritis dissecans.

The patellar compression test is performed by having the patient lie supine with the knee extended. The examiner holds the superior end of the patella firmly against the femur, preventing it from moving proximally, while the patient contracts the quadriceps (Fig. 2-11). Pain is considered indicative of patella femoral pain syndrome. It is important to ask the patient if this is the type of pain they have been experiencing, as the test may be overly sensitive, and identify subclinical patellofemoral pathology which is not the source of knee pain that brought them to the doctor.

An acute knee injury during sports with a hemarthrosis should raise the suspicion of internal derangement such as ACL tear, meniscal injury, articular cartilage injury, patellar dislocation, or bone bruise. Physical examination in this setting should include stability testing with Lachman test, pivot shift test, anterior-posterior drawer, varus-valgus stability, and posterolateral dial testing. Meniscal pathology can be assessed with McMurray maneuvers, joint line tenderness, and pain with terminal flexion/extension. Although an ACL tear is suspected, a twisting injury with a pop and swelling can often be patellofemoral instability. Examine the patellofemoral joint by assessing tracking, tilt, medial tenderness, and apprehension. An MRI may be indicated to confirm the diagnosis or guide treatment, but should not be used in lieu of careful physical examination.

> **THE GURU SAYS...**
>
> A Salter Harris I fracture will be tender on both sides of the distal femur and usually accompanied by a large effusion. An MCL tear may have localized swelling and tenderness only on the medial side.
>
> HANK CHAMBERS

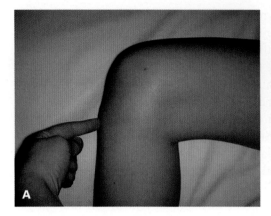 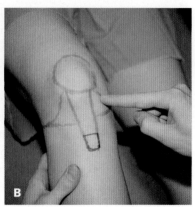

Figure 2-10 The point of maximal tenderness is often easy to identify in the subcutaneous structures of the knee. These photos demonstrate the different points of maximal tenderness in Osgood-Schlatter disease with tibial tubercle tenderness (**A**) versus a medial meniscal tear with joint line tenderness (**B**).

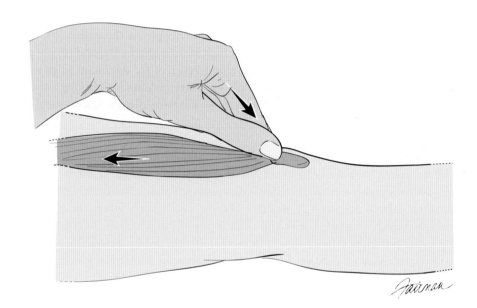

Figure 2-11 In the patella grind test, the examiner holds the superior end of the patella firmly against the femur, preventing it from moving proximally, while the patient contracts the quadriceps. Pain is considered indicative of patellofemoral syndrome, though the test may be overly sensitive.

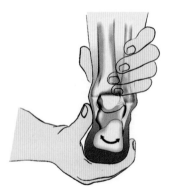

RW.Williams

Figure 2-12 Subtalar motion may be simply evaluated by observing passive motion of the heel in the prone patient. Have one hand cup heel in palm, while the other holds leg above ankle.

Foot and Ankle

Inspection of the foot and ankle occurs during gait as well as at rest. A cavus foot or claw toes should immediately cause you to think that the patient has an associated neurologic disorder until proven otherwise. If the pes cavus is unilateral, it may be associated with a tethered spinal cord. Look for redness or callosities over the talar head, fifth metatarsal head or other bony prominences. Look at the shoes, as patterns of shoe ware may provide a clue to abnormal foot position.

Observe the position of the hindfoot. The Achilles tendon and hindfoot should be in a neutral to slightly valgus position when standing, and when the child stands on their toes, the heel should invert into slight varus. If the first metatarsal is pronated or plantarflexed, it will cause the hindfoot to roll into varus with weight bearing. The Coleman block test is classically described for assessment of hindfoot mobility; however, we have found a much simpler test preferable: With the child prone and the knees flexed to 90°, grasp the tibia with one hand and cup the heel with the other hand. Observe hindfoot motion while moving the heel into a varus and valgus positions (Fig. 2-12).

In a patient with a pes planus deformity, the arch should be evaluated with the child standing, standing on their toes, and in a non–weight bearing position. If the arch is flat when standing but re-creates when the child is on their toes or non–weight bearing, this by definition is a flexible flat foot. Almost all babies have flat feet from the significant subcutaneous fat in this region and the arch will increase from birth to about 10 years of age. Beware that a child with a rigid flat foot may have a tarsal coalition. Subtalar motion may be assessed by stabilizing the tibia with one hand, while cupping the heel with the other hand and moving the hindfoot from side to side. This is a deceptively difficult examination as motion at the ankle joint may be mistaken for subtalar motion.

It is important to remember that a valgus heel and flat foot may be secondary to a valgus ankle. Palpation of the ankle should reveal that the lateral malleolus is more distal than the medial malleolus. If not, consider fibular hemimelia or other anomalies. Remember to test ankle dorsiflexion with the foot in maximum supination to lock the subtalar joint and prevent midfoot motion from giving the appearance of ankle dorsiflexion. Also, begin to test ankle dorsiflexion with the knee bent to relieve the pull of the gastrocnemius, then with the knee straight. The decrease in the amount of dorsiflexion achieved with the knee extended, compared to that with the knee flexed, represents the contribution of the medial and lateral gastrocnemius muscles to the equinus contracture. It is important to remember that lack of ankle dorsiflexion and increased muscle tone are present in many neuromuscular disorders.

Do not forget that otherwise normal children with a leg length discrepancy will often develop ankle equinus on the short leg from chronic toe walking, which should not be confused with an underlying neurologic condition. Conversely, children with cerebral palsy with spastic hemiplegia usually have a short leg on the effected side, with the equinus resulting primarily from muscle spasticity, not the leg length discrepancy.

Examination of a deformed foot in the newborn may present a few challenges. A longitudinal deficiency of the tibia may give the appearance of a clubfoot. A rather significant amount of metatarsus adductus should not be too concerning as long as the foot is passively correctable. A key finding that helps differentiate metatarsus adductus from a congenital clubfoot deformity is that the clubfoot cannot be dorsiflexed past neutral.

Spine

Perhaps the easiest pitfall in the physical examination of the spine is to not have the patient sufficiently unclothed out of respect for their modesty. No more than bottom underwear and either a bikini top or gown that opens to the back should be worn. Inspection of the skin for lesions (neurofibromatosis) and the feet for deformities are important, as well as observing a child bend naturally without being encumbered by half pulled up T shirts. No examination of the spine is complete unless the feet have been inspected (Fig. 2-13).

When inspecting the back the presence of a midline defect or a hairy patch may suggest an underlying spinal dysraphism. Hairy patches tend to be overdiagnosed by eager residents and medical students. The real thing is usually unequivocal (Fig. 2-14). Dimples above the gluteal cleft (butt crack) may be indicative of underlying spinal pathology and may warrant an MRI (Fig. 2-15). Small dimples within the gluteal cleft are less concerning in an otherwise normal child. A unilateral pes cavus deformity may be the only detectable clinical finding in a patient with a tethered spinal cord.

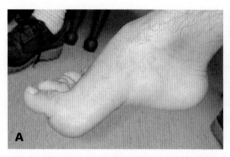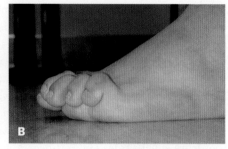

Figure 2-13 No examination of the spine is complete until the shoes and socks have been removed. A cavus foot (**A**) or claw toes (**B**) indicates underlying neurologic pathology may be present.

With the child standing, asymmetry of the shoulder blades and waist should be evaluated. Comparison of the space between the patient's arms and waist for side-to-side symmetry is particularly sensitive in the identification scoliosis in the standing position. To perform the Adams forward bending test, have the child standing in front of the examiner facing away from the examiner. The examiner's head should be at back level, which usually means the examiner sits on a stool. Ask the child to place their hands together, as this ensures that any observed shoulder asymmetry is not due to one hand reaching further downward than the other. Then ask the child to bend forwards as if trying to touch their toes. Rotational asymmetry can be appreciated on forward bending and correlates with curvature of the spine. A scoliometer can be used to quantitate asymmetry on forward bending. Scoliometer measurements over 7° typically warrant further evaluation with referral or X-rays.

A potential pitfall in the Adams forward bending test is a false positive test because of a leg length discrepancy. Remember to first assess the leg lengths by placing your fingers on the child's iliac crests when sitting behind the child. If one leg is significantly longer, this will give the appearance of an ipsilateral lumbar fullness during the Adams forward bending test. Equalizing leg lengths with a block prior can then allow for an accurate Adams forward bending test. A red flag in this test is if the child consistently bends or "lists" off to one side when asked to bend forwards. This may be indicative of a serious underlying spinal pathology (Fig. 2-16).

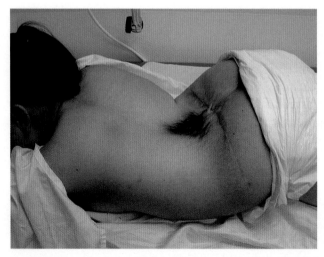

Figure 2-14 A true hairy patch (one with enough hair to braid) is associated with underlying spinal pathology.

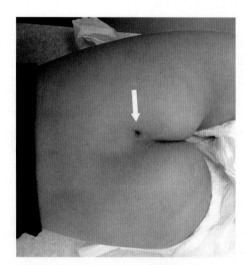

Figure 2-15 A dimple (*arrow*) above the gluteal cleft may be associated with spinal dysraphism.

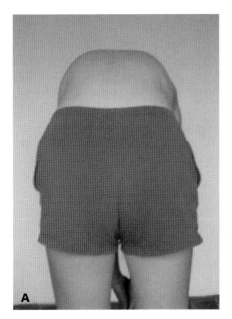
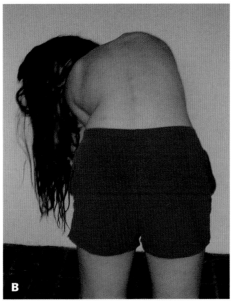

Figure 2-16 When a child repeatedly bends to one side, or "lists" when bending forward in the Adam's forward bending test, this may indicate underlying spinal pathology. **A**: Child bending normally. **B**: Child listing to the left.

With the child in the Adams forward bending position, observe from the side as well if sagittal alignment is of concern. A sharp angulation is indicative of Scheuermann kyphosis. We have seen many children with Scheuermann kyphosis successfully hide their deformity when standing up, only to be revealed when bending forward (Fig. 2-17).

When evaluating a child for back pain, do not forget to have the child bending backward when standing as well as forward. Localized pain in the lower lumbar region with back extension may be indicative of spondylolysis or spondylolisthesis.

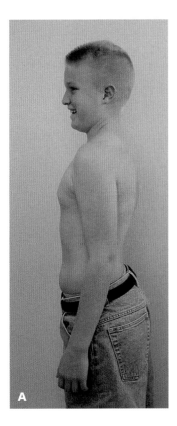
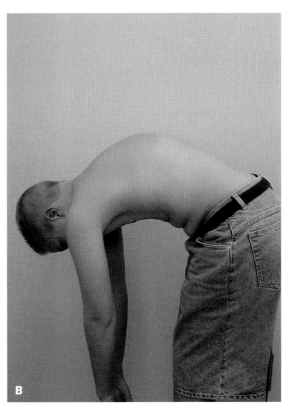

Figure 2-17 A: Child with Scheuermann kyphosis who smiles as he believes he is escaping detection. **B**: Forward bending test shows sharp kyphotic angulation. Radiographs confirmed Scheuermann kyphosis.

This may be more pronounced in unilateral spondylolysis with single leg standing extension on the ipsilateral side. Palpation of the back is often quite illuminating when a patient's chief complaint is back pain. When a child complains of tenderness to palpation that seems out of proportion or not physiological, a repeat palpation of the back when the child's attention is diverted may fail to produce the same reaction. Although children seek secondary gain less frequently than adults, this finding suggests secondary gain or other psychological forces should be considered.

An additional test that is quite helpful in the evaluation of a patient with back pain is the "finger test." When asked to show the doctor where the back hurts, if the child points with one finger to a specific, repeatable location, this suggests underlying pathology (spondylolysis, tumor, etc.). When a child motions over a large area of the back, particularly a transverse distribution across the lumbar spine, adult-type mechanical low-back pain is more likely (Fig. 2-18).

In terms of the cervical spine, inspection of head position may reveal the traditional cock robin position of torticollis in which the head is tilted in one direction and rotated in the opposite direction. Inspection of the head and neck should be performed looking for webbing of the neck, plagiocephaly, and a low-set hairline, as is seen in Klippel-Feil syndrome, in addition to palpation of the potentially tight sternocleidomastoid muscle, as is seen in congenital muscular torticollis.

One of the most important parts of the physical examination of the spine is the neurologic examination. This may be performed relatively quickly and should be considered in a patient with any spinal complaint. To perform a brief neurologic examination (Table 2-2), first have the child walk on their toes, walk on their heels, and jump up and down on one foot at the time. Sit on a stool next to the child who sits on the edge of the examination table with her legs hanging off. Inspect the feet for deformities, and sharply (rapidly) dorsiflex each ankle to test for clonus and

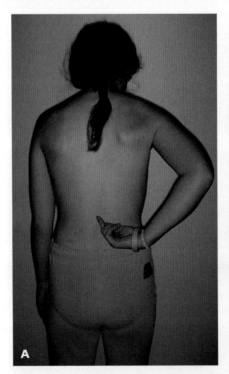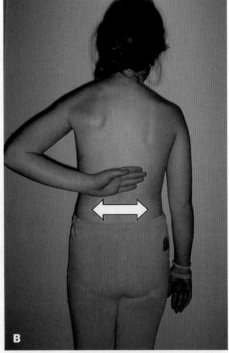

Figure 2-18 A: Positive finger test. Child points with finger to one repeatable location as the source of back pain. This raises the suspicion of underlying spinal pathology.
B: Nonlocalized back pain, especially transversely distributed over the lumbar region, is more likely to be adult style musculoskeletal back pain.

TABLE 2-2 60-Second Neurologic Examination
● Hop on each foot, one at a time
● Walk on heels
● Reflexes
● Foot inspection and dorsiflexion to assess muscle tone and clonus
● Sensation
● Popliteal angle

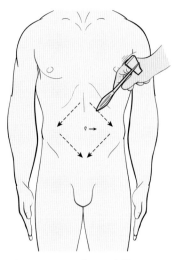

Figure 2-19 The umbilicus reflex is positive when the umbilicus moves asymmetrically in response to lightly stroking the adjacent skin with a sharp object. This may indicate an underlying syrinx. In the setting of scoliosis, this finding justifies an MRI.

assess muscle tone. Test the patella tendon and Achilles tendon reflexes. This can usually be done with the examiner's fingers, as many children do not appreciate being hit with a hammer. If the patella tendon reflexes are not forthcoming, a useful trick is to ask the child to gently push against your finger placed aver the anterior ankle while tapping the patella tendon. This slight amount of quadriceps contraction is usually sufficient to encourage a reflex at the next attempt.

Next, position the child supine on the examining table. The abdominal reflexes are assessed by lightly stroking the skin to the side of the umbilicus and observing for any movement of the umbilicus in the direction of the stimulus. The test is positive when the movement is asymmetrical, and a positive abdominal reflex may be the only detectable clinical finding in a patient with scoliosis secondary to syringomyelia (Fig. 2-19).

In a brief neurologic examination, sensation to light touch should be tested in the following dermatomes: L3, medial knee; L4, medial malleolus; L5, dorsum of big toe; and S1, plantar and lateral aspect of the foot. Lightly touch each area on both legs simultaneously and ask the child if it feels normal and the same on both sides.

And last but certainly not least, assess the popliteal angle. The popliteal angle may be thought of as the ESR of the spine examination, in that it is very sensitive to underlying spinal pathology such as a spondylolisthesis or tethered spinal cord, but not very specific. The reason why varied spinal pathologies may lead to a final common pathway of hamstring tightness is open to speculation. With the child supine flex one hip to 90° with the knee bent, then slowly extend the knee as far as is comfortable. The angle between the tibia and vertical is the popliteal angle. An angle over 50° to 60° may be considered abnormal, and the cause of hamstring tightness should be sought (Fig. 2-20).

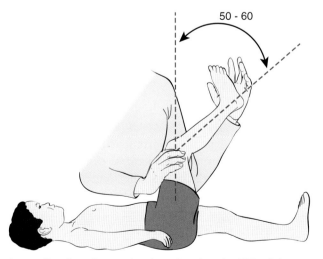

50 - 60

Figure 2-20 The popliteal angle may be thought of as the ESR of the neurologic examination. It is very sensitive for nerve root irritation, but not specific. It may be considered positive if the angle is greater than 50° to 60°.

Shoulder

Pathology about the shoulder is less common in children than other areas of the body. Particular attention should be paid to the height of the scapula, as a high riding scapula may be indicative of a Sprengel deformity. When elevating the shoulder to 180°, the normal ratio of glenohumeral to scapulothoracic motion is 2:1. If the scapula is elevated and does not appear to be abducting in a normal fashion, consider the possibility of a Sprengel deformity. Young children can be so flexible and thin that their humeral head can be palpated in the axilla during full shoulder elevation; this is not pathologic if the patient is flexible. If a diagnosis of a brachial plexus injury is suspected, pay careful attention to the amount of shoulder external rotation present, as this is often limited following a brachial plexus injury involving the C5 and C6 nerve roots.

Sports shoulder disorders include anterior instability, multidirectional instability, internal impingement, and SLAP tears. Stability can be tested by load and shift testing, anterior apprehension in the abducted–externally rotated position, and sulcus sign. Make sure to assess for generalized ligamentous laxity and baseline stability of the contralateral shoulder. Internal impingement in the throwing athlete is characterized by unilateral findings of a tight posterior capsule with decreased cross body adduction and GIRD with decreased internal rotation.

Elbow and Forearm

A normal carrying angle of 5° to 15° valgus may be expected. Following healing of a fracture adjacent to the elbow joint, the carrying angle may be compared to the contralateral side. Normal elbow hyperextension is quite common in children and teenage girls. A child who lacks full elbow extension should be considered to have serious pathology (e.g., OCD, AVN, arthritis, infection, occult fracture) until proven otherwise. It even has been said that there cannot be anything seriously wrong with an elbow if it will fully extend. To assess elbow flexion, ask the patient to touch their shoulder with their fingers. Approximately 125° of elbow flexion is required to perform this task, and it is better tolerated in young children than use of the goniometer.

Pronation and supination of approximately 80° to 90° should be expected. Limited forearm rotation most often results from a fracture; however, careful attention to the radial head is warranted. Early recognition of a dislocated radial head may avoid later problems. A prominent radial head may be indicative of a congenital radial head dislocation, or an unrecognized Monteggia fracture-dislocation.

Hand

The most common reason a pediatric orthopaedist examines a child's hand is to assess nerve function. A careful preoperative examination of nerve function prior to fracture treatment may help keep the surgeon out of trouble. The most commonly damaged nerve in a supracondylar fracture of the distal humerus is the anterior interosseous branch of the median nerve. To test this nerve, ask the child to make an "O" with their index finger and thumb. Active interphalangeal flexion of the thumb and index finger confirms that the nerve is intact (Fig. 2-21).

Ulnar nerve function is particularly important to test prior to performing a closed reduction and crossed pinning of a distal humeral supracondylar fracture if using a medial pin is planned. Motor function of the ulnar nerve can be tested by

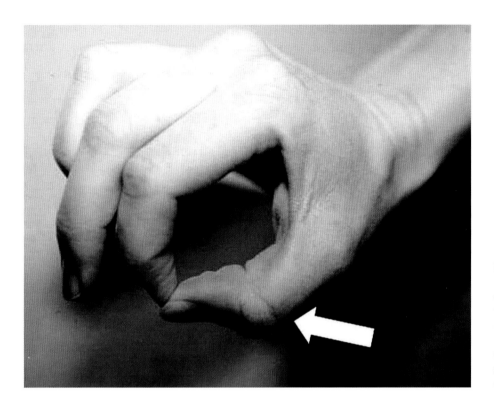

Figure 2-21 Active interphalangeal flexion of the thumb and index finger confirms that the anterior interosseous branch of the median nerve is intact (*arrow*). This is the most commonly damaged nerve in a supracondylar fracture of the distal humerus.

asking the child to cross their fingers. Young apprehensive children seem to find this test difficult. If a child can be convinced to pinch something between their thumb and index finger, the examiner may palpate a contraction of the muscle belly of the first dorsal interosseous muscle and confirm motor function of the ulnar nerve.

Testing sensation of a child with the needle should be avoided as future examinations may be severely compromised. In the preverbal or uncooperative child, soaking the hand in a wet cloth for a few minutes will produce skin wrinkling if the skin sensory nerves are intact. This may substitute for a sensory examination. To evaluate the sensory component of a nerve in an older child, it is accurate and painless to test two-point discrimination using a paper clip, comparing the injured side with the uninjured side.

Staying Out of Trouble With the Pediatric Orthopaedic Examination

* Examine the area of chief complaint last, so you don't forget the other parts (except for hip dysplasia).
* Ortalani and Barlow tests may be negative in a child with a dislocated hip by the age of 3 months.
* If a baby is crying, high-quality provocative tests of the hip are impossible.
* The single most useful examination in the evaluation of an older child's hip is prone internal rotation.
* In a child presenting with knee or leg pain, the most important pitfall to avoid is to remember to examine the hips.
* A cavus foot or claw toes should immediately cause you to think that the patient has an associated neurologic disorder until proved otherwise.

SOURCES OF WISDOM

1. Diab M. Physical examination in adolescent idiopathic scoliosis. *Neurosurg Clin North Am.* 2007; 18(2):229-236.
2. Foster H, Kay L, May C, Rapley T. Pediatric regional examination of the musculoskeletal system: a practice- and consensus-based approach. *Arthritis Care Res.* 2011;63(11):1503-1510.
3. Gunner KB, Scott AC. Evaluation of a child with a limp. *J Pediatr Health Care.* 2001;15(1):38-40.
4. Khamis S, Carmeli E. Relationship and significance of gait deviations associated with limb length discrepancy: a systematic review. *Gait Posture.* 2017;57:115-123.
5. MacDonald J, Stuart E, Rodenberg R. Musculoskeletal low back pain in school-aged children: a review. *JAMA Pediatr.* 2017;171(3):280-287.
6. Price BD, Price CT. A simple demonstration of hindfoot flexibility in the cavovarus foot. *J Pediatr Orthop.* 1997;17(1):18-19.
7. Rose SA, Ounpuu S, DeLuca PA. Strategies for the assessment of pediatric gait in the clinical setting. *Phys Ther.* 1991;71(12):961-980.
8. Schwend RM, Shaw BA, Segal LS. Evaluation and treatment of developmental hip dysplasia in the newborn and infant. *Pediatr Clin North Am.* 2014;61(6):1095-1107.

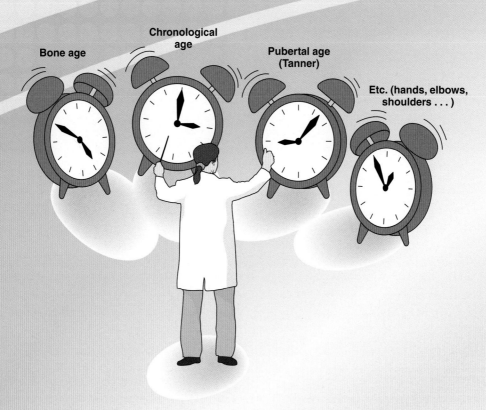

Adapted with permission from Alain Diméglio, MD.

Chapter 3

The Growing Child

MICHAEL G. VITALE, MD, MPH, JOHN M. (JACK) FLYNN, MD, and DAVID L. SKAGGS, MD, MMM

Gurus: Alain Diméglio, MD and James O. Sanders, MD

General Considerations

To stay out of trouble when treating orthopaedic problems in the growing child, it is important to have a practical understanding of normal growth and development. We do not need to be developmental pediatricians but need to be able to recognize when something is amiss. The pediatric orthopaedic surgeon is often the first to evaluate the child with subtle developmental delays or alternations in growth that may signal an underlying problem. While this chapter will provide an overview of important aspects of growth and development, more specific aspects of growth as they pertain to the spine, leg length discrepancy, and limb alignment are covered in those chapters.

It is important to recognize that the definition of "normal" depends on whether or not you are dealing with an underlying condition. Normal size and normal motor milestones are different for children with Down syndrome, achondroplasia, or Marfan syndrome. In some cases, specific growth charts have been made for these conditions. While our primary role is to treat the musculoskeletal consequence of problems with growth and development, we can help families by having a high level of suspicion and referring these families to their primary care provider, geneticist, or other pediatric specialist.

Recording height and weight is important and not only for the EMR! While growth is fastest in the first 3 years of life and then again at puberty, steady increase in height and weight is expected regardless of age in the skeletally immature child. Any child that is losing weight (not on purpose) over a few months could be showing signs of trouble. Tracking changes in height is especially useful in guiding treatment decisions in the adolescent with scoliosis. Knowing the timing of the growth peak provides valuable information on the likelihood of progression of scoliosis to a magnitude requiring spinal arthrodesis[1] (Table 3-1). Likewise, orthopaedists who are monitoring leg length inequalities find a growth chart or electronic equivalent valuable.

PHYSIS: "FRIEND OR FOE"

Think about what a tough job the physis has! In order to end up with a fully grown, "straight," and symmetric body, hundreds of physes need to perform perfectly over many years. In a way it is amazing that growth disturbances don't happen more often. The physis can be both friend and foe and can at times keep us out of trouble but at other times do the opposite.

Orthopaedic surgeons caring for children also need to have a good understanding of the percentage of growth that is contributed by each physis (Fig. 3-1). Such knowledge of normal growth and development helps the orthopaedic surgeon time epiphysiodesis and understand the potential effects of a traumatic growth arrest.

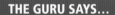

THE GURU SAYS...

Human growth and development is the product of more than 300 growth plates working in the shadow of bones in perfect synchronization.

ALAIN DIMÉGLIO

TABLE 3-1 Useful Guides for Childhood Stature and Growth
• By the age of 5 y, birth height has usually doubled and the child is about 60% of adult height.
• Arm span should be nearly equal to standing height.
• The head is disproportionately large at birth.
• In the lower extremity, most growth is around the knee; the opposite is true for the upper extremity where most growth comes from the proximal humerus and wrist.
• Skeletal maturity varies considerably, so it is critical to consider bone age rather than chronological age especially around adolescence!

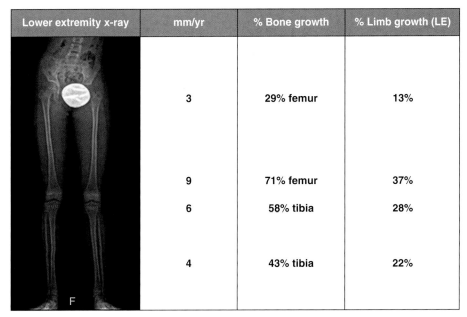

Lower extremity x-ray	mm/yr	% Bone growth	% Limb growth (LE)
	3	29% femur	13%
	9	71% femur	37%
	6	58% tibia	28%
	4	43% tibia	22%

Figure 3-1 Percentage contribution of femoral and tibial physes to lower extremity growth. (Adapted with permission from Hubbard EW, Liu RW, Iobst CA. Understanding skeletal growth and predicting limb-length inequality in pediatric patients. *J Am Acad Orthop Surg.* 2019;27(9):312-319. Copyright © 2019 by the American Academy of Orthopaedic Surgeons.)

While physeal injuries are covered in detail in other chapters in this book, a few general principles will help us stay out of trouble. For example, an understanding of the normal pattern of physeal ossification centers is helpful in diagnosing occult fractures of the elbow and other areas. Fractures of the distal femoral physis result in a 30% to 50% chance of growth arrest, and these patients need careful follow-up. On the other hand, proximal humerus fractures rarely result in significant problems with growth and alignment.

When considering whether to do an epiphysiodesis to treat leg length discrepancy, it is important to understand growth remaining in the opposite leg. The multiplier method allows for a quick calculation of the predicted limb length discrepancy at skeletal maturity, without the need to plot graphs, and is based on as few as one or two measurements. This method is independent of generation, height, socioeconomic class, ethnicity, and race. Paley et al. verified the accuracy of this method clinically by evaluating patients who had been managed with limb-lengthening or epiphysiodesis.[2-4] And, yes, there is an app for that!

Special Considerations for Different Age Groups

THE INFANT

The typical infant is born with flexion contractures. The hips are generally externally rotated. Genu varum and flat feet are normal. On the other hand, asymmetry of any kind should prompt attention. Be alert for possible handedness before the age of 1 year as it may be a sign of hemiplegia or any other unilateral problem. The orthopaedist caring for infants and toddlers should be generally familiar with a series of milestones that can help quickly identify a child who is lagging behind (Table 3-2). Such an understanding of milestones can have an important role in managing a potential musculoskeletal problem, and counseling families as to whether further investigation is needed. A consult with a developmental pediatrician should be if a child is falling short of developmental milestones.

THE GURU SAYS...

The age-based multiplier overall works very well. However, because children into their adolescent growth spurt at different times, the variability gives age-based multipliers a wide variance during this phase of growth. Skeletal maturity becomes a much more reliable method once the child enters a growth spurt.

JAMES SANDERS

THE GURU SAYS...

At birth, the newborn is hypertonic with archaic reflexes. The trunk makes up 70% of the standing height and the lower limb 30%.

ALAIN DIMÉGLIO

TABLE 3-2 Key Motor Milestones to Keep the Orthopaedist Out of Trouble	
Age	**Achievement**
2 mo	Good head control in prone position; partial head control in supine position
3 mo	Loss of grasp primitive
4 mo	Good head control in supine position; rolls over prone to supine
6 mo	When prone, lifts head and chest with weight on hands; sits with support
	Loss of Moro primitive reflex
	Loss of asymmetric and symmetric tonic neck primitive reflex
8 mo	Sits independently; reaches for toys
10 mo	Crawls; stands holding onto furniture
	Loss of neck-righting primitive reflex
12 mo	Walks independently or with hand support
	Gain of parachute postural reflex
18 mo	Developing handedness
2 y	Jumps; knows full name
3 y	Goes upstairs alternating feet; stands momentarily on one foot; knows age and gender
4 y	Hops on one foot; throws ball overhand
5 y	Skips; dresses independently

It's important to understand the difference between a deformation and a malformation. Malformations, such as syndactyly or proximal focal femoral deficiency (PFFD), are defects in organ development that occur early in fetal life. Deformations are changes in the limbs trunk, head, or neck caused by mechanical force over time. During the rapid period of fetal growth, such a force can lead to a deformation such as a calcaneovalgus foot or metatarsus adductus. Unlike malformations, deformations can be corrected by gentle manual forces.

THE TODDLER

Children generally start walking by the age of 14 months and a delay in walking past 18 months is generally considered a developmental delay. While evaluation of developmental delay requires a multidisciplinary team, the orthopaedic surgeon often sees these kids early on. Birth history and early asymmetry in physical examination can be clues prompting further subspecialty evaluation. Orthopaedists are often consulted because a toddler is "clumsy." It's tempting to brush off such complaints, explaining that the child is accident-prone or that clumsiness is common in all children during periods of rapid growth. While these observations are true, it is particularly important to be vigilant for the child whose clumsiness is increasing during their toddler years. Increasing clumsiness or frank loss of milestones are not normal and should prompt a broader workup.

Bowlegs turn to knock-knees over the first 3 or 4 years of life. Normal lower extremity development starts with a period of physiological genu varum, which is most obvious in the new walker before the age of 18 months. Expect genu valgum to be maximal at 36 to 42 months of age and to spontaneously correct as the child approaches 5 years of age. Having a handout with these expected norms can reassure anxious parents.

Maturation of the nervous system in the first few years of life allows the development of a more efficient gait pattern. Early gait is characterized by a wide base of support, higher cadence to allow more time in stance versus single leg swing, and less reciprocal arm swing, or holding the arms up for balance. These immature gait characteristics should diminish by 3 years of age.

THE GURU SAYS...

When changes outside of age-appropriate values in mechanical axis of the lower limb are seen, one must look for causes. Always keep in mind that you have to look for a subtle neurological disorder! Look for a discrete spasticity of the lower limb! Behind a genu varum, search for a chondrodystrophy or rickets.

ALAIN DIMÉGLIO

THE SCHOOL-AGED CHILD

By the time children enter grade school, their gait has matured into a near adult-like pattern, and their lower extremity limb alignment should be approaching normals for adults. Be alert to asymmetries of size. At this age, children sometimes present with limb asymmetry. While this can be a limb length inequality, it can also be an asymmetry in limb girth. While leg length discrepancy is common and usually benign, discrepancies in girth, tone, and range of motion should prompt some concern. A rule of thumb is to accept 1 to 2 cm larger thigh circumference in the dominant leg.

At this age, lower extremity height accounts for about 35% of adult height, and this increases to 50% by maturity. It's normal for young children to have proportionately longer torsos! Again, in the school age child, be alert to clumsiness or a decrease in motor abilities. The classic example is the 5- or 6-year-old boy who is having trouble climbing the stairs as the first manifestation of Duchenne muscular dystrophy. Understanding proportional growth in children can help in counseling of families and in keeping the orthopaedist out of trouble. One valuable rule of thumb for leg length inequalities[5] is that if growth inhibition stays constant in a short limb, a limb length inequality in a girl of 3 and a boy of 4 years of age will be twice as large at maturity. Again, the multiplier method can be very helpful in predicting ultimate leg lengths in this age group.

THE ADOLESCENT

Humans are one of the few species that goes through an adolescent growth spurt, but this can occur over a broad range of age. In this age group, we really want to know when a child is going through peak height velocity (PHV, also called peak growth age), but it's not necessarily so obvious. Chronological age correlates with skeletal age within 6 months in only about 50% of children. Dr. Skaggs says, "I agree with Kasser, who found find bone age by the Gruelich and Pyle Atlas to be so variable as to not be worthwhile, especially around adolescence."[6]

Secondary Sex Characteristics

Girls develop secondary sex characteristic and attain peak height velocity about 1.5 years prior to boys. Breast budding is the first sign of puberty in girls and occurs about one year before peak height velocity. Menarche occurs about 2 years later, and most girls have achieved 95% of their adult height at that point. The first appearance of puberty in boys is testicular enlargement with pubic hair developing soon after. This occurs about 1.5 years before peak height velocity and about 3 to 3.5 years before the attainment of adult height[7] (Fig. 3-2)

While menarche, the development of secondary sex characteristics, the Risser sign, and triradiate closure provide some information regarding skeletal maturity, they all occur relatively late in development and have limited usefulness. The triradiate cartilage closure indicates that the adolescent is two-thirds of the way through the most rapid phase of growth. At menarche in girls and the first shaving episode in boys, the adolescent will generally be at Risser I, past peak growth. So we need ways to assess growth before they are obvious looking at the child's body, and several radiographic options can be useful. Although the Risser sign was historically used as a routine maturity assessment tool of adolescents with scoliosis, it evolves too late in the growth process and is unreliable compared to other methods of skeletal maturity assessment. Sanders staging of the digital physis has been shown to be much more accurate, reliable, and useful in the prediction of spine growth and scoliosis progression.[8,9]

> **THE GURU SAYS...**
>
> Although the age of entering the adolescent growth spurt varies significantly from child to child, once this process starts, maturity is very standardized from child to child. Bone age, which is really not an age but a maturity indicator, becomes tightly correlated to where the child is in their growth spurt.
>
> JAMES SANDERS

> **THE GURU SAYS...**
>
> When children enter their adolescent growth spurt, they're between 80% and 85% of their adult height and 2 years prior to their peak height velocity. At the peak height velocity, they have reached 90% of their adult height, 92% of their adult limb length, and 87% of their adult spine height. Rapid growth continues for proximally 2 more years and total growth for 3.5 years beyond their peak height velocity.
>
> JAMES SANDERS

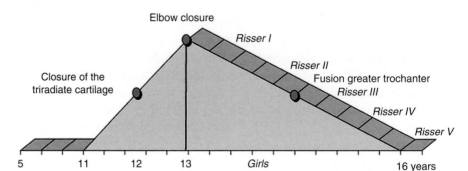

Figure 3-2 Relative timing of various growth milestones according to Dimeglio. Note that peak growth rate has passed by Risser 1. (Reprinted with permission from Diméglio A. Growth in pediatric orthopaedics. In: Morrissy RT, Weinstein SL, eds. *Lovell and Winter's Pediatric Orthopaedics*. Vol. 1. 6th ed. Philadelphia, PA: Lippincott Williams & Wilkins; 2006:35-66. Figure 2-5A.)

Dr. Vitale says, "I find using Sanders simplified classification of digital physeal closure (Sanders Scale) the most useful and easiest way to understand where a child is in growth. I keep a chart in every exam room but it really becomes second nature over time."[10] Figure 3-3 depicts the relative timing of peak growth in the context of various skeletal maturity schemas.

Understanding growth and development is a prerequisite to give optimal counsel about risks of progression of scoliosis, the potential efficacy of bracing, and timing of cessation of bracing. This will be discussed in more detail in the chapter about adolescent idiopathic scoliosis.[11,12]

Slipped Capital Femoral Epiphysis

Growth and skeletal maturation play a key role in the pathogenesis of slipped capital femoral epiphysis (SCFE). Loder et al. studied the radiographs of 30 children and concluded that there is a uniform skeletal age or "narrow window" during which epiphyseal slipping occurs, regardless of the child's chronologic age.[13] Another recent studied showed that in 83 children with slipped capital femoral epiphysis, 95% of boys and 83% of girls presented with their SCFE during the accelerating phase of puberty.[14] The triradiate cartilage was still open at the time of diagnosis in 65% of boys and 64% of girls. These investigators determined that once the triradiate cartilage is closed, there is only a 4% chance of a contralateral SCFE.

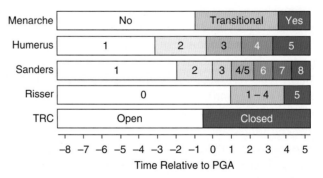

Figure 3-3 Peak growth age (PGA) (in years) in relation to various skeletal maturity systems. (Reprinted with permission from Li DT, Cui JJ, DeVries S, et al. Humeral head ossification predicts peak height velocity timing and percentage of growth remaining in children. *J Pediatr Orthop.* 2018;38(9):e546-e550.)

Adolescents often develop transient muscle contractures during this most rapid period of growth and development. Such muscle contractures cause a tremendous amount of trouble for adolescent athletes, particularly any muscle that crosses or attaches to the rapidly growing femur. Contractures of the quadriceps, hamstrings, and gastrocs are normal, but can cause a host of symptoms such as patellofemoral pain and heel problems, but remember that isolated progressive hamstring contractures are a spine problem until proved otherwise.

Staying Out of Trouble With the Growing Child

* The definition of "normal" depends on whether or not you are dealing with an underlying condition. Normal size and normal motor milestones are different for children with Down syndrome, achondroplasia, or Marfan syndrome.

* Look at the growth chart. Lack of normal growth over a 6-month period represents a significant deviation from normal, and evaluation by an endocrinologist should be considered.

* It is tempting to brush off a complaint of "clumsiness." It is particularly important to be vigilant for the child whose clumsiness is increasing during their toddler years. The parents may be bringing you a child showing the first manifestations of a disorder such as muscular dystrophy.

* Digital epiphyseal staging as described by Sanders is much more reliable than Risser sign in assessing the most rapid period of growth and in making decisions about scoliosis treatment.

* In SCFE, there is a uniform skeletal age or "narrow window" during which epiphyseal slipping occurs, regardless of the child's chronologic age. Once the triradiate cartilage is closed, there is only a 4% chance of a contralateral SCFE.

SOURCES OF WISDOM

1. Little DG, Song KM, Katz D, Herring JA. Relationship of peak height velocity to other maturity indicators in idiopathic scoliosis in girls. *J Bone Joint Surg Am.* 2000;82:685-693.
2. Paley D, Bhave A, Herzenberg JE, Bowen JR. Multiplier method for predicting limb-length discrepancy. *J Bone Joint Surg Am.* 2000;82A:1432-1446.
3. Aguilar JA, Paley D, Paley J, et al. Clinical validation of the multiplier method for predicting limb length at maturity, part I. *J Pediatr Orthop.* 2005;25:186-191.
4. Aguilar JA, Paley D, Paley J, et al. Clinical validation of the multiplier method for predicting limb length discrepancy and outcome of epiphysiodesis, part II. *J Pediatr Orthop.* 2005;25:192-196.
5. Diméglio A. Growth in pediatric orthopaedics. Morrissy RT, Weinstein SL, eds. *Lovell and Winter's Pediatric Orthopaedics.* Vol. 1. 6th ed. Philadelphia, PA: Lippincott Williams & Wilkins; 2006:35-66.
6. Kasser JR, Jenkins R. Accuracy of leg length prediction in children younger than 10 years of age. *Clin Orthop Relat Res.* 1997;338:9-13.
7. Dimeglio A. Growth in pediatric orthopaedics. *J Pediatr Orthop.* 2001;21:549-555.
8. Vira S, Husain Q, Jalai C, et al. The interobserver and intraobserver reliability of the Sanders classification versus the Risser stage. *J Pediatr Orthop.* 2017;37(4):e246-e249.
9. Hung AL, Shi B, Chow SK, et al. Validation study of the thumb ossification composite index (toci) in idiopathic scoliosis: a stage-to-stage correlation with classic Tanner-Whitehouse and Sanders simplified skeletal maturity systems. *J Bone Joint Surg Am.* 2018;100(13):88.
10. Li DT, Cui JJ, DeVries S, et al. Humeral head ossification predicts peak height velocity timing and percentage of growth remaining in children. *J Pediatr Orthop.* 2018;38(9):e546-e550.
11. Minkara A, Bainton N, Tanaka M, et al. High risk of mismatch between Sanders and Risser staging in adolescent idiopathic scoliosis: are we guiding treatment using the wrong classification? *J Pediatr Orthop.* 2020;40(2):60-64.

12. Jackson TJ, Miller D, Nelson S, et al. Two for one: a change in hand positioning during low-dose spinal stereoradiography allows for concurrent, reliable Sanders skeletal maturity staging. *Spine Deform*. 2018;6(4):391-396.

13. Loder RT, Farley FA, Herzenberg JE, et al. Narrow window of bone age in children with slipped capital femoral epiphyses. *J Pediatr Orthop*. 1993;13:290-293.

14. Puylaert D, Dimeglio A, Bentahar T. Staging puberty in slipped capital femoral epiphysis: importance of the triradiate cartilage. *J Pediatr Orthop*. 2004;24:144-147.

FOR FURTHER ENLIGHTENMENT

Iobst C. Growth of the musculoskeletal system. In: Martus J, ed. *Orthopedic Knowledge Update: Pediatrics*. 5th ed. Rosemont, IL: American Academy of Orthopaedic Surgery; 2016:59-68.

Lowrey GH. *Growth and Development in Children*. 6th ed. Chicago, IL: Mosby-Year Book; 1973.

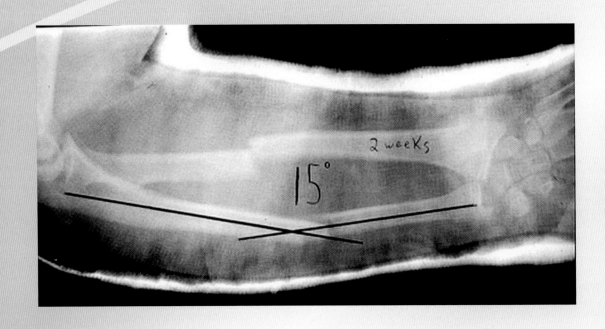

Chapter 4

Casts and Casting

KENNETH J. NOONAN, MD, MHCDS

Gurus: Matthew A. Halanski, MD and Benjamin J. Shore, MD

General Considerations

A lot has changed in orthopaedics over the past 50 years. Our specialty has morphed from one where traction and cast immobilization played a large role in managing patients of all ages for trauma, congenital conditions, and the aftermath of polio. We have witnessed advances in internal fixation, intraoperative imaging, and surgical techniques. For example, adult femur fractures are now treated with intramedullary fixation and are no longer treated with weeks of traction followed by walking spica casts. Simply put, we are no longer managing many adult fractures with closed methods. Even in children, advances in fixation have decreased our dependency on external methods of stabilization. Furthermore, changes in health care delivery have left casting to technicians and nurses (and who can do a great job), but this leaves even fewer opportunities for residents to learn the art of casting. There will always be a role for cast and splint immobilization, and in pediatric orthopaedics the need for these measures is not likely to change. While over 90% of adult forearm fractures are treated with surgery, 90% of pediatric forearm fractures are treated with reduction and cast immobilization. This is due in part to the remodeling potential of pediatric bones, where acceptable alignment rather than exact anatomic reduction is sufficient for many fractures. Similarly, joint stiffness is not typically a long-term problem for children treated with a cast.

Although casting is often viewed as "conservative" treatment, the physician and family should recognize that this does not imply that this treatment is without potential complications and pitfalls. The lay population have seen casts on other people's kids their whole lives and are biased to think that nothing wrong could happen to their kid. Although the true incidence of cast complications is unknown, a litigation history of a large multispecialty multilocation pediatric group showed that casts were the number one cause of litigation. When using a cast, it's important that a frank discussion of the risks and pitfalls of casting be explained to patients and families. I explain that cast sores occur in 1 per 100 patients and that together we have to be vigilant in preventing them. At the very least, this is important for protecting oneself from litigious and angry parents who can't understand why their child got a sore from a cast. Yet more importantly, we need to educate them that pain in high-risk areas such as the heel, dorsum of the foot and ankle, popliteal fossa, patella, and olecranon may be an impending sore. Stay out of trouble and tell them where the incision is on the child's extremity, if they have pain anywhere else they need to come in. **ORTHOPAEDICS 101: There are no hypochondriacs in casts.** If a child in a cast develops pain under the cast that persists longer than 12 hours, the cast needs to be removed or windowed and the skin inspected. This should be explained clearly to all parents and caregivers.

Certain pediatric patients may be at a higher risk for cast complications. Discerning problems in the very young or developmentally delayed may be quite difficult, and cast sores can occur despite appropriate and careful application. Many of these patients have comorbidities such as spasticity, malnutrition, altered sensation, and poor communication which increase difficulty of developing, detecting, and articulating cast problems.

Problems with casts can arise when they are used to obtain reductions; some of these can be minor and some can be limb threatening (Fig. 4-1). Fundamentally, when it comes to fracture care, its critical to remember that "reduction," whether it be open or closed, is not the same as stabilization, which is what casts and

THE GURU SAYS...

Consider an informed consent with cast application, a practice that is common in other countries, like Australia.

MATTHEW HALANSKI

THE GURU SAYS...

In nonverbal children or families with limited medical knowledge, marking the toes in a cast with an indelible marker is good technique to help guide parents on when to return for re-evaluation.

BENJAMIN SHORE

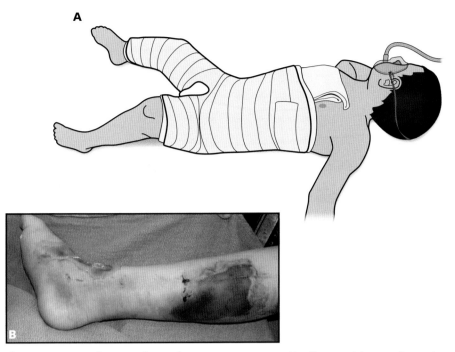

Figure 4-1 A: In the past, femur fractures were treated by first applying a spica cast to all portions except the broken femur. When these portions were hard, the fracture was reduced by applying traction through the casted lower leg; the thigh portion was the last part to be incorporated. **B:** Although apparently a simple method, a series of patients (including the one pictured) developed compartment syndrome in the leg. Lesson: *Using a cast to reduce a fracture is dangerous.* (Used with the permission of the University of Wisconsin Division of Pediatric Orthopaedics.)

splints do. If you need a cast to obtain a reduction, you need a different plan or an implant. Similarly, if you chose an implant that requires a cast to maintain a reduction, one should consider a more stable implant. A good example is the 10-year-old with a femur fracture that undergoes flexible nailing and the surgeon is concerned about stability and uses a long leg cast that ends at the fracture site. (The long lever arm of the cast actually makes it more unstable.) In this situation, a spica cast would be a *better* external immobilization method, yet a plate or a locked nail is likely the *best* choice for this fracture. *Nobody* likes spica casting.

Where does cast wedging for trauma come into play? Casts can be wedged with good results if done within certain time limits depending on the location of the fracture, the bone that is angulated, and the age of the patient. It is reasonable to consider cast wedging within 10 days for distal radius fractures; 14 days for both bone forearm fractures (Figs. 4-2 and 4-3); and 3 weeks for femur and tibia fractures. The reason cast wedging is acceptable is because we are not trying to *obtain* a reduction we are trying to *restore* a reduction that was lost in the cast. Where you can hurt a child is when you try to wedge an unreduced fracture acutely or try to wedge a fracture that will not move because it has "flexible" rod in it, or when the fracture is beyond the time windows outlined above (Fig. 4-4). Many of these fractures are very sticky and hard to move; in addition, radiographs of the fracture through cast material often hide signs of healing.

> **THE GURU SAYS...**
>
> When performing an "opening wedge" to realign fracture, it must be done slowly and gradually. Typically we use two cast spreaders to create space and use a cork spacer to facilitate our wedge. If the child is in pain after wedging we need to be concerned about creating a pressure ulcer or compartment syndrome. Often good practice is to keep a child in clinic for 30 minutes after wedging to make sure they are comfortable before sending home.
>
> BENJAMIN SHORE

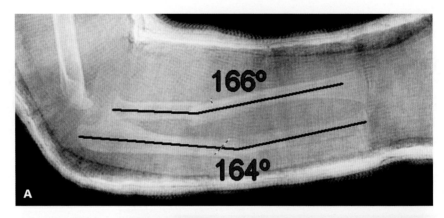

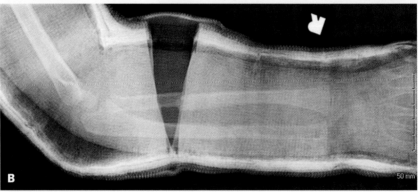

Figure 4-2 A: This 5-year-old boy was 10 days out from a both bone forearm fracture that had sagged into an unacceptable ulnar bow as the swelling decreased. **B:** Cast wedging restored the alignment. Be aware of the contralateral side of the cast; there is subtle buckling of the plaster, which can cause a pressure ulcer on the opposite side of the wedge. (Used with the permission of the University of Wisconsin Division of Pediatric Orthopaedics).

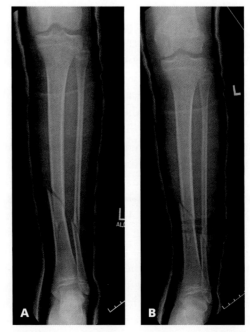

Figure 4-3 A: A 10-year-old girl with a tibia and fibula fracture treated with a long leg cast. Initial visit demonstrated valgus angulation. **B:** Angulation was corrected with an opening wedge cork spacer of about 1.5 cm.

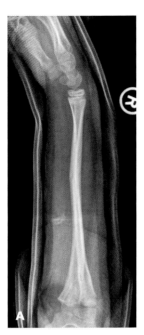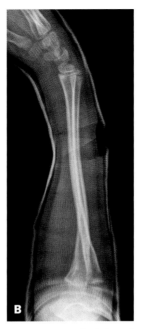

Figure 4-4 You cannot wedge a greenstick fracture. If you feel that the angulation needs to be corrected this needs to be done with a closed reduction and not wedging of the cast. **A:** This child with a greenstick forearm fracture had acceptable alignment; yet the provider was bullied into improving it by anxious parents. **B:** The child had his cast wedged without improvement of alignment. Note the fulcrum on the skin on the volar surface. This child developed a Volkmann ischemic contracture as a result of the compartment syndrome that ensued from this.

When wedging, the clinician needs to ensure that no excessive focal pressure is exerted at the bridge causing a pressure ulcer or nerve compression. A disadvantage of a "closing wedge" is that it may pinch soft tissue.

What about using casts to stretch joints and correct deformity that is not trauma related? The answer is "maybe," but be careful! In casting clubfeet, you get into trouble when you apply a cast in a position of correction beyond that which you obtain with manipulation. It is not uncommon to lengthen the hamstrings of a child with cerebral palsy who also has a knee flexion contracture. One can apply a long leg cast than do serial wedging to stretch the knee. Even if extra padding is placed on the heel and the knee, sores can happen—*be careful* (Fig. 4-5).

Pitfalls in Cast Application

It is important to have ready and in easy access the needed padding (cast lining and stockinette), water (lukewarm, not hot), cast material (plaster and fiberglass in rolls and reinforcing slabs), and needed instruments (C-arm imaging and X-rays clearly visible in line of sight, scissors, cast saws, spreaders etc.). This is key as cast application is a timely undertaking with materials that cure and harden in a short period, and the application may depend on a short window of time available for comfort or sedation of the child. It is further recognized that all needed personnel need to be ready, and this will ideally include a sedation team and child life specialists, in addition to the one to three people needed to apply a cast.

MATERIAL SELECTION

The two main choices for cast application are plaster of Paris and synthetic cast material like fiberglass. Plaster of Paris is cheaper and allows one to intimately

> **THE GURU SAYS...**
>
> If using a long leg cast to gradually stretch out a knee flexion contracture, removing the cast around the heel often can help prevent complications, but make sure there is not an edge to the cast putting pressure on soft tissue.
>
> BENJAMIN SHORE

> **THE GURU SAYS...**
>
> Consider casting to be an extension of your soul. Residents should put their initials on their casts to allow for feedback when patients return to the cast room.
>
> BENJAMIN SHORE

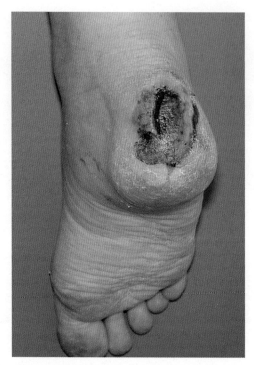

Figure 4-5 Heel ulcer that occurred during stretching cast for knee flexion contracture in a patient with spastic diplegia. (Used with the permission of the University of Wisconsin Division of Pediatric Orthopaedics.)

mold the material to the extremity being treated. It is also twice as heavy and not nearly as strong as fiberglass. There are different rates at which plaster can cure; the faster curing plasters tend to be much more exothermic and can lead to potential cast burns. Dip water temperatures of 50°C and thicknesses of 24 ply can yield temperatures high enough to cause burns. Placing a curing plaster cast on pillows can also lead to high temperatures in the area of pillow contact; these temperatures can be high enough to cause thermal damage. Overwrapping a curing plaster cast with fiberglass can also insulate and direct the heat back into the limb (Fig. 4-6). Fiberglass tape is commonly used and has several benefits in comparison to plaster such as being light weight, radiolucent, waterproof, and having lower peak temperatures of curing. The peak temperature of curing rarely exceeds 45°C, and thus, the risk of thermal injury from synthetic fiberglass tape is substantially less than plaster.

PROBLEMS WITH PADDING

Stockinette or liner may be applied against the skin, under the cast and cast padding. Although not essential, these liners minimize skin irritation; allow nice well-padded and polished edges to the cast to be applied. They also minimize the tendency of some children to "pick out" their cast padding. These liners are made of cotton, water-friendly synthetic materials such as polyester, sliver-impregnated cotton (to minimize bacterial growth), or Gore-Tex (W.L. Gore & Associates; Newark, Delaware). Some in the care of children who require spica cast application favor water-permeable liners such as Gore-Tex. In addition to being more convenient for patients, these newer synthetic materials have been shown to minimize skin irritation.

Ideally, the limb should be held in the desired position of immobilization prior to padding application. A common pitfall is when casting material is applied for a

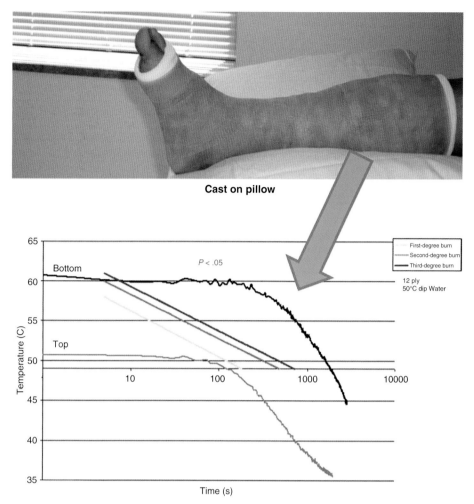

Cast on pillow

Figure 4-6 Recipe for disaster: Short leg plaster cast is covered with fiberglass and placed on a pillow while curing. Research has shown that this combination can yield temperatures high enough to burn the patient. (Used with the permission of the University of Wisconsin Division of Pediatric Orthopaedics.)

short leg cast with the ankle in less than 90° of ankle flexion; if the ankle is then flexed to 90° during the application or curing of the cast, the material will bunch up and will impinge on the dorsum of the ankle. Stay out of trouble by not using circumferential gauze under perioperative casts, which can become tourniquets as they shrink from dried blood combined with the limb swelling. It's better to cover wounds with noncircumferential sterile 4 × 4s and then wrap with cotton rolls, which can stretch or tear with swelling.

Pressure sores are not necessarily prevented by extra cotton padding; in fact, extra padding can lead to loss of reduction as swelling goes down, which can lead to shear forces and subsequent sores. Cast padding should be applied between three and five layers thick over the limb being casted. Bony prominences and cast edges should be additionally padded to prevent irritation yet allow a cast to be molded to fit snugly without undue pressure. The heel, malleoli, patella, anterior superior iliac spine (ASIS), and olecranon are areas that may require additional padding. The use of foam or felt padding in such areas may help decrease the incidence of pressure sores.

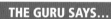 **THE GURU SAYS...**

While I cannot confirm, in the early part of the 20th century, plaster was applied directly to the skin with a perfect mold without any padding. I wouldn't recommend that now, but it shows that molding is probably more critical than padding.

MATTHEW HALANSKI

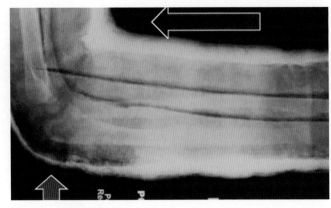

Figure 4-7 Classic example of excessive plaster in the concavity (blue arrow) and minimal plaster along convexity (red arrow). (Used with the permission of the University of Wisconsin Division of Pediatric Orthopaedics.)

THE GURU SAYS...

Plaster can be applied without gloves. While it is almost a rite of orthopaedic passage to walk around the hospital looking like a drywall installer, don't forget your gloves when applying fiberglass.

MATTHEW HALANSKI

PITFALLS IN CAST APPLICATION AND MOLDING

Plaster is dipped in water appropriate in temperature, some water is squeezed out, and then the plaster is progressively applied to the limb with circumferential wraps that overlap by 50%. Avoid wrapping too tight by taking tucks as you wrap around the convexities of a limb. **ORTHOPAEDICS 101: When wrapping any type of cast material (cotton roll, fiberglass, or plaster), there is a natural tendency to have excessive material in the concavities of a joint** (Fig. 4-7). We have seen burns from curing plaster in front of the ankle when the plaster becomes inadvertently too thick (Fig. 4-8). Stay out of trouble by keeping plaster uniform by using splints in back of the ankle and elbow and then incorporating with circumferential plaster (Fig. 4-9). Although similar problems wrapping fiberglass around convexities can occur, the relative strength of the material does not seem to lead to the same problems as plaster. One problem unique to fiberglass casting is inadvertent tightness that sometimes occurs as a result of the increased tackiness of

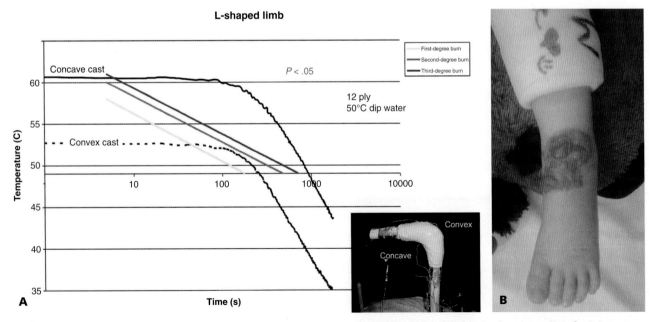

Figure 4-8 A: Research has shown that temperatures can get high enough to burn the skin in the concavity of a joint undergoing plaster application. **B:** Full-thickness burn over the anterior ankle from a plaster cast. (Used with the permission of the University of Wisconsin Division of Pediatric Orthopaedics.)

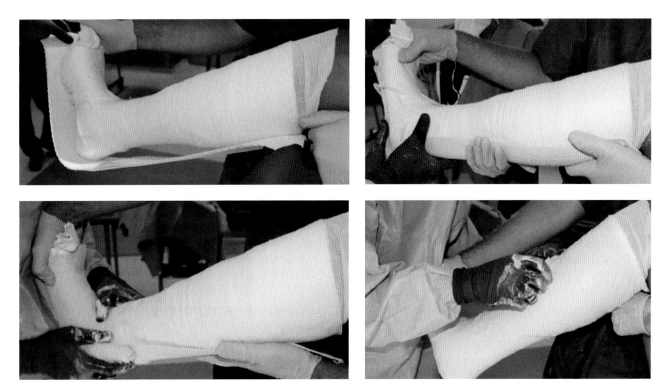

Figure 4-9 After the cotton has been applied to this short leg cast, a posterior plaster slab splint is applied then incorporated with circumferential plaster wraps. With this methodology, concave overwrapping is decreased. (Used with the permission of the University of Wisconsin Division of Pediatric Orthopaedics.)

the material as the roll is unwound. This can increase in older fiberglass that is more challenging to unroll. To avoid this, fiberglass should be applied in a stretch relaxation manner; the fiberglass roll is lifted off of the limb (in contradistinction to plaster which stays in contact); unrolled first then wrapped around the limb (Fig. 4-10). Difficulty exists when wrapping a wide roll into a concavity (anterior elbow or ankle), as the fiberglass can only lay flat if pulled too tight. Small relaxing cuts in the fiberglass may be needed, as fiberglass does not tuck as easily as plaster of Paris. Remember that fiberglass begins to cure as it exposed to air; don't open the package until you need it.

Plaster goes through stages of curing until it reaches full hardness 24 hours later. It's convenient to frame discussions about the stages of plaster molding as the initial stage, terminal stage, and final hardness. Initially as the plaster is being applied, it's critical to mold the plaster wraps together to incorporate the gypsum and the cotton fabric together to increase the strength of the cast. Merely wrapping plaster without incorporating it is a recipe for failure. Your hands and fingers should constantly be rubbing and incorporating the material in this initial phase, and you don't have to worry too much about pressure points, as the cast material is too soft to remain permanently deformed. We teach the residents that if you see fibers after wrapping the plaster you aren't molding enough! As the plaster begins to cure, however, you will notice that the material will become warm and firm and does not spring back. This is the terminal stage, when your final mold is produced, and this also the time where fingertips and pointy objects can leave permanent plaster indentations, which can lead pressure sores (Fig. 4-11). The same stages of initial and terminal molding also apply to fiberglass, yet less initial molding is required to incorporate the fiberglass, as it tends to cure faster. Both fiberglass and plaster can get divots during the terminal molding stages, and the cast should be held with open palms and not

> **THE GURU SAYS...**
> Residents often do not mold long enough. Moldings should occur until after a plaster cast is warm and after a fiberglass cast becomes warm and sticky. You will know when that is by the sounds of your hand sticking to the cast like you're walking through old soda on the movie theater floor.
> MATTHEW HALANSKI

> **THE GURU SAYS...**
> Fiberglass tends to have more memory and wants to "bounce" back after molding, so often the mold needs to be held longer with fiberglass until there is no doubt that it has set.
> BENJAMIN SHORE

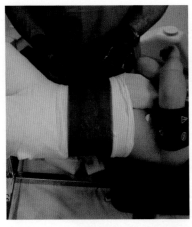
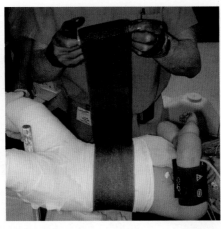
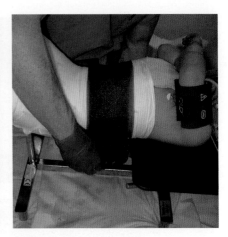

Figure 4-10 Stretch relax fiberglass application can decrease tightness. Unwinding the fiberglass and then wrapping the fiberglass will overcome the adhesive nature of the fiberglass roll as it is applied. (Used with the permission of the University of Wisconsin Division of Pediatric Orthopaedics.)

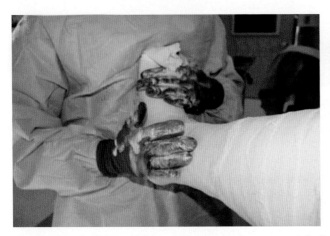
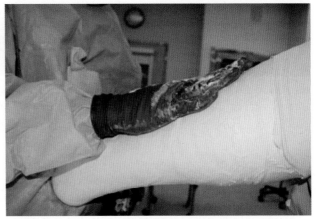

Figure 4-11 In the terminal molding stage, the surgeon's belly is a good place to support the foot in neutral while final molding is performed with the flat of the hand to avoid pressure spots. (Used with the permission of the University of Wisconsin Division of Pediatric Orthopaedics.)

fingertips. When you are done applying a plaster leg cast (and its cool), rest it on a pillow with the heel hanging free (Fig. 4-12). Even though plaster appears hard, it can deform gradually over the next several hours until it fully hardens. It's a good idea to tell patients to abstain from weight bearing on a plaster cast for 24 hours.

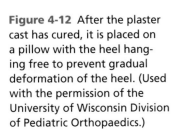

Figure 4-12 After the plaster cast has cured, it is placed on a pillow with the heel hanging free to prevent gradual deformation of the heel. (Used with the permission of the University of Wisconsin Division of Pediatric Orthopaedics.)

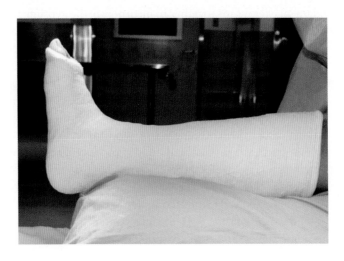

Pro Tips for Dealing With Casts

- Families and patients may be tempted to alleviate itching by sticking things down the cast. We tell families to avoid getting anything down in the cast, yet we have seen food, toys, writing utensils, money, and other items have been found down casts. We recommend a hair dryer on a cool setting to help with itching. Any patient with a suspected foreign body down the cast should have the cast removed and skin inspected (Fig. 4-13).
- A bar or wooden stick is sometimes used between the legs for a Petrie cast or to strengthen a spica cast. Do not apply the bar until the fiberglass or plaster is fully hard, as this can cause a divot when it's fastened down. Also, do not apply the bar until after the spica cast is trimmed; if you think cutting out the crotch of a spica cast is difficult, try doing it after you put the bar on.
- When you use a long leg cast in which the knee is flexed, teach nurses and family to keep a pillow under calf and the knee to support the leg. Without this, all of the weight goes to the heel and pressure sores can ensue.
- The good resident looks at the postreduction radiograph and checks alignment of the bone but also scrutinizes their cast for wrinkles, poor fit, and poor mold (Figs. 4-15 and 4-16).
- It can be difficult to apply a good cast simultaneously across two joints. As an example, it's a good idea to reduce and immobilize the wrist fracture and then extend it above the elbow after the wrist portion is set (Fig. 4-17).

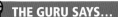

THE GURU SAYS...

Placing additional padding proximal to the calcaneus over the Achilles tendon can help to allow the heel to float inside the cast. This can be useful for patients in a long leg cast in knee extension with or without spasticity.

Be aware of using a cylinder cast with limited knee flexion in a nonverbal or delayed child, as the cast often slides down and creates pressure on the Achilles tendon (Fig. 4-14). A supracondylar mold is critical to prevent a straight-legged cast from slipping down, but consider including the foot to prevent pressure ulceration at Achilles.

BENJAMIN SHORE

Dr. Skaggs Adds

Any time you think a cast may need to be split to allow for swelling, consider putting foam directly on the skin and fiberglass on top of that. This combination will allow for swelling, have more strength than a split cast, and avoid the danger of cast burns splitting a cast (Fig. 4-18).

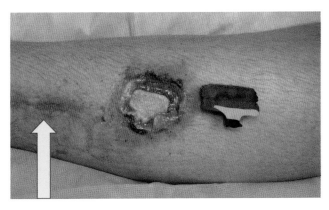

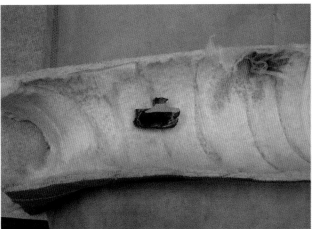

Figure 4-13 This is an emotional moment for all involved. Bobby is happy his long-lost tank has been found in his cast. Dad is nauseated from the full-thickness pressure sore. The third-year resident is angry that he injured Bobby with a cast saw (arrow). (Used with the permission of the University of Wisconsin Division of Pediatric Orthopaedics.)

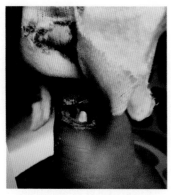

Figure 4-14 Achilles pressure ulcer from cylinder cast in autistic child. (Courtesy of Benjamin Shore, MD.)

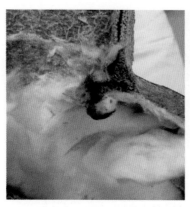
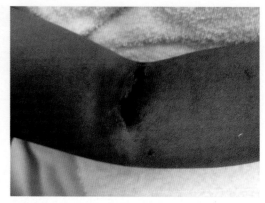

Figure 4-15 In this case, the fiberglass crease in the antecubital fossa was not noticed. (Courtesy of Jeff Sawyer, MD, Campbell Clinic.)

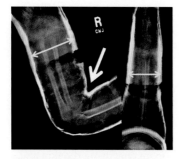

Figure 4-16 Our resident is happy that his cast is cylindrical with a cast index (width to depth ratio) that is about 0.7 (optimal) and the fractures are nicely aligned after the wedging. Hopefully they will have noticed that this fiberglass wrinkle (arrow) could lead to a bad sore, so they should replace the cast or removed the wrinkle. (Used with the permission of the University of Wisconsin Division of Pediatric Orthopaedics.)

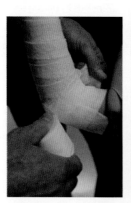
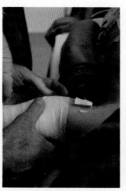
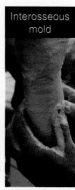
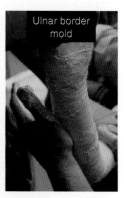

Figure 4-17 Cotton padding is applied up the entire arm in this boy with a distal both bone forearm fracture. In order to prevent problems, the team casts and molds the forearm fracture first. Once this portion hardens, it will be extended up the arm. (Used with the permission of the University of Wisconsin Division of Pediatric Orthopaedics.)

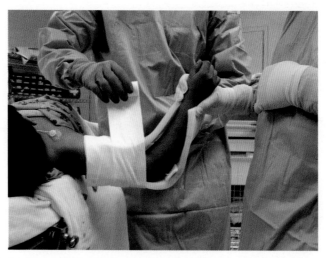

Figure 4-18 Sterile foam placed directly on skin with no underlying circumferential bandages allows for swelling under the cast.

PITFALLS IN CAST SPLITTING AND REMOVAL

Casts often need to be split and spread prophylactically before swelling peaks. Cast saw injuries are a large source of morbidity and can lead to painful lawsuits (Fig. 4-19). Injury to the child is likely a combination of mechanical and thermal injury.

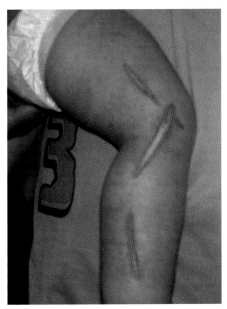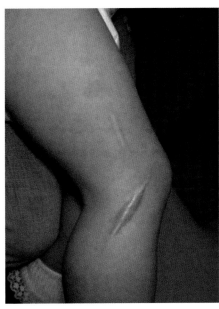

Figure 4-19 This baby had her clubfoot cast removed by an inexperienced resident who was unfamiliar with the technique of cast saw removal and was unaware of the relatively thin padding that is used with the Ponseti method. (Used with the permission of the University of Wisconsin Division of Pediatric Orthopaedics.)

Stay Out of Trouble When Splitting a Cast

* Remember that cast saws *can* cut or burn children; showing the parents that the cast saw won't cut your hand is not the same for the child who can't pull away in time. *It happens a lot.*

* If you are wondering whether a cast should be split, do it, and do it when the child is still sedated or under anesthesia, *but make sure you leave enough time for the cast to cure first.* (Splitting a cast at 2 am with a screaming child and a sleep-deprived mom standing nearby is never pleasant.)

* Residents and other learners should have adequate training before using a cast saw.

* Do not attempt to split a plaster cast until its fully cured. We have shown that when you are in a hurry and try to split a wet cast you are more likely to injure the patient. These casts are ready when they are warm and after 12 minutes. Fiberglass can be cut once it is hard.

(continued)

Dr. Skaggs Adds

Commit to making cast saw burns "never events." Assign someone the important task of making certain a cast saw guard is located next to every cast saw in the hospital and checking this on a regular basis. I cannot recall seeing a cast saw burn occur when a cast guard was used.

Stay Out of Trouble When Splitting a Cast *(continued)*

* Plan to univalve a cast opposite the side the bone is expected to displace. For example, split the wrist cast on the volar surface for dorsally displaced fractures.

* Make sure that the cast saw blade is sharp. Dull saw blades can get very hot. Check blade frequently, and cool in water if necessary.

* Use cast saw guards at all possible opportunities (Fig. 4-20).

* Cast saws should not be slid along the cast. Cut the material by pushing and withdrawing, with your finger bracing the saw off of the cast (Fig. 4-21).

* Simply cutting a cast will not decrease swelling, the cast needs to be spread and held open. Plan to cut the cotton padding and to bivalve casts if extreme swelling is expected. Commercially available wedges can keep the cast open; make sure the wedges are not pushed down as this can lead to a pressure sore (Fig. 4-22).

THE GURU SAYS...

Forget "cutting" a cast off. Think instead of "perforating" the cast. Cutting brings to mind use of a circular saw that is dragged along a board. Cast saw injuries occur when a hot oscillating blade remains in contact with the skin too long or pulls the skin tight so that the skin cannot oscillate with the blade. By "perforating" the cast, blade to skin contact time is minimal and skin is not pulled tight. When using a cast saw, consider rotating your wrist so different parts of the circular cast saw are in contact with the skin, thereby decreasing the heat and increasing the chance of using a sharp edge of the cast saw. Listen for the pitch change associated with completely perforating the plaster or fiberglass; train you ear to hear this and respond to it.

BENJAMIN SHORE

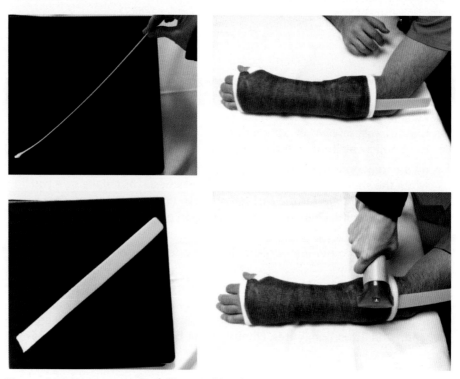

Figure 4-20 To stay out of trouble, use thin plastic saw guards wherever possible. (Courtesy of David Skaggs, MD, Children's Orthopaedic Center, Los Angeles.)

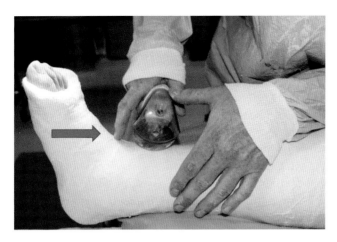

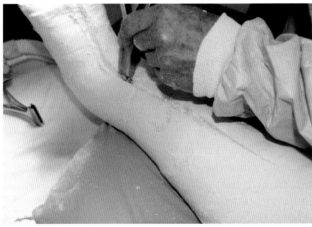

Figure 4-21 Correct use of a cast saw. The surgeon is using two hands to brace the saw, and his index finger acts as a guard from plunging. Just splitting a cast does not decrease pressure; it needs to be spread with a cast spreader. (Used with the permission of the University of Wisconsin Division of Pediatric Orthopaedics.)

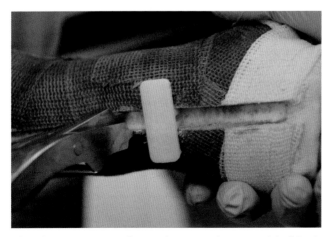

Figure 4-22 After the cast is cut and spread, cast wedges are critical for keeping the cast wedged open. Fiberglass casts have a propensity to spring back after being spread. Once the wedge is in place, make sure it isn't pushing on the soft tissues. (Used with the permission of the University of Wisconsin Division of Pediatric Orthopaedics.)

Long Arm Cast Application

Fracture reduction and long arm cast application is best done in a setting in which the child is adequately sedated and in which enough qualified personnel can apply the cast under fluoroscopic guidance, although this may not be possible in many locations. Fracture reduction technique may consist of longitudinal traction, manipulation re-creating the deformity, reducing the fracture and placing the intact periosteum on tension, and three-point molding in completely displaced fractures at the same level in the forearm.

Longitudinal traction is used with an assistant while a thin layer of cast padding is applied. Alternatively, the fingers could be placed in finger traps with the elbow flexed just short of 90° and with weights from the distal humerus. Individual strips of cast padding are placed and torn with tension to fit intimately on the posterior elbow thus avoiding too much anterior padding.

Padding is rolled high in the axilla to ensure enough padding for the proximal trim line (see Fig. 4-17). After padding is applied to the entire arm a small splint of five layers of plaster of Paris is fashioned to fit into the first web space (Fig. 4-23) and then incorporated with sequential layers of plaster; we find that this method allows for a better fit in the hand. Plaster is pushed and unrolled up the arm to the elbow without lifting the plaster roll off of the arm unless tucks are needed in the concavity. We prefer to apply plaster of Paris or fiberglass to a limb in stages by focusing and immobilizing one joint at a time; for long arm casts, we apply and mold the wrist and forearm and we extend the cast up over the elbow after the material has hardened. Once enough plaster is applied, the initial mold to incorporate the layers is started by rubbing the arm circumferentially. As the plaster begins to harden, terminal molding of the arm is performed under fluoroscopy by flattening the plaster over the apex of the deformity, molding the ulnar border with the flat of the hand (see Fig. 4-17), and finally with some interosseous molding that will make the cast flatter and less cylindrical in cross section. Fluoroscopy images are obtained as the short arm portion hardens before extending the cast up the humerus. If acceptable reduction is apparent, the antecubital fossa is inspected closely to detect and trim back cast material which may be too high and which could lead to neurovascular compromise. This

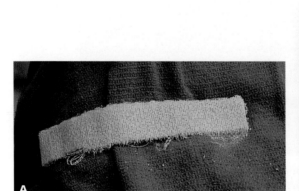
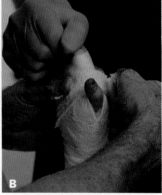

Figure 4-23 A small strip of plaster **(A)** works well in the web space of the thumb and index finger **(B)**. (Used with the permission of the University of Wisconsin Division of Pediatric Orthopaedics.)

method of applying the cast in two stages has the potential downside of edges of the short arm cast digging into soft tissue proximally, so this must be avoided. As the cast is extended up the humerus, a small posterior splint can be applied to elbow convexity to decrease the tendency to fill the concavity of the elbow with thick exothermic plaster. The humerus portion is molded terminally by flattening the posterior humerus and molding along the supracondylar ridges. Plain radiographs are then obtained while the child is still sedated, and if alignment is good, the forearm cast is univalved and spread. In general, the cast should be univalved and spread on the side of the arm which is opposite the direction of initial displacement; a fracture with a propensity for dorsal displacement should be split volarly and a fracture with a propensity for volar displacement should be split and spread along the dorsal surface.

Long Leg Cast Application

The short leg cast is applied first with goals of fully immobilizing the lower leg and keeping the ankle at 90° while avoiding complications from pressure points. After applying proximal and distal stockinette, the ankle is held at 90° and the limb is wrapped with cotton padding. To avoid excessive plaster of Paris cast material over the anterior ankle, a posterior splint of five layers thick is measured, applied, and then overwrapped with plaster rolls (see Fig. 4-9). The ankle can be held at 90° by the surgeon's torso, and the plaster is carefully molded around the malleoli and the pretibial crest. Some fractures require less than 90° of equinus at the ankle to hold the reduction; great care with ankle padding is necessary in these situations. Once the short leg portion has hardened the upper thigh is wrapped with padding and the knee (held in the chosen degree of flexion), and thigh is overwrapped with cast material. Care is needed to make sure the posterior trim line of the short leg cast is not too high and which could be compressing in the popliteal fossa. The anterior knee portion can be reinforced with a splint and thus further decreasing the cast load in the popliteal fossa. Finally, a medial and lateral supracondylar mold (similar to that in long arm cast) can be used to support the weight of the cast and prevent distal migration. Plaster long leg casts can be heavy, as such we will use an all fiberglass cast or consider a composite cast whereby the short leg portion is molded with plaster of Paris, and then when hardened, the proximal portion is placed with fiberglass.

The cast should be hard and well cured before cutting; bivalving a wet cast will weaken it, and the foot can drift into equinus. The cooled cast can be supported on a pillow with the ankle hanging free (see Fig. 4-12). Once hardened, the cast can be univalved and spread anteriorly if needed to accommodate swelling; if significant swelling is expected, then the cast can be bivalved and spread with release of the cotton padding.

Spica Cast Application

Spica casts can be applied from infants to adolescents and the type of cast can vary according to the clinical problem. For length-stable femur fractures in toddlers and small children, the clinician may choose a single leg walking spica for which the hip and knee will be flexed 30° (Fig. 4-24). For more severe fractures, one could use a standard one and half spica. In subtrochanteric fractures, the hip

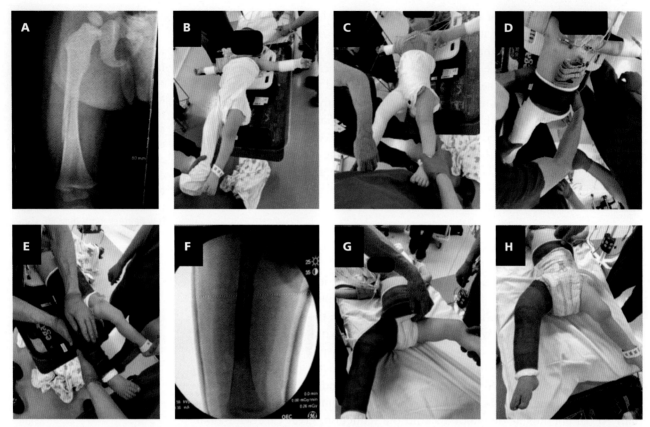

Figure 4-24 **A:** Single-leg spica cast is a good option for length stable fractures in smaller children. **B:** Gore-Tex pantaloon is applied to the affected leg as the child is positioned on the spica table. **C:** With an abdominal spacer in place, cotton is applied. **D:** Casting begins on the thorax and the abdomen and is extended down the leg. **E:** Femur fractures tend to drift into procurvatum and varus, and thus, anterior and lateral molds are developed. **F:** Fluoroscopic images show good alignment. **G:** The child has an abdominal pad placed under the cast against the perineum to immediately absorb urine and feces. *This is critical* to avoid cast sores. **H:** A diaper is then placed over the cast and the pad. (Used with the permission of the University of Wisconsin Division of Pediatric Orthopaedics.)

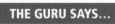
THE GURU SAYS...

While not an absolute requirement, consider endotracheal tube intubation for these cases, as an laryngeal mask airway can easily become dislodged moving on and off the spica table.

BENJAMIN SHORE

will need to be flexed 90° (Fig. 4-25) to account for the pull of the psoas muscle. In general, we include the foot in neuromuscular patients who are prone to develop an equinus contracture and whose distal tibia is osteoporotic and prone to fracture at the level of the distal trim line.

The location where the cast is applied can vary according to age and clinical problem. For instance, infants and most children with painful injuries will require sedation and application in the supine position on a spica table. In contrast, a single leg spica cast can be used as an adjunct to internal fixation for femur fracture in large children or adolescents. These latter casts can be applied in a supine or even a standing position with a compliant and comfortable patient. Because of the size of the casts, most spica casts are constructed with synthetic cast material; plaster of Paris still has utility in small infants where a more intimate mold is used and where it's hard to conform fiberglass rolls.

Spica cast application in children is performed on a well-padded spica table that should be firmly attached to the OR bed or cart; one person should be responsible for managing the torso and making sure the child does not fall off the table; one to two assistants will support the legs while the anesthesia team manages the head and airway—this leaves the last of a four- to five-person team to apply the cast. Before placing the child on the spica table, a waterproof pantaloon or stockinette is applied to the torso and legs. To have room for food

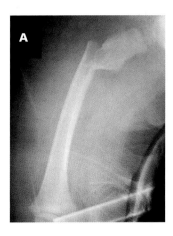
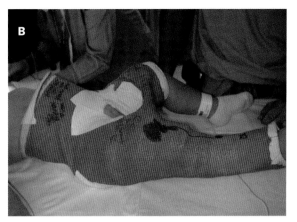
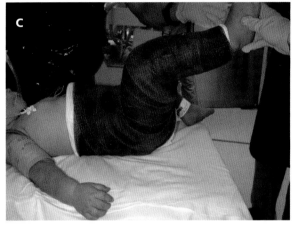
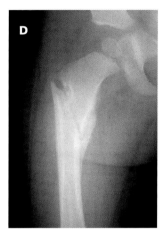

Figure 4-25 **A, B:** This 3-year-old with a proximal intertrochanteric fracture was treated with a standard 1 and ½ spica cast with the hip flexed 30°. The proximal femur was malreduced, likely as a result of pull from the psoas tendon. **C:** Ten days after injury, the child was revised to a 90/90 hip spica cast. **D:** Six weeks later, the fracture has healed anatomically. (Used with the permission of the University of Wisconsin Division of Pediatric Orthopaedics.)

and respiration; place a 2- to 3-inch thick towel or other pad on the stomach and under the liner or stockinette, that will be removed when the cast is dry. The child is lifted onto the table, and three to six thicknesses of padding are applied, with more at bony prominences such as over the patella and heels. It is also wise to completely cover the perineum with padding and high over the thorax; it is extremely hard to add padding once the cast material is applied. After padding is appropriately applied, the thorax is wrapped with synthetic cast material (see Fig. 4-10) and extended down over the uninjured thigh for a standard spica. Care is needed to cover the "intern's triangle" (Fig. 4-26), the posterior area of the cast at the junction of the thigh, buttock, and thorax.

Once the uninjured leg portion is hardened, the injured leg is casted from proximal to distal. We recommend casting from the thorax, over the hip and to the distal thigh and then extending over the knee and onto the distal leg as soon as the hip and thigh portion is firm; once the knee and leg portion is hardened, the cast can be extended down to include the foot and ankle for those patients who need it. Care must be taken not to apply a short leg cast first and then use it to apply traction across the femur, as this is associated with soft tissue problems and compartment syndrome (see Fig. 4-1).

THE GURU SAYS...

I like to incorporate posterior splints of fiberglass into the cast as it is rolled in this area. I have found this often increases the rigidity of the cast to the point a Petrie bar is not needed. Typically, three splints are applied: one from trochanter to trochanter and one splint each that wraps from pubic tubercle under the ischium to the ischial tuberosity and posteriorly wraps to the contralateral leg.

BENJAMIN SHORE

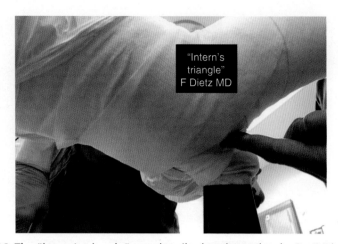

Figure 4-26 The "intern's triangle" was described to the author by Dr. F. Dietz, a skilled pediatric orthopaedist. This is the posterior junction of the thigh that is not visualized and is easily overlooked during spica cast application. Care must be taken to make sure there is enough padding and cast material in this structurally important area. (Used with the permission of the University of Wisconsin Division of Pediatric Orthopaedics.)

Once the cast is hardened, the perineal region is trimmed and patient is removed from the spica table. The abdominal pad is removed, and in some children, a hole over the abdomen can be cut for further room. Next appropriate radiographs are obtained, and the trim lines are padded by rolling back the under padding and lining and incorporated with trim fiberglass. The decision to apply a bar from leg to leg is made based on the structural integrity of the cast. Usually, this is not needed in small children and infants. Should a bar be needed, then it is wise to wait until the cast is fully cured and the chance of a pressure sore is decreased. Non–toilet-trained infants and children need to have an absorbent pad (small diaper, abdominal pad, or sanitary napkin) placed in the perineal region and then a diaper is placed over this (see Fig. 4-24). Simply placing a diaper over the cast will not absorb the waste material, as the diaper will not be in contact before the waste tracks under the cast (Fig. 4-27).

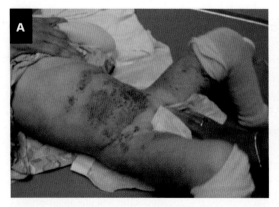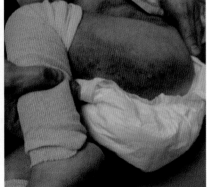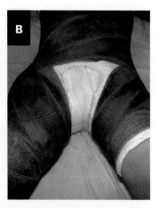

Figure 4-27 A: This poor child had horrific contact dermatitis from urine and feces. The family was not properly taught to perform mandatory spica care. **B:** We tell families to tuck an adsorbent pad under the cast adjacent to the perineum and *then* apply the diaper. Simply placing a diaper will not prevent urine from tracking up the cast. Families are instructed to change the pad that is next to the skin and the diaper every 2 to 3 hours. The families cannot leave the hospital until seen by an orthopaedic cast technician who is armed with pictures like this and who will bring the fear of God on them. (Used with the permission of the University of Wisconsin Division of Pediatric Orthopaedics.)

Doozies

Eleanor Roosevelt once said, "Learn from the mistakes of others. You can't live long enough to make them all yourself." In the interest of learning from examples of poor casts and pitfalls (and providing entertainment value), we show some doozies in Figures 4-28 to 4-34.

Text continues on Page 68

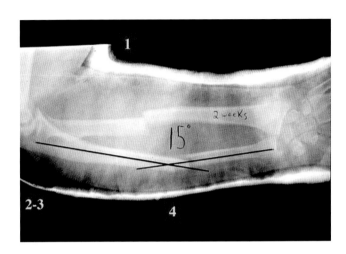

Figure 4-28 What four errors do you see here? *Survey says:* (1) Too much concave cast material. (2, 3) Too much padding and not enough convex plaster. (4) A bowed ulnar border allows the arm to sink into the cast. (Used with the permission of the University of Wisconsin Division of Pediatric Orthopaedics.)

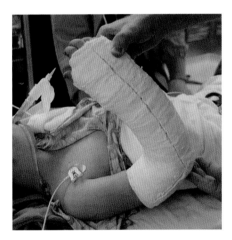
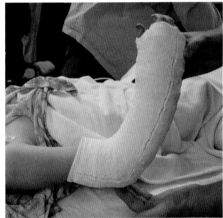
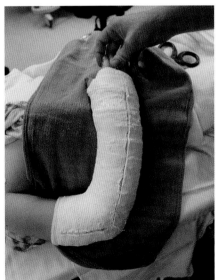
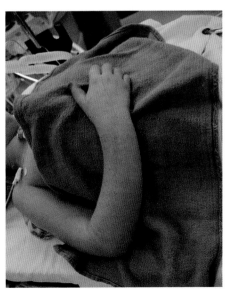

Figure 4-29 This "long" arm cast hardly immobilizes the elbow. The 4 pounds of plaster applied and the bent cast resulted in a bent arm. A better cast would go higher, would be lighter, and would be better molded. (Used with the permission of the University of Wisconsin Division of Pediatric Orthopaedics.)

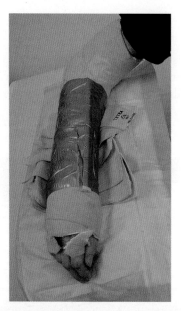

Figure 4-30 This is one for the DIY (do it yourself) crowd. The intern who applied this cast failed to work to mold the plaster together and the cast quickly fell apart. In the initial molding stage, it is important to incorporate the gypsum and the fabric fibers for cast strength. Although duct tape and wooden sticks seemed to work, they're not recommended at most modern children's hospitals. (Used with the permission of the University of Wisconsin Division of Pediatric Orthopaedics.)

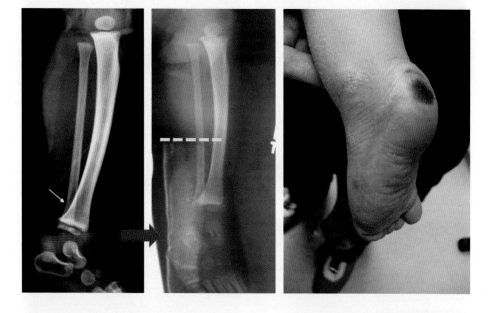

Figure 4-31 What could go wrong with a toddler's fracture? This patient with a minimal fracture had a short posterior splint (yellow line) applied that migrated distally and led to posterior pressure on the heel (red line). (Used with the permission of the University of Wisconsin Division of Pediatric Orthopaedics.)

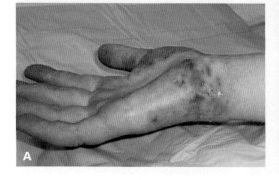
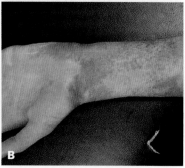

Figure 4-32 Just because the fiberglass cast and differing cast paddings (**A:** Gore-Tex, **B:** other synthetic padding) are "waterproof" does not mean the skin will do well if constantly wet. (Used with the permission of the University of Wisconsin Division of Pediatric Orthopaedics.)

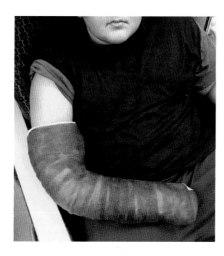
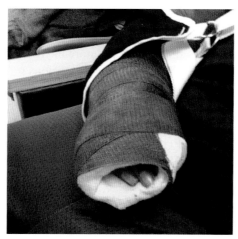

Figure 4-33 The "dreaded banana" cast that slides down the arm with the "disappearing fingers sign." Too much padding. The cast doesn't go high enough. The elbow is not at 90°. The forearm portion weighs more than the patient. For this resident, the last time he saw a "mold," he was inspecting his running shoes. (Courtesy of David Skaggs, MD, Children's Orthopaedic Center, Los Angeles)

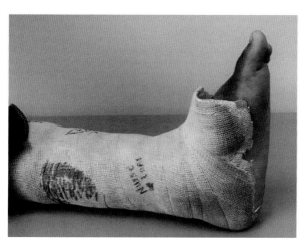
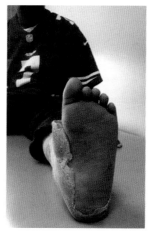

Figure 4-34 Some youth football players consider protected weight bearing more of a suggestion as opposed to a medical recommendation. (Used with the permission of the University of Wisconsin Division of Pediatric Orthopaedics.)

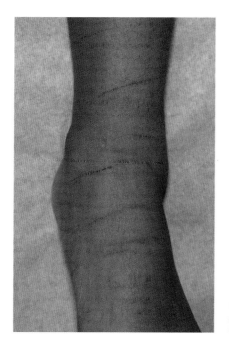
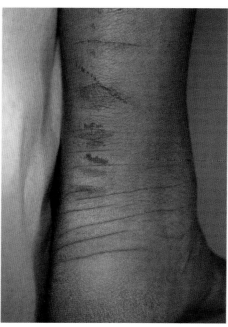

Figure 4-35 This child sprained her ankle and had an Ace bandage applied. Stay out of trouble and consider an Ace bandage as simply a brown covering that should be applied without any tension. (Used with the permission of the University of Wisconsin Division of Pediatric Orthopaedics.)

Conclusion

Fractures in children are more likely to be treated with a cast than with surgery. In our minds, the many complications result from inappropriate use of the cast or splint to *obtain* correction; in contrast, the cast or splint should be used to *maintain* reduction achieved either open or closed. Tight casts and bandages (Fig. 4-35) can cause compartment syndrome. Problems such as tight casts, wet casts leading to infection, foreign objects in casts, and pressure ulcers are not uncommon. It is important to educate parents that small children may not adequately communicate problems occurring under a cast.

Staying Out of Trouble With Casts and Casting

* Remember that cast application is a common cause for iatrogenic injury and legal action.
* Cast and splint application is an art form and that proper training and experience is needed to avoid injuring patients.
* Get help when applying large casts in younger patients. Immobilize one joint at a time.
* There are no hypochondriacs in casts.
* Involve your patients and their families in cast education. To help avoid problems, they need to know the following:
  * Casts can harm the patient
  * How to assess blood flow and decrease swelling with elevation
  * Where the potential sites of pressure sores occur
  * General cast care
  * Objects should not be stuck into the cast
* If you are thinking about using a cast to obtain a reduction, you are in dangerous waters and your bilge just broke. Consider another method to affect the reduction. Casts and splints are designed to *maintain* reduction.
* Plaster can burn your patient; avoid hot water and thick material.
* Cast molding—not cast padding—helps to prevent cast sores.
* Proper training is needed to cut or split a cast.
  * You can cut someone easily.
  * Is the blade sharp?
  * Is the material hard enough? (Wait 10 minutes for plaster.)
* When you assess a reduction with X-rays, look at the cast in addition to the bones. Does it fit well? Is it too thick in areas?

Acknowledgment

This chapter is dedicated to Fred Dietz, MD, a good friend, a master in cast application, and an even better doctor.

FOR FURTHER ENLIGHTENMENT

Ansari MZ, Swarup S, Ghani R, Tovey P. Oscillating saw injuries during removal of plaster. *Eur J Emerg Med*. 1998;5(1):37-39.

Bingold AC. On splitting plasters. *J Bone Joint Surg Br*. 1979;61B(3):294-295.

Cannaway JK, Hunter JR. Thermal effects of casting materials. *Clin Orthop*. 1983;181:191-195.

Davids JR, Frick SL, Skewes E, Blackhurst DW. Skin surface pressure beneath an above-the knee cast: plaster casts compared with fiberglass casts. *J Bone Joint Surg*. 1997;79-A(4):565-569.

DeMaio M, McHale K, Lenhart M, et al. Plaster: our orthopaedic heritage: AAOS exhibit selection. *J Bone Joint Surg Am*. 2012;94(20):e152.

Gannaway JK, Hunter JR. Thermal effects of casting materials. *Clin Orthop Relat Res*. 1983;181:191-195.

Garfin SR, Mubarak SJ, Evans KL, et al. Quantification of intracompartmental pressure and volume under plaster casts. *J Bone Joint Surg Am*. 1981;63-A(3):449-453.

Halanski M, Noonan KJ. Cast and splint immobilization: complications. *J Am Acad Orthop Surg*. 2008;16(1):30-40.

Halanski MA, Halanski AD, Oza A, et al. Thermal injury with contemporary cast-application techniques and methods to circumvent morbidity. *J Bone Joint Surg Am*. 2007;89(11):2369-2377.

Halanski MA. How to avoid cast saw complications. *J Pediatr Orthop*. 2016;36(suppl 1):S1-S5.

Hawkins BJ, Bays BN. Catastrophic complication of simple cast treatment: case report. *J Trauma*. 1993;34:760-762.

Killian JT, White S, Lenning L. Cast-saw burns: comparison of technique versus material versus saws. *J Pediatr Orthop*. 1999;19(5):683-687.

Kowalski KL, Pitcher JD, Bickley B. Evaluation of fiberglass versus plaster of Paris for immobilization of fractures of the arm and leg. *Military Med*. 2001;167:657-661.

Kruse RW, Fracchia M, Boos M, Guille JT, Bowen JR. Gore tex fabric as a cast underliner in children. *J Ped Orthop*. 1991;11:786-787.

Lavalette R, Pope MH, Dickstein H. Setting temperatures of plaster casts: the influence of technical variables. *J Bone Joint Surg Am*. 1982;64(6):907-911.

Lindeque BG, Shuler FD, Bates CM. Skin temperatures generated following plaster splint application. *Orthopedics*. 2013;36(5):364-367.

Marson BM, Keenan MAE. Skin surface pressures under short leg casts. *J Orthop Trauma*. 1993;7(3):275-278.

Monroe KC, Sund SA, Nemeth BA, et al. Cast-saw injuries: assessing blade-to-skin contact during cast removal: does experience or education matter? *Phys Sportsmed*. 2014;42(1):36-44.

Mubarak SJ, Frick S, Sink E, Rathjen K, Noonan KJ. Volkmann contracture and compartment syndromes after femur fractures in children treated with 90/90 spica casts. *J Pediatr Orthop*. 2006;26:567-572.

Pope MH, Callahan G, Lavalette R. Setting temperatures of synthetic casts. *J Bone Joint Surg Am*. 1985;67(2):262-426.

Puddy AC, Sunkin JA, Aden JK, et al. Cast saw burns: evaluation of simple techniques for reducing the risk of thermal injury. *J Pediatr Orthop*. 2014;34(8):e63-e66.

Shore BJ, Hutchinson S, Harris M, et al. Epidemiology and prevention of cast saw injuries: results of a quality improvement program at a single institution. *J Bone Joint Surg Am*. 2014;96(4):e31.

Shuler FD, Grisafi FN. Cast-saw burns: evaluation of skin, cast, and blade temperatures generated during cast removal. *J Bone Joint Surg Am*. 2008;90(12):2626-2630.

Steiner SRH, Gendi K, Halanski MA, Noonan KJ. Efficiency and safety: the best time to valve a plaster cast. *J Bone Joint Surg Am*. 2018;100(8):e49.

Stork NC, Lenhart RL, Nemeth BA, et al. To cast, to saw, and not to injure: can safety strips decrease cast saw injuries? *Clin Orthop Relat Res*. 2016;474(7):1543-1552.

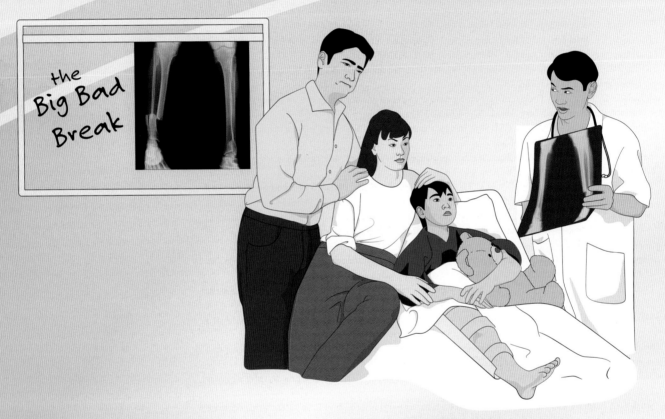

the Big Bad Break

From the outset, position the injury as the enemy you and the family are partnering to beat.

Chapter 5

Caring for the Injured Child

JOHN M. (JACK) FLYNN, MD and DAVID L. SKAGGS, MD, MMM

Guru: Steven Frick, MD

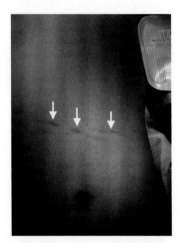

Figure 5-1 A seatbelt sign may be subtle, as in this example of horizontal ecchymosis in the setting of a soft tissue Chance fracture. In this case, the injury was missed on the initial radiology reading, and the clinical picture helped make the diagnosis. (Used with permission of the Children's Orthopaedic Center, Los Angeles.)

Caring for injured children is central to the mission of pediatric orthopaedics. Someday, they may invent a drug or genetic treatment that completely cures a syndrome or genetic deficiency that causes musculoskeletal deformity or disease. But they will never stop kids from hurting themselves: jumping out of trees, tackling friends on the trampoline, or skateboarding down the hill through traffic. **NEWSFLASH! The pediatric orthopaedist who treats injuries will never go out of business.** Understanding and avoiding the common pitfalls in caring for the injured child is central to the wisdom a pediatric orthopaedist gains over the years in practice.

Trauma is the leading cause of mortality in children. The outcome from the injuries is primarily related to the severity and management of the head and musculoskeletal injuries. It's important to listen carefully to the story of the injury (from the child and from the family whenever possible). Most pediatric fractures are isolated injuries, but be on the lookout for associated injuries on initial evaluation, especially after high falls, bike and vehicle crashes, and kids hit by cars. Recognize that certain injuries are sentinels for other types of injuries. Examples of this include rib fractures, pelvic fractures, facial injuries, and a lap belt sign (Fig. 5-1) on the anterior aspect of the abdomen or chest.

The value of mobilizing injured children is increasingly being appreciated, especially by busy families not prepared for their 5-year-old to be in a spica cast for 6 weeks. The vast majority of pediatric fractures can be treated successfully with cast immobilization. However, in the 21st century, we've seen a dramatic paradigm shift to internal fixation of pediatric fractures, often with improved outcomes, but not always with improved outcomes. Essential to the art of pediatric orthopaedics is understanding where surgery for a fracture gives a better outcome and where surgery just gives a temporarily better X-ray.

In an era in which families share stories and X-rays on social media and families Google an injury as soon as the emergency department (ED) doc gives it a name, there is often parental pressure to "put the puzzle back together perfectly" in the operating room. They may not want to deal with a spica cast for 6 weeks when Dr. Google says that maybe their 2-year-old could have a metal plate put on the femur, making the X-ray perfect, and have their toddler walking in a few days. All it takes is that rare infection, or intraoperative complication, or that second operation to remove the plate from the 2-year-old femur, before the seasoned orthopedist knows to use her judgment and convince the family that nature does a better job healing the fracture than a surgeon. **NEWSFLASH! With operative treatment of fractures in young children, just because you can, doesn't mean you should.**

A major source of trouble in caring for multiply injured children results from the family's perspective and expectations. When they arrive with their injured child, the family may be overwhelmed and shocked by the traumatic event. The relationship with the health care team is quickly established. As the surgeon, you may find yourself cast in one of two lights: part of the problem or part of the solution. Some families quickly look for someone to blame for the calamity, and if there is no one outside the hospital, they look for someone inside the hospital—and who better than the surgeon, the captain of the ship. The surgeon becomes solely responsible for "making it all like it was before the accident" and anything different is grounds for a malpractice suit. To stay out of trouble, use those first few minutes with the family to establish the optimal relationship—a partnership that is you and the family against the injury (Fig. 5-2).

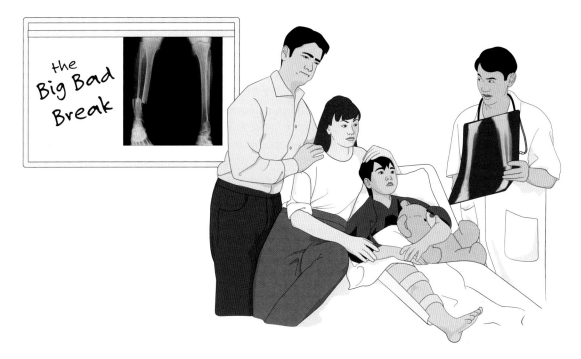

Figure 5-2 From the outset, position the injury as the enemy you and the family are partnering to beat.

It is fair for you to describe the extent of the problem in graphic detail, the outcome if untreated, the prolonged length of recovery (yes, many children do limp for a year or more after a serious lower extremity injury), and the numerous complications that have been described in the literature. Remember: you've been summoned to rescue this child and the family from the injury. The injury is not your fault. You are going into battle against it. It is wise to paint the worst possible picture, offer reassurance that often things go much better than that, and then at each stage express relief that the treatment and the healing is going fairly well. An example might be a Salter-Harris II distal femur fracture: explain that it is the fastest-growing growth plate that will give much of the remaining leg length in the teenager, and that studies have shown a growth arrest rate ranging from 30% to 40%, and surgery does not necessarily change this because the growth plate was damaged at the moment of injury. Then in the months that follow, as the fracture heals and the boy returns the soccer field, and there is no growth arrest, the family will feel blessed and appreciative, and you will be a hero. When rescuing a child from their injury, begin dark and end sunny; it's best for everyone involved. The more untrusting the family, the more you should see them, both inpatient and outpatient. After many weekly clinic visits, such families often thank you, rather than complain about the hassle of such close follow-up.

There are certain anatomic and physiologic differences that make a child's injury unique and may alter treatment. Ligaments may attach to the epiphysis. Because the ligaments are stronger than the physis, a force to such a joint leads to physeal injury rather than ligamentous disruption.

Plastic deformation is an important and unique type of fracture in children. Plastic deformation can lead to loss of motion or deformity, such as in a diaphyseal forearm fracture, or make reduction of an associate fracture difficult, such as in a type III Monteggia fracture. The ulnar border should be "ruler straight." A plastically deformed fibula can challenge tibia fracture reduction. Plastic deformation

THE GURU SAYS...

Challenging patients and families may make you want to skip post-op rounds or frequent office visits; resist the urge. Take on the challenge and win them over with concern for their child, honesty about how things are going, and a promise to them that you will go through this stressful, uncertain experience with them.

STEVE FRICK

THE GURU SAYS...

Know your teammates and communicate. Don't assume they know what you know about musculoskeletal trauma and the potential for significant blood loss. Use the preoperative time-out as an opportunity to voice your concerns. Assume the worst and be prepared.

STEVE FRICK

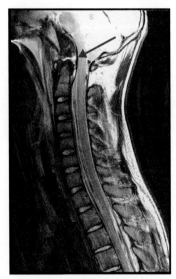

Figure 5-3 MRI is an important tool to avoid trouble when caring for a child with a possible occult cervical spine injury. MRI is particularly valuable to clear the cervical spine of a child who cannot cooperate with voluntary flexion and extension radiographs. This image allowed the diagnosis of ligamentous disruption at the occipitocervical junction (red arrow).

THE GURU SAYS...

Expose the zone of injury completely, irrigate thoroughly, define all relevant local anatomy (especially arteries/nerves that cannot be debrided), and seek and remove nonviable tissue. Knowing what to take and what to leave is likely the most important thing in open fracture management; take your time and be thoughtful.

STEVE FRICK

can be improved with operative reduction using a slow, steady (and significant) force, particularly in the forearm.

The two primary causes of death in pediatric trauma victims are head injury and intraabdominal hemorrhage. One of the most important ways to stay out of trouble as an orthopaedist caring for severely injured children is establishing a good relationship with your trauma team. Children have a smaller blood volume and become hypovolemic quite quickly. This is particularly problematic in femur fractures associated with splenic injury or other internal bleeding. Because of their amazing ability to compensate with an increased pulse, children may not show a drop in blood pressure due to hypovolemia until they are in a very critical range; this insight may be lost on the junior anesthesia resident covering your trauma case, so stay alert. Blood loss is easily underestimated because most pediatric trauma is blunt and the bleeding is internal. Partnering with a general surgeon and a neurosurgeon and using a careful physical examination with liberal use of imaging (Fig. 5-3) are valuable ways to optimally collaborate care when there are both skeletal injuries and multiple internal injuries.

Open fractures are relatively common in pediatric high-energy trauma. The most common areas are the forearm and tibia or an open fracture of the foot and ankle when the foot is run over by a car (Fig. 5-4). As in adults, the wound should be inspected once in the ED, classified, and covered with betadine gauze. Repeated evaluation of these wounds can lead to increased blood loss and the risk of nosocomial infections. Antibiotics and tetanus should also be given upon arrival in the ED. The key to reducing the infection rate in open fractures is the quality of the operative debridement, and how quickly appropriate antibiotics are given after arrival in the ED; the days of feeling obligated to treat a routine open fracture in the middle of the night are long gone. Although there may be other reasons to rush an open fracture to the OR, such as a neurovascular injury, soft tissue injury, or severe contamination, many clean open fractures in children can have their operative debridement within 24 hours with no increased risk of infection. Because of the better microvascular supply, soft tissue injuries seem to recover much better in children. To stay out of trouble, leave questionably damaged tissue at the first debridement and reassess at a second operation. In many cases, more extensive soft tissue coverage can be avoided if the surgeon is conservative in the initial debridement of a child's soft tissue.

Some hope to make life easier by going one step further: washing out the fracture in the ED, putting on a cast, and sending the family home. This is a recipe for disaster. Experienced pediatric orthopaedic trauma experts know that even open fractures with tiny wounds can have dirt inside the medullary canal of the bone, or fragments of grass or clothing pulled under the skin. Some of us have amputated a limb for gas gangrene caused by a failure to perform proper fracture debridement. A squirt of betadine by the ED resident is not enough. Open fractures need a careful, thorough open debridement under optimal conditions in the OR. Research studies that advocate for the "ED betadine squirt" will always be underpowered. Do the right thing for the child and get that fracture clean on Day 1.

Compartment syndrome creates lots of trouble in children because its diagnosis is more difficult. It can be harder to differentiate normal trauma pain from abnormal compartment pain in children. Look for a rise in the 3 A's: anxiety, agitation, and analgesic needs. It's tough to walk into the hospital room of a 5-year-old and say, "Hold still, I'm going to stick your leg a few times with this big needle to test the swelling" (Fig. 5-5). Maybe you get one stick, but you won't get two! If the scene is concerning (injury, 3 A's, tense feeling compartments), go to the OR, where you can get accurate measurements under optimal circumstances. If the compartments feel tense, there is a better than 90% chance it will be compartment syndrome. And in that remaining 10%, it is "impending compartment syndrome," and you will likely do the releases anyway. Finally, be alert that compartment syndrome may be quite delayed in children. Although the reason for this delay is not established (tissue compliance? better vascularity?), the first diagnosis is often 20 to 40 hours after fracture. Even when a compartment syndrome is diagnosed this late in children, the results are often good, with lower risk of devitalized muscle and other complications seen in adults.

To stay out of trouble, don't underestimate the extent that a child can recover from severe multitrauma, particularly head and spinal cord injury. The orthopaedist may be reluctant to operate on a child with severe closed head injury given the fact that fracture alignment seems to be the least of the child's problems. The inexperienced orthopaedist may expect that the child's chance of survival is low and allow the injuries to go untreated. The same surgeon may then have to face this child's malunion in his office 6 weeks later, when the child walks in with his physical therapist and parents. Operative stabilization may be necessary if spasticity develops in the days following head injury. Because the healing rates are faster with head injury, the decision for stabilization should be made early.

Physeal Fractures and Growth Arrest

Approximately 25% of all pediatric fractures are physeal fractures. To stay out of trouble, counsel the parents at your first discussion with them about the risk of growth arrest. Current statistics indicate that the risk of growth arrest is about 30% to 40% in the distal femur, 25% to 30% in the distal tibia, about 60% for the distal ulna, and about 4% for the distal radius. Physeal fractures tend to heal more quickly than

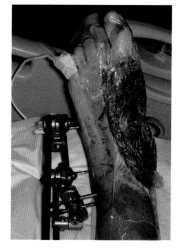

Figure 5-4 This patient had soft tissue loss down to bone across the ankle joint and foot from "road drag." The ankle is stabilized at 90° with an external fixator while a wound VAC provides immediate treatment for soft tissue loss. (Used with permission of the Children's Orthopaedic Center, Los Angeles.)

THE GURU SAYS...

Patients with long bone fractures and traumatic brain injury are often excellent candidates for use of external fixation because of its associated low blood loss, ability to be rapidly applied, and maintenance of length and alignment.

STEVE FRICK

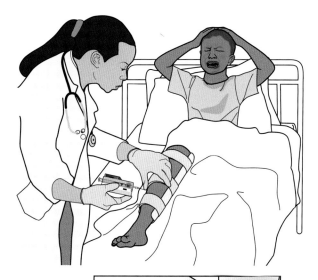

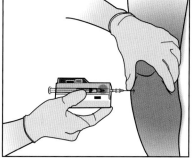

Figure 5-5 This is not going to go well. Do it in the OR.

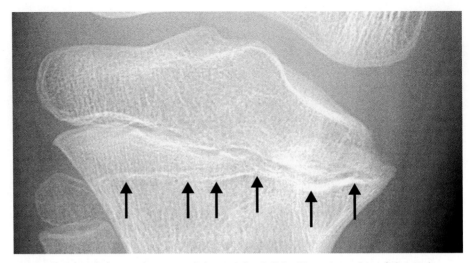

Figure 5-6 Medial growth arrest of the proximal tibia. Note the value of the Park-Harris growth arrest line in making this diagnosis (arrows).

THE GURU SAYS...

This means schedule follow-up in the clinic with an X-ray on arrival to check your reduction in 3 days. Even if the reduction is partially lost, most of the time it is best to await remodeling and see if late osteotomy is needed.

STEVE FRICK

metaphyseal and diaphyseal fractures. Therefore, the window for remanipulation of a physeal fracture is quite short. Most experts agree that a physeal fracture should not be subject to manipulative reduction more than 3 to 5 days after injury.

To stay out of trouble, physeal fractures at locations at high risk for physeal arrest should be followed for 6 to 12 months beyond healing. The Park-Harris line is valuable (Fig. 5-6). MRI can typically demonstrate a physeal arrest by approximately 6 months after injury. Beware of the occult physeal fracture; these are complete physeal fractures that are barely displaced on initial presenting radiographs. The typical case is a distal femoral physeal fracture that is dismissed as a sprain. An uninformed radiologist may read the radiographs as normal. Physical examination is essential in these cases. Be aware that physes adjacent to diaphyseal fractures (the distal femoral physis adjacent to an ipsilateral tibial shaft fracture) may sustain an unrecognized injury.

Child Abuse

THE GURU SAYS...

For every childhood fracture ask yourself these questions:
1. Does the stated mechanism match the fracture I see? (Consider child abuse).
2. Is this bone normal? (Consider pathologic fracture.)

STEVE FRICK

Missing child abuse may cost the child his or her life and the orthopaedist his or her license to practice. To stay out of trouble, the orthopaedist should get a social worker, pediatricians, and other appropriate experts and consultants involved if nonaccidental injury is a possibility. The history should include a thorough discussion of how the child was hurt and who was present at the time of injury. Family history of osteogenesis imperfecta or other multiple-fracture problems should be sought. About 95% of children can be diagnosed with osteogenesis imperfecta based on a family history and a physical examination of the child. The physical examination of a child suspicious for nonaccidental injury should include a full evaluation of the skin, trunk, and other parts of the body, in addition to the particular injured limb. Remember that the age of the child is a very important consideration in nonaccidental injury (Fig. 5-7). Abuse is the cause of about 60% of fractures in children younger than 1 year and approximately 90% of fractures in children younger than 6 months. Nearly half of all femur fractures that occur in children before walking age are due to nonaccidental injury. There is no "pathognomonic fracture pattern" in abuse. Rather, the age of the child, the overall injury pattern, the stated mechanism of injury, and pertinent psychosocial factors must all be considered in each case.

Classically, corner fractures, especially of the distal femur, and multiple rib fractures, skull fractures, or fractures in multiple stage of healing are considered highly suggestive of nonaccidental injury. Important: chart your history, examination, and assessment expecting that your words will be read aloud by lawyers in court.

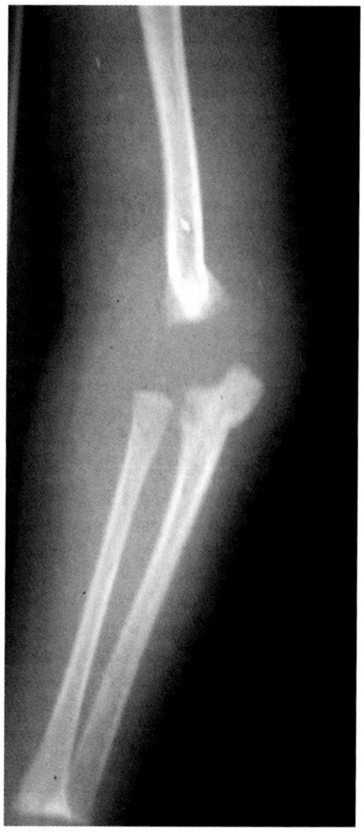

Staying Out of Trouble With the Injured Child

* Recognize that certain injuries are sentinels for associated injuries. Examples of this include rib fractures, pelvic fractures, facial injuries, and a lap belt sign on the anterior aspect of the abdomen or chest.

* Upon first meeting the family, use the first few minutes to establish the optimal relationship: a partnership, you and the family against the injuries.

* Present a comprehensive list of risks and complications caused by each injury. Don't let the family take a great result for granted.

* The more untrusting the family, the more you should see them, both inpatient and outpatient.

* In complex high-energy trauma, partnering with a general surgeon and a neurosurgeon and using a careful physical examination and liberal use of imaging are valuable ways to optimally collaborate care when there are both skeletal injuries and multiple internal injuries.

* Compartment syndrome in kids is often signaled by the 3 A's: anxiety, agitation, and increased analgesic requirements.

* Be alert that compartment syndrome may be quite delayed in children. Although the reason for this delay is not clear, the first diagnosis is often 20 to 40 hours after fracture.

* Don't underestimate the extent that a child can recover from severe multitrauma, particularly head and spinal cord injury. Treat fractures expecting recovery.

* The orthopaedist should get a social worker, pediatricians, and other appropriate experts and consultants involved as soon as nonaccidental injury is suspected.

* Worsening pain in a cast means that the cast should be removed and the limb should be examined.

* Postreduction radiographs should be examined closely for signs of potential cast trouble. At the joint creases, particularly the anterior aspect of the ankle and elbow, look for creases in the cast that may result in skin breakdown.

Figure 5-7 Understanding mechanism of injury is essential. This "floating elbow"—a combination of a distal humeral epiphyseal fracture and a Monteggia fracture—is caused by hyperextension, such as when a child falls on an outstretched hand. However, this 3-month-old does not even have the reflex yet to break a fall with an outstretched hand. Understanding the mechanism produces the conclusion that this injury resulted when someone (in this case a parent) forcibly hyperextended the baby's arm in anger.

Dr. Noonan Adds

There are no hypochondriacs in casts.

FOR FURTHER ENLIGHTENMENT

Flynn J, Bashyal R, Yeger-McKeever M, et al. Acute traumatic compartment syndrome of the leg in children: diagnosis and outcome. *J Bone Joint Surg.* 2011;93:937-941.

Hresko MT, Kasser JR. Physeal arrest about the knee associated with non-physeal fractures in the lower extremity. *J Bone Joint Surg Am.* 1989;71:698-703.

Kocher MS, Kasser JR. Orthopaedic aspects of child abuse. *J Am Acad Orthop Surg.* 2000;8:10-20.

Leaman L, Hennrikus W, Bresnahan J. Identifying non-accidental fractures in children aged <2 years. *J Child Orthop.* 2016;10:335-341.

Skaggs DL, Friend L, Alman B, et al. The effect of surgical delay on acute infection following 554 open fractures in children. *J Bone Joint Surg Am.* 2005;87A:8-12.

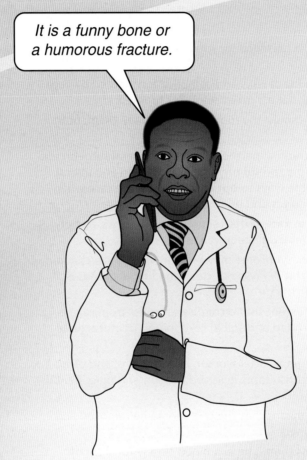

Beware! About 50% of radiograph interpretations of elbow fractures in children by emergency department physicians are incorrect.[1] Don't trust the phone call; insist on seeing the X-ray. (From Shrader MW, Campbell MD, Jacofsky DJ. Accuracy of emergency room physicians' interpretation of elbow fractures in children. *Orthopedics*. 2008;31(12).)

Chapter 6

Trauma About the Elbow I: Overview, Supracondylar and Transphyseal Fractures

DAVID L. SKAGGS, MD, MMM

Gurus: Martin J. Herman, MD and Steven Frick, MD

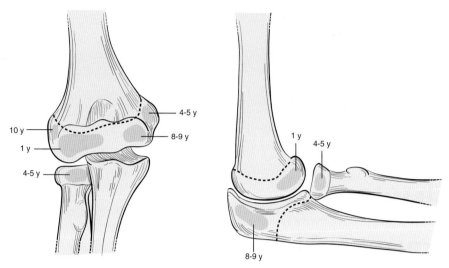

Figure 6-1 Secondary ossification centers of the elbow, with range of ages of appearance.

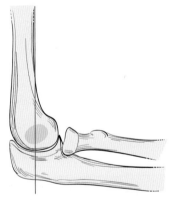

Figure 6-2 In the normal elbow, a line drawn down the anterior humeral line will be in the middle third of the capitellum in children of age 5 years and older. In children younger than 5 years, the line will always touch the capitellum in a normal elbow, but it may not be in the middle third.[2] (Reprinted with permission from Ryan DD, Lightdale-Miric NR, Joiner ER, et al. Variability of the anterior humeral line in normal pediatric elbows. *J Pediatr Orthop.* 2016;36(2):e14-e16.)

Elbow fractures in children present the practicing orthopaedist with many opportunities to get in trouble. A thorough understanding of the anatomy and development of the immature elbow helps one stay out of trouble.

Anatomy and Imaging

The secondary centers of ossification of the bones about the elbow appear in a relatively predictable order, which may serve as landmarks to define the anatomy of the largely cartilaginous elbow during early childhood (Fig. 6-1). Easily remembered mnemonics aid in remembering the order of ossification; however, in our age of political correctness, the most memorable ones may only be passed on verbally to trusted confidents. As a fracture line in pediatric elbows may travel through unossified cartilage, one often must rely on the relationship between the ossification centers and visible bone to define the injury on radiographs. The radial head, the trochlea, and the olecranon may appear as multiple ossification centers, which may be mistaken for a fracture.

To stay out of trouble, get into the habit of establishing the four following anatomic relationships in every radiograph of a child's elbow:

1. *The anterior humeral line intersects the capitellum.* If the center of the capitellum is posterior to this line, an extension-type supracondylar fracture, or a transphyseal fracture, is likely seen more commonly in the very young. If the capitellum is anterior to the line, the less common flexion-type supracondylar fracture or transphyseal fracture is likely (Fig. 6-2).[2] One must be certain that the X-ray is a true lateral view of the distal humerus because any rotation will make the capitellum appear posterior.

2. *The radius usually points to the capitellum in all views* (Figs. 6-3 and 6-4). If it doesn't, a lateral condyle fracture, a radial neck fracture, a Monteggia fracture-dislocation or equivalent lesion, or an elbow dislocation should be considered. While traditional teaching has been that a line drawn along the radial shaft *always* points to the capitellum, in reality this line misses the ossific nucleus in about one in seven normal children's elbow X-rays.[3]

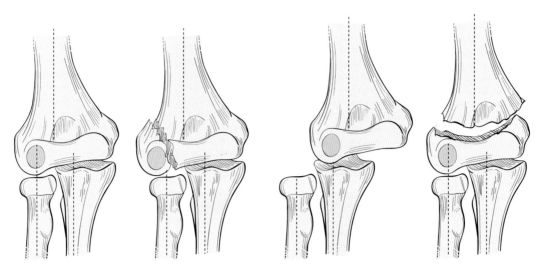

Figure 6-3 Relationship between the radius and capitellum, and the ulna and humerus, in normal and injured elbows, as visualized on an AP radiograph.

3. *The humeral capitellar (Baumann) angle should be in valgus (95% of normal elbows have an angle of at least 10°)* (Fig. 6-5). Baumann angle is a relatively sensitive indicator of varus angulation of the distal humerus and is primarily useful in assessing angulation or reduction in supracondylar and transphyseal fractures. Angulation of the humerus to the X-ray cassette or the X-ray beam to the humerus in the sagittal plane can lead to significant measurement errors of this angle, so if there is a question, repeat the X-ray with a true AP of the distal humerus.

4. *In radiographs of a normal elbow, the long axis of the ulna should be parallel and slightly medial to the long axis of the humerus on a true AP view* (see Fig. 6-3). If not, and the radial head and capitellum remain in correct alignment, a transphyseal injury or displaced supracondylar fracture should be considered. If the radius is no longer pointing to the capitellum, a lateral condyle fracture and an elbow dislocation must be considered.

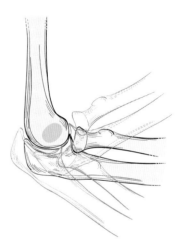

Figure 6-4 The radius usually points to the capitellum in all radiographic views.

Occult fractures about a child's elbow are easy to miss. A lateral radiograph of a normal elbow flexed at 90° may show a small anterior fat pad bulging from the shallow coronoid fossa; this is a normal finding and of no clinical significance. Do not waste brain power thinking or talking about anterior fat pads. In contrast, if an elevated posterior fat pad is visible, but no fracture is appreciated on initial radiographs, an occult fracture is likely present, and the child's arm should be protected on the assumption that it is fractured.[4]

Growth and Remodeling

The distal humerus physis provides 20% of growth and the proximal 80%. As there is very little growth about the elbow, there is very little remodeling potential, even in the plane of motion. Have a low threshold for surgery on elbow fractures; if in doubt, your default should be to fix elbow fractures anatomically.

In contrast, because there is lots of growth about the proximal humerus and distal radius, we can predict remodeling in children who have years of remaining growth in fractures of the distal radius and proximal humerus. It is thought provoking that the opposite pattern is true of the lower extremity, with the most active growth about the distal femur, which is the most common site of bone tumors. Why are we designed this way?

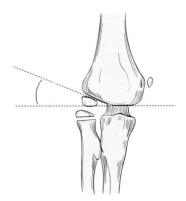

Figure 6-5 Baumann angle is variable, but is usually at least 10°.

Routine use of comparison radiographs of the uninjured elbow have generally not proved useful in improving diagnostic accuracy by orthopaedic surgeons. However, if doubt remains, comparison views may be helpful in individual cases.

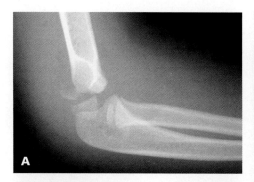

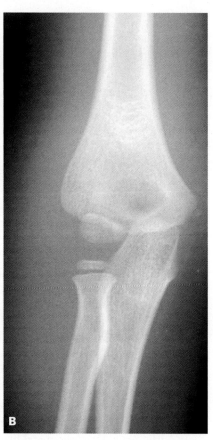

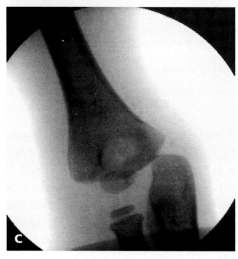

Figure 6-6 A Salter II fracture of the distal humerus may be mistaken for a lateral condyle fracture prior to the ossification of the trochlea and medial epicondyle. Lateral elbow radiograph of a 4-year-old boy who fell down the stairs. Preservation of the anatomic relationship of the radius to capitellum in all views and medial translation of the capitellum on the intraoperative imaging help make this diagnosis. (Used with permission of the Children's Orthopaedic Center, Los Angeles.)

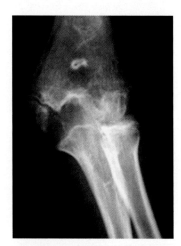

Figure 6-7 Avascular necrosis of the trochlea following posterior open reduction of a supracondylar humerus fracture. Patient has severely limited motion and pain. At this point, there is no good treatment option. (Used with permission of the Children's Orthopaedic Center, Los Angeles.)

An arthrogram and/or live fluoroscopic imaging, or even MRI, will sometimes help to establish a diagnosis when plain radiographs are inconclusive. For example, prior to ossification of the trochlea and medial epicondyle, a lateral condyle fracture may appear identical to Salter II fracture on a plain AP radiographs (Fig. 6-6). These particular two fractures may at times be clinically differentiated by the location of maximal swelling, which is on the side where the periosteum is torn. The periosteum is torn opposite the Thurston Holland fragment in a Salter II fracture (medial) or on the lateral side of a lateral condyle fracture.

While collateral circulation about the elbow is generally rich, the capitellum and the lateral portion of the trochlea rely on end arteries entering posteriorly. Avoid the potentially catastrophic iatrogenic complication of avascular necrosis of the trochlea by avoiding posterior dissection of the distal humerus (Fig. 6-7).

Physical Examination

The two most important aspects of the physical examination are the neurovascular and soft tissue assessments (Fig. 6-8). The neurologic examination of a young child with an injured elbow is difficult yet essential, as the rate of neurological injury or vascular compromise is around 15% for displaced supracondylar fractures (Fig. 6-9). A thorough preoperative evaluation helps avoid the uncomfortable and dangerous situation of finding vascular compromise or a neurologic deficit postreduction without knowing the prereduction status. It is rarely necessary, but if sensation cannot be established by standard techniques, soaking a child's hand in a wet washcloth will cause wrinkling in areas that have sensory nerves intact, while the skin with complete loss of afferent innervation will remain smooth.[5]

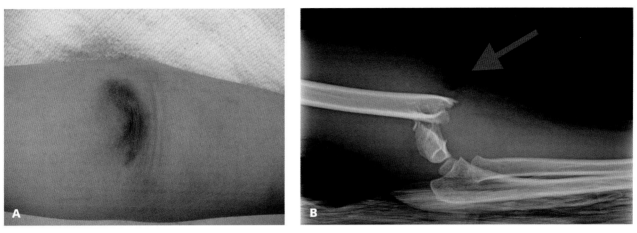

Figure 6-8 A: Skin puckering and antecubital ecchymosis are both red flags that timely surgery is required. **B:** Skin puckering signifies the distal humerus has torn through the brachialis, and almost tore through the skin, but is stuck in the dermis (arrow).

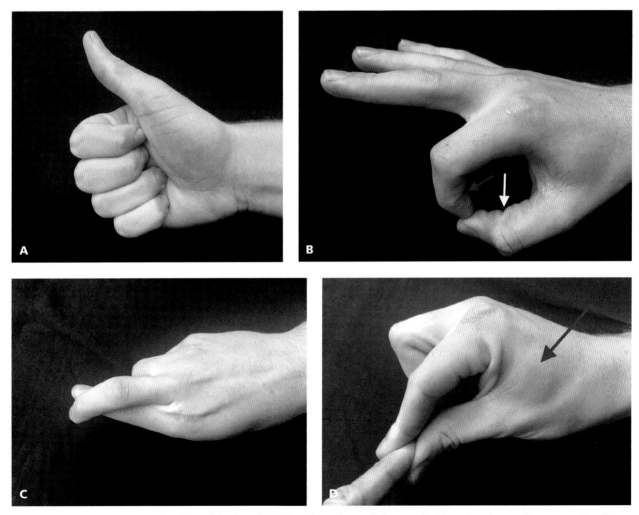

Figure 6-9 Motor nerve examination of the hand. **A:** Thumb up for radial nerve. **B:** Okay sign for median nerve. Confirm distal interphalangeal (DIP) flexion of index finger (red arrow) and IP flexion of thumb (white arrow). **C:** Crossing fingers for ulnar nerve. **D:** Preoperative assessment in a scared injured child can be challenging. However, even young children will usually pinch an examiner's finger, allowing the examiner to palpate contraction of the first dorsal interosseous muscle (arrow) and confirm ulnar motor function. (Used with permission of the Children's Orthopaedic Center, Los Angeles.)

Supracondylar Fractures

Supracondylar humerus fractures are the most common fracture in children requiring surgery. Although common, these fractures are notorious for complications and litigation.

TIMING

Often, reduction and pinning of a supracondylar fracture can safely wait until the morning. Studies report that mean delays of 8 to 21 hours in the treatment of supracondylar humerus fractures do not increase the risk of complications or need for an open reduction. These studies must be interpreted with a great deal of caution, as they are retrospective. One interpretation of these studies is that orthopaedic surgeons' clinical judgment in determining which fractures needed urgent treatment was correct, and we should therefore continue to have a high vigilance for fractures at risk. Most type II and III fractures without undue swelling, skin puckering from the proximal fragment, significant vascular impairment, or signs of compartment syndrome do not require urgent surgery. Children awaiting surgery may have their arms splinted in 20° to 45° of elbow flexion, elevated, and checked every hour or two by someone capable of recognizing signs of trouble.

One of the best ways to stay out of trouble with these potentially problematic fractures is with a timely and careful evaluation.

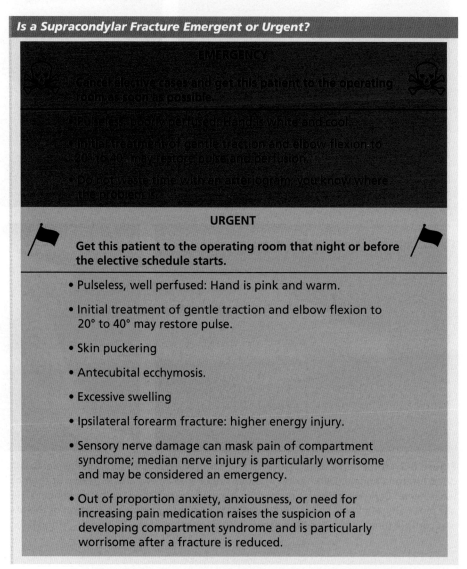

Is a Supracondylar Fracture Emergent or Urgent?

☠ **EMERGENCY** ☠

Cancel elective cases and get this patient to the operating room as soon as possible.

- Pulseless, poorly perfused: Hand is white and cool.
- Initial treatment of gentle traction and elbow flexion to 20° to 40° may restore pulse and perfusion.
- Do not waste time with an arteriogram; you know where the problem is.

URGENT

Get this patient to the operating room that night or before the elective schedule starts.

- Pulseless, well perfused: Hand is pink and warm.

- Initial treatment of gentle traction and elbow flexion to 20° to 40° may restore pulse.

- Skin puckering

- Antecubital ecchymosis.

- Excessive swelling

- Ipsilateral forearm fracture: higher energy injury.

- Sensory nerve damage can mask pain of compartment syndrome; median nerve injury is particularly worrisome and may be considered an emergency.

- Out of proportion anxiety, anxiousness, or need for increasing pain medication raises the suspicion of a developing compartment syndrome and is particularly worrisome after a fracture is reduced.

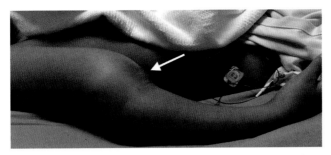

Figure 6-10 Gentle traction flexion can help improve circulation and take pressure off soft tissues at risk (arrow). (Used with permission of the Children's Orthopaedic Center, Los Angeles.)

VASCULAR COMPROMISE

Up to 20% of displaced supracondylar fractures present with an absent pulse. To clarify your thinking, consider three clinical scenarios:

- Hand well-perfused (pink and warm), radial pulse present
- Hand well-perfused (pink and warm), radial pulse absent
- Hand poorly perfused (white and cool), radial pulse absent

A child with a poorly perfused, pulseless hand requires emergent treatment. Vascular compromise is often positional, with the proximal fragment causing occlusion the brachial artery (Figs. 6-10 and 6-11). Gentle traction and placement of the elbow in 20° to 40° of flexion should not be delayed. Most frequently a child with a poorly perfused, pulseless hand, whose arm was splinted in full elbow extension will have significant improvement in vascular perfusion with this maneuver. Note that this maneuver is *not* an attempt to anatomically reduce the fracture, as iatrogenic injury to neurovascular structures is possible. Arteriograms generally have no role in preoperative evaluation of the pulseless supracondylar fracture, as they delay treatment and rarely contribute useful information.

Following a closed reduction of the fracture with a poorly perfused, pulseless hand, perfusion usually returns. If the hand remains poorly perfused and pulseless, operative exploration of the brachial artery is indicated. An anterior approach is best when the purpose of the approach is for arterial exploration. The secret to the anterior approach is the lacertus fibrosus (Fig. 6-12). (Fully extend your own

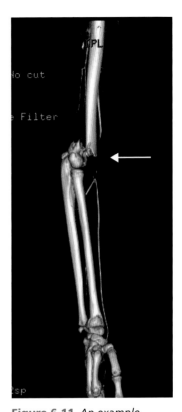

Figure 6-11 *An example of what not to do.* This 10-year-old with a pulseless, poorly perfused hand presented to a community hospital with the elbow splinted in full extension. An angiogram was performed in this position, which did not provide any useful information, and delayed the patient's care without benefit. We know the arterial flow is stopped over the sharp bone fragment; we don't need a study to prove that. *What should have been done?* Gentle traction and flexion of the elbow should have been done when the patient was first seen. When that maneuver was done many hours later, the pulse and perfusion immediately returned. Keeping the child's elbow in full extension prevented the pulse and perfusion from returning to normal and increased the risk of a compartment syndrome. (Used with permission of the Children's Orthopaedic Center, Los Angeles.)

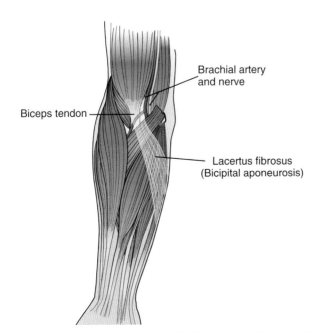

Brachial artery and nerve

Biceps tendon

Lacertus fibrosus (Bicipital aponeurosis)

Figure 6-12 The key to the anterior approach is the lacertus fibrosus. (Used with permission of the Children's Orthopaedic Center, Los Angeles.)

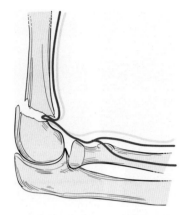

Figure 6-13 Brachial artery and median nerve may be trapped at the fracture site. If a reduction feels rubbery, and a gap at the fracture site is seen on imaging, entrapment is possible, especially in the setting of vascular compromise or median nerve or anterior interosseous (AIN) injury.

THE GURU SAYS...

Additional information provided by assessment of the presence and quality of a Doppler signal in the radial artery at the wrist is helpful in assessing perfusion. If all is quiet, call for a vascular surgeon's opinion. If you hear a good signal, plan for careful observation.

STEVE FRICK

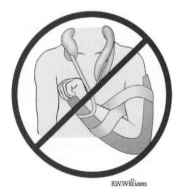

R.W.Williams

Figure 6-14 Avoid casting supracondylar fracture beyond 90° as this position increases compartment pressures and decreases perfusion to the hand and forearm.

elbow and use your other hand to feel the lacertus fibrosus just medial to the bicep tendon in the antecubital fossa; it has a sharp fascial edge.) After making a transverse skin incision, place a clamp just under the lacertus fibrosus, cut it, and the brachial artery and nerve lie just medial to the biceps tendon in a normal elbow. If they are not there, dissect proximally until you find them. Many times the brachial artery itself is not trapped in the fracture site, but soft tissue adjacent to the artery is trapped, tethering the artery just enough to stop flow (Fig. 6-13). If the hand is still poorly perfused after exploration and removal of an entrapped or tethered artery from fracture site, a general or vascular surgical consult is wise.

If, following closed reduction, the hand is pulseless but warm and well perfused, management is controversial. Some favor arterial exploration and repair if needed at that time. With such excellent collateral circulation about the elbow, close in-hospital observation of at least 48 hours and mild elevation is usually sufficient, with an understanding that if the hand loses perfusion, or there are signs of compartment syndrome, an urgent return to the operating room will be necessary.

If during a closed reduction, one feels "rubbery" reduction, it could signify entrapped median nerve or brachial artery, particularly if these structures are compromised preoperatively. In this case, consider proceeding with an open reduction from an anterior approach—there is very little chance that an open reduction will cause harm.

THE GURU SAYS...

If the reduction feels rubbery, careful assessment of your reduction fluoroscopically is helpful. Any gap at the fracture is bad and may signal an entrapped nerve or artery; open and take a look. "Mind the gap" is not just for the London Tube.

STEVE FRICK

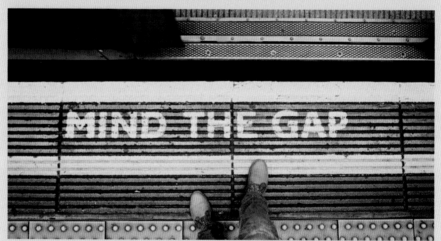

COMPARTMENT SYNDROME

With proper vigilance, compartment syndrome should be very infrequent. A great way to minimize the risk of compartment syndrome is to avoid elbow flexion greater than 90° in any supracondylar fracture (Fig. 6-14). With the predictable efficacy and safety of closed reduction and pin fixation, elbow hyperflexion should no longer be used to hold a fracture reduction. As a general rule, if an elbow needs to be held in more than 90° of flexion to keep the fracture reduced, using Kirschner wires (K-wires) to maintain the reduction is probably safer. In a child with a supracondylar fracture, as elbow flexion increases, forearm compartment pressures increase dramatically[6] and brachial artery flow decreases.[7]

Particular presentations deserve special attention. If the elbow is excessively swollen, perhaps with anterior skin tenting suggesting significant soft-tissue injuries, treatment should be urgent to prevent compartment syndrome and soft tissue injury. Patients with a concomitant forearm fracture should be closely watched for compartment syndrome as well. Particularly in children, soft findings such as paresthesias are difficult to interpret, and worsening pain is the most valuable sign of developing compartment syndrome. As in adults, follow the golden rule for staying out of trouble: if you are thinking about compartment syndrome, you should probably measure compartment pressures or release the compartments. One may want to consider avoiding narcotics for pain management to better follow an examination in children at high risk for compartment syndrome.

A situation that has resulted in lawsuits is a compartment syndrome that is initially unrecognized in the setting of a median nerve injury. Any child with impaired sensation, either from local nerve injury or decreased mental status, should be closely evaluated for compartment syndrome. In these situations, consider a posterior splint or a bivalved cast so the anterior section can be removed allowing palpation and monitoring of the volar compartment of the forearm for tightness from swelling.

NEUROLOGIC INJURY

Nerve damage at the time of injury should be observed; it usually improves within 3 months. One exception to this is an open fracture, where exploration of the nerve should be considered if it would not require extensive dissection. An iatrogenic ulnar nerve palsy following fixation with a medial pin most often resolves within 4 months, but removal of the medial pin upon recognition of the nerve injury is probably a good idea. If the surgeon chooses to remove the medial pin before the fracture is healed, loss of fracture reduction is a potential pitfall. Thus, medial pin removal in a potentially unstable fracture should occur in the operating room only after an additional lateral pin has been placed to ensure maintenance of fracture reduction after medial pin removal.

Loss of median nerve function after surgical reduction should raise the concern that the nerve may be trapped or tethered at the fracture site, and timely exploration is indicated (see Fig. 6-13).

TREATMENT

A type I supracondylar fracture can be treated in a long arm cast for about 3 weeks. It has been recommended that to reduce and maintain reduction of a type II extension supracondylar fracture without pins, the elbow must be flexed to at least 120°. While good results are certainly possible with this technique, it is more predictable to perform a closed reduction and pinning of any displaced supracondylar fracture (see Fig. 6-14). Anecdotally, it appears that more malpractice suits are generated from malreduction of type II fractures than of type III fractures. As there is relatively little growth in the distal humerus, significant remodeling cannot be relied upon, even in the plane of motion. Stay out of trouble by pinning type II fractures.

One type of supracondylar fracture deserves special mention—the apparently minimally displaced fracture with medial comminution or impaction and a change in Baumann angle. This fracture pattern is easy to mistake for a type I fracture and treat nonoperatively, which would result in cubitus varus (Fig. 6-15). Operative reduction can usually be achieved by applying a significant valgus force

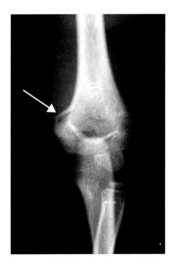

Figure 6-15 Look for medial comminution, which is indicative of the fracture being in varus and usually requires operative reduction and pinning.

THE GURU SAYS...

A fracture with buckling of the medial column is known as the "osteotomy generator." Avoid later need for osteotomy by prompt recognition and reduction with pinning.

STEVE FRICK

THE GURU SAYS...

Achieving stable fracture fixation of a type III supracondylar is a surgical priority. While the child is being anesthetized, I map out on a simple schematic of my ideal pin configuration for lateral pins (I have not used a medial pin in many years) and tape it to the imaging monitor. It reinforces the concepts of bicortical placement, adequate pin spread and two-column fixation and looks something like this:

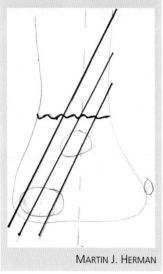

MARTIN J. HERMAN

on a fully extended elbow, followed by flexion, pronation (to maintain tension across the medial column), and pinning. Beware that you may have to push so hard into valgus that you will be afraid of breaking something in order to reduce the fracture.

Type III fractures should be reduced and pinned. The criteria for accepting a closed reduction are as follows:

1. Baumann angle is restored.
2. The anterior humeral line intersects the capitellum.
3. The medial and lateral columns have substantial contact.

A few millimeters of translation is acceptable. A fair amount of rotation is also acceptable, as the shoulder joint can make up for it. Open reductions should be done to remove interposed tissue, and only after a very patient effort at closed reduction has failed. While many orthopaedic surgeons have more experience with a lateral approach, this often leaves an unsightly and very visible scar. Consider becoming proficient in using the anterior approach (see Fig. 6-12).

CUBITUS VARUS

Cubitus varus is a function of inadequate reduction in the frontal plane. It does not occur as a result of a medial growth arrest, as there is too little growth in the distal humerus to cause this deformity within months of injury. After pinning, full extension of the arm is often not possible as pins are in the olecranon fossa, so the clinical examination may be unreliable. There is no way to avoid this complication other than being strict in obtaining and carefully scrutinizing adequate quality imaging confirming the fracture is not in cubitus varus (Baumann angle is at least 10°).

OPTIMAL PIN CONFIGURATION

Following publication of the first edition of this text, the question of cross pins versus lateral-entry pins is less controversial following the publication of multiple studies and meta-analysis in favor of lateral entry pins.[8-10] Iatrogenic injury of the ulnar nerve by medial pins has been reported in 5% to 6% in two large series of operatively treated supracondylar fractures. This complication is predictably avoided by eschewing the use of a medial pin.

The important technical points for successful lateral entry pin fixation are as follows (Fig. 6-16):

1. Maximize separation of the pins at the fracture site.
2. Engage the medial and lateral columns proximal to the fracture.
3. Engage sufficient bone in proximal and distal fragments.
4. Have a low threshold to use a third lateral pin if there is concern over fracture stability or pin placement following the placement of two lateral pins.

A review of supracondylar fractures pinned with lateral pins that lost reduction revealed the cause was always secondary to errors in pin placement, such as pins crossing or immediately adjacent to each other at the fracture site (Fig. 6-17). No failures were identified in cases fixed with three lateral pins.[11]

If the surgeon chooses to use a medial pin, avoiding injury to the ulnar nerve is a complex issue. One thing that is certain is to avoid placing a medial pin when the elbow is flexed. In children younger than 5 years, when the elbow is flexed more than 90°, the ulnar nerve migrated over, or even anterior

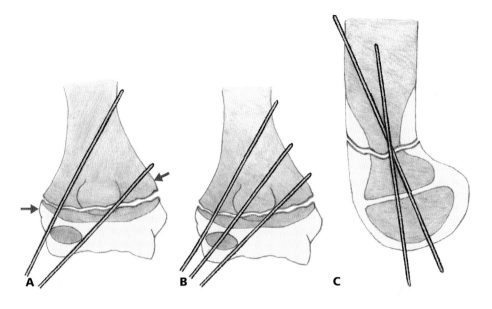

Figure 6-16 Proper positioning of two or three lateral entry pins. A potential pitfall is to have insufficient bone purchase (arrows). (Reprinted with permission from Skaggs DL, Cluck MW, Mostofi A, et al. Lateral-entry pin fixation in the management of supracondylar fractures in children. *J Bone Joint Surg Am.* 2004;86-A(4): 702-707. Copyright © 2004 by The Journal of Bone and Joint Surgery, Incorporated.)

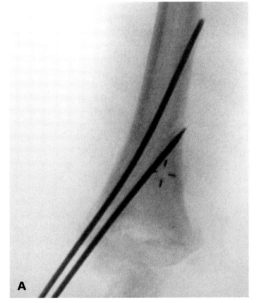

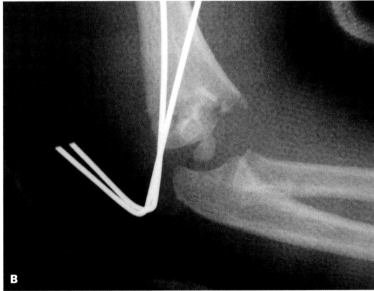

Figure 6-17 A: Intraoperative radiograph showing that pins are so close that they biomechanically function as one, allowing loss of reduction. **B:** Postoperative loss of reduction.

to, the medical epicondyle in 61% of children.[12] Unfortunately, even making an incision over the medial epicondyle to make certain the ulnar nerve is not directly injured by a pin does not ensure protection of the nerve.[13] We have found a medial pin to be necessary every decade or so in cases of a very oblique fracture pattern. If an iatrogenic ulnar nerve injury occurs, it is rare for the nerve to be directly penetrated by a pin. More commonly soft tissue around the nerve pinches the nerve. Thus, even if direct penetration of the ulnar nerve is avoided, simply placing a medial epicondyle entry pin adjacent to the nerve may cause injury.

THE GURU SAYS...

My most important operating room pearls when setting up to pin supracondylar fractures:

1. The image intensifier of a C-arm (round head) that has been turned 180° with the machine's base placed at the foot of the bed. For very small children, place the child's torso, head, and fractured arm onto a hand table to enable a good image of the elbow without tugging the head off the bed.
2. Room set-up is critical (Fig. 6-18). The surgeon and assistant should both be able to easily view the imaging monitor without turning their heads.
3. You only have to remember one size of K-wire: 0.062 mm. These are adequately sized for most children.

MARTIN J. HERMAN

THE GURU SAYS...

Four steps to reducing a supracondylar fracture, gently performed without sweating:

1. Apply traction under AP fluoroscopic view.
2. Correct medial-lateral translation.
3. Correct any varus-valgus angulation.
4. Flex elbow while pushing olecranon anteriorly with thumb.

STEVE FRICK

SURGICAL TECHNIQUE

As supracondylar humerus fractures are so common, and so predisposed to trouble, a detailed discussion of surgical technique is warranted. Traction is applied in line with the humerus, with the elbow in slight flexion. Avoid traction in full extension as this may cause tethering of neurovascular structures over the proximal fragment and *never* re-create the deformity by hyperextending the elbow like one does for a distal radius. If there is suspicion that the proximal fragment has pierced through the brachialis muscle, persistent, gradual traction of the slightly flexed elbow for a full minute will often reward you with a palpable freeing of the proximal fragment retracting through the brachialis. Alternatively, the proximal to distal "milking" maneuver over the brachialis may achieve the same end.[14] Freeing the proximal fragment from soft tissue entrapment is essential for an anatomic reduction and worth the time invested. For the reduction maneuver, hyperflex the elbow while pushing in an anterior direction on the olecranon. Keep the elbow hyperflexed during fluoroscopic assessment.

If anatomic reduction is elusive, repeat the reduction with forearm pronation, and then again with supination, to see if one works better than the other. If Bauman angle is not clearly at least 10°, or medial comminution remains, repeat the reduction while stressing the arm in valgus. When the reduction is acceptable, surgeons who like to relax, such as myself, may tape the arm with Coban in the hyperflexed, reduced position to securely maintain reduction. Lateral entry pins are placed by

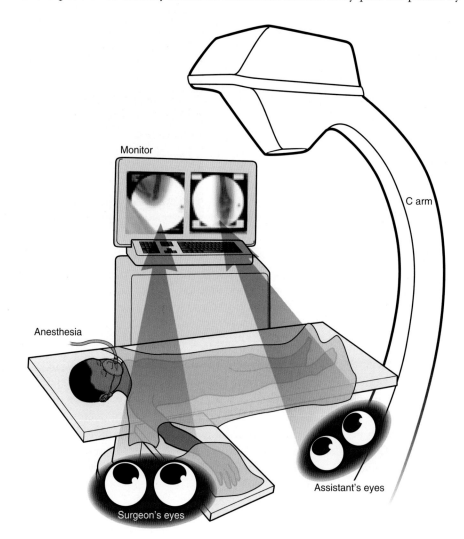

Figure 6-18 Operating room setup for pinning supracondylar fractures. The surgeon and assistant should both be able to easily view the imaging monitor without turning their heads.

the above technique, being certain to go through proximal cortex, and pin position is assessed with AP and lateral imaging. The arm is then straightened, and Baumann angle is again assessed with AP imaging. The arm is then subjected to varus, valgus, internal to external rotation, and flexion-extension stress under live imaging to assess stability. If there is any question of stability, place a third or even fourth lateral pin, then reassess stability by stressing the fracture under live imaging. Pins sometimes skive off the cortex up the medullary canal of the humerus. When this occurs, try to shove the pin against the cortex with extra force and speed; this is usually enough for it to catch. If this fails, try a thicker pin such as 2 mm.

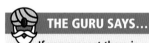

THE GURU SAYS...

Remember that the case is not over after the pins go in! Test stability of the fixation by stressing the fracture under live fluoroscopy, carefully bend and cut the pins so that the skin is not tented, and apply a well-padded long arm splint or bivalved cast. At our place, postoperative analgesia is provided adequately by acetaminophen or ibuprofen to avoid the side effects of narcotic medications.[15] The child's pain level and neurovascular status should be assessed carefully and documented prior to discharge.

MARTIN J. HERMAN

Pulse and perfusion is assessed, and the arm is casted in about 30° to 70° of elbow flexion depending on swelling, but no less than 30° of extension greater than the amount of flexion at which the pulse disappears. Pins can be bent 90° outside the skin to help prevent subcutaneous migration, with the skin protected by sterile felt or petroleum jelly impregnated gauze. Foam padding placed directly on skin, with no underlying circumferential bandaging, allows for swelling and obviates the need for splitting the cast (Fig. 6-19).[16] Fiberglass is stronger and lighter than plaster, and it allows for better postoperative radiographs.

Occasionally, one faces the challenge of a type IV fracture with so little intact periosteum that the distal fragment can be moved into flexion and extension. This is usually not recognized until you are in the operating room with patient asleep, so it is wise to think this through ahead of time. A potential pitfall is to create this situation iatrogenically by an overly enthusiastic reduction, in which the posterior periosteum is torn, as the hapless surgeon feels the fracture fragment move from extension to flexion. Using the surgical technique described in the next section for flexion-type supracondylar fractures, these completely unstable fractures can often be treated without the need for an open reduction.

THE GURU SAYS...

If you suspect there is potential for a type III fracture to convert to a type IV fracture, don't do the case on top of the C arm. Attach a solid arm board so you can rotate the C-arm from AP to lateral position easily.

STEVE FRICK

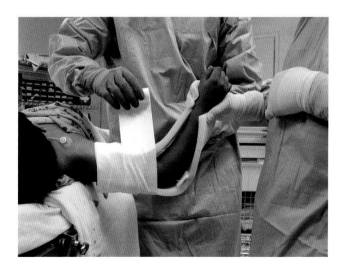

Figure 6-19 Sterile foam placed directly on skin with no underlying circumferential bandages allows for swelling under the cast. (Used with permission of the Children's Orthopaedic Center, Los Angeles.)

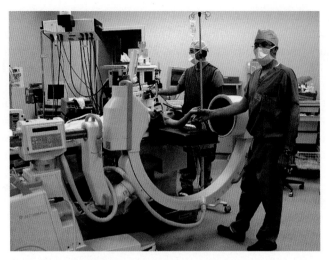

Figure 6-20 Positioning of the C-arm for a lateral image of the elbow for a completely unstable or flexion-type supracondylar fracture. (Used with permission of the Children's Orthopaedic Center, Los Angeles.)

FLEXION-TYPE SUPRACONDYLAR FRACTURES

While flexion-type supracondylar fractures are relatively rare injuries, closed reduction and pinning of these injuries is technically more challenging than in extension-type fractures. To reduce the fracture, the elbow is extended. However, in an extended position, K-wires are more difficult to place. In addition, when attempting to view the lateral image of the elbow, fracture reduction can be lost if the arm is rotated. These difficulties have led to the belief that open reduction is usually necessary.

These fractures can usually be closed reduced. It is helpful to first place two lateral entry pins in the distal fragment before the fracture is reduced. To confirm fracture reduction, rotate the image machine between AP and lateral positions instead of rotating the arm. This can be accomplished by positioning the fluoroscopy unit parallel to the operating table and rotating the C-arm. First confirm fracture reduction in the AP plane. Then rotate the C-arm for a lateral view (Fig. 6-20). Reduce the fracture in the sagittal plane, and then drive the pins across the fracture site. Kelly Flynn recently reported that if there was an associated ulnar nerve palsy, the rate of performing an open reduction was 60%.[17]

> ### THE GURU SAYS...
>
> Flexion supracondylar fractures may seem like a simple variation of the standard extension supracondylar fracture, but they are not. Keeping in mind a few differences from supracondylar fractures that will keep you out of trouble:
> 1. Position the arm on a hand table so orthogonal views are easily obtained by rotating the C-arm not the child's arm.
> 2. Use a full prep and drape because the rate of opening is higher compared to supracondylar fractures; always try closed reduction first, because it is surprisingly easier than you think.
> 3. Place a bump under the distal humerus just proximal to the fracture; fracture reduction is done by applying gentle posterior translation while extending the elbow (the opposite of a supracondylar reduction); at 75° to 80° of elbow flexion, reduction is usually acceptable.
> 4. Drill a pin (or two) into the distal fragment prior to reduction. Cross the fracture site with the pins after reduction is achieved, and then complete your fixation.
> 5. The ulnar nerve may be an obstacle to reduction; open reduction is best accomplished through a medial approach.
>
> MARTIN J. HERMAN

Transphyseal Fractures of the Distal Humerus

Transphyseal fractures, or Salter I fractures, of the distal humerus (Fig. 6-21) are much less common than supracondylar fractures, although the similarities warrant inclusion in this chapter. There are two notable opportunities for trouble with transphyseal fractures: making the diagnosis and missing child abuse. These injuries tend to occur in children younger than 4 years, when the majority of the distal humerus is unossified. Prior to ossification of the capitellum, the appearance of a transphyseal fracture on plain radiograph is indistinguishable from an elbow dislocation (see Fig. 6-3). Elbow dislocation in this age group is exceedingly rare, so any time one is considering the diagnosis of an elbow dislocation in a younger child, remember it is much more likely to be a transphyseal fracture. An arthrogram will highlight the cartilage and assist in the diagnosis, reduction, and pinning (Fig. 6-22).

Treatment is similar to that of supracondylar fractures as described above, with a few exceptions. If the fracture presents late with callus already present or is already healed to the point where gentle reduction is not possible, avoid open reduction or forceful manipulation, either of which may injure the physis. Accept the position of the fracture and perform a supracondylar osteotomy in the future, if needed. Because of the wider surface area at the level of the physis, this fracture is inherently more stable than supracondylar fractures. A small amount of translation will remodel, but varus/valgus angulation will not.

The mechanism of physeal failure is believed to be rotatory shear, consistent with the fracture's association with child abuse and birth injuries. Pay careful attention to the plausibility of the parent's description of how the fracture occurred with concern for child abuse. In addition, a careful physical examination to uncover other injuries is warranted (Fig. 6-23).

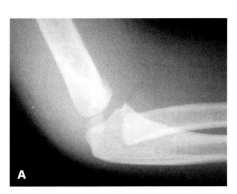
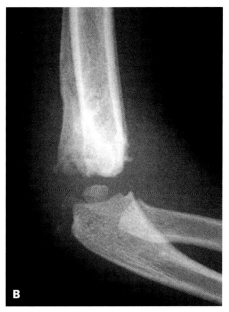

Figure 6-21 Unrecognized acute transphyseal fracture. **A:** This radiograph was considered normal at initial medical contact. Note that the capitellum is posterior to the anterior humeral line. **B:** Same patient 2 months after injury.

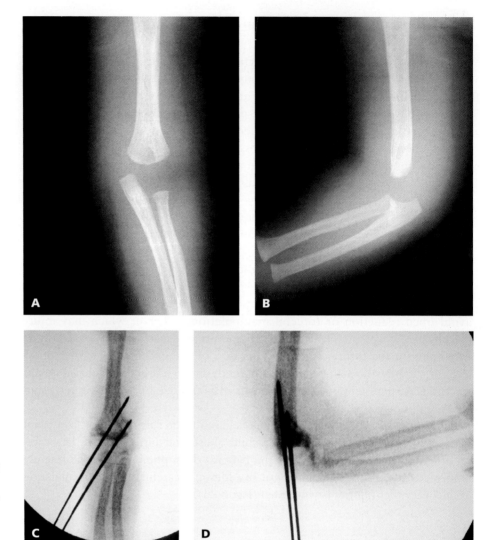

Figure 6-22 A: Anteroposterior radiograph of a 4-month-old boy. As there are no secondary ossification centers visible, a diagnostic pitfall is to call this an elbow dislocation. **B:** The lateral view may be similarly misinterpreted as an elbow dislocation. **C, D:** Arthrography confirms diagnosis of transphyseal fracture and aids in visualization of fracture during reduction and pinning.

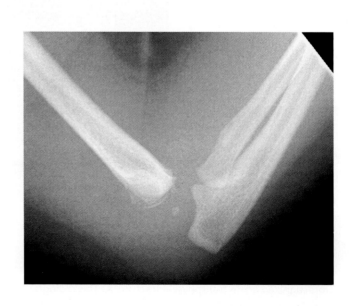

Figure 6-23 Lateral elbow radiograph in a 3-month-old child at initial presentation for medical care for an acute "swollen elbow" demonstrates a transphyseal fracture. Child abuse is suspected from presence of fracture callus, suggesting a delay in seeking medical care.

Staying Out of Trouble With Trauma About the Elbow

For every pediatric elbow X-ray, verify three points:

* The anterior humeral line intersects the capitellum.

* The radius points to the capitellum in every view.

* Baumann angle is in valgus.

For supracondylar fractures:

* A pulseless, poorly perfused hand needs an urgent reduction, not an arteriogram.

* If an elbow needs to be held in more than 90° of flexion to keep the fracture reduced, using K-wires to maintain the reduction is probably safer.

* If in doubt as to fix a type II fracture, fix it. The chances of a good outcome achieved safely are quite high.

* Have a low threshold to place a third lateral entry pin.

SOURCES OF WISDOM

1. Shrader MW, Campbell MD, Jacofsky DJ. Accuracy of emergency room physicians' interpretation of elbow fractures in children. *Orthopedics*. 2008;31(12).

2. Ryan DD, Lightdale-Miric NR, Joiner ER, et al. Variability of the anterior humeral line in normal pediatric elbows. *J Pediatr Orthop*. 2016;36(2):e14-e16.

3. Ramirez RN, Ryan DO, Williams J, et al. A line drawn along the radial shaft misses the capitellum in 16% of radiographs of normal elbows. *J Pediatr Orthop*. 2014;34(8):763-767.

4. Skaggs DL, Mirzayan R. The posterior fat pad sign in association with occult fracture of the elbow in children. *J Bone Joint Surg Am*. 1999;81(10):1429-1433.

5. Phelps PE, Walker E. Comparison of the finger wrinkling test results to established sensory tests in peripheral nerve injury. *Am J Occup Ther*. 1977;31(9):565-572.

6. Battaglia TC, Armstrong DG, Schwend RM. Factors affecting forearm compartment pressures in children with supracondylar fractures of the humerus. *J Pediatr Orthop*. 2002;22(4):431-439.

7. Mapes RC, Hennrikus WL. The effect of elbow position on the radial pulse measured by Doppler ultrasounography after surgical treatment of supracondylar elbow fractures in children. *J Pediatr Orthop*. 1998;18(4):441-444.

8. Slobogean BL, Jackman H, Tennant S, et al. Iatrogenic ulnar nerve injury after the surgical treatment of displaced supracondylar fractures of the humerus: number needed to harm, a systematic review. *J Pediatr Orthop*. 2010;30(5):430-436.

9. Babal JC, Mehlman CT, Klein G. Nerve injuries associated with pediatric supracondylar humeral fractures: a meta-analysis. *J Pediatr Orthop*. 2010;30(3):253-263.

10. Woratanarat P, Angsanuntsukh C, Rattanasiri S, et al. Meta-analysis of pinning in supracondylar fracture of the humerus in children. *J Orthop Trauma*. 2012;26(1):48-53.

11. Skaggs DL, Cluck MW, Mostofi A, et al. Lateral-entry pin fixation in the management of supracondylar fractures in children. *J Bone Joint Surg Am*. 2004;86(4):702-707.

12. Zaltz I, Waters PM, Kasser JR. Ulnar nerve instability in children. *J Pediatr Orthop*. 1996;16(5):567-569.

13. Skaggs DL, Hale J, Kay RM, et al. Operative treatment of supracondylar fractures of the humerus in children: the consequence of pin placement. *J Bone Joint Surg Am*. 2001;83(5):735-740.

14. Archibeck MJ, Scott SM, Peters CL. Brachialis muscle entrapment in displaced supracondylar humerus fractures: a technique of closed reduction and report of initial results. *J Pediatr Orthop*. 1997;17(3):298-302.

15. Swanson C, Chang K, Schleyer E, et al. Post-operative pain control after supracondylar humerus fracture fixation. *J Pediatr Orthop*. 2012;32(5):452-455.

16. Seehausen DA, Kay RM, Ryan DD, Skaggs DL. Foam padding in casts accommodates soft tissue swelling and provides circumferential strength after fixation of supracondylar humerus fractures. *J Pediatr Orthop*. 2015;35(1):24-27.

17. Flynn K, Shah AS, Brusalis CM, et al. Flexion-type supracondylar humeral fractures: ulnar nerve injury increases risk of open reduction. *J Bone Joint Surg Am*. 2017;99(17):1485-1487.

FOR FURTHER ENLIGHTENMENT

Lee SS, Mahar AT, Miesen D, Newton PO. Displaced pediatric supracondylar humerus fractures: biomechanical analysis of percutaneous pinning techniques. *J Pediatr Orthop.* 2002;22:440-443.

Mehlman CT, Strub WM, Roy DR, et al. The effect of surgical timing on the perioperative complications of treatment of supracondylar humeral fractures in children. *J Bone Joint Surg Am.* 2001;83:323-327.

Rasool MN. Ulnar nerve injury after K-wire fixation of supracondylar humerus fractures in children. *J Pediatr Orthop.* 1998;18(5):686-690.

Shaw BA, Kasser JR, Emans JB, Rand FF. Management of vascular injuries in displaced supracondylar humerus fractures without arteriography. *J Orthop Trauma.* 1998;4(1):25-29.

Zaltz I, Waters PM, Kasser JR. Ulnar nerve instability in children. *J Pediatr Orthop.* 1996;16(5):567-569.

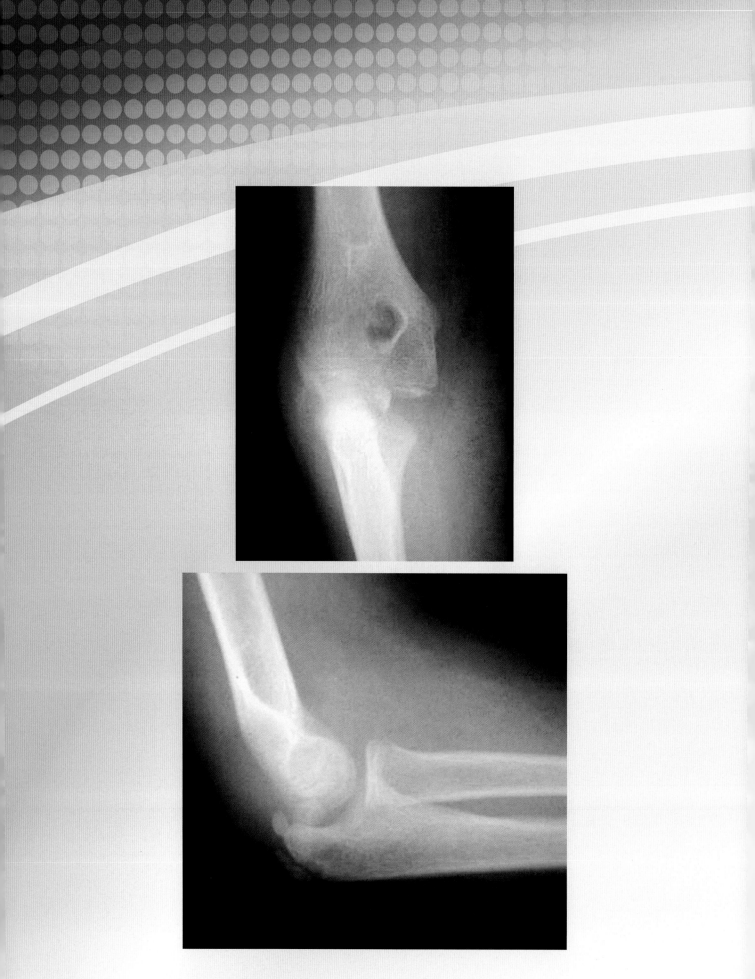

Chapter 7

Trauma About the Elbow II: Other Fractures

JOHN M. (JACK) FLYNN, MD

Guru: Jeffrey R. Sawyer, MD

Lateral Condylar Fractures

Fractures of the lateral condyle of the distal humerus are the second most common fracture about the elbow in children after supracondylar fractures, and have a well-earned reputation for trouble: nonunion, malunion, cubitus varus, and persistent loss of motion. Fortunately, these problems usually are avoidable if the fracture is recognized in a timely fashion and treated with sound principles. To stay out of trouble, remember that in most cases, this is a torn-off block of cartilage with a bit of bone inside, so healing is slower than a metaphyseal fracture (like a supracondylar), articular congruity must be assured, and thoughtful fixation is even more important when dealing with a ball of cartilage. Soft tissue injury (torn/punctured muscle) is typically less severe than with supracondylar fractures, and acute associated neurovascular injury is rare.

DIAGNOSIS

Lateral condylar fractures are sometimes missed, or the fracture displacement is underestimated, on standard AP and lateral radiographs of the elbow (particularly by urgent care center doctors, who apparently are supposed to know everything about everything; Fig. 7-1). Because the plane of a lateral condylar fracture is oblique from anterior lateral to posterior medial, an internal oblique view of the elbow is usually best to show the largest amount of displacement (Fig. 7-2). Sometimes the metaphyseal fragment is such a thin sliver of bone that the fracture is missed completely. Another pitfall in diagnosis is confusing a less common Salter II fracture of the distal humerus with a lateral condylar fracture.

> **THE GURU SAYS...**
>
> Make it a habit to really study the AP and the lateral radiographs for every fracture but especially with pediatric elbow trauma. You won't see this one unless you are intentionally looking for it, and this fracture can be bad if missed.
>
> JEFFREY R. SAWYER

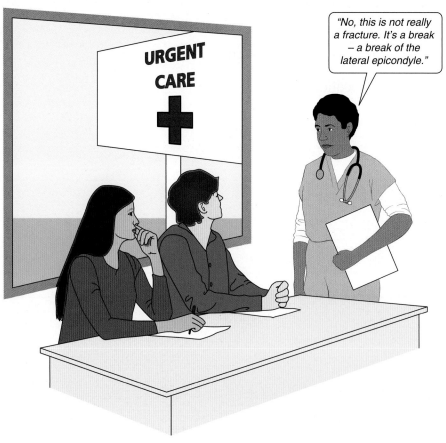

Figure 7-1 Urgent care center does struggle diagnosing pediatric elbow fractures.

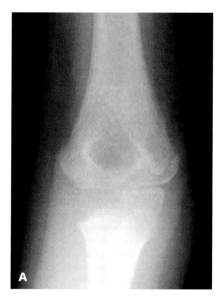 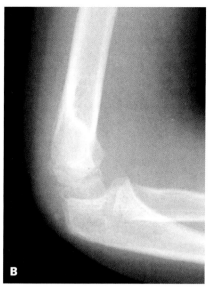 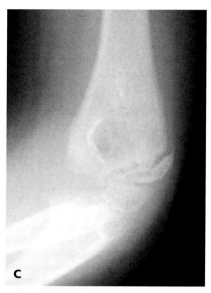

Figure 7-2 A: AP view of a lateral condyle fracture demonstrating less than 2 mm displacement. **B:** Lateral view of a lateral condyle fracture demonstrating less than 2 mm of displacement. **C:** Oblique view, looking at the lateral side of the elbow tangentially, showing greater than 2 mm of displacement. Without this radiograph, one may have assumed there was less than 2 mm of displacement, and treated the fracture nonoperatively.

The radiographic appearance of a Salter II fracture with a lateral metaphyseal fragment may be similar to that of a lateral condylar fracture before ossification of the trochlea (see Fig. 6-6 in Chapter 6). Physical examination can be helpful. With a lateral condylar fracture, swelling and tenderness are predominantly on the lateral side of the elbow, while a Salter II fracture has more swelling medially, where the periosteum is torn, and not laterally, where the periosteum is intact. In addition, tenderness is more diffuse with a Salter II fracture.

TREATMENT

Some wisdom in treating a lateral condylar fracture can be gained by considering the biomechanics. These fractures resemble a tearing injury: the child lands from a fall and instead of the elbow hyperextending (supracondylar fracture), a high-energy varus force is applied. The lateral metaphyseal bone and cartilage "tear." Sometimes this tear stops in the midline cartilage (Fig. 7-3A), and sometimes it propagates into the joint (Fig. 7-3B). With still more force, it can tear the entire lateral piece off and spin it around (Fig. 7-3C). Rarely, there can even be an associated elbow dislocation. If the amount of maximal fracture displacement on all radiographs is 2 mm or less, and the fracture line does not extend through the trochlear cartilage, cast immobilization for 6 weeks will be successful. To stay out of trouble, pay special attention to fractures extending into the epiphysis: if initial displacement is less than 2 mm, apply a cast but image the fracture weekly for 3 weeks to be certain displacement has not occurred. To allow better radiographic visualization of the fracture, fiberglass rather than plaster casting is helpful, but do not hesitate to remove the cast to get good quality radiographs. **NEWSFLASH! If a minimally displaced lateral condylar fracture is so unstable that you are concerned about removing the cast for a good X-ray, it probably should be pinned.**

Stay out of trouble by treating fractures with more than 2 mm of displacement with operative reduction and internal fixation. If a medial hinge is in question, an arthrogram can help. **NEWSFLASH! Arthrograms of pediatric elbow fractures should be done by injecting the dye into the olecranon fossa, not the fracture**

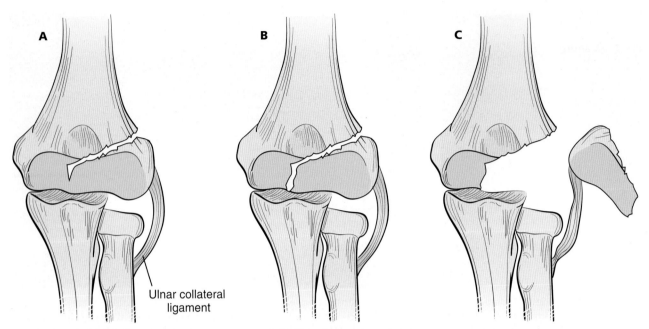

Ulnar collateral
ligament

Figure 7-3 A: A lateral condyle fracture may be completely through the ossified portion of the distal metaphysis, but not enter into the joint. This fracture pattern presumably occurs because of the flexible nature of the cartilaginous epiphysis. **B:** Other times, the fracture crosses the joint. **C:** With enough force, the entire lateral piece can be broken off and spun around.

THE GURU SAYS...

Follow the traumatic rent whenever possible. The proximal dissection usually is done by the fracture itself. Use the radial head as your limit for distal exposure and the posterior interosseous nerve will be protected.

With widely displaced fractures, the distal fragment may be so rotated that it is difficult and a little disorienting at first to determine how to reduce it. Remember that the articular surface may be just under the capsular incision and is at risk for iatrogenic injury. Use the concave surface of the capitellum to orient yourself.

JEFFREY R. SAWYER

site (Fig. 7-4). Fractures with a medial hinge and more than 2 mm of displacement often can be reduced closed, then pinned in place successfully. Reduction is achieved with the elbow in extension and a valgus force applied, but holding that position and force while pinning can be frustrating, even with the best assistant. To decrease your frustration and increase your pinning joy, put towel roll under the distal humerus. If the articular surface is displaced, open the fracture site and get a perfect articular reduction.

In little elbows, the distance from the fracture to the posterior interosseous nerve and brachial artery is short.

Fortunately, once you've dissected through superficial fascia, a traumatic rent in the wrist extensor muscle mass is usually present, which gets you to the fracture site with very little sharp dissection below the skin. This opening may be enlarged

Figure 7-4 A: Lateral view of elbow with fluoroscopy in which an arthrogram is being performed by placing a needle into the olecranon fossa from a posterior approach. **B:** Anterior-posterior view of an arthrogram of the same elbow. This demonstrates that the articular surface is intact, so the fracture does not extend into the joint. Most frequently, closed pinning is sufficient when the articular surface is intact.

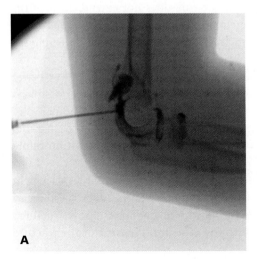

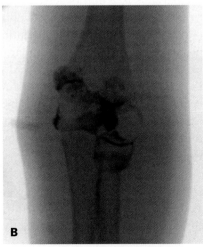

to visualize the fracture site and remove hematoma. To minimize the chances of osteonecrosis, soft tissue attachments on the posterior portion of the fracture fragment should not be detached, as the only blood supply to the lateral trochlea and capitellum enter in the posterior nonarticular portion.

Anatomic reduction of the articular surface is performed and verified under direct visualization (a headlight can be helpful). If reduction is challenging, try some dorsiflexion of the wrist to relax the wrist extensors attached to the distal fragment. Two smooth pins are placed percutaneously (just posterior to the incision) in a divergent trajectory—the same one you would use for divergent pinning of a supracondylar fracture. To stay out of trouble, avoid a lower pin that is parallel to the joint, and usually only in cartilage (cartilage doesn't pin well, does it?) and the wrong trajectory for the fracture plane (Fig. 7-5). **ORTHOPAEDICS 101: Fixation is best when it is perpendicular to the plane of the fracture.**

Unlike supracondylar fractures, which nearly always heal in 3 weeks, lateral condylar fractures should be casted with the pins in for 4 weeks, then remove the cast, image, remove the pins, and then cast for an additional 2 weeks. With all that cartilage, give a lateral condyle a solid 6 weeks of cast protection. A potential complication with these intra-articular pins is pin site infection with a subsequent septic elbow, so carefully weigh the benefits versus risks of leaving pins in longer than 4 weeks, and certainly examine the pin sites if you choose to leave the pins in longer.

Despite the usual excellent results with reduction and pin fixation, some have experimented with using a screw to hold the fragment in place. This is a path to unnecessary trouble, especially in young children (<8 years of age), who usually get great results with simple pin fixation. In young children, the fracture fragment is mostly cartilage, and it is small. So, some try a single screw to compress this cartilage fragment in place. As you might expect, the cartilage fragment rotates on that single screw axis, creating a malunion machine. In addition, screw fixation should not be through the olecranon fossa (a joint is a bad place for threads), so it must be up the lateral column, which demands a trajectory starting on the lateral edge of the fragment (not much bone there). Screw fixation is valuable in delayed unions and malunions and in older children (>10 years of age) with very large bone fragments. Otherwise, the pediatric fracture surgeon is actually looking for

> **THE GURU SAYS...**
>
> This is a deep dark hole, and it is difficult to see. Headlamps or lighted suction tips that are used in ENT can be helpful. Usually, only one person will have a good view of the fracture due to the depth, lighting, and position of retractors, so get your head out of the way from time to time for others to see.
>
> JEFFREY R. SAWYER

> **THE GURU SAYS...**
>
> No shortcuts. There usually is some plastic deformation of the metaphysis. While easier to reduce than the joint itself, relying solely on the metaphyseal reduction can lead to joint malunion when plastic deformation present.
>
> Dorsiflexing the wrist can help relax the extensor musculature and make the distal fragment more mobile.
>
> JEFFREY R. SAWYER

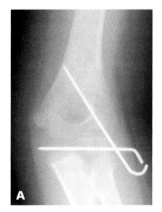 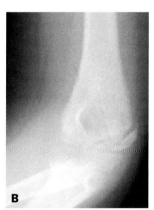 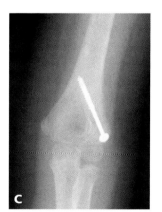 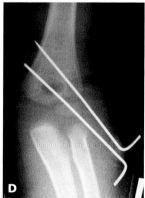

Figure 7-5 A: Anteroposterior radiograph demonstrating the horizontal pin failing to engage ossific bone in the proximal to the fracture. **B:** Ten weeks after surgery, the patient has elbow pain and stiffness, and the radiograph demonstrates a lack of union. **C:** Rigid fixation with a compression screw was used at time of second surgery to allow early motion. Screw should be only in the lateral column and not in the olecranon fossa or terminal elbow extension would be compromised. **D:** The ideal pin configuration for a lateral condyle fracture. Both pins are perpendicular to the plane of the fracture, and both engage to far cortex. The lower pin has four cortices thanks to the olecranon fossa. The fracture is perfectly reduced. These pins were pulled in the office at 4 weeks, and then the fracture was casted for 2 additional weeks with a perfect result. A screw cannot do better than this and would be removed with a second anesthetic.

trouble when they abandon the successful divergent pin strategy for a fresh fracture in young children.

LATE PRESENTATION

Traditional teaching suggests that open reduction should not be performed in fractures seen later than 3 weeks, as the risk of poor results from stiffness and osteonecrosis increases. However, if one carefully avoids posterior dissection to maintain blood supply of the distal fragment, good results with open reduction of lateral condylar fractures can be achieved.

A key approach to avoiding trouble in the treatment of *late* lateral condylar fractures is to not necessarily aim for anatomic reduction; it is preferable to fix it where it lies with no posterior stripping. This technique has been described as "metaphyseal osteosynthesis in situ" in the past. These fractures are similar to a slipped capital femoral epiphysis in that respect. Consider rigid fixation with a screws or screws in compression in late cases to maximize healing and early ROM, while remembering to avoid the olecranon fossa.

OTHER TROUBLE

Lateral condylar fractures heal more slowly than other fractures the pediatric orthopaedist is accustomed to treating. Be patient. It can be 10 or even 12 weeks before solid union. Look on the lateral radiograph for the first signs of healing—a wisp of periosteal new bone from fragment to metaphysis is a great sign that healing is under way. Lateral overgrowth from new bone can give the appearance of cubitus varus—but it is not. Warn parents ahead of time that they may see a lateral prominence when the cast comes off and the arm is atrophied. In some cases, lateral overgrowth is clear (Fig. 7-6). Either way, assure parents it is rarely severe enough to require treatment. Posterior osseous spurs may occur with both operative and nonoperative treatment. These seldom cause any problem other than parental concern over the radiographs (Fig. 7-7). Persistent elbow stiffness is more common following lateral condylar fractures than supracondylar fractures; prepare the family, use physical therapy (PT) after healing, and set expectations that return to sports may be a few months after injury.

> ### THE GURU SAYS...
>
> Overgrowth can occur from fractures treated operatively or nonoperatively. Tell the parents ahead of time, every time, about this. If it does not occur, everyone is happy. If it occurs, you will look like a prophet and they will trust you that function will be fine. If you don't tell them and it occurs, it is more difficult to gain their trust that all will be fine.
>
> JEFFREY R. SAWYER

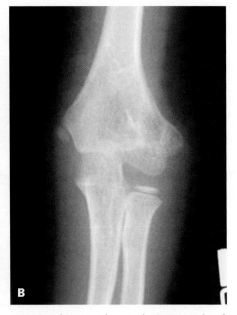

Figure 7-6 A: X-ray at time of injury confirms previously normal growth. **B:** Example of lateral overgrowth following operative treatment of a lateral condyle fracture.

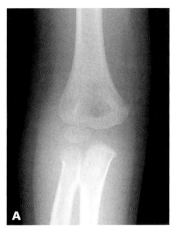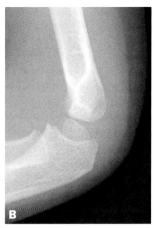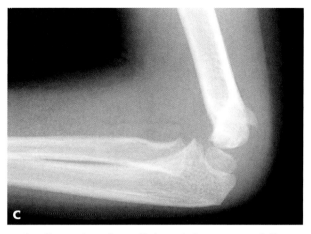

Figure 7-7 A: Anteroposterior radiograph at time of injury. **B:** Lateral radiograph at time of injury. **C:** Osseous spur following treatment with casting for a minimally displaced lateral condyle fracture.

Medial Epicondylar Fractures

One key to staying out of trouble in the evaluation of medial epicondylar fractures is ruling out concomitant injury, as up to 50% of these fractures may be associated with an elbow dislocation. Simple fractures of the medial epicondyle are extra-articular injuries with limited soft tissue injury, thus an elevated posterior fat pad should not be present in an isolated medial epicondylar fracture. If an elevated posterior fat pad is seen, have a high index of suspicion for associated injuries, such as a reduced elbow dislocation. Gross instability of the elbow or significant swelling of the joint suggests other injuries, such as an intraarticular medial condylar fracture and an elbow dislocation.

A potential pitfall is to miss a medial epicondylar fracture (associated with an elbow dislocation) where the epicondyle has become incarcerated in the joint, which occurs in about 15% of cases. It may be quite difficult to see the fracture fragment in the joint, but one should become suspicious if the ossification center for the medial epicondyle is not appreciated after the ossification centers for the trochlea and/or olecranon are present.

TREATMENT

There is little controversy that minimally displaced (<5 mm) fractures not associated with elbow dislocation are best managed with 3 weeks in a cast. However, medial condylar fractures displaced than 5 mm or associated with elbow dislocation or in the elbow of a throwing athlete (especially when the injury occurred with throwing) are best treated with reduction, screw fixation, and early mobilization. Operative fixation and early mobilization also are of value to upper extremity weight-bearing athletes, such as gymnasts. A challenge that is hotly debated is how to determine actual displacement. Because of its anatomic attachments to the medial ligamentous complex, a displaced medial epicondylar fracture usually displaces anteriorly in a way that actual displacement from its anatomic home is difficult to appreciate on standard AP and lateral radiographs. A CT scan of the elbow can be valuable in equivocal cases (although CT of every medial epicondylar injury should not be standard of care).

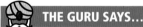 **THE GURU SAYS...**

Emphasize to the parents that this is an elbow dislocation (stiffness problem) with an associated medial epicondyle fracture and not the other way around (fracture problem). The ultimate determinant of outcome is the elbow dislocation and the potential for long-term elbow stiffness.

JEFFREY R. SAWYER

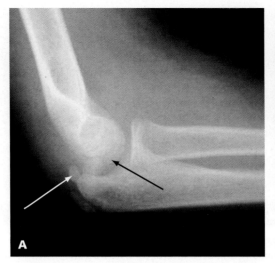
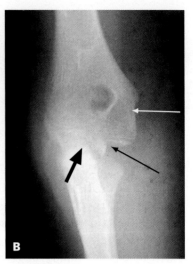

Figure 7-8 A: An incarcerated fragment may be removed at times with closed means by open-view of elbow demonstrating an incarcerated medial epicondyle (*black arrow*) following spontaneous reduction of a dislocated elbow. Note that the olecranon apophysis is ossified (*white arrow*), suggesting the child is skeletally mature enough that the medial epicondyle should be ossified and visible on the AP view. **B:** Anteroposterior view of same elbow. Note that the trochlea is beginning to ossify (*thin black arrow*), suggesting the medial epicondyle should be visible, but is absent from its anatomic position (*white arrow*). The mystery is solved by identifying the medial epicondyle in the joint (*thick black arrow*).

THE GURU SAYS...

Force yourself to identify the medial epicondyle on every adolescent patient you are called to see for an elbow dislocation. These are often missed. Look for the "empty epicondyle sign" on the radiograph with the elbow dislocated. Not only will you make the diagnosis of an associated medial epicondyle fracture, but you can compare this to the radiograph with the elbow reduced to determine if the fragment is entrapped or not.

If you have any doubts, a contralateral elbow film or limited-cut CT scan through the elbow can confirm the diagnosis.

JEFFREY R. SAWYER

THE GURU SAYS...

While it is not necessary to fully expose or transpose the ulnar nerve, it is usually pretty easy to find it in a layer of fat just proximal to the fracture site. Once it is identified, it can be fully protected during the procedure. Gentle handling of the nerve is essential because it may be partially injured/stretched at the time of the elbow dislocation. Knowing and documenting in the record that the nerve is not entrapped by direct vision will be very helpful to you and the patient if they wake with an ulnar nerve palsy.

For comminuted fractures, which are very rare, or iatrogenic fracture of the epicondyle fragment, a suture repair with a suture anchor in the proximal humeral fracture bed can provide some stability.

Consider a hinged elbow brace rather than a cast and early ROM for compliant patients with stable fixation.

JEFFREY R. SAWYER

A pitfall is to miss a medial epicondylar fracture incarcerated within the elbow joint following either spontaneous or supervised reduction of a dislocated elbow. Be particularly vigilant when an older child or young teenager presents a couple days after injury and reports having had an elbow dislocation reduced at an urgent care center or community hospital emergency room. Look closely to be certain that there is a medial condyle in its home on the medial side of the metaphysis, and not in the joint. Contralateral elbow X-rays often come with that child. We see several children each year who have an incarcerated epicondyle that has been there for several days, and it can cause a lot of damage to the articular cartilage. Stay out of trouble by looking for the incarcerated medial epicondylar fracture in the joint (Fig. 7-8).

An incarcerated fragment can sometimes be removed by opening the elbow with valgus stress, while extending the wrist to place tension across the wrist flexors whose origin are on the epicondyle; however, an open reduction usually is required When an open reduction is chosen, consider rigid fixation with a screw to allow early motion.

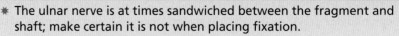

Staying Out of Trouble in the Operative Treatment of Medial Epicondylar Fractures

* The ulnar nerve is at times sandwiched between the fragment and shaft; make certain it is not when placing fixation.
* If using a screw, place the screw up the medial column and not across the olecranon fossa, which will limit elbow extension.

(continued)

Staying Out of Trouble in the Operative Treatment of Medial Epicondylar Fractures *(continued)*

✳ Be aware of the perils of cannulated screw systems, especially in older kids with hard bone.
  ✳ The guidewire can bend and then be sheared off by the cannulated drill.
  ✳ The screw can skirt along the posterior cortex (or any other cortex) and the bone is so hard that the threads can shear off, causing a pigtail of metal to lodge in the bone—that requires a long explanation to the parents.
  ✳ Overdrill if bone seems too hard.
  ✳ Be careful not to fragment the piece with the last crank of the screw.

Olecranon Fractures

There are three potential pitfalls to avoid with olecranon fractures in children. The first is missing another fracture, as more than half of all olecranon fractures are associated with another fracture about the elbow. The second pitfall to avoid is failing to recognize displacement of the fracture during the course of treatment by cast immobilization. Particularly at risk for displacement is the flexion-type fracture in which the posterior portion of the olecranon fails in tension and the fracture line extends to the articular surface. If complete, this fracture is potentially unstable because the torn posterior periosteum cannot function as a tension band, and the pull of the biceps and triceps may further displace the fracture over time. If closed treatment is chosen, good quality radiographs at about 1 week after injury are indicated to assess possible displacement. The third pitfall is failure to recognize the type of olecranon fracture that is almost pathognomonic for osteogenesis imperfecta. This fracture is an avulsion of the proximal ulnar metaphysis and, following one fracture, is eventually bilateral in 70% of children with osteogenesis imperfecta. Most fractures require operative treatment, and refracture is not uncommon (Fig. 7-9). In a normal child with an olecranon fracture, the risk of elbow loss of

THE GURU SAYS...

Force yourself to look at the relationship between the radial head and capitellum in every pediatric elbow trauma radiograph you see. The olecranon fracture is readily seen, and the accompanying radial head dislocation (Monteggia) can be missed.

JEFFREY R. SAWYER

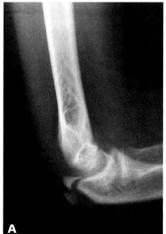
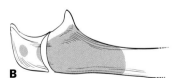

Figure 7-9 A: Lateral radiograph of a 12-year-old boy with type IA osteogenesis imperfecta demonstrating a characteristic olecranon fracture seen in children with osteogenesis imperfecta. **B:** Drawing shows characteristic fracture pattern involving the olecranon observed in children with osteogenesis imperfecta. (**A:** Reprinted with permission from Zionts LE, Moon CN. Olecranon apophysis fractures in children with osteogenesis imperfecta revisited. *J Pediatr Orthop.* 2002;22(6):745-750.)

motion is not as severe as in adults, so we usually place the child in a long arm cast following open reduction and internal fixation of olecranon fractures. A fiber-wire tension band works very well, and the Kirschner wires (K-wires) can be left percutaneous. This technique obviates the need for return to the operating room for implant removal.

Proximal Radial Fractures

The biggest problem with proximal radial fractures is loss of motion (especially supination and pronation), despite optimal treatment. Alert the family that motion loss is common after the radiocapitellar joint is injured, and prepare them for months of stiffness, especially if the fracture is intra-articular.

DIAGNOSIS

As with olecranon fractures, associated injuries are common with proximal radial fractures, and missing a second fracture or dislocation is a potential pitfall. A valgus injury may cause an associated medial epicondylar avulsion or olecranon fracture. Proximal radial fractures also are associated with posterior elbow dislocations, with the radial head displacing anteriorly if the fracture occurs during the dislocation, or posteriorly if the fracture occurs during relocation. Fractures of the proximal radius in children tend to involve the metaphyseal neck or, less commonly, the physis (Salter type I or II), rather than the head as seen in adults.

Subtle proximal radial fractures may be easily overlooked on radiographs, with only one cortex in one radiograph showing too sharp of an angle where there should be a gentle curve. A subtle radial neck fracture may be present without elevation of the posterior fat pad (as it may be extracapsular). There are two potential areas of radiographic confusion. First, the radial head is normally angulated up to 15° valgus and, thus, is not necessarily perpendicular to the diaphysis of the radius. Second, a bipartite ossification center may be mistaken for a fracture. The physical examination is often quite helpful in diagnosing subtle fractures, as tenderness is well localized in isolated, nondisplaced fractures. Pronation and supination usually are more painful than elbow flexion and extension when a proximal radial fracture is present.

TREATMENT

The primary goal of treatment is preservation of pronation and supination. The importance of early motion and physical therapy should be discussed with the family at the first visit to help ensure compliance. Good results can be expected in fractures with less than 30° of angulation and less than 3 mm of translation. **NEWSFLASH! The key to staying out of trouble is to really focus on motion, not millimeters or degrees of angulation.** One particularly effective reduction method is the Israeli technique: flex the elbow to 90°, forcibly pronate the forearm, and apply direct pressure over the radial head with your thumb. After reduction, with the patients under sedation in the ED or in the operating room, the surgeon must assure that the reduction is stable and pronation and supination are returned to normal. Document the range of motion examination after reduction. If there is block to pronation and supination, indirect or open reduction methods are necessary. Percutaneous manipulation with K-wires is effective in most cases where the fragment is primarily angulated (of course, it doesn't work if the fragment is flipped 180° in the joint).

THE GURU SAYS...

Start with an à la carte approach, from least invasive and lowest risk of stiffness (closed reduction and casting) to most invasive and highest risk of stiffness (open reduction internal fixation [ORIF]). Start with closed reduction, then percutaneous reduction/pinning, and finally ORIF. If ORIF is performed, consider using a small proximal radial plate to allow early ROM.

Explain to the parents that closed reduction with slight malalignment is better than open reduction with perfect anatomic alignment. If open reduction is performed, especially in older patients, some loss of forearm rotation and elbow extension is to be expected.

JEFFREY R. SAWYER

Staying Out of Trouble With Percutaneous K-Wire Fixation of Proximal Radial Fractures

✳ Insert the K-wire into the skin at least 8 cm distal to the radial head to allow a proximally directed force that frees the fracture fragment.

✳ Use a blunt and a fairly large-diameter K-wire (a tiny skin incision facilitates entry).

✳ Rotate the forearm until the maximal displacement of the fracture is seen and perform the reduction using that view.

✳ Be careful not to injure the posterior interosseous nerve, with supination of the forearm bringing the nerve posteriorly and under less tension (Fig. 7-10). If percutaneous reduction with a K-wire is inadequate, try inserting a Freer elevator to lever the fragment in place (Fig. 7-11). In a very young child prior to robust ossification of the radial head, an arthrogram may help in visualization and manipulation of the proximal radius (Fig. 7-12).

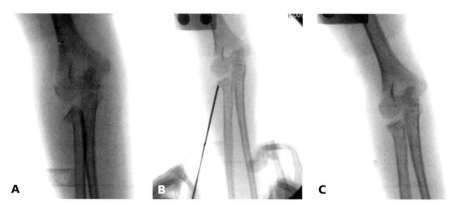

Figure 7-10 A: Displaced radial neck fracture in an 11-year-old girl. Attempts at closed reduction have failed. Rotate the forearm until the maximal displacement of the fracture is seen, and keep this position to visualize the reduction. **B:** A 2.4-mm Kirschner wire (K-wire) is inserted proximal to fracture, and then the blunt end of the wire is used to push the fracture fragment free. **C:** Final image showing near anatomic reduction. At this point, the patient had 80° of pronation and supination.

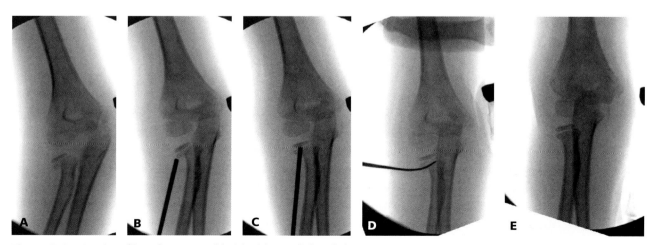

Figure 7-11 A: Injury film of a 6-year-old girl with a radial neck fracture. **B:** Attempting percutaneous reduction with a Kirschner wire (K-wire). **C:** Even when using the blunt end of the K-wire, the K-wire may become lodged in the bone, with incomplete reduction. **D:** Through a 4-mm incision a freer elevator can be used to lever the fracture fragment into place. **E:** Reduction with minimal dissection was possible.

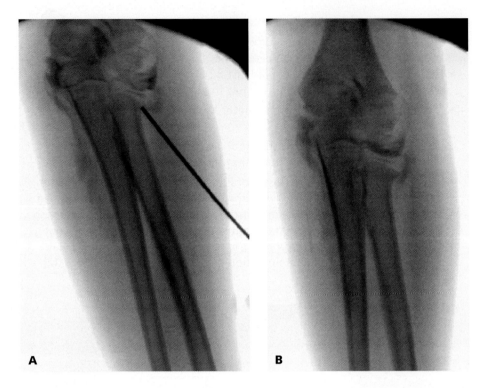

Figure 7-12 A: In the young child with little ossification of the radial head, an arthrogram may prove useful in visualizing the proximal radius during reduction. **B:** Following reduction.

If open reduction is needed, the fracture should always be fixed or nonunion is a very high risk. Excision of the radial head as initial treatment in the immature skeleton should be avoided at all costs, because synostosis, cubitus valgus, and ulnar deviation of the wrist may develop.

Elbow Dislocations

Elbow dislocations are relatively uncommon in children, but there are a few pitfalls to watch out for.

Over half of posterior elbow dislocations are associated with other fractures, most commonly the medial epicondyle, radial head and neck, and the coronoid process. Following a stable reduction of a dislocated elbow, expect a fairly large arc of motion without severe pain; if there is no motion or severe pain with little motion, look for a fracture, particularly an incarcerated medial epicondylar fracture (see Fig. 7-8).

Nerves can become entrapped during reduction, so careful pre- and postreduction neurologic examinations are essential. Any postreduction nerve deficit not recognized before reduction should be considered an entrapped nerve until proven otherwise with an MRI or surgical exploration.

Elbow dislocations in young children are particularly rare, because the physes tend to fail before the ligaments. Before ossification of the capitellum, an injury with the radiographic appearance of an elbow dislocation is most likely a transphyseal fracture, which usually requires pinning. The diagnosis can be confirmed with an intraoperative arthrogram (see Fig. 6-21 in Chapter 6). For further discussion of transphyseal injuries, see Chapter 6.

THE GURU SAYS...

While elbow dislocations in skeletally immature patients can occur, they should be considered to have an associated medial epicondyle fracture until proven otherwise.

JEFFREY R. SAWYER

Staying Out of Trouble With Elbow Trauma

Lateral Condylar Fractures

✳ Lateral condylar fractures are intra-articular and need anatomic reduction for union and long-term good outcome. Expect the healing process to be at least twice as long as a supracondylar fracture.

✳ Get an internal oblique radiographs to make the most accurate measurement of fracture displacement.

✳ When performing a reduction, don't kill the blood supply by dissecting posteriorly.

✳ Have a low threshold for radiographs out of plaster if loss of reduction is suspected.

Other Fractures

✳ Fix medial epicondylar fractures if they are more than 5 mm displaced, especially when associated with elbow dislocation or in overhead or upper extremity weight-bearing athletes.

✳ Be sure that you've restored pronation and supination after reduction of a proximal radial fracture.

✳ If you open a proximal radial fracture for reduction, you must fix it or risk nonunion.

✳ With olecranon and proximal radial fractures, as well as elbow dislocations, look for associated injuries.

FOR FURTHER ENLIGHTENMENT

Beck JJ, Bowen RE, Silva M. What's new in pediatric medial epicondyle fractures? *J Pediatr Orthop.* 2018;38(4):e202-e206.

Cruz AI Jr, Steere JT, Lawrence JT. Medial epicondyle fractures in the pediatric overhead athlete. *J Pediatr Orthop.* 2016;36(suppl 1):S56-S62.

De Mattos CB, Ramski DE, Kushare IV, et al. Radial neck fractures in children and adolescents: an examination of operative and nonoperative treatment and outcomes. *J Pediatr Orthop.* 2016;36(1):6-12.

Knapik DM, Fausett CL, Gilmore A, Liu RW. Outcomes of nonoperative pediatric medial humeral epicondyle fractures with and without associated elbow dislocation. *J Pediatr Orthop.* 2017;37(4):e224-e228.

Knapik DM, Gilmore A, Liu RW. Conservative management of minimally displaced (≤2 mm) fractures of the lateral humeral condyle in pediatric patients: a systematic review. *J Pediatr Orthop.* 2017;37(2):e83-e87.

Pace JL, Arkader A, Sousa T, et al. Incidence, risk factors, and definition for nonunion in pediatric lateral condyle fractures. *J Pediatr Orthop.* 2018;38(5):e257-e261.

Pannu GS, Eberson CP, Abzug J, et al. Common errors in the management of pediatric supracondylar humerus fractures and lateral condyle fractures. *Instr Course Lect.* 2016;65:385-397.

Zimmerman RM, Kalish LA, Hresko MT, et al. Surgical management of pediatric radial neck fractures. *J Bone Joint Surg Am.* 2013;95(20):1825-1832.

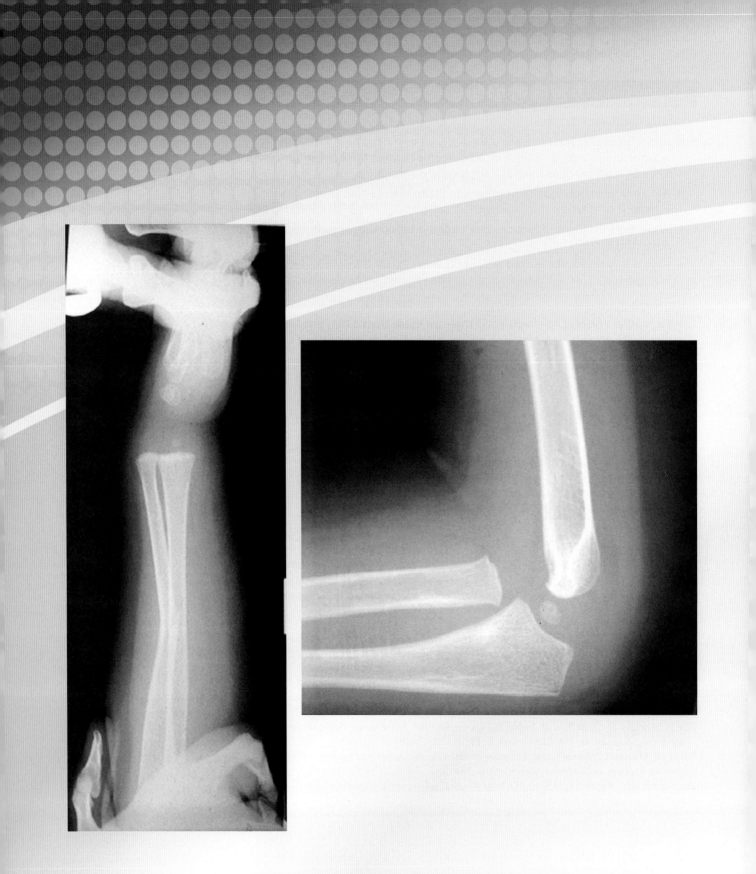

Chapter 8

Hand, Wrist, and Forearm Injuries

KENNETH J. NOONAN, MD, MHCDS

Guru: Donald Bae, MD

General Principles

Hand, wrist, and forearm injuries are among the most common injuries sustained by children. Although not life-threatening and usually not debilitating, they may be a frequent source of management trouble due to the sheer volume seen by most orthopaedists caring for children. Most injuries can be treated successfully and will heal uneventfully; however, careful attention to certain principles of diagnosis and management is critical to a consistently good outcome. In hand injuries, 75% create no problems, but 25% need careful diagnosis and treatment. To stay out of trouble, the orthopaedist must promptly recognize and treat problem fractures early.

Hand and Wrist Injuries

Although a pediatric orthopaedist or a general orthopaedist caring for children can handle the vast majority of hand injuries in children, it is important to know which cases should be transferred directly to a hand surgeon.

Physeal injuries represent 10% to 40% of all hand fractures. Fortunately, growth arrest is very rare. To stay out of trouble, it is important to recognize that an apparent "tendon disruption" may instead be a physeal fracture in a young child (Fig. 8-1). The flexor digitorum profundus inserts onto the distal phalanx and the flexor digitorum superficialis inserts onto the middle phalanx. The extensor tendons insert onto the epiphysis of the distal phalanges.

Evaluation of the pediatric hand can be challenging. It's always a good idea to exam the uninjured hand first in order to gain trust. Questions should be general and with simple queries such as if the fingers feel sleepy or if they feel the same as the uninjured side. The tenodesis concept is critical to the examination. The orthopaedist should check the digital cascade at rest and with tenodesis wrist motion. This maneuver will call attention to the diagnosis of malrotated fractures and flexor tendon injuries. Fingers that don't extend or flex with wrist flexion may indicate an occult tendon injury.

The orthopaedist should assess for the extent of open injuries, which can be subtle in the hand. Radiographs of a bleeding nail bed injury are needed to rule out an open growth plate fracture of the distal phalanx. Neurologic examination can be very difficult in children. One clue to a possible nerve injury is excessive bleeding from a wound around the area of the digital nerve, as the digital artery and nerve are often lacerated together. To stay out of trouble in assessing a nerve, it is helpful to do the "wrinkle test." Immerse the digit in warm water for about 5

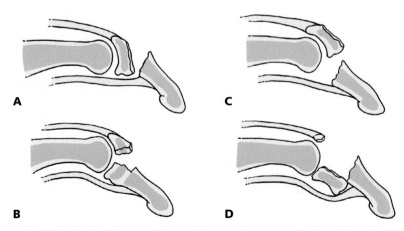

Figure 8-1 What looks like a tendon avulsion can be a growth plate injury in children.

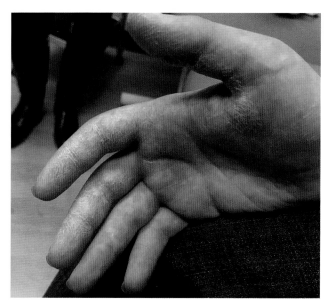

Figure 8-2 This child has a median nerve palsy following a supracondylar humerus fracture. In addition to altered sensation in the median nerve distribution and weakened thenar function, his skin is dry with abnormal sweat pattern in the same distribution. (Used with the permission of the University of Wisconsin Division of Pediatric Orthopaedics.)

minutes. Denervated digits will not have any wrinkling of the volar skin, and over time, they will have altered sweat patterns (Fig. 8-2).

Radiographs of the injured palm and wrist should include an AP, lateral, and oblique views. More complex imaging is rarely needed. Evaluating an injured digit is done best by asking the radiology technician to focus on the finger as opposed to ordering hand films. A true lateral of the injured digit may be very valuable as opposed to a lateral of the hand, often with overlapping fingers that are nondiagnostic.

The treatment of any hand injury begins with proper pain control. Digital blocks are very effective for phalangeal fractures and nail bed injuries. To stay out of trouble, do not use epinephrine for digital block, as it may lead to distal ischemia. Also, never inject a circular weal around the digit as the circulation of the digit can be compromised.

Nail Bed Injuries

Nail bed injuries in children are common and can easily be missed. Plain radiographs should be obtained to assess for a concomitant fracture and the germinal matrix can be entrapped in the physeal fracture (the Seymour fracture; Fig. 8-3). The nail should be removed if it is not already off and can be placed in iodine solution for later use. Finger tourniquets can be helpful for visualization and eponychium incisions will allow you to extract the germinal matrix. The wound should be irrigated just like an open fracture. When you repair a nail bed in a child, use loupes and use #6-0 absorbable chromic suture. Stent the nail bed repair with Xeroform or the sterilized nail (if using the nail, put a hole in it to allow drainage).

Distal Phalangeal Injuries

Just like adults, children can jam their finger and suffer a "mallet finger" injury. As opposed to adults (where the extensor tendon is torn), forced flexion of the distal phalanx can result in a Salter Harris I or II injury with the extensor tendon

---

THE GURU SAYS...

The warm water immersion test is extremely helpful in younger children. Remember, two-point discrimination and other threshold sensory testing can only be reliably done in patients over 5 to 7 years of age.
DONALD BAE

THE GURU SAYS...

Avoid the temptation to accept suboptimal radiographs! Orthogonal views of the affected digit should be obtained when evaluating finger/thumb injuries.
DONALD BAE

THE GURU SAYS...

Remember, a Seymour fracture is an open fracture—the wound is just hidden beneath the nail plate. To adequately irrigate and debride the open wound, as well as remove interposed soft tissue to reduce the fracture, you need to remove the nail plate.
DONALD BAE

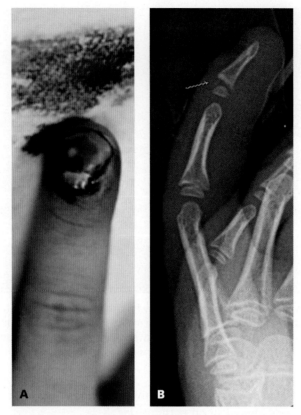

Figure 8-3 Seymour fracture. The bleeding from the nail fold is directly adjacent to the widened growth plate seen on the radiograph. This is an open fracture and their may be interposed nail bed in the fracture.

attached to the epiphysis while the profundus tendon flexes the distal piece. "Jersey finger" injuries usually occur in adolescents near skeletal maturity. The classic example is a football player whose finger gets caught in an opposing player's jersey, leading to a profundus tendon avulsion.

AP, lateral, and oblique radiographs should be obtained to look for avulsion fractures entrapped in the pulley system or in the palm. To stay out of trouble, surgical intervention, within 7 to 10 days after injury, is usually required to reattach the tendon after a jersey finger injury.

Distal fingertip amputations and avulsions can be gruesome injuries, brought in by nauseated parents. If the parent brings the amputated part, it is important to assess its quality to decide whether replantation or a composite graft is warranted. When faced with a fingertip amputation you can offer the patient three choices based on the injury: (1) dressing changes for very distal injuries; (2) a composite grafting of the amputated part; or (3) replantation if the amputation is proximal to the DIP joint and the amputated part is in good condition.

Fractures of the Proximal and Middle Phalanx

Fractures of the proximal and middle phalanx in children can generally be managed successfully, but do present a few specific sources of trouble. Overall, most proximal and middle phalangeal fractures can be treated with nonoperative management utilizing reduction and casting for 3 to 4 weeks.

One important cause of problems is failure to recognize a rotational deformity (Fig. 8-4). All children should have splints removed, and an examination for rotational malalignment as described above is critical. Phalangeal neck

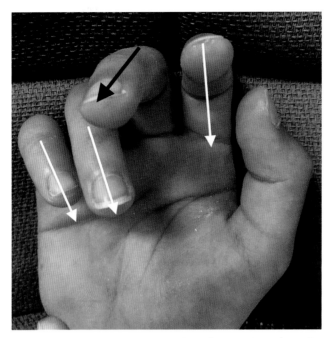

Figure 8-4 The long finger has a proximal phalanx fracture in malrotation (*black arrow*). The other unaffected fingers more or less point in the same direction (*white arrows*) when they are flexed. (Used with permission of Dr. Nina Lightdale-Meric and the Children's Orthopaedic Center, Los Angeles.)

fractures are small injuries with big problems if not fully appreciated on true lateral radiographs. These fractures need closed reduction and percutaneous pinning. If the articular surface is allowed to heal in a dorsally displaced position, the child will have a permanent loss in flexion. Displaced intra-articular fractures can also lead to joint stiffness if not similarly reduced and pinned. Coronally angulated Salter-Harris (extra octave fracture) proximal phalangeal fractures of the small finger can remodel with growth severe angulated fractures will still require reduction.

Finger Dislocations

Although finger dislocations in young children are relatively rare, these injuries are not uncommon in the teenage athlete. To stay out of trouble, look for areas of open injury and do a good prereduction neurovascular examination. If the joint is irreducible, it is possible that there is an interposed ligament or volar plate hindering reduction. Open reduction may be necessary. After an injury to the volar plate, it is important to move the joint early. Do not do extension block splinting because you risk contracture of the child's PIP joint.

Fractures of the Metacarpals

In children, the most common site of metacarpal fracture is the neck. Most can be treated with closed reduction and splinting. The physis in the metacarpal is distal, often very near the site of fracture, and remodeling will often correct the residual

THE GURU SAYS...

For phalangeal neck fractures, try this trick: Take the lateral X-ray and turn it upside down, imagining the PIP joint is the elbow joint and the phalangeal neck fracture similar to a supracondylar humerus fracture. Just like Gartland type II and III supracondylar humerus fractures, displaced phalangeal neck fractures merit closed reduction and pin fixation to preserve joint motion and function.

DONALD BAE

THE GURU SAYS...

Beware the nondisplaced unicondylar fracture of the phalanx. These injuries may be unstable, so careful serial radiographic follow-up is needed, and if there's any displacement resulting in articular incongruity, go the OR for reduction and fixation!

DONALD BAE

THE GURU SAYS...

The collateral ligaments of the MCP joint are loose in extension and taut in flexion. For closed reduction of proximal phalangeal physeal fractures, flex the MCP joint prior to correcting the angulation to maximize your ability to reduce the fracture. In these specific cases, you have to bend it to straighten it!

DONALD BAE

THE GURU SAYS...

Open reduction of irreducible or "complex" MCP dislocations may be performed via dorsal or volar approaches. Consider going dorsal to avoid the volar neurovascular bundles. And in young children, beware of an osteochondral shear fracture that may not have been apparent on the injury radiographs!

DONALD BAE

deformity in young children. In those that don't remodel, the malunion in the plane of joint motion is better tolerated than in the coronal plane.

Metacarpal shaft fractures must be evaluated carefully for malrotation. When the child makes a fist, all fingers should point to the scaphoid and all nail beds should be parallel. Unstable fractures with residual rotational malalignment may require closed reduction and percutaneous pinning. Fractures at the base of the finger metacarpals are infrequent in children. They are usually the result of high-energy trauma. In these cases, a CT scan is valuable. These injuries will often require either closed reduction and percutaneous pinning or open reduction and internal fixation.

Fractures at the base of the thumb metacarpal can present as simple transverse fractures or intra-articular fractures. Salter-Harris type III and IV fractures at the base most closely resemble the adult Bennett fracture. Fractures at the base of the thumb without intra-articular extension can be treated with closed reduction and immobilization. There is great remodeling potential at the base of the thumb because the fracture is juxtaphyseal and the carpal metacarpal joint has universal motion; angulation of up to 20° can be accepted.

Ulnar collateral ligament injuries of the thumb (a.k.a., gamekeeper's thumb) are typically encountered in adolescents rather than young children. Similar to other injuries, the ulnar collateral ligament will be stronger than the adjacent bone, resulting in a Salter-Harris III avulsion fracture rather than ligament disruption. This is a "gamekeeper's equivalent" and requires open reduction and internal fixation if displaced.

Fractures of the Carpal Bones

In general, fractures of the carpal bones in young children are exceedingly rare. The most common is a scaphoid fracture. Be alert to the fact that the scapholunate space may be physiologically wider in an immature child as there is unossified cartilage. This should not be mistaken for a perilunate injury. Comparison views will help define the normal space for the child that presents to you. To stay out of trouble with carpal bone injuries, any patient with pain in the snuffbox should be treated using a thumb spica cast for 10 to 14 days, even if the radiographs are negative. If still tender, MRI is now thought to be the best diagnostic test if there is a question of a scaphoid fracture and X-rays are equivocal. Proximal pole scaphoid fractures are rare but have a high risk of avascular necrosis (AVN). Distal pole fractures seem to heal with no problem. Fractures at the scaphoid waist are similar risks as in adults.

Fractures of the Forearm

FRACTURES OF THE DISTAL RADIUS AND ULNA

Fractures of the distal radius and ulna are exceedingly common in children. The keys to staying out of trouble include understanding remodeling, avoiding overtreatment, putting your reductions in good casts, and being alert for associated injuries. Remodeling is greatest in young children, in fractures near a rapidly growing physis, in fractures that are in the plane of motion of the adjacent joint, and in fractures with greater amounts of angulation. Typically, the child can correct about 10° of apex-volar angulation for each year of growth remaining. Radial-ward angulation of the distal radius, caused by the pull of the brachioradialis, corrects more slowly. Bayonet apposition remodels reliably in younger children, especially those younger than about 8 years.

Physeal Injuries

Physeal injuries of the distal radius are the most common growth plate injury in children. To stay out of trouble, evaluate for open injuries, especially subtle pinpoint openings on the volar skin. Higher energy injuries, such as when a teenager falls rollerblading, can lead to neuropraxia of the median nerve, or even acute carpal tunnel syndrome or compartment syndrome[1] (Fig. 8-5). To stay out of trouble, do a careful nerve examination and get these fractures reduced as quickly as is practical. The easiest injury to miss is the *second* injury, so be certain to evaluate the elbow and hand carefully when confronted with a distal radius fracture (Fig. 8-6).

Minimally displaced fractures are often placed in a splint and an Ace wrap in the emergency department and sent on to an orthopaedist office for management. **NEWSFLASH! There are few things more dangerous than an inexperienced resident with an Ace bandage.** A tight Ace wrap can be trouble (Fig. 8-7). Children will shift in the splint, or play with their Ace wrap, which can become rolled and cause a tourniquet-like effect. The Ace wrap can create a row of blisters at the seams between the Ace wrap or create a tremendous amount of swelling distally.

Displaced fractures can be reduced under conscious sedation at the time of injury. It is a general principle to avoid reductions or rereductions of physeal injuries later than approximately 10 days following injury, in order to avoid growth arrest. Open or closed reduction with Kirschner wire (K-wire) fixation

> ### THE GURU SAYS...
> Sometimes it is hard to know how much more growth a child or adolescent has. One trick is to look at the thumb metacarpal physis, which is usually captured on AP wrist X-rays! If the thumb metacarpal physis is open, the patient has two or more years of growth remaining, and therefore remodeling potential.
> DONALD BAE

> ### THE GURU SAYS...
> Remodeling is powerful, but remember the radius and ulna don't spin as they grow longer! Therefore, one cannot expect remodeling of rotational malalignment.
> DONALD BAE

> ### THE GURU SAYS...
> It's especially important to look at the wrist for a possible concomitant scaphoid fracture. Don't lose the forest for the trees!
> DONALD BAE

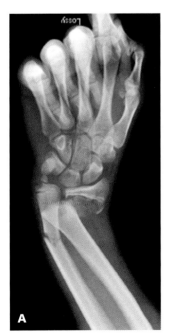 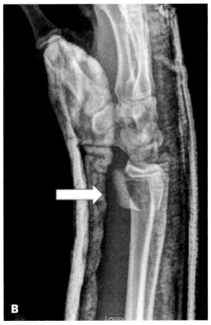 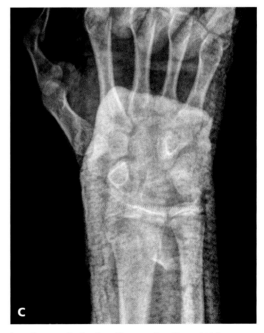

Figure 8-5 This 14-year-old snowboarder was "catching some sweet air" when he stuck the landing and suffered this comminuted distal radius fracture. After reduction, he developed a compartment syndrome with an acute carpal tunnel syndrome as a result of the large volar bone fragment. (Used with the permission of the University of Wisconsin Division of Pediatric Orthopaedics.)

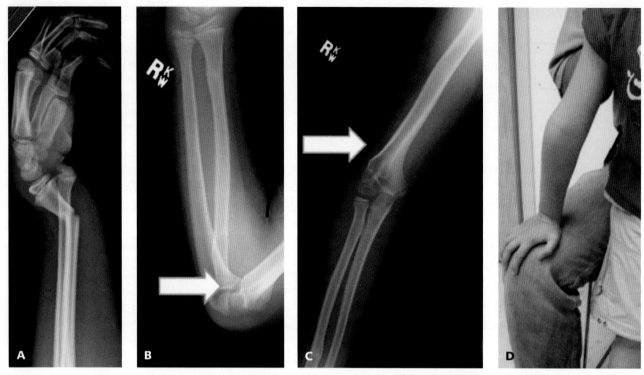

Figure 8-6 An 8-year-old boy fell and fractured his right wrist and underwent closed reduction and long arm casting. The family was pleased his wrist healed well but wondered why his elbow was crooked. In retrospect, he also had a type 2 supracondylar fracture that healed in a varus and extension. The treating team would have stayed out of trouble if they examined the joint above the fracture. (Used with the permission of the University of Wisconsin Division of Pediatric Orthopaedics.)

> **THE GURU SAYS...**
>
> Often one well-placed pin and a cast are sufficient if the reduction is anatomic. You don't always need to put multiple pins across the physis.
>
> DONALD BAE

> **THE GURU SAYS...**
>
> Physeal fractures that cross the resting zone of the physis (Salter-Harris III and IV fractures) are more challenging. These injuries have a higher growth arrest rate (up to 40%!) and require anatomic reduction to restore articular congruity.
>
> DONALD BAE

is used in special circumstances.[2] To stay out of trouble with distal radius pinning, care should be taken to avoid the radial sensory nerve and the extensor tendons. Most agree that smooth K-wires across the physis are not a significant risk for growth arrest.[3]

Up to 30° to 40° of dorsal angulation at the site of a distal radial physeal fracture will remodel satisfactorily in a child with more than 3 years of growth remaining (Fig. 8-8). Of course, this should not be the goal at the first reduction. However, if an 8-year-old returns to your office with 30° of angulation 10 days later, that can be accepted with an excellent result. The risk of growth arrest from a distal radius physeal fracture is considered to be 4%. However, the rate of growth arrest of a distal ulnar physeal fracture is 60%.[4] Stay out of trouble by looking for radiographic growth arrest for a year after any ulnar physeal injury and in any patient whose radial physeal fracture underwent reduction.

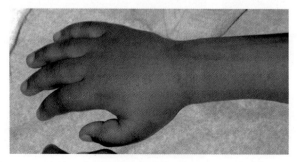

Figure 8-7 This 5-year-old boy had a distal radius fracture, which was splinted in the emergency department 2 days prior to presentation. As often occurs, the Ace wrap rolled up around his wrist, creating a tourniquet effect and leading to dramatic hand swelling. His mother was more concerned about the hand than the wrist fracture. Fortunately, it was only 2 days.

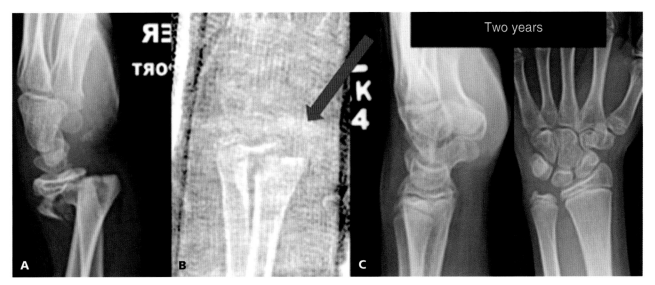

Figure 8-8 This 12-year-old boy had a displaced physeal injury of the wrist that underwent reduction to about 50% trans-lation *(arrow)*. The treating physician knew he could get in trouble if he tried another reduction. After 2 years, the wrist was fully remodeled without signs of arrest. (Used with the permission of the University of Wisconsin Division of Pediatric Orthopedics.)

Metaphyseal Distal Radius and Ulnar Fractures

To stay out of trouble with these fractures, the clinician has to primarily under-stand which fractures have to be reduced and what aspects of displacement need to be reduced. As mentioned, a complete bayonet opposed radius fracture does not have to be reduced as long as angulation is acceptable. Putting a child through the pain and risk of a reduction is not justified to make an X-ray look pretty. Conversely, the adept clinician knows that 15° of dorsal angulation in an 8-year-old will remodel, but it won't in a 14-year-old boy who is skeletally mature and who looks old enough to have a mortgage.

Nondisplaced or minimally displaced distal radial metaphyseal fractures can be treated in many ways with a good result. Some orthopaedists use splints and Ace wraps, some use removal Velcro splints, and many cast: in our experience, the least trouble occurs when a well-padded short arm cast is used.

For completely displaced fractures requiring closed reduction, it is important to understand how the thick pediatric periosteum can hurt you and help you. Distal radius fractures in children have tremendous remodeling potential, and this is due in great part to the biologically active periosteum. Mechanically speak-ing, the intact dorsal periosteum in a volarly angulated fracture can help hold your reduction. However, the periosteum can also hurt your reduction in fractures with bayonet apposition. In this instance, the proximal fragment can buttonhole through the periosteum, making reduction difficult (Fig. 8-9). In bayonet fractures with obliquity, it would be necessary to hyperdistract the fracture to translate the distal fragment volarly; the tough periosteum may make this almost impossible even for the strongest orthopaedic resident. Bayonet apposition in an 8-year-old is fine as long as angulation is minimal.

Once adequate conscious sedation is obtained, the fracture is reduced by re-creation of the deformity, which may lead to fainting by one or both par-ents (usually dad) who should remain seated during the event. To avoid loss of reduction (Fig. 8-10), a well-molded cast with a dorsal mold over the distal

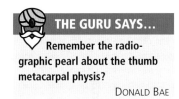

THE GURU SAYS...

Remember the radio-graphic pearl about the thumb metacarpal physis?

DONALD BAE

Dr. Skaggs Adds

One of the few things in pediatric orthopaedics with support from multiple ran-domized prospective trials is the use of a short arm casts for distal third forearm fractures. I find it curious how many doctors still prefer a long arm cast, despite how much more comfortable a short arm cast is for the patient. It might be different, if it were the doctors wearing the casts.[5,6]

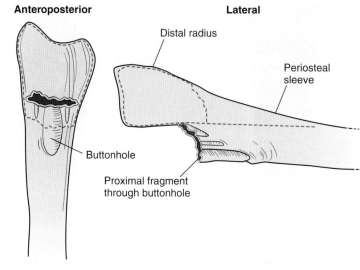

Anteroposterior

Lateral

Distal radius

Periosteal sleeve

Buttonhole

Proximal fragment through buttonhole

Figure 8-9 In bayonet opposed fractures, the proximal fragment can buttonhole through the periosteum and make anatomic reduction impossible. (Adapted with permission from Noonan KJ, Price CT. Forearm and distal radius fractures in children. *J Am Acad Orthop Surg.* 1998;6(3):146-156. Copyright © 1998 by American Academy of Orthopaedic Surgeons.)

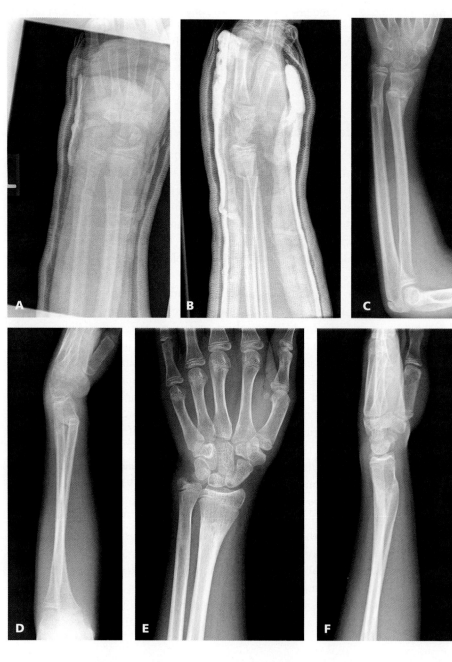

Figure 8-10 This case illustrates the trouble from a bad cast and the need to avoid overtreatment. This 12-year-old boy sustained a high-energy distal radius and ulna fracture. **A, B:** AP and lateral radiographs after reduction. The reduction is satisfactory, but the cast predicts trouble: there is no mold on the distal radius, either dorsally or radially. A prefabricated splint was used, rather than plaster splints. Predictably, he lost reduction. **C, D:** The boy neglected to follow up until 7 weeks after injury, when he presented with an ugly arm and angulation that textbooks say is unacceptable for a 12-year-old. Mom wanted some corrective surgery "as soon as possible." Instead, education was offered. **E, F:** Six months after injury: dramatically better, but not yet good enough. He still lacked about 10° of pronation and supination. Mom no longer wanted surgery; in fact, she probably won't bring him back for further follow-up.

radius. The less experienced resident will often put pressure over the carpus during reduction and casting. To stay out of trouble, the radial styloid should be palpated and this will quickly orient one to the location of the metaphyseal fragment. The cast should be oval so that the anterior-posterior diameter is less than 0.7 of the radioulnar diameter (this has been called the cast index). Extreme pronation and supination should be avoided, as it is thought to increase compartment pressures. A long arm cast is used for completely displaced fractures. A follow-up X-ray is often done about 5 to 7 days after reduction. Isolated distal radius fractures have a propensity to displace dorsally in a cast. The savvy resident knows that in a 4-year-old, this is not a major risk, yet in the mature patient, this may not remodel.

In children younger than 10 years, up to 30° of dorsal angulation or 20° of radial-ward angulation will yield a good result. One way to stay out of trouble with parents is to put a chart up in your office or cast room that shows progressive radiographs of a distal radius fracture remodeling over the course of several months (Fig. 8-11).

This will help to decrease anxiety in parents when the parents see the crooked bone on radiograph. It will also help you avoid the temptation to overtreat these injuries. When a displaced distal radial metaphyseal fracture occurs with a displaced ipsilateral supracondylar fracture, stay out of trouble by pinning both.[7,8] Growth arrest is possible after a metaphyseal fracture of the distal radius, so at least one later follow-up visit may be advisable.[9]

If a patient is going to the operating room because they have an ipsilateral supracondylar humerus fracture, or they have massive swelling and at are risk for compartment syndrome, or the reduction attempt failed, or the patient has had loss of reduction at the first follow-up period or because safe sedation is not possible, or if the helicopter parent demands their child be taken to the operating room, the child should be pinned.

In many cases, the child will return to clinic and there is a loss of reduction, which could be slight or significant, depending on patient maturity and degree of reangulation. These patients can be nicely managed by replacing the likely loose cast with a more intimate fitting fiberglass cast and then having it wedged. Rereduction in the operating room is possible for fractures less than 2 weeks old; attempts at reduction after this time period may be impossible and potentially dangerous (Fig. 8-12).

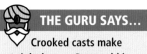

THE GURU SAYS...

Crooked casts make straight bones. Cast mold is critically important!

DONALD BAE

THE GURU SAYS...

Approximately, a third of fractures will displace late in cast. Careful early follow-up is needed, and if deformity recurs beyond what would be anticipated to remodel with growth, the fracture may be rereduced with or without internal fixation to maintain stability.

DONALD BAE

THE GURU SAYS...

Beware the floating elbow! When pinning, my preference is to reduce and pin the radius first, then address the elbow. After the wrist is pinned, you can still manipulate the elbow through the proximal forearm. In addition, once the elbow pins are in, it may not be easy to extend the elbow, making the radius reduction, pinning, and intraoperative imaging more challenging.

DONALD BAE

Injury casted   Early healing   7 months later

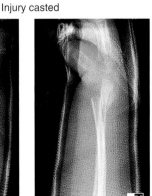
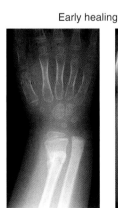
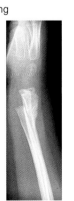
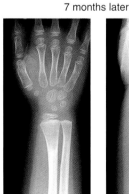
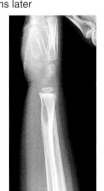

Figure 8-11 Many pediatric orthopaedic practices hang a chart such as this one in their cast room to reassure parents and avoid overtreatment of distal radius fractures. (From Children's Hospital of Philadelphia.)

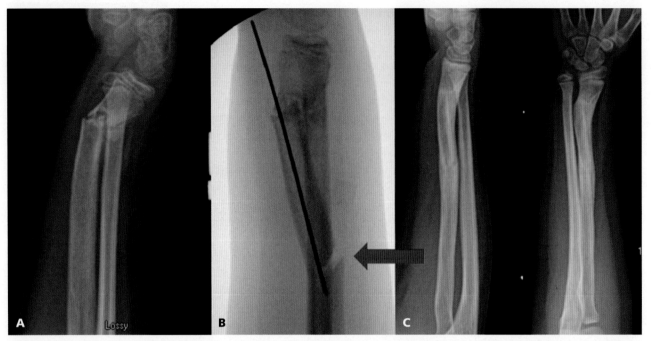

Figure 8-12 A: This 11-year-old girl had a malunited distal radius fracture that the treating surgeon decided to attempt closed osteoclasis at 6 weeks. Unfortunately, the distal radius did not move much but the osteopenic radial shaft did. **B:** To stay out of even more trouble, the treating physician should not have attempted closed osteoclasis after 2 weeks, regardless of the menacing appearance of the mother. **C:** Follow-up X-rays at 5 months from the original fracture show that the distal radius has already begun to straighten out. (Used with the permission of the University of Wisconsin Division of Pediatric Orthopaedics.)

> **THE GURU SAYS...**
>
> Careful inspection of the lateral radiograph will often show that the distal ulnar epiphysis has displaced with the distal radius. This is *not* a Galeazzi fracture, just a displaced distal forearm fracture.
>
> DONALD BAE

Galeazzi Fracture

A Galeazzi fracture is a distal radius fracture with disruption of the triangular fibrocartilage complex (TFCC). These are very rare injuries in children. In children, the TFCC is rarely torn; instead, the distal ulnar physis is fractured and displaced (an equivalent injury). Remember the 60% physeal arrest rate of displaced distal ulnar physeal fractures. Most Galeazzi fractures can be treated with closed reduction and a long arm cast for about 6 weeks, with the forearm in slight supination. Open reduction and pinning are rarely necessary in pediatric Galeazzi fractures except in cases of interposed periosteum or the extensor carpi ulnaris or flexor carpi ulnaris tendon.

FRACTURES OF THE SHAFTS OF THE RADIUS AND ULNA

Despite the fact that 90% of both bone forearm fractures (BBFFs) are treated with casting, they do require more consideration and attention to detail than distal radius and ulna fractures which have greater remodeling potential. **NEWSFLASH! Proximal fractures and fractures in which the radius is broken more proximally than the ulna are inherently more difficult to treat.** When you see this pattern, it's time to get your game face on (Fig. 8-13). In addition, a significant malunion of a forearm diaphyseal fracture will lead to permanent loss of pronation and supination, and sometimes an unsightly curvature or prominence in the forearm. To stay out of trouble, understand that many of these fractures, especially greenstick

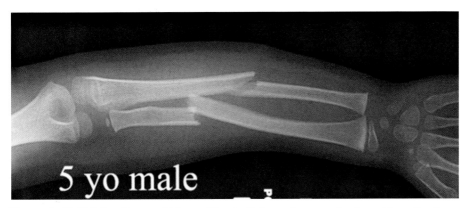

Figure 8-13 This is a 5-year-old boy with a both bone forearm fracture. His radius is broken proximal to his ulna. When faced with this injury, the treating physician should recognize dark clouds on the horizon. (Used with the permission of the University of Wisconsin Division of Pediatric Orthopaedics.)

injuries, are rotational injuries and are reduced with derotation of the forearm in the direction of the apex of the deformity. Apex volar angulation is reduced with rotating the palm volarly (pronation); apex dorsal angulation is reduced with rotating the palm dorsally (supination). The age-old dictum that one needs to complete greenstick fractures during the reduction is just that: old.

Although upper extremity compartment syndrome is rare, the most common cause in children today is a forearm fracture (and no longer supracondylar fractures treated with flexion, which lead to Volkmann ischemic contracture). Don't be fooled by pseudo-Volkmann contracture due to tethering of the flexor digitorum profundus to fractures of the ulna. One report described seven cases, detected 2 days to 16 years after closed reductions of fractures of the shafts of the radius and ulna. The children did not have nerve palsies or undue pain after the reductions. Normal length, excursion, and function of the flexor digitorum profundus were restored by untethering the muscle and its tendons from the ulnar fracture by early manipulation or by late localized myotenolysis. The passive range of motion of all fingers should be routinely checked immediately after closed reductions of fractures of the radius and ulna. If muscle tethering is detected, the fracture is remanipulated to release the muscle. If the muscle is still tethered, then surgical release, through a small incision, is recommended.[10]

Another key source of problems is missing a second subtle injury. The most common and most important oversight is the missed Monteggia fracture, especially in the apparently isolated ulna injury. To stay out of trouble, the orthopaedist should insist on two views of the entire forearm at right angles to one another, as well as dedicated films of the elbow, to be assured that the radiocapitellar relationship is satisfactory (Fig. 8-14). **ORTHOPAEDICS 101: Every joint above and below a long bone injury must be examined and radiographed.**

Most fractures are managed with closed reduction and long arm cast application. The successful clinician will remember that the acceptable limits of reduction for all proximal fractures are less than 10°. Children younger than 9 or 10 years can accept 15° of angulation at the midportion of the forearm, but 10° remains the cutoff for patients older than that. Remember that true angulation is only in one plane even if it is detected on orthogonal X-rays. The true magnitude of angulation is at least as great as the largest measure and can be resolved with the ancient orthopaedist Pythagoras and his theorem.

Rotation is difficult to assess but malrotation of greater than 30° will likely to lead to decreased forearm rotation. One can suspect malrotation when the

THE GURU SAYS...

Remember the rule of thumbs, which will help you remember how to derotate greenstick fractures: Point the thumb toward the apex of fracture angulation during reduction of a rotational greenstick forearm fracture. For example, for apex volar angulation, the thumb points volarly, pronating the forearm!

DONALD BAE

THE GURU SAYS...

Most children feel better, not worse, after forearm fracture reduction. In cases of worsening or escalating pain after forearm fracture reduction, think about compartment syndrome, muscle incarceration, or nerve injury... all of which may require surgical intervention!

DONALD BAE

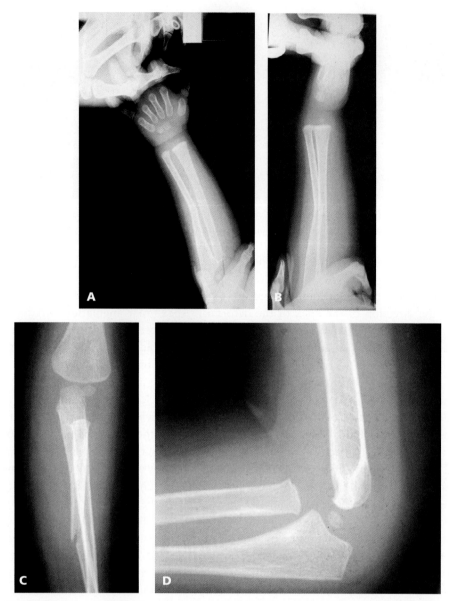

Figure 8-14 A missed Monteggia fracture presented 2 weeks after injury. **A, B:** The radiographic images done at the outside hospital showed only a greenstick fracture of the ulna, as mom's hand covering the elbow and the dislocated radial head. **C, D:** Suspecting a Monteggia fracture, we removed the cast and obtained good elbow images, revealing the dislocated radial head.

proximal and distal diameters of the bone at the fracture site are different. Malrotation can be confirmed if the bicipital tuberosity and the radial styloid are not 180° to each other on an AP forearm radiograph, or if the coronoid process and the ulnar styloid are not 180° opposite to each other on the lateral forearm film.

In all angulated or displaced radius and ulna diaphyseal fractures, manipulative closed reduction under conscious sedation or general anesthesia should be performed. Diaphyseal fractures in children require 6 weeks of immobilization, at a minimum. In older children, 8 weeks may be necessary. Similar to distal radius fractures, BBFF can slowly lose reduction as the swelling decreases in the cast. To stay out of trouble, the patient should be seen at 7 and 14 days for radiographs. Unacceptable progressive alignment can be managed with cast wedging (Fig. 8-15) in the clinic or closed reduction in the OR up to 3 weeks from injury.

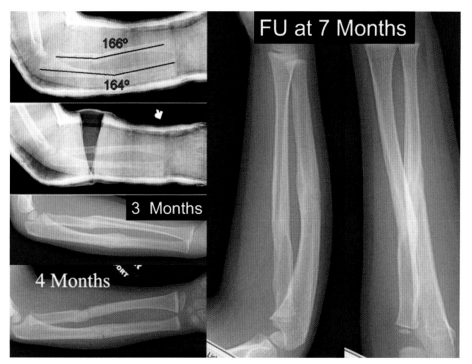

Figure 8-15 Our 5-year-old boy from Figure 8-13 has sagged into unacceptable alignment at 2 weeks. His cast was wedged and excellent alignment was noted at 3 months. Unfortunately, he was not given a protective splint, and he refractured his arm at 4 months. **ORTHOPAEDICS 101: Never give a kid with an even break, an even break.** Recasting led to an acceptable alignment at 7 months. Parents were given a laminated card with the clinic number for future fractures. (Used with the permission of the University of Wisconsin Division of Pediatric Orthopaedics.)

Remember extension casting is an excellent method for those patients that require repeat manipulation in the operating room and is especially effective for very proximal BBFF (Fig. 8-16).

To stay out of even more trouble, warn families that diaphyseal forearm fractures are among the rare fractures in children that are at risk for refracture. Refracture seems to be a risk in proximal fractures, greenstick fractures and in the first 3 months after cast removal. One study of 768 children with displaced forearm fractures requiring reduction found a refracture incidence of 4.9%.[11] The median time to refracture was 8 weeks after discontinuing cast immobilization. The authors found that diaphyseal fractures were eight times more likely to refracture than metaphyseal fractures, and that the risk of refracture was inversely proportional to the duration of cast immobilization. Cast immobilization for a minimum of 6 weeks reduces the risk of refracture by a factor of between four and six. Midshaft forearm fractures are at risk of refracture for 16 weeks from cast removal.

Plastic deformation of the forearm can be a source of trouble. In young children in whom there is no cosmetic deformity with a full range of motion, casting without reduction is acceptable. However, if the arm appears bowed or motion is lost, reduction should be attempted in the operating room. A great amount of force must be applied at a very slow rate over a long period of time to correct plastic deformation.[12] After reduction, a long arm cast is used for 4 to 6 weeks. Again, beware of the plastically deformed ulna that distracts your attention from an associated radial head dislocation.

THE GURU SAYS...

Extension casts like to slide off the arm, so try these two tricks: (1) adding a thumb spica component to the cast and (2) placing a D-ring on the distal forearm with a sling or cuff around the neck.

DONALD BAE

THE GURU SAYS...

Reduction of plastically deformed bones takes great and sustained force! If a reduction is needed, consider doing it in the operating room under general anesthesia. This will also facilitate placement of a well-molded cast.

DONALD BAE

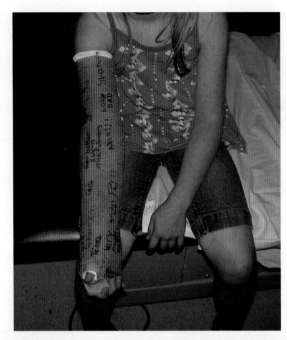

Figure 8-16 Extension cast is a great solution for the proximal both bone forearm fracture (BBFF) that requires rereduction. (Used with the permission of the University of Wisconsin Division of Pediatric Orthopaedics.)

Operative fixation of BBFF is needed in about 10% of cases. Implants can include plates that may require later removal and usually have larger scaring. Intramedullary K-wires or titanium nails are increasingly used to stabilize one or both bones of pediatric diaphyseal forearm fractures. Although the long-term outcome is similar between both implants, most pediatric orthopaedists prefer this method as this is a load-sharing device and the scaring is less extensive. In addition, removal of the implant is much easier. Some have found good success with hybrid fixation (Fig. 8-17). Despite the different options, the best way to stay out of trouble is to use the method that works best in your hands.

The preferred entry site for IM fixation of the ulna is proximal in most cases. For the radius, the best entry site is on the radial side of the radius, with caution to avoid injury to the radial nerve or the thumb extensor tendons. Flexible nailing of the radius is the hardest bone to successfully instrument with this technique.

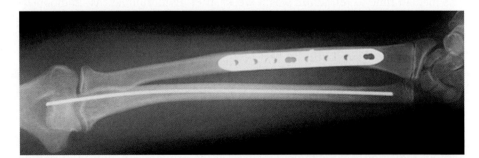

Figure 8-17 This 14-year-old football player underwent hybrid fixation for a both bone forearm fracture (BBFF). The treating physician preferred an ulnar rod that would not irritate the skin as a plate would, and it may provide some protection against fracture around the plate with future athletic adventures. (Used with the permission of the University of Wisconsin Division of Pediatric Orthopaedics.)

Staying Out of Trouble With IM Fixation of the Ulna

✳ Instrument the radius before the ulna, because it can be impossible to translate a broken radius after the ulna is stabilized.

✳ Distal radius fractures that are rodded through the radial styloid can radially deviate when the rod is not contoured at this location (Fig. 8-18). **ORTHOPAEDICS 101: No matter which bone needs rodding (femur, tibia, radius etc), IM fixation at these locations can lead to malalignment if the rod is not contoured at the entry site of a proximal fragment or if it is not centered in the metaphysis of the distal fragment.**

✳ Single bone fixation, usually with an ulnar intramedullary K-wire, is often a simple solution, especially for fractures in the 8- to 12-year-old age range. As children approach maturity, adult style plating allowing rapid mobilization is usually the best way to stay out of trouble.

✳ Use a small diameter nail (1.5-2.0 mm) in the radius. Prebending the radial nail prior to insertion can help restore radial bow and facilitate nail passage. The tip of the nail may need to be cut off as the offset will make the functional diameter of the nail greater than the actual diameter.

✳ Don't make multiple passes in an attempt to get the intramedullary wire across the fracture site. If you don't get the wire across in three attempts, it is safer to open the fracture.[13] Multiple missed passes in a swollen forearm increase the risk for compartment syndrome.

✳ In cases of delayed rodding (greater than 10 days) the immature callus can make it impossible to reduce the fracture for IM fixation. Have a low threshold for opening the fracture site.

✳ Refractures may be best managed by IM fixation; despite saying this, the successful surgeon will recognize that the medullary canal is usually filled with old bone and thus open nailing with drilling of the canal prior to nail placement will significantly decrease the rate of intraoperative profanity.

THE GURU SAYS...

Converting to open reduction via a small incision during IM fixation is a sign of experience, not failure!

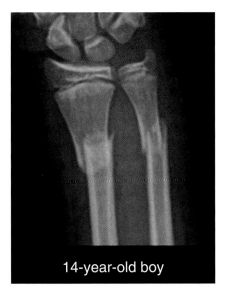
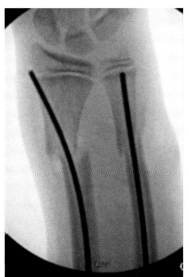
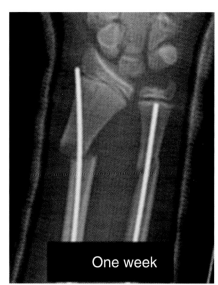

14-year-old boy

One week

Figure 8-18 A 14-year-old boy with a distal both bone forearm fracture (BBFF) was treated with flexible nailing, and he developed radial deviation. To stay out of trouble, the treating surgeon should have deformed the distal rod to accommodate the oblique entry into the distal radius. (Used with the permission of the University of Wisconsin Division of Pediatric Orthopaedics.)

MONTEGGIA FRACTURES

Although Monteggia fractures (Fig. 8-19) represent less than 1% of all pediatric forearm fractures, they receive great attention because they create so much trouble. Most of these injuries occur in children younger than 10 years. Many "isolated radial head dislocations" that walk into your office as routine visits were probably missed traumatic lesions rather than congenital dislocations.[14] To stay out of trouble, high-quality radiographs are mandatory to manage Monteggia fractures successfully. The views should include the whole forearm, as well as isolated elbow radiographs. The ulna should be "ruler straight"[15] (Fig. 8-20). A line drawn down the shaft of the radius should point to the center of the capitellum. Be sure to assess this after initial reduction and at each follow-up, as late dislocation of the radial head has been reported.[16] Remember, there is normal angulation of the proximal ulna in children, and the proximal radial neck can angulate up to about 12° of valgus. Also, a careful neurologic examination is essential, as up to 20% of Monteggia fractures present with nerve palsy. The most common scenario is a posterior interosseous nerve palsy associated with a Bado type III lesion.

If the diaphyseal fracture is either plastic deformation or an incomplete fracture, closed reduction is possible with an initial attempt at closed reduction with conscious sedation or general anesthesia. If the injury is acute, a very satisfying reduction radial reduction "clunk" is usually felt as the orthopaedist realigns the ulna shaft. Type I fractures are reduced with forearm supination and complete elbow flexion, but they should not be casted in hyperflexion. A well-molded long-arm cast at 90° for about 4 to 6 weeks is satisfactory. For type II fractures are rare in children, the fractures are reduced with elbow extension. This can be

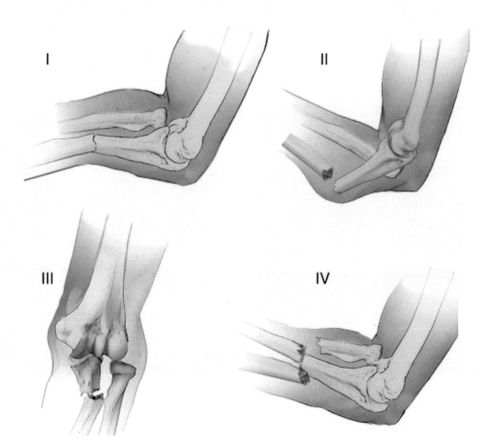

Figure 8-19 Four types of Monteggia fractures, as described by Bado. (Reprinted with permission from Shah AS, Waters PM. Reconstruction for missed Monteggia lesion. In: Flynn JM, Sankar WN, eds. *Operative Techniques in Pediatric Orthopaedic Surgery*. 2nd ed. Philadelphia, PA: Wolters Kluwer; 2016:69-80. Figure 9-6.)

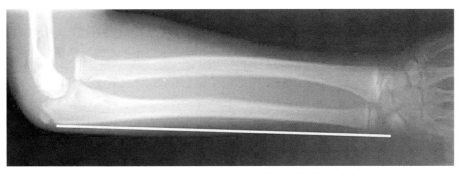

Figure 8-20 The ulna should be "ruler straight." This radial head dislocation is associated with plastic deformation of the ulna (anterior bowing). Many of the children who present with "isolated" or "congenital" radial head dislocations actually had a Monteggia fracture of equivalent. (Reprinted with permission from Price CT, Flynn JF. Management of fractures. In: Morrissy RT, Weinstein SL, eds. *Lovell and Winter's Pediatric Orthopaedics*. 6th ed. Philadelphia, PA: Lippincott Williams & Wilkins; 2006.)

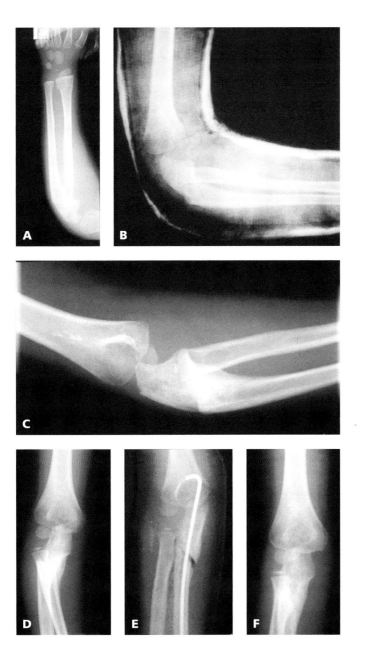

Figure 8-21 Getting out of trouble: an ulnar osteotomy to salvage a missed Monteggia fracture. **A:** Trouble: the focus was on the distal radius, so the radial head dislocation was missed. **B:** More trouble: they thought to get an elbow radiograph, but the cast obscured the radial head dislocation, so it was missed. The family presents for a second opinion a few weeks after injury. **C, D:** The ulna is healed, and the radial head is out. After an ulnar osteotomy and intramedullary fixation with a Steinmann pin, the radial head was reduced and stable. **E:** The radiocapitellar joint was not opened. **F:** Six months later, all better.

a difficult position to maintain in a long arm cast. Often fixation of the ulna is necessary for stability. Type III fractures are the second most common pattern in children require a correction of the varus angulation in order to reduce the radial head. Type IV fractures are very difficult to treat with a simple closed reduction. Often, the radial shaft fracture must be internally fixed with either a plate or a wire in order to successfully reduce the radial head (Fig. 8-21). For complete fractures, the problem is instability in the cast. As such, intramedullary ulna fixation for short oblique or transverse fractures is preferred, open reduction and internal fixation with screws and/or plates is chosen for long oblique fractures of the ulna.

Very close postinjury and postsurgical follow-up is mandatory in Monteggia fractures. To stay out of trouble during the follow-up period, immobilize the Monteggia fracture in a cast with only thin fiberglass at the elbow. In this way, you will be able to visualize the elbow joint clearly without obscuring plaster. If there is any question about the relationship of the radius and capitellum during the postoperative period one could consider a CT scan (more radiation) or an MRI (more expensive). Alternatively, it may be better to take the cast off and get good X-rays and risk loss of reduction, than to continue to cast a malaligned radiocapitellar joint obscured by cast material.

Complications with Monteggia fractures include compartment syndrome, failure of recognition, failure of initial reduction, loss of reduction, nerve injury, late stiffness, radial head avascular necrosis, and radial ulnar synostosis. If a Monteggia fracture is missed, late reconstruction involves restoring ulnar length and alignment and an open reduction of the radial head, often with angular ligament reconstruction.[17] Even in the best of hands, results of late reconstruction are often disappointing if more than 6 to 12 months has elapsed since the injury.[18]

FRACTURES OF THE PROXIMAL RADIUS

In children, intra-articular radial head fractures are unusual, but metaphyseal proximal radial neck fractures are not. The savvy resident who never gets in trouble with these injuries knows that most of these injuries result from a valgus injury to the elbow and this mechanism can also break the proximal ulna or pull off the medial epicondyle. **ORTHOPAEDICS 101: Avoid the hubristic phenomenon known as "satisfaction of search"—the tendency to stop looking for other fractures once you find one.**

As the radial head's relationship with the capitellum is critical in maintaining forearm rotation, optimal reduction of angulation—and more important, translation—offers the best chance of a good functional result. Proximal radius fractures cause a remarkable amount of trouble, especially persistent loss of motion after injury. Even compartment syndrome has been reported after these troublesome injuries.[19] Pay careful attention to the radial nerve on the initial neurovascular examination. An attempt should be made to reduce displaced proximal radius fractures under conscious sedation or general anesthesia. This can be aided by injecting a local anesthetic into the radiocapitellar joint and evacuating the hematoma prior to reduction. After an attempt at closed reduction, up to 30° of angulation and 3 mm of translation can be accepted. If reduction under conscious sedation fails, additional attempts should be made with fluoroscopic guidance in the operating room.

To stay out of trouble, attempt a variety of different maneuvers to reduce a proximal radius fracture before resorting to open reduction. Many of the complications described in the literature for radial head and neck fractures are the result of open reduction. Of course, these are probably the worst proximal radius fractures, but it is clear that once you open these injuries you are inviting a lot of trouble. A recent prospective multicenter study concluded that the restricted use of open interventions may be the key to improving results.[20] Before opening a radial head or neck fracture, attempt reduction with the elbow extended in a valgus force, attempt closed reduction with the Israeli technique (flexion and pronation), and attempt a reduction aided by percutaneous manipulation using a small K-wire or an awl.

To stay out of trouble with the percutaneous manipulation maneuver, be certain you understand where the posterior interosseous nerve is. There are reports of radial nerve injury using this technique (Fig. 8-22). If you open a proximal radius fracture, it is wise to stabilize the fracture after reduction with an intramedullary rod passed retrograde from the radial styloid into the radial head. To support this concept, one study reviewed nine cases of radial neck nonunion.[21] The authors concluded that the severity of initial fracture displacement and inadequate fixation technique contributed to radial neck nonunion. Healing of the nonunion did not necessarily lead to improvement of clinical symptoms.

To stay out of trouble with radial head and neck fractures, be sure to warn families at the time of injury that loss of motion is common, regardless of treatment. These fractures should not be immobilized for more than about 3 to 4 weeks.

FRACTURES OF THE PROXIMAL ULNA

Olecranon fractures are relatively uncommon in children. Most are minimally displaced and involve the metaphysis without significant articular disruption. Be alert that an olecranon sleeve fracture may be the first presentation of mild osteogenesis imperfecta[22] (Fig. 8-23). Also be aware that the fracture may have had a much more disruptive effect on the articular surface than is seen on plain radiographs.[23,24] Displaced intra-articular olecranon fractures are managed with open reduction and internal fixation, using either a tension band technique or compression fixation with an interfragmentary screw. In children, the tension band can be a strong permanent suture rather than a wire. The K-wires can be placed percutaneously. This technique can allow you to remove the K-wires in the clinic and leave the suture, saving the child a hardware removal in the late postoperative period. To stay out of trouble, use a large nonabsorbable suture.

> **THE GURU SAYS...**
> Think of the treatment of radial neck fractures like a ladder: move on to more invasive techniques only if simpler, less invasive maneuvers fail. The steps of the ladder include closed reduction, percutaneous pin–assisted reduction, Metaizeau technique, and finally open reduction.
> DONALD BAE

> **THE GURU SAYS...**
> Another option is to use oblique K-wires passed from the rim of the radial head distally and obliquely across the fracture to stabilize these injuries.
> DONALD BAE

> **THE GURU SAYS...**
> Consider immobilizing nondisplaced olecranon fractures in less than 90° flexion. Excessive flexion causes traction on the proximal apophysis, which may lead to displacement!
> DONALD BAE

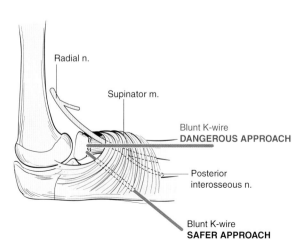

Figure 8-22 The position of the radial nerve is adjacent to a joystick pin or awl.

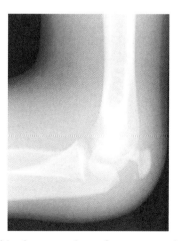

Figure 8-23 This olecranon sleeve fracture was the first presentation of mild osteogenesis imperfecta in this child. (Reprinted with permission from Price CT, Flynn JF. Management of fractures. In: Morrissy RT, Weinstein SL, eds. *Lovell and Winter's Pediatric Orthopaedics*. 6th ed. Philadelphia: Lippincott Williams & Wilkins; 2006.)

Staying Out of Trouble with Hand, Wrist, and Forearm Injuries

Hand Injuries

* 75% of finger fractures create no problems, but 25% need prompt treatment.
* A "tendon disruption" may instead be a physeal fracture in a young child.
* In assessing a nerve, the "wrinkle test" is helpful in young children.
* Check the digital cascade at rest and with tenodesis wrist motion.
* Get a true lateral of the injured digit.
* Beware of germinal matrix entrapped in the distal phalanx physis.
* Be aware that a jersey finger can be dismissed as a jammed finger.
* MRI is the best test to find an occult scaphoid fracture.
* After an injury to the volar plate, move the joint early. Do not do extension block splinting because you risk contracture of the child's PIP joint.

Fractures of the Distal Radius and Ulna

* Understand remodeling to avoid overtreatment.
* Be alert that high-energy distal radial physeal fractures can lead to acute carpal tunnel syndrome.
* Look for a "second injury" elsewhere in the injured upper extremity.
* With distal radius pinning, care should be taken to avoid the radial sensory nerve and the extensor tendons.
* To avoid a loss of reduction, a well made cast (oval, three-point mold) is essential to maintaining reduction. Bad casts are a big source of trouble in these fractures.
* Put up a remodeling fracture poster in your cast room to calm anxious parents and save them second-opinion trips.
* Growth arrest is 60% for the distal ulna: counsel families as to that fact.

Radius and Ulnar Shaft and Monteggia Fractures

* A significant malunion of a forearm diaphyseal fracture will lead to permanent loss of pronation and supination.
* The most common cause of upper extremity compartment syndrome today is forearm fractures.
* Watch out for the occult Monteggia fracture.
* Insist on two views of the entire forearm at right angles to one another, as well as dedicated films of the elbow to be assured that the radiocapitellar relationship is satisfactory.
* Don't make multiple passes in an attempt to get the intramedullary wire across the fracture site. If you don't get the wire across in three attempts, it is safer to open the fracture.
* To manage Monteggia fractures successfully, radiograph views should include the whole forearm, as well as isolated elbow radiographs. The ulna should be "ruler straight."
* If there is any question about the relationship of the radius and capitellum during the postoperative period, it is better to take the cast off to get good radiographs and risk loss of reduction rather than to continue to cast a malaligned radiocapitellar joint obscured by plaster.
* The key to managing Monteggia fractures lies in ulnar stability.

Staying Out of Trouble with Hand, Wrist, and Forearm Injuries (continued)

Fractures of the Proximal Radius and Ulna

✴ Pay careful attention to the radial nerve on the initial neurovascular examination.

✴ Attempt a variety of different maneuvers to reduce a proximal radius fracture before resorting to open reduction.

✴ With the percutaneous manipulation maneuver for radial head fractures, be certain to avoid the posterior interosseous nerve.

✴ With radial head and neck fractures, be sure to warn families at the time of injury that loss of motion is a problem. These fractures should not be immobilized for more than about 3 to 4 weeks.

✴ An olecranon sleeve fracture may be the first presentation of mild osteogenesis imperfecta.

✴ In children, the tension band can be a strong permanent suture rather than a wire (and don't use absorbable suture).

SOURCES OF WISDOM

1. Santoro V, Mara J. Compartmental syndrome complicating Salter-Harris type II distal radius fracture. *Clin Orthop Relat Res*. 1988;(233):226-229.
2. Kadiyala RK, Waters PM. Upper extremity pediatric compartment syndromes. *Hand Clin*. 1998;14(3):467-475.
3. Choi KY, Chan WS, Lam TP, et al. Percutaneous Kirschner-wire pinning for severely displaced distal radial fractures in children: a report of 157 cases. *J Bone Joint Surg Br*. 1995;77(5):797-801.
4. Ray TD, Tessler RH, Dell PC. Traumatic ulnar physeal arrest after distal forearm fractures in children. *J Pediatr Orthop*. 1996;16(2):195-200.
5. Bohm ER, Bubbar V, Yong Hing K, Dzus A. Above and below-the-elbow plaster casts for distal forearm fractures in children: a randomized controlled trial. *J Bone Joint Surg Am*. 2006;88(1):1-8.
6. Webb GR, Galpin RD, Armstrong DG. Comparison of short and long arm plaster casts for displaced fractures in the distal third of the forearm in children. *J Bone Joint Surg Am*. 2006;88(1):9-17.
7. Ring D, Waters PM, Hotchkiss RN, et al. Pediatric floating elbow. *J Pediatr Orthop*. 2001;21(4):456-459.
8. Roposch A, Reis M, Molina M, et al. Supracondylar fractures of the humerus associated with ipsilateral forearm fractures in children: a report of forty-seven cases. *J Pediatr Orthop*. 2001;21(3):307-312.
9. Tang CW, Kay RM, Skaggs DL. Growth arrest of the distal radius following a metaphyseal fracture: case report and review of the literature. *J Pediatr Orthop B*. 2002;11(1):89-92.
10. Deeney VF, Kaye JJ, Geary SP, et al. Pseudo-Volkmann's contracture due to tethering of flexor digitorum profundus to fractures of the ulna in children. *J Pediatr Orthop*. 1998;18(4):437-440.
11. Bould M, Bannister GC. Refractures of the radius and ulna in children. *Injury*. 1999;30(9):583-586.
12. Sanders WE, Heckman JD. Traumatic plastic deformation of the radius and ulna: a closed method of correction of deformity. *Clin Orthop Relat Res*. 1984;(188):58-67.
13. Yuan PS, Pring ME, Gaynor TP, et al. Compartment syndrome following intramedullary fixation of pediatric forearm fractures. *J Pediatr Orthop*. 2004;24(4):370-375.
14. Kemnitz S, De Schrijver F, De Smet L. Radial head dislocation with plastic deformation of the ulna in children: a rare and frequently missed condition. *Acta Orthop Belg*. 2000;66(4):359-362.
15. Lincoln TL, Mubarak SJ. "Isolated" traumatic radial-head dislocation. *J Pediatr Orthop*. 1994;14(4):454-457.
16. Weisman DS, Rang M, Cole WG. Tardy displacement of traumatic radial head dislocation in childhood. *J Pediatr Orthop*. 1999;19(4):523-526.
17. Ring D, Waters PM. Operative fixation of Monteggia fractures in children. *J Bone Joint Surg Br*. 1996;78(5):734-739.
18. Rodgers WB, Waters PM, Hall JE. Chronic Monteggia lesions in children: complications and results of reconstruction. *J Bone Joint Surg Am*. 1996;78(9):1322-1329.
19. Peters CL, Scott SM. Compartment syndrome in the forearm following fractures of the radial head or neck in children. *J Bone Joint Surg Am*. 1995;77(7):1070-1074.
20. Schmittenbecher PP, Haevernick B, Herold A, et al. Treatment decision, method of osteosynthesis, and outcome in radial neck fractures in children: a multicenter study. *J Pediatr Orthop*. 2005;25(1):45-50.

21. Waters PM, Stewart SL. Radial neck fracture nonunion in children. *J Pediatr Orthop.* 2001;21(5):570-576.

22. Zionts LE, Moon CN. Olecranon apophysis fractures in children with osteogenesis imperfecta revisited. *J Pediatr Orthop.* 2002;22(6):745-750.

23. Gaddy BC, Strecker WB, Schoenecker PL. Surgical treatment of displaced olecranon fractures in children. *J Pediatr Orthop.* 1997;17(3):321-324.

24. Song KS, Jeon SH. Osteochondral flap fracture of the olecranon with dislocation of the elbow in a child: a case report. *J Orthop Trauma.* 2003;17(3):229-231.

FOR FURTHER ENLIGHTENMENT

Dicke TE, Nunley JA. Distal forearm fractures in children: complications and surgical indications. *Orthop Clin North Am.* 1993;24(2):333-440.

Graves SC, Canale ST. Fractures of the olecranon in children: long-term follow-up. *J Pediatr Orthop.* 1993;13(2):239-241.

Kay S, Smith C, Oppenheim WL. Both-bone midshaft forearm fractures in children. *J Pediatr Orthop.* 1986;6(3):306-310.

Nelson OA, Buchanan JR, Harrison CS. Distal ulnar growth arrest. *J Hand Surg Am.* 1984;9(2):164-170.

Noonan KJ, Price CT. Forearm and distal radius fractures in children. *J Am Acad Orthop Surg.* 1998;6(3):146-156.

Ring D, Jupiter JB, Waters PM. Monteggia fractures in children and adults. *J Am Acad Orthop Surg.* 1998;6(4):215-224.

Wilkins KE. Changes in the management of Monteggia fractures. *J Pediatr Orthop.* 2002;22(4):548-554.

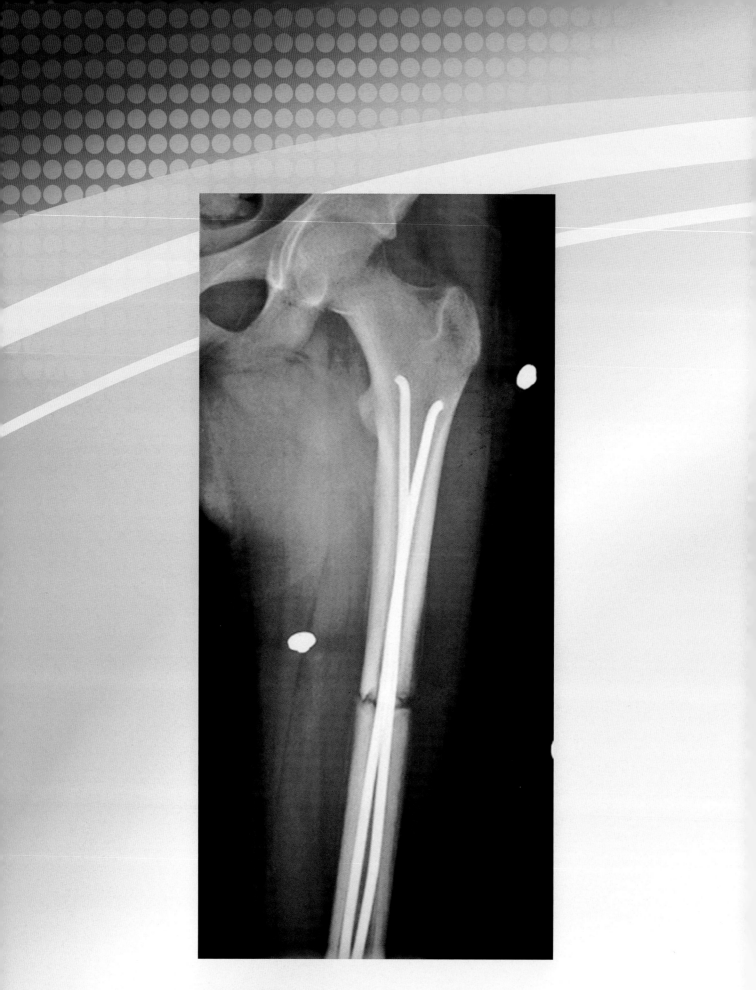

Chapter 9

Trauma About the Pelvis, Hip, and Femur

JOHN M. (JACK) FLYNN, MD

Guru: Martin J. Herman, MD

Fractures to the pelvis, hip, and femur in children usually result from significant trauma. Although low-energy hip and femur fractures are seen, as the treating surgeon you are usually assuming care of a child whose body has been subjected to significant force. Perhaps the most important guideline for staying out of trouble with these fractures is to look for injuries to other organ systems. In many cases, help from a traumatologist will best serve you and the child. Although we have grouped pelvis, hip, and femur fractures together anatomically, the management philosophy of these injuries is quite different: the vast majority of pediatric pelvic fractures are treated without surgical intervention, while most pediatric hip and femur fractures are optimally managed with surgery.

Pelvic Fractures

If the triradiate cartilage is open in your trauma patient, you are dealing with a pediatric pelvis. Compared to adults, the pediatric pelvic fracture patterns are different; internal fixation is rarely necessary, but the associated injuries are the major cause of morbidity and mortality. In the adult literature, the pelvis is often compared to the ring of a pretzel. A break in the ring in one location generally indicates a break in a second location (either through the ligaments, or through another part of the bony ring). In children, think of the pelvis as a soft Philadelphia-style pretzel. The ring can indent, or it can break in one place or in two or more places. The abdominal and pelvic contents are not as well protected in kids as in adults. The ligaments tend to be stronger than bone, so CT scans (to define ligamentous disruption) play a smaller role than in adults. Look for iliac wing fractures rather than sacroiliac joint disruption, and pubic rami fractures rather than pubic symphysis disruption. Most importantly, work with your trauma surgeon to rule out abdominal, urologic, chest, and head injuries (Fig. 9-1). For this reason, almost all children with a pelvic fracture are evaluated with an MRI.

Although most children with a pelvic fracture do well, leg length discrepancy, nerve palsies, heterotopic ossification, and triradiate cartilage growth arrests have been the most frequently reported problems. Sacral nerve root injuries have been reported after pediatric sacral fractures. There are also isolated reports of common sciatic nerve injury after pediatric pelvic fractures. A careful neurologic examination at presentation is essential. Heterotopic ossification occurs occasionally, but is rarely disabling. Therefore, counsel parents about the risk of persistent hip stiffness after a severe hip or pelvic fracture. Displaced acetabular fractures through the triradiate cartilage are rare injuries. Like any growth plate fracture, early anatomic alignment is recommended. Families should be counseled at the time of injury about triradiate cartilage growth arrest and the possibility of later acetabular dysplasia.

In summary, most children with a pelvic fracture recover well from their bone injuries. Their hospital course and rehabilitation is often dominated by associated injuries. On occasion, a child may have an adult-type injury or may present with hemodynamic instability. In these rare cases, adult principles of external fixation, possibly augmented by internal fixation, should be utilized to close and stabilize the pelvic ring.

Follow pelvic fractures for a year after injury to ensure there is no triradiate cartilage growth arrest, leg length inequality, heterotopic ossification, or other potential long-term problem.

THE GURU SAYS...

In my mind, these are the two most important keys to successful management of displaced pelvic ring and acetabular fractures in children and adolescents:

- Manage these injuries identically to equivalent injuries in adults. Remodeling will occur to some degree but cannot guarantee great results in all cases.
- Check your ego at the scrub sink. Enlist an adult trauma colleague to help with operative management of these injuries, regardless of the child's age and size. Together you can restore the anatomy and achieve stable fixation while also taking into consideration prevention of growth disturbance of the pelvis and acetabulum.

MARTIN J. HERMAN

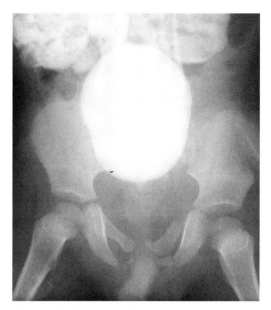

Figure 9-1 Like a soft pretzel, the pelvis of a young child can absorb considerable force, bending, or breaking in just one place. In this child, who was run over by a car, the apparently minor bony injury belies the tremendous force that impacted the pelvis—and more important—its visceral contents. This child didn't need plates and screws; he needed a trauma surgeon and a urologist.

Hip Fractures

Pediatric femoral neck fractures cause a lot of trouble. On your first encounter with the parents, you should counsel extensively about the long list of risks that have been so well described. These injuries often occur in children who fall from heights or are struck by vehicles. Search for other injuries before focusing on the femoral neck. Results reported since the advent of intraoperative fluoroscopic imaging and stable internal fixation are far superior to the old, classic series of reports of pinning (good for elbows, not for hips). Early anatomic reduction, stable internal fixation with screws, and 4 to 6 weeks in a spica cast (for the young child where the physis is not crossed by the screws) is the best way to stay out of trouble. Early capsular decompression may reduce the risk of femoral head necrosis, and there is little morbidity from adding this to the treatment plan. In teenagers, you can use the same principles as in adults and cross the growth plate with stable fixation (just as you would fix a slipped capital femoral epiphysis [SCFE]). This allows them to be partial weight bearing without cast immobilization.

Avascular necrosis (AVN) is the primary cause of poor results after a pediatric femoral neck fracture (Fig. 9-2). The risk of AVN is related to fracture type: the closer the fracture to the proximal femoral epiphysis, the more likely it will result in AVN. There is not yet convincing evidence to support the notion that AVN can be consistently prevented after a pediatric femoral neck fracture. However, prompt anatomic reduction and internal fixation, perhaps with capsulotomy or aspiration of the fracture hematoma, is the best the orthopaedic surgeon can offer the child with a femoral neck fracture. AVN may take 12 months or more to manifest itself. Good quality AP and frog-lateral radiographs up to 2 years after injury are recommended. An MRI may also delineate the AVN, although artifact from the screws can make its interpretation difficult as well.

THE GURU SAYS...

While proximal femoral growth is important, stable fixation of pediatric hip fractures trumps physeal growth every time. Cross the physis with screws or wires if it is needed to guarantee that your anatomic reduction holds and reliable healing occurs.

MARTIN J. HERMAN

THE GURU SAYS...

Use of a one-legged spica cast to supplement fixation is not a sign of failure. The smart surgeon will protect less-stable constructs with a spica cast, especially in younger children and unreliable patients such as those with special needs regardless of age.

MARTIN J. HERMAN

THE GURU SAYS...

Avascular necrosis occurs after *all* types of pediatric hip fractures. Make families aware of the potential seriousness of this complication during the preoperative discussion.

MARTIN J. HERMAN

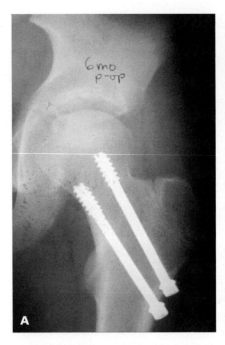
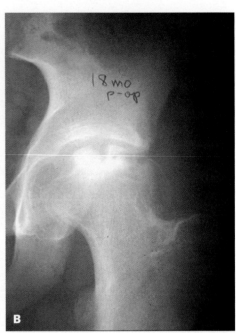

Figure 9-2 A: Plain radiograph taken 6 months after screw implantation. **B:** Plain radiographs taken after screw removal at 18 months shows avascular necrosis of the femoral head.

Coxa vara has been reported in up to 30% of pediatric femoral neck series published over the last century (Fig. 9-3). Many believe that modern imaging and fixation have markedly reduced this complication. Probably the most important cause of coxa vara is malunion. AVN or damage to the physis in the proximal femur can also cause coxa vara. Many children will tolerate a neck shaft angle down to 120° and still function at a very high level. Especially in younger children, some improvement of the neck shaft angle over time may be noted. If an older child (>8 years old) has a persistent abductor lurch more than 2 years after injury and a neck shaft angle less than 110°, a valgus osteotomy may be helpful.

Premature physeal closure has been reported in up to 28% of pediatric femoral neck fractures (Fig. 9-4). In most cases, AVN is the culprit. Although an

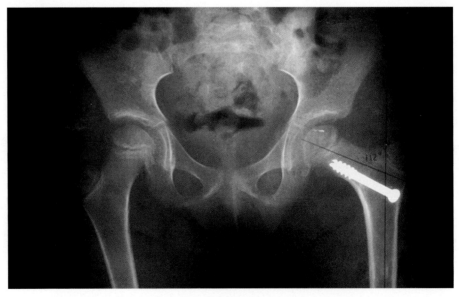

Figure 9-3 Plain radiograph showing coxa vara 2 years after surgery.

abductor lurch and altered hip mechanics are common, functionally important leg length inequality is rarely seen, except when there is physeal arrest in very young children. In cases of leg length inequality, a contralateral epiphysiodesis can be performed.

The incidence of nonunion in pediatric femoral neck fractures is about 5% to 10% (Fig. 9-5). If there is persistent pain and no evidence of healing by 3 months after injury, a nonunion should be suspected. Operative treatment is recommended, with removal of initial internal fixation, repeat internal fixation and possibly a subtrochanteric valgus osteotomy.

Traumatic Hip Dislocation

Pediatric traumatic hip dislocations come in two varieties: toddlers/young children who have dislocation with trivial trauma; and older children/teens with hip dislocation, often with significant trauma. In younger children, closed reduction is generally easy, associated injuries are unusual, and AVN is rare. Traumatic hip dislocation in older children presents much more trouble (Fig. 9-6).

In older children, hip dislocations are usually seen in athletic injuries, or in pedestrian or motor vehicle accidents. Staying out of trouble requires recognizing that the injury has occurred (sometimes spontaneous reduction may be unrecognized), being sure the reduction is done early and produces an anatomic reconstitution of the joint, and using an MRI or CT scan, if necessary, to assure that there is no interposed tissue after reduction (Figs. 9-7 and 9-8).

Hip dislocation with spontaneous reduction is seen in football, soccer (Fig. 9-9), track, or any other running and jumping sport. Consider this possibility when presented with a teenage athlete who experienced sudden hip pain during sports and has persistent groin pain or other associated symptoms a few days later. Use a careful physical examination and good quality radiographs to be

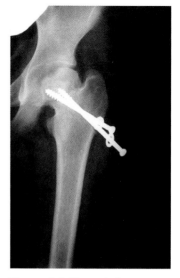

Figure 9-4 Physeal closure after type II femoral neck fracture.

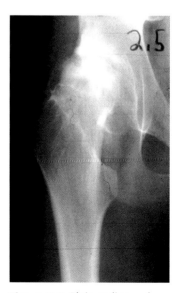

Figure 9-6 Plain radiograph showing patient 2.5 years after hip dislocation.

THE GURU SAYS...

Postreduction imaging with a CT alone may miss osteochondral injuries of the head and acetabulum. Consider MRI after reduction, especially for younger children.

MARTIN J. HERMAN

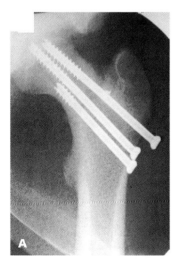
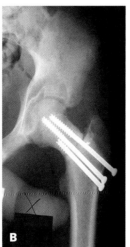
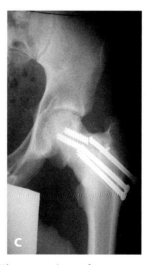

Figure 9-5 **A:** Plain radiographs taken after screw fixation. There are signs of a struggle: note the small metal fragment adjacent to the most superior screw, indicating that a prior attempt with a screw here was hampered by unraveling of the thread on the dense bone. The screws are not parallel, probably holding the fracture in some distraction. **B:** Plain radiograph 3 months later shows early nonunion. The boy was lost to follow-up for 2 years. **C:** When he returned, he was healed because the screws broke. He had coxa vara with a limp and a small leg length inequality.

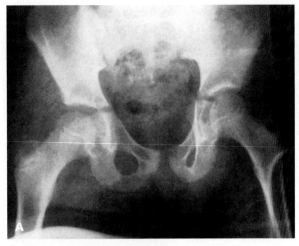
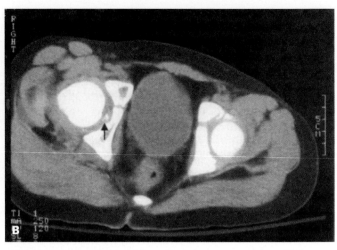

Figure 9-7 A: Plain radiograph of a 12-year-old boy who sustained a traumatic hip dislocation. **B:** CT scans showed labrum, capsule, and cartilage (*arrow*) from posterior wall interposed. (Reprinted with permission from Price CT, Pyevich MT, Knapp DR, et al. Traumatic hip dislocation with spontaneous incomplete reduction: a diagnostic trap. *J Orthop Trauma.* 2002;16(10):730-735.)

THE GURU SAYS...

Prior to attempting a closed reduction, carefully search for evidence of an occult fracture in the proximal femur. Scrutinize the injury radiographs and CT for signs of a physeal or femoral neck fracture, and consider gently moving the proximal femur under live fluoroscopy before force is applied. Abandon attempts at closed reduction if one is suspected.

MARTIN J. HERMAN

certain that the hip is reduced, stable, and not affected by tissue interposed in the joint. If there is persistent pain or any sign of joint space widening, or possible fragments seen on the X-ray in the vicinity of the femoral epiphysis, an MRI is recommended. Sometimes a widened joint space without radiographic density is the only sign of an interposed capsule or labrum.

In the adolescent with a dislocated hip, the femoral epiphysis can be unstable. Before going to the operating room to reduce a dislocated hip in a teenage patient with an open proximal physis, warn the parents that there may be an unrecognized fracture at the proximal femoral physis. Displacement may occur through the physis, giving the appearance of an acute SCFE, at the time of attempted closed reduction. It may be best to perform the reduction in the operating room with maximum relaxation and pain control. AVN after traumatic hip dislocations

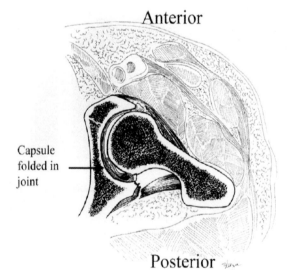

Figure 9-8 Be suspicious of potential hip dislocation with spontaneous reduction; there may be tissue in the joint, as seen on this artist's rendering. Check CT or MRI. (Reprinted with permission from Price CT, Pyevich MT, Knapp DR, et al. Traumatic hip dislocation with spontaneous incomplete reduction: a diagnostic trap. *J Orthop Trauma.* 2002;16(10):730-735.)

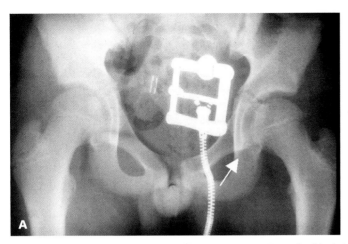
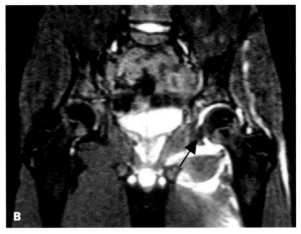

Figure 9-9 A: Plain radiograph taken at presentation of a hip injury (*arrow*) acquired while playing soccer. **B:** MRI scans showed the presence of interposed tissue (*arrow*). (Reprinted with permission from Price CT, Pyevich MT, Knapp DR, et al. Traumatic hip dislocation with spontaneous incomplete reduction: a diagnostic trap. *J Orthop Trauma.* 2002;16(10):730-735.)

is seen most commonly in older children and teenagers. It is probably related to the severity of the initial trauma. As for femoral neck fractures, reduction within 6 hours after injury may be beneficial in preventing AVN.

Femur Fractures

In general, pediatric femur fractures are much more forgiving than their adult counterparts. In children, particularly very young children, the periosteum is thick, remodeling potential is excellent, and small leg length differences may correct spontaneously. However, treatment decisions are often complex due to concern about damaging the physis or the blood supply to the proximal femoral epiphysis. In adults, decision-making is simple: you slam down an intramedullary nail, interlock it, and move on. In children, several options offer a variety of risks and benefits. Different fracture patterns and clinical situations may dictate that the best option is either a walking spica cast, a traditional spica cast, flexible intramedullary nailing, submuscular plating or trochanteric entry IM nailing; in rare circumstance, external fixation can be used temporarily.

To stay out of trouble, there are several important management principles that should be heeded. First, although most pediatric femur fractures heal without any long-term sequelae (often regardless of treatment method), complications are a frequent source of bad outcomes and professional liability claims. Second, pediatric femur fractures are managed with an age-based algorithm, which is further informed in some cases by the child's weight or the length instability of the fracture (Table 9-1). Third, infants who present with femur fractures should be evaluated carefully for the possibility of nonaccidental injury. This is a source of potentially great danger for the child, agony for the family, and significant trouble for the medical team. Surround yourself and the child with experts in this clinical scenario.

To avoid trouble with pediatric femur fractures, follow accepted standards of alignment and shortening (Table 9-2). Remember that the alignment and shortening recommendations are age-based and reflect acceptable standards abstracted from several retrospective series. Understand that many children do

THE GURU SAYS...

While closed reduction of traumatic dislocations in the ED under sedation is dramatic and satisfying, consider performing closed reduction of these injuries in children and adolescents in the OR with the patient intubated and his or her muscles relaxed.

MARTIN J. HERMAN

TABLE 9-1 Management by Fracture Classification

Class	Treatment	Example
1	It will heal itself; don't make things worse for child or caregivers.	Infant (Pavlik harness), GMFCS V cerebral palsy patient (well-padded cast)
2	Nonoperative management, but watch closely	6-month-old to 5-year-old (spica cast or walking spica)
3	Operative better than nonoperative management; load-sharing implant	6- to 12-year-old (elastic nails)
4	Operative, rigid fixation	Teen or heavy 10- to 12-year-old, or fracture pattern that cannot be treated with elastic nails in younger patient (trochanteric entry nail or plate)
5	Limb at risk. Aggressive operative management; may need staged treatment. Associated injuries may take precedent initially	

GMFCS, Gross Motor Function Classification System.

well functionally—even when these standards are exceeded—but that may be difficult to explain in a courtroom setting. Regarding acceptable angulation, accept less around the knee than around the hip. Even 5° or 10° of angulation in the distal femur of a teenager can cause trouble. In general, families tend to be more forgiving when an injured side is longer after a fracture rather than when the injured side is shorter after a fracture. Although you should counsel extensively about the concept of overgrowth and remodeling in pediatric femur fractures, it is wise to achieve the best possible alignment with the safest clinical method and then deal with potential overgrowth later.

Spica casting may be the "most conservative" way to treat a pediatric fracture, but it is an art and can cause a remarkable amount of trouble in even the best, most experienced hands. The long-term results are excellent with this method but the first 6 months can be very tough on the child and family (especially in the child older than 4 years). To reduce the burden on the family, use a walking spica on children with between the ages of 6 months and 5 years old with less than 2 cm of shortening. Apply the first section of the cast so that it includes the foot, ankle, and calf, and goes just above the knee. Using this first step, there is less risk that you will put excessive pressure or force on the popliteal fossa or peroneal nerve as the rest of the cast is applied (Fig. 9-10). Shortening is less likely if the hip and knee are flexed to 90°. A valgus mold should be made laterally—femoral shaft fractures treated with casting always drift into varus (Fig. 9-11). Ensure that there is enough padding over bony prominences and along the path that your cast saw will take at the time of removal. In bigger, stronger children connecting the legs with a bar will prevent failure of the cast at the hip. Generally, it is best to leave the foot out of the cast. When it is time to remove the cast, take an X-ray in the cast first to assure that there is satisfactory callus. Be very careful about cast saw burns. The blade becomes extremely hot, especially in the area of the hip. Stop

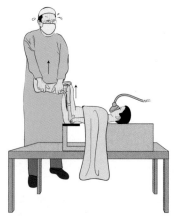

Figure 9-10 The dangers of pulling upward on the calf when applying a spica cast. This upward pull, which is used to reduce the fracture, can be dangerous, because it puts pressure on the gastrocnemius muscle and the other posterior leg structures, such as the popliteal artery and femoral vein.

TABLE 9-2 Femur Fractures: Acceptable Alignment at Union

	2-10 y old	≥11 y old
Varus/valgus angle	<15°	≤5°-10°
Anterior/posterior angle	≤20°	≤10°
Malrotation	≤30°	≤30°

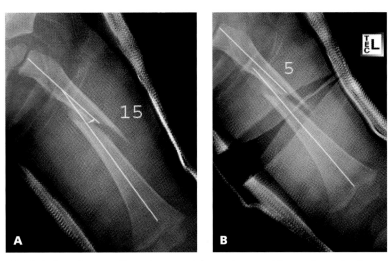

Figure 9-11 A: Despite a well-made cast with a valgus mold exactly at the fracture site, this toddler's femur fracture drifted into varus about 10 days after injury. **B:** The cast was wedged in clinic with nice correction.

frequently to allow the cast saw to cool. After the cast is removed, avoid the temptation to send the child immediately to physical therapy. Most children fresh out of a spica cast do not like to have a therapist manipulating their joints. Tell the parents that the child is restricted to "stroller and carrying" for a week or so. Physical therapy is rarely necessary, but you should warn the family that the child is going to walk with an asymmetric date (they may want to call it a limp) for up to a year after the injury.

THE GURU SAYS...

Spica casting remains my treatment of choice for *most* femoral shaft fractures in children between the ages of 6 months and 5 years. Application of a good, safe spica cast is an art that requires appropriate help and expertise. In our place, this is best done in the OR. But remember that successful care of this fracture only *begins* in the OR.

- While waterproof liners reduce skin complications, the best way to have the cast survive 4 to 6 weeks of wear is to have the parents carefully instructed prior to discharge in care of the child, especially for patients who are still in diapers.
- Safe transportation of a child in a spica requires a specialized car seat. Consider this when placing the cast; wide hip abduction and extension of the hip and knee make fitting of a car seat more difficult. Also, alert your discharge planners on admission to avoid delays in securing the car seat because they can be expensive and hard to come by.
- Be prepared in the postoperative period to wedge or even replace the cast. Many reasons make this necessary but loss of reduction and cast soilage are the most common. While it is extra work and sometimes inconvenient, you—and the parents—will not regret it.

MARTIN J. HERMAN

Flexible intramedullary nailing has become the standard of care for most pediatric femur fractures in children between the ages of 6 and 12 years, unless the fracture is very high energy with excessive risk of shortening, or the 10- to 12-year-old is very obese (greater than 50 kg). The principles outlined by the French pioneers are important: there should be symmetry of nail entry site, nail size, and nail length in order to have two opposing internal splints that stabilize the fracture. These implants allow rapid mobilization; they are good at holding length and alignment while a large amount of callus is formed (Fig. 9-12). There is minimal risk of AVN, physeal injury, and refracture with these implants.

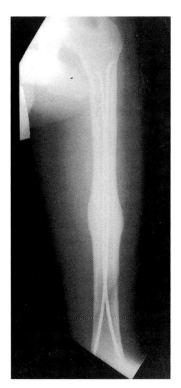

Figure 9-12 Flexible nails have several advantages, including rapid mobilization, maintaining length and alignment, good callus formation, and minimal risk for avascular necrosis, physeal injury, and refracture.

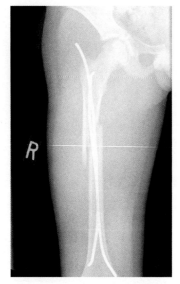

Figure 9-13 Injuries such as this long oblique proximal femur fracture can be managed very successfully with titanium nails, but the surgeon may have to alter technique and aftercare to get the best result. In this case, a proximal lateral entry was used, along with a distal medial entry, creating an excellent internal splint. A single leg "walking spica" was used for 4 weeks to prevent shortening or excessive angulation.

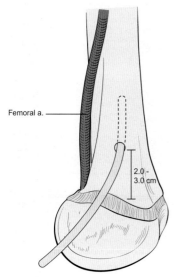

Figure 9-14 The nails are generally placed retrograde, with a starting point about 2.5 cm above the distal femoral physis.

Long spiral fractures, comminuted fractures, and proximal (Fig. 9-13) and distal fractures can be treated with elastic intramedullary nailing; however, in some cases alternative fixation methods are better, or supplemental immobilization should be used after the elastic nailing.

A few technical tips are worth noting to stay out of trouble with titanium elastic nailing. The nails are generally placed retrograde, with a starting point about 2.5 cm above the distal femoral physis (Fig. 9-14). Avoid any deep dissection in the area of the distal femoral physis to minimize the chance of growth arrest, and posterior to the femur, as vascular injury may result. The tip of the titanium elastic nail is sharp enough to penetrate the cortical bone in the area of the distal femoral metaphysis (Fig. 9-15); image frequently if you meet resistance as the nail is started up the canal. Leave only 1 to 1.5 cm of nail outside the bone and don't bend the nail tip away from the metaphysis (Fig. 9-16). The most frequent complication of these devices is soft-tissue irritation by the distal, extraosseous portion of the nail. Be certain that rotation and distraction are eliminated before leaving the operating room. There are a few cases of delayed union or nonunion that resulted when tight-fitting titanium elastic nails held the fracture site distracted in the first couple of months after surgery (Fig. 9-17). In most centers, titanium elastic nails are removed once the fracture is healed. Once the fracture line is gone, the nails can be removed, but protect the child in a knee immobilizer for at least a month or two after nail removal in order to avoid refracture through the nail entry site.

> ### THE GURU SAYS...
>
> Despite more than 20 years of experience with flexible intramedullary nail fixation of femur fractures, I am still humbled by it at times, often because I tried to "get away with" using them in less than ideal situations. Failing to adequately assess length stability of a particular fracture pattern, using flexible nails in children heavier than 110 pounds or so, and fixating very proximal or distal fractures remain the "snakes in the grass." Until we have an app that predicts construct stability, my suggestions to avoid reoperation include
>
> - Carefully scrutinize injury radiographs and examine the fracture fragments under fluoroscopy in multiple planes so that "occult" comminution or the extent of obliquity can be judged.
> - After fixation, stress the construct in multiple planes, including under compression across the fracture. While this is not foolproof, length-instability or inadequate fixation can often be judged. In many cases, applying a supplemental a one-legged spica cast for 3 or 4 weeks has allowed me to "get away with" some less than ideal constructs.
> - Always have Plan B ready in the room and don't be too proud to go to it, even if the flexible nails are in, remove them and proceed. Plan B may include locked intramedullary devices for children older than 9 years, submuscular plates, and in the extreme, old school external fixation or even application of traction.
>
> MARTIN J. HERMAN

A wide variety of well-designed trochanteric entry nails are now available for use in the adolescent or very heavy preadolescent. It is wise to lock proximally and distally in order to avoid rotational malunion. A relatively small diameter nail (9 mm) works for most of these fractures and obviates the need for excessive reaming. Avoid nail designs that require excessive amount of reaming of the

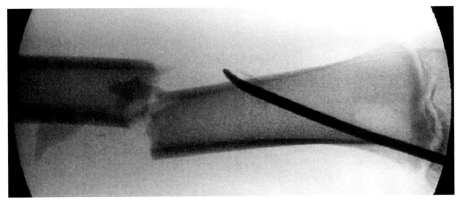

Figure 9-15 To avoid trouble with titanium elastic nailing, image frequently during nail passage.

proximal entry site, which can be particularly problematic in the young heavy kids who have not yet developed a large intertrochanteric area. Some centers prefer submuscular plating to trochanteric entry nailing. Both are highly successful treatment methods for length unstable fractures. This is a case where the surgeon must decide what is best in their hands.

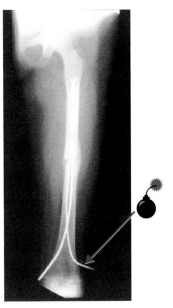

Figure 9-16 To avoid irritation, leave only 1 to 1.5 cm of nail out distally and don't bend the tip away from the bone.

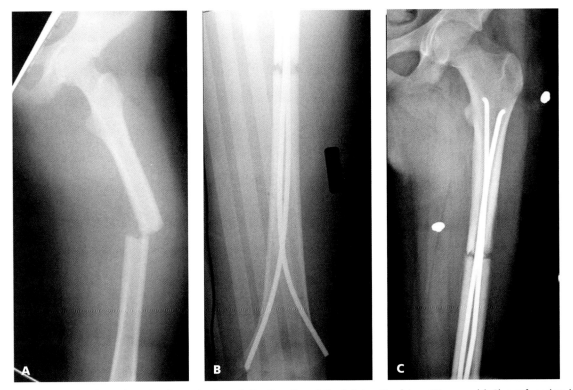

Figure 9-17 Delayed union after titanium elastic nail fixation (in a bit of distraction) in a 14-year-old. She refused to bear weight because of distal nail irritation of the knee. The nail tips in the dense metaphyseal bone held the fracture in distraction, leading to a nonunion at 1 year. A locked trochanteric entry nail (the revision solution here) could have had the same problem if fixed in distraction.

Staying Out of Trouble With Trauma About the Pelvis, Hip, or Femur

Pelvic Fractures

* Search for associated trauma.

* Counsel at presentation: leg length discrepancy, heterotopic ossification.

* Perform a thorough neurologic examination at presentation.

* Follow patient for at least 1 year.

Hip Fractures

* Counsel at presentation: AVN, coxa vara, growth arrest.

* Early, anatomic reduction. Do a capsulotomy.

* Use screws, not Kirschner wires (K-wires) or spica cast alone.

* If your screws are not across the physis, use a spica for a few weeks after internal fixation.

* Follow patient for at least 2 years.

Femur Fractures

* Counsel at presentation: Leg length discrepancy, limping for up to 1 year.

* Consider child abuse, especially in children younger than 1 year.

* Follow standards for length and alignment.

* Spica: Don't use excessive traction on leg and protect popliteal fossa.

* Titanium elastic nailing: symmetrical configuration, no excessive bend at entry, no distraction/rotation, knee immobilizer (stable fracture), one-leg spica (unstable fracture) for 4 to 6 weeks. Be careful with bigger, older kids (especially >11 years old, >50 kg)

* Intramedullary nail: Stay out of the piriformis fossa (Fig. 9-18).

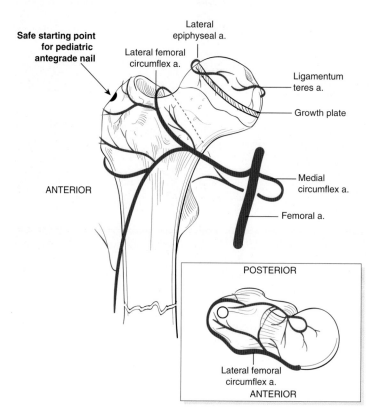

Figure 9-18 To avoid trouble when using solid intramedullary nails and to avoid avascular necrosis ensure no awl in the piriformis fossa, a trochanteric starting point, and use smaller diameter nails.

FOR FURTHER ENLIGHTENMENT

Flynn JM, Curatolo E. Pediatric femoral shaft fractures: a system for decision making. *Instr Course Lect*. 2015;64:453-460.

Flynn JM, Garner MR, Jones KJ, et al. The treatment of low-energy femoral shaft fractures: a prospective study comparing the "walking spica" with the traditional spica cast. *J Bone Joint Surg Am*. 2011;93:2196-2202.

Mubarak SJ, Frick S, Sink E, et al. Volkmann contracture and compartment syndromes after femur fractures in children treated with 90/90 spica casts. *J Pediatr Orthop*. 2006;26:567-572.

Patterson JT, Tangtiphaiboontana J, Pandya NK. Management of pediatric femoral neck fracture. *J Am Acad Orthop Surg*. 2018;26:411-419.

Price CT, Pyevich MT, Knapp DR, et al. Traumatic hip dislocation with spontaneous incomplete reduction: a diagnostic trap. *J Orthop Trauma*. 2002;16:730-735.

Silber JS, Flynn JM, Koffler KM, et al. Analysis of the cause, classification, and associated injuries of 166 consecutive pediatric pelvic fractures. *J Pediatr Orthop*. 2001;21:446-450.

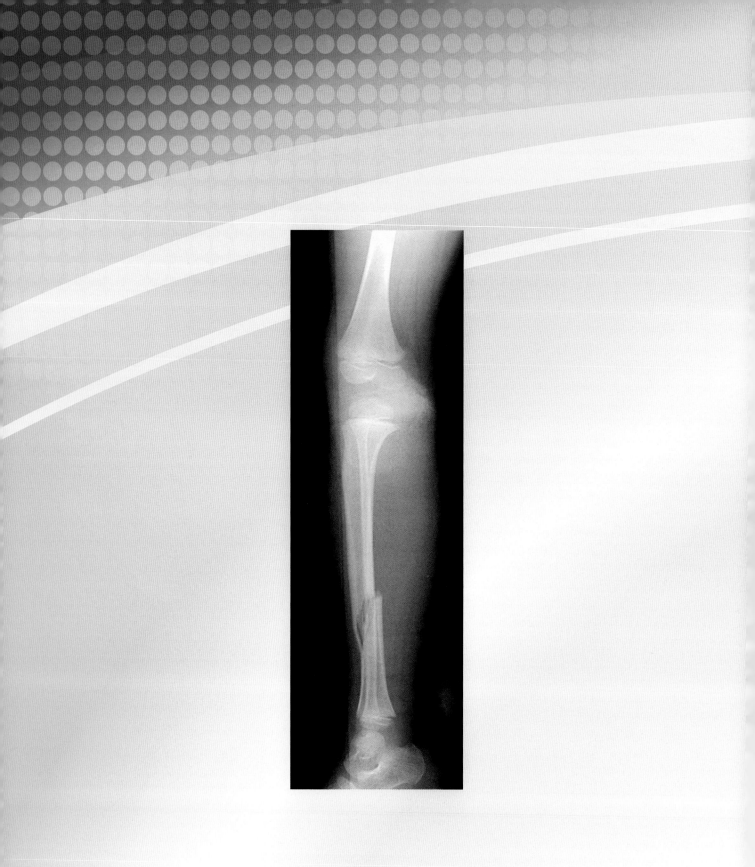

Chapter 10

Trauma About the Knee, Tibia, and Foot

MININDER S. KOCHER, MD, MPH

Guru: Kevin G. Shea, MD

Knee

PATELLA SLEEVE FRACTURES

In this injury unique to children, the extreme distal or proximal pole of the patella, together with a significant sleeve of articular cartilage, periosteum, and retinaculum is pulled off the remaining main body of the patella (Fig. 10-1). The easiest pitfall in this fracture is to miss it at initial presentation (Fig. 10-2), as there may only be a hint of ossified bone on initial radiographs. The clinical picture at presentation usually includes a palpable defect at the affected patella pole and an inability to fully extend the knee or perform a straight leg raise.

Any significant displacement should be operatively fixed, as there may be significant articular cartilage avulsion not appreciated on plain radiographs. If displacement is questionable, flexion/extension lateral films should be made in superior and inferior sleeve avulsion fractures to assess intrinsic soft tissue stability. Widening of the fracture gap with lateral radiographs in flexion usually indicates a need for surgical stabilization.[1] MRI can be useful as a small bony fragment of the inferior pole on X-ray may include a large patellar articular cartilage component appreciate on MRI.

During surgery, retinacular repair is performed. If necessary, sutures securing the patella tendon or quadriceps tendon may be passed through drill holes through the patella for fixation. A nonoperative, or inadequate operative repair may progress to further displacement during healing or rehabilitation (Fig. 10-3). A patella sleeve fracture should not be confused with Sinding-Johansson-Larsen disease, which is a chronic overuse injury that may be thought of as an Osgood-Schlatter (OGS) disease of the other side of the patella tendon.

> **THE GURU SAYS...**
>
> The threshold for obtaining the MRI should be low, as these images can facilitate early diagnosis and treatment.
>
> KEVIN G. SHEA

> **THE GURU SAYS...**
>
> The use of suture anchors for repair may not be preferred, as the strength of repair through drill holes is much higher.
>
> KEVIN G. SHEA

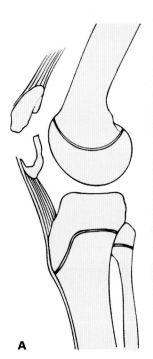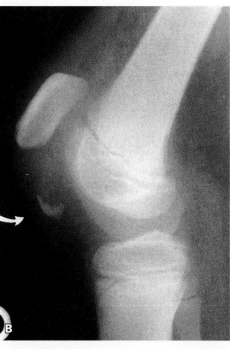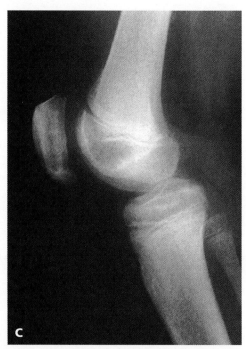

Figure 10-1 Sleeve fracture of the patella. **A:** A small segment of the distal pole of the patella is avulsed with a relatively large portion of the articular surface. **B:** On lateral view, the small osseous portion of the displaced fragment is visible, but the cartilaginous portion is not seen. **C:** Healed sleeve fracture after open reduction and internal fixation. (Reprinted with permission from Sponseller PD, Stanitski CL. Fractures and dislocations about the knee. In: Beaty JH, Kasser JR, eds. *Rockwood & Wilkins' Fractures in Children.* 5th ed. Philadelphia, PA: Lippincott Williams & Wilkins; 2001:981.)

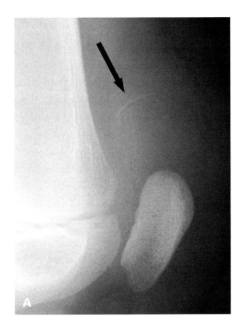
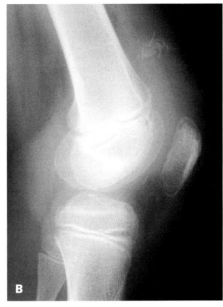

Figure 10-2 A: Patella sleeve fracture of the superior pole. This was missed in the emergency department. **B:** Two weeks later, ossification makes fracture more visible on radiographs. Surgical reconstruction at this stage is more involved.

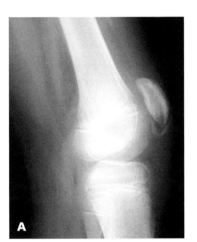
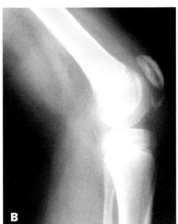
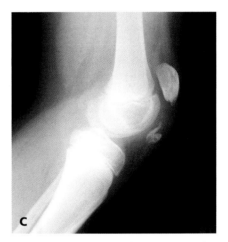

Figure 10-3 A: Six-week postoperative radiograph, lateral view, demonstrating migration of fracture fragment. **B:** Three-month postoperative radiograph of the same patient. **C:** One year postoperative radiograph of the same patient.

Staying Out of Trouble With Surgical Repair of Patella Sleeve Fractures

* When repairing the retinaculum, place all the sutures first without tying them. If the sutures are tied as they are placed, it becomes increasingly difficult to visualize the torn retinaculum and fracture.

* If closing the gap of the extensor mechanism is difficult:
  * Consider letting down the tourniquet, which may be tethering the quadriceps.
  * If the fracture is not acute, quadriceps contraction may have occurred, in which case judicious musculotendinous lengthening of the quadriceps complex may be needed.

* Late recognition of patella sleeve fractures is not uncommon. Consider this diagnosis in any trauma patient who does not have full active extension of their knee.

THE GURU SAYS...

If drill holes are placed on the patella for suture repair, consider using a small drill, rather than a beath pin, to place the drill hole. The use of a drill may avoid the excessive heat which can be generated by the use of beath pins during drilling in dense patellar bone. After placing the drill hole, a beath pin can be used to pass the sutures through the patella.

KEVIN G. SHEA

DISTAL FEMORAL PHYSEAL FRACTURES

The first pitfall in these fractures is missing the diagnosis. In the mature skeleton, ligaments usually fail before bone when a bending stress is applied across the knee joint, so following a severe valgus stress across the knee a medial collateral ligament (MCL) injury may occur (Fig. 10-4). As the collateral ligaments originate on the epiphysis, in an immature skeleton, the physis will fail in tension and the knee will fall into valgus though a Salter I or II fracture (Fig. 10-5). A Salter I fracture may be non-displaced and not radiographically obvious. If suspicious of a type I distal femoral undisplaced fracture, the width of the physis is often greater than the contralateral physis on X-ray. Clinically, there should be tenderness about the physis, which is near the superior pole of the patella on either side of the knee, and the knee may be unstable to valgus or varus stress. A stress view radiograph or MRI can confirm the diagnosis; however, the need for either test has been questioned as the initial treatment for both an MCL injury and a nondisplaced distal femoral Salter I fracture is immobilization. Repeat radiographic and clinical examination at 10 to 14 days should help clarify the diagnosis.[2] It is important to make a diagnosis at some point, because Salter fractures about the knee require follow-up for evaluation of possible growth plate injury.

The most common sequelae to distal femoral physeal injuries is growth disturbance, either total arrest which leads to shortening, or partial arrest leading to angular deformity. Angular deformity following distal femoral physeal injury is reported in 18% to 51% of recent series.[3-6] Growth injuries usually occur at the time of injury, and not a result of mismanagement. Stay out of trouble, and depositions, by informing parents *before* a growth disturbance occurs that the chances are nearly 50% this problem will occur in their child, and that surgery,

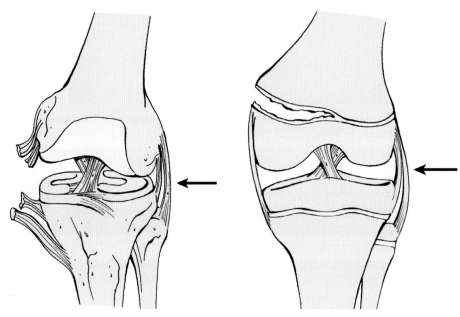

Figure 10-4 Injury pattern with closed growth plates. In the mature skeleton, ligaments usually fail before bone when a bending stress is applied across the knee joint, so following a severe valgus stress across the knee a medial collateral ligament (MCL) injury may occur. Black arrow is direction of force.

Figure 10-5 Injury pattern with open growth plates. As the collateral ligaments originate on the epiphysis, in an immature skeleton, the physis will fail in tension and the knee will fall into valgus, though a Salter I or II fracture. Black arrow is direction of force.

including stopping the growth of the "normal" side may be needed in the future. While these injuries cannot be prevented, one thing we can do is to follow children with physeal injuries about the knee for at least 1 year closely. A growth disturbance which is identified early may be treated with either a contralateral epiphysiodesis (near the end of growth) or a Langensköld procedure. An angular deformity recognized late may require an osteotomy. An MRI with sequences chosen to highlight cartilage can aid in the early diagnosis of a physeal bar formation. One mechanism of injury that lies in wait to trap an unsuspecting orthopaedic surgeon is an unrecognized physeal injury in association with nonphyseal fractures in the femur or tibia. Hresko et al reported on seven children who had a physeal arrest about the knee in association with nonphyseal fractures in the lower extremity.[7]

In terms of treatment, one should strive for anatomic reduction of these fractures. Series have reported rates of 43% to 70% of distal femoral fractures treated without internal fixation have displaced.[8,9] Unless a fracture is truly nondisplaced and stable, stay out of trouble by providing internal fixation. To avoid further injury to the physis, reduction should be 90% traction and 10% manipulation, preferably in the operating room with maximal relaxation. Salter I fractures may be stabilized by smooth Kirschner wires (K-wires). Wires should not cross at the fracture, but one should attempt to have the K-wires maximally separated at the fracture line. Clinical experience and animal studies have demonstrated that crossing the physis with smooth K-wires of the size commonly used should not cause a growth disturbance.[10] Anteriorly displaced Salter I fractures deserve special mention. Previous texts have recommended closed reduction and casting with the knee in a flexed position; however, this treatment may lead to knee stiffness and makes evaluation of frontal plane alignment quite difficult. Stay out of trouble by pinning these fractures and providing immobilization in near full extension. Of course the knee should not be immobilized in extension until the fracture has been reduced, or vascular occlusion or peroneal nerve injury may result.

A potential pitfall using intra-articular K-wires is the possibility of a superficial pin tract infection progressing to a septic knee joint. Early fracture healing usually allows these pins to be pulled at 3 or 4 weeks, which helps prevent this complication. Continued protected immobilization is still indicated until clinical healing. In thin children, pins may be brought out of the skin proximal to the fracture site, and thus not be intra-articular. Salter II fractures may often be closed reduced and fixed with cannulated screws in compression across the metaphyseal fragment.

Regardless of the local stability of fracture fixation about the distal femur or proximal tibia, immobilize the entire leg to prevent the long lever arms of the tibia and femur from displacing the fracture. Series report 20% loss of reduction of these fractures. In children with short and/or wide thighs, consider extending immobilization proximally to include the waist.

Associated ligament injuries may occur at time of injury and should be evaluated following fracture fixation and again following fracture healing. Knee stiffness can be expected in about 25% of patients, so the surgeon should warn parents ahead of time, as well as consider early physical therapy. Fortunately, while peroneal nerve and popliteal artery injuries may occur with distal femoral physeal fractures, they are not common. Dr. Chad Price reminds us of the "satisfaction of search" pitfall.[11] This describes a situation in which the detection of one radiographic abnormality interferes with that of others—once one fracture is found, you are satisfied and stop looking (Fig. 10-6).

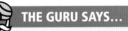

THE GURU SAYS...

For distal femur fractures, use of stiffer smooth K-wires may help maintain fracture reduction. Burying the pins subcutaneously may lower the risk of pin track infection.

KEVIN G. SHEA

THE GURU SAYS...

Static and dynamic stretching devices, such as splints or braces, may be helpful to address some knee stiffness after these injuries.

KEVIN G. SHEA

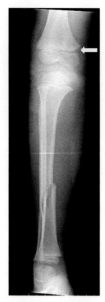

Figure 10-6 AP radiograph of a 5-year-old boy in a stroller who was struck by a car. The Salter I fracture of the distal femoral physis was not recognized, and the child was initially treated with a short leg cast. This is an example of falling into the trap of "satisfaction of search." When the first fracture is noted, human nature is to feel satisfied and not view the remainder of the radiograph with necessary diligence.

THE GURU SAYS...

Avulsion of the extensor mechanism may require distinct repair of the patella tendon, in addition to screw fixation of the bone tuberosity displacement. The screws used for fracture reduction may also be used to anchor the sutures of the soft tissue repair. Use of partially threaded screws will allow these to act as "anchor points" for the sutures of the soft tissue repair. Use of suture anchors may also be an option to anchor the soft tissue repair.

KEVIN G. SHEA

DISTAL FEMORAL METAPHYSEAL FRACTURE

This injury is mentioned only to avoid the pitfall of trying to treat a displaced fracture with casting without fixation. The gastrocnemius muscle attaches to the distal femur, thus pulling the distal femur into flexion. This tempts the surgeon to cast reduce and cast this fracture in knee flexion. However, if the knee is casted in flexion, exact alignment of varus/valgus positioning is nearly impossible to verify. Unfortunately, once the knee is extended after fracture healing, the full extent of varus or valgus malalignment becomes apparent. Avoid this complication by providing fixation, often with K-wires, cannulated screws, flexible IM nails, or an external fixator for displaced distal femoral metaphyseal fractures.

Tibia

See Chapter 14, The Pediatric Athlete, for tibial spine fractures.

TIBIAL TUBERCLE FRACTURES

Tibial tubercle fractures occur almost exclusively in boys, and usually during jumping sports such as basketball. This fracture occurs along the apophysis deep to the tibial tubercle, and should not be confused with Osgood-Schlatter disease (Table 10-1), although preexisting OGS symptoms may be present.

This fracture tends to occur in adolescents near the end of growth, so growth disturbance is usually not a problem. The fracture may extend into the joint (type III), in which case anatomic reduction is needed and associated intra-articular injuries such as meniscus or ligamentous injuries should be searched for. Beware that some active knee extension may still be present through retinacular fibers, so active knee extension does not rule out a tibial tubercle fracture. Type IV fractures that occur up the apophysis, across the physis, and then down the posterior metaphysis are particularly unstable and usually require surgical screw stabilization[12] (Fig. 10-7).

Tibial tubercle fractures may involve extensive soft tissue avulsion requiring repair as well Sleeve avulsion fractures of the tibial tuberosity extending over the anterior metaphyseal area of the tibia has been recently described.[13] These injuries are similar to patellar sleeve fractures, in that initial radiographs may show no more than small subchondral fragments of bone. Davidson and Letts report fixation of the type V sleeve avulsion fracture is challenging because of a lack of a large bony fragment.[13] They recommend fixation with small-diameter screws and heavy nonabsorbable sutures between the intact periosteum or bone and the large avulsed segment of periosteum.

The most common complication following fracture healing is prominent hardware requiring removal. The use of multiple smaller screws (4.5 mm instead of 7.3 mm) may help minimize this complication. The most serious complication of this fracture is compartment syndrome.[14,15] Because this fracture is associated with relatively low-energy trauma, compartment syndrome may not be on the radar screen of the unknowing surgeon. Compartment syndrome occurs presumably

TABLE 10-1 Do Not Confuse a Tibial Tubercle Fracture With Osgood-Schlatter Disease		
	Tibial Tubercle Fracture	**Osgood-Schlatter Disease**
Location of pathology	Deep to tibial tubercle, fracture along apophysis continuous with proximal tibial physis	Superficial to tibial tubercle, at insertion of patella tendon into tubercle
Temporal	Acute	Chronic
Ambulatory	Unusual	Yes, limp may be present
Patella alta	Present with displaced fractures	No

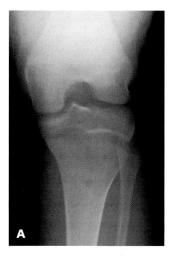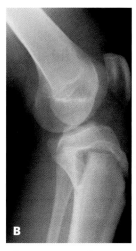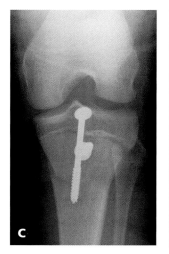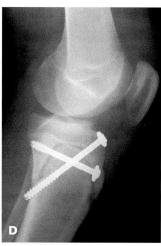

Figure 10-7 Type 4 tibial tubercle fractures are often very unstable. **A, B:** Preoperative. **C, D:** Postoperative fixation.

because of tearing of anterior tibial recurrent vessels, which fan out at the tubercle but retract into the anterior compartment when torn (Fig. 10-8). Close monitoring is necessary for patients treated nonoperatively, and careful inspection, possibly with prophylactic anterior fasciotomy, is recommended for patients treated operatively.

PROXIMAL TIBIAL PHYSEAL FRACTURES

This fracture is uncommon but can be associated with lots of trouble. In contrast to the distal femoral physis, the proximal tibial physis has intrinsic anatomic stability from the proximal fibula, an overhanging tibial tubercle, and the medial collateral ligament (MCL) extending beyond the physis to insert into the upper metaphysis. Because of this protection, separation of the proximal tibial epiphysis is relatively rare and requires significant force.

The most serious injury associated with proximal tibia physeal fracture is vascular compromise. The popliteal artery is tethered by its major branches to the posterior surface of the proximal tibial epiphysis, with anterior tibial artery passing forward just proximal to the interosseous membrane. A hyperextension injury that results in posterior displacement of the upper end of the metaphysis may stretch and tear the bound popliteal artery (Fig. 10-9). It is important to remember, that even a fracture that appears minimally displaced at presentation in an emergency department, may have had significantly more displacement at the time of injury, particularly in motor vehicle accidents (Fig. 10-10).

Compartment syndrome may occur following proximal tibial physeal fractures because of mechanical blockage of the vascular structures from a displaced fracture following the injury or damage to the popliteal artery at time of injury, including an intimal tear that may not be clinically significant at presentation. It is important to remember in this injury that even a small posterior displacement of the metaphysis may obstruct popliteal blood flow as the artery is tethered anteriorly against the metaphysis by the anterior tibial artery (Fig. 10-11).

Most patients with proximal tibial physeal fractures have associated ligamentous injuries, primarily anterior and valgus laxity. I suspect that these are underrecognized injuries and recommend assessment of ligaments by physical exam following operative fixation and fracture healing.

Although the intact proximal tibial epiphysis is inherently stable, separations of the proximal tibial epiphysis may be surprisingly unstable. There should be no hesitation to provide fixation with K-wires or cannulated screws if there is any question about stability of fracture reduction.

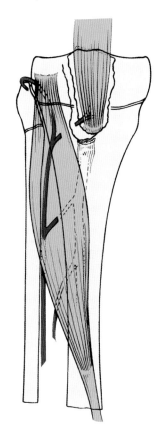

Figure 10-8 Probable mechanism of development of compartment syndrome after tibial tubercle avulsion. The anterior tibial recurrent artery, and possibly its branches, are torn and retract into the anterior compartment musculature. (Reprinted with permission from Sponseller PD, Stanitski CL. Fractures and dislocations about the knee. In: Beaty JH, Kasser JR, eds. *Rockwood and Wilkins' Fractures in Children.* 5th ed. Philadelphia: Lippincott Williams & Wilkins; 2001:981.)

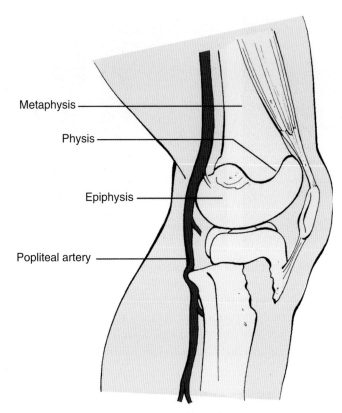

Figure 10-9 Posterior displacement of the epiphysis following fracture-separation at the time of injury can cause arterial injury. In addition, a posteriorly displaced fragment can cause persistent arterial occlusion by direct pressure.

Children who have sustained physeal injury to the proximal tibial physis should be monitored for evidence of growth arrest or development of a physeal bar for at least 2 years. Families should be counseled early of the signficant risk of secondary physeal arrest and deformity which may require future treatment.

OSTEOCHONDRAL FRACTURES

These fractures may be difficult to appreciate on plane radiographs and are usually associated with patellar dislocations. MRI or arthroscopy may be helpful for diagnosis. Despite the fact that these fractures involve articular cartilage, they do not always require surgery if they are in non–weight-bearing area and stuck in synovium out of the way of weight-bearing surfaces. Sometimes, however, these fragments can involve larger portions of the medial patellar facet or lateral trochlear groove and require fixation. This can be done arthroscopically or may require arthrotomy. Fixation devices include bioabsorbable tacks and headless (metal or bioabsorbable) screws. Recent studies suggest that even fragments that appear grossly as "cartilage only" may heal in pediatric patients.[16]

PROXIMAL TIBIAL METAPHYSEAL FRACTURES (COZEN FRACTURES)

It has been proposed that a fracture of the proximal tibial metaphysis without a fibula fracture may develop a valgus deformity over half the time.[17] Maximum valgus occurs about 1 year following injury. A 15-year follow-up of seven patients with this fracture demonstrated a mean of 8° of improvement of the proximal tibia valgus from the point of maximal deformity. Less well known is that every patient had a limb length discrepancy (mean = 9 mm) at time of last follow-up.

THE GURU SAYS...

While some of these fragments may have large, stellate contusion/cartilage damage patterns, many of these fragments are repairable. For larger fragments from the patella, the repair can be performed through a smaller medial arthrotomy, in which the patella is rotated 90° to the trochlea, rather than fully everted. In most cases, this smaller arthrotomy approach without full patella rotation/exposure allows for excellent visualization of the fracture through a significantly smaller incision.

KEVIN G. SHEA

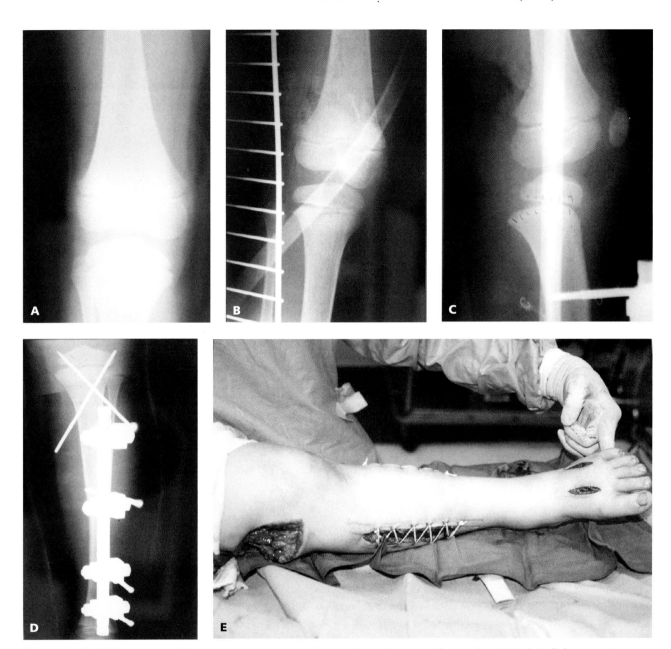

Figure 10-10 Child on back of bicycle struck by car sustained ipsilateral proximal femoral and tibial shaft fracture. **A, B:** proximal tibial physeal fracture on initial radiographs were not appreciated. **C:** Following external fixation of the tibial diaphyseal fracture, a Salter-Harris type I fracture of the proximal tibial physeal is evident. **D:** Closed reduction and Kirschner wire (K-wire) fixation were used to treat the proximal tibial physeal fracture. **E:** Compartment syndrome occurred, which is associated with proximal physeal fractures of the tibia. In this case, the contribution of concomitant injuries to the compartment syndrome is difficult to discern.

These fractures have developed notoriety as growth disturbances.[17] Patients may correct the valgus by developing a "serpentine" tibia: the lower portion of the tibia becomes varisized, resulting in an S-shaped tibia.

It is common sense to try to cast these fractures in no valgus, and even a little varus if possible. It is unclear, and probably unlikely, that anatomic operative reduction will prevent future valgus.[18] Stay out of trouble by expecting varus remodeling to be sufficient in most patients, and wait at least 2 or 3 years after injury before considering intervention in most cases. Valgus deformity has been shown to recur following early osteotomies.[19] However, if malalignment does not remodel over time, joint degeneration of the lateral compartment requiring an

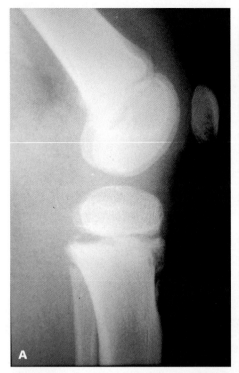
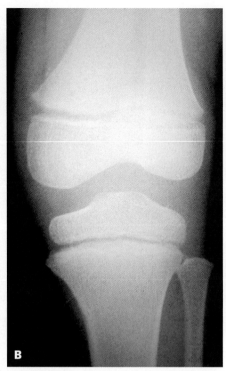
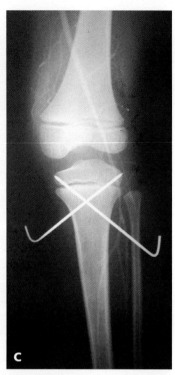

Figure 10-11 A: Lateral radiograph demonstrating minimal posterior displacement of a Salter-Harris I fracture of the proximal tibia. **B:** No significant displacement is noted on the AP radiograph. **C:** Although angiogram demonstrates good flow past the fracture site, a compartment syndrome developed.

osteotomy has been reported.[17] In the rare case where intervention for the valgus deformity is necessary, we recommend consideration of staple hemiepiphysiodesis in children with growth remaining (Fig. 10-12).

TIBIAL SHAFT FRACTURES

Most tibial shaft fractures in children heal well with casting, though loss of reduction is common in unstable fractures. Fractures may be manipulated up to 2 or 3 weeks when the callous is "sticky" with good results. **NEWSFLASH! Following wedging a cast for a malaligned tibia fracture, be cognizant of potential for pressure sores as there is little soft tissue in this region, especially in thin children.**

Isolated Tibial Shaft Fractures

One third of fractures of the tibial shaft, with the fibula, intact tend to drift into varus and/or posterior angulation over the first 3 weeks and deserve close monitoring during this time.[20] The initial cast should attempt to mold maximum valgus, and especially in lower third fractures consider casting the foot in equinus to prevent posterior angulation. Residual or recurrent varus and posterior angulation of 10° or less has been shown to correct spontaneously with growth and remodeling.[20] We would observe for remodeling a fracture with even more deformity in younger children prior to recommending open realignment or osteotomy.

Tibia and Fibula Shaft Fractures

These fractures tend to be the result of higher-energy injuries than tibia fractures alone. While many may be managed by casting alone, unstable fractures my require fixation. Unlike adults, stabilization with K-wires alone is frequently sufficient for many fractures, including open fractures. Wires may be left out of the skin and removed in about 4 weeks in clinic after early callous formation.

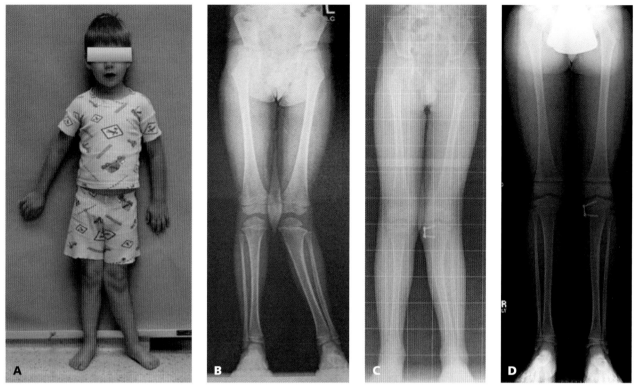

Figure 10-12 Cozen fracture. **A, B:** Proximal tibial metaphyseal fractures without a fibula fracture may develop valgus deformity. **C, D:** This typically resolves with observation but occasionally requires osteotomy or hemiepiphysiodesis if it does not resolve.

Initial experience with flexible intramedullary nails in the tibia fractures is quite encouraging and applicable for most fracture patterns, except truly length unstable fractures. For open fractures, IM nails avoid the soft-tissue tethering of external fixation, and keep the plastic surgeons happy by maximizing their access to the wound. In some cases, only one IM nail may be used (Fig. 10-13). Flexible nails may be left out of skin and removed in clinic after callus formation. External fixation (a.k.a. nonunion generators) may be indicated in length unstable fractures, and those near joints. Rigid IM rods as used in adult tibia fractures should be avoided in skeletally immature patients due to the risk of injury to the tibial tubercle apophysis and resultant hyperextension deformity.

Staying Out of Trouble With Tibia and Fibula Shaft Fractures

✳ Remember to set fracture in correct rotational alignment by evaluating and matching the other side. This is especially easy to forget when casts are placed in the emergency department under questionable sedation.

✳ **Distal tibia fractures:** Unlike adults, children casted in ankle equinus td not develop ankle stiffness. Lower tibial fractures tend to drift into apex posterior angulation, which will be exacerbated by an ankle casted in neutral and improved by an ankle casted in equinus.

✳ **Open fractures:** For open fractures with small soft tissue openings, beware of forceful irrigation (i.e., jet lavage) forcing fluid into compartments and causing a compartment syndrome.

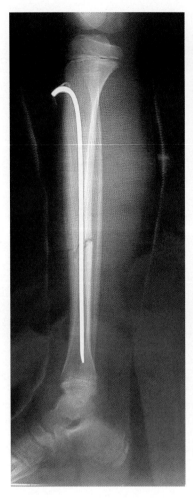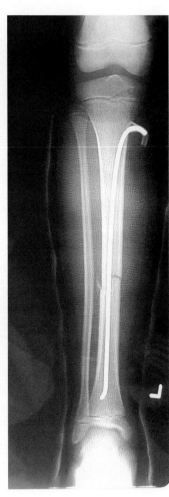

Figure 10-13 Example of a tibia fracture that was not stable to closed reduction treated with a single intramedullary rod left out of the skin proximally. The rod was removed in the office at 4 weeks following injury, at which time adequate callus formation stabilized the fracture.

THE GURU SAYS...

Localized pain in the distal tibia, subtle swelling, or an area of palpable warmth of the leg, may indicate a radiographically invisible toddler's fracture. In some cases, the diagnosis can be made with physical examination. A history of clear trauma may be helpful for confirming the diagnosis, but in many cases, an observed trauma event is not part of the history.

KEVIN G. SHEA

Toddler's Fracture

An oblique, nondisplaced fracture of the tibia, with the fibula intact, often results from a young child falling while running. The big pitfall here is missing the fracture (Fig. 10-14; see also Fig. 13-3 in Chapter 13). At times, in addition to standard AP and lateral views, oblique views may be needed to see a nondisplaced spiral fracture of the tibia. If the surgeon is convinced there is localized pain in the tibia (which may be difficult in a toddler), and the child is not walking, many recommend treatment for a presumed toddler's fracture. Always beware of the possibility of infection, and counsel the family that if the symptoms are worsening despite casting, return for reevaluation soon. **ORTHOPAEDICS 101: If a child will not walk but will crawl, chances are good that the pathology is distal to the knee.**

DISTAL TIBIAL AND ANKLE FRACTURES

There are a number of classification schemes of pediatric ankle fractures which we find confusing and not particularly helpful (Fig. 10-15). To stay out of trouble with pediatric ankle fractures be aggressive in treating Salter fractures that enter the joint (Salter III and IV). These fractures have been reported to have up to a 38% rate of premature physeal closure even with modern treatment methods. These fractures tend to do poorly with closed treatment,[21] and degenerative changes are common these fractures healing in a nonanatomic position. Any displacement of at least 2 mm should be treated with anatomic reduction and

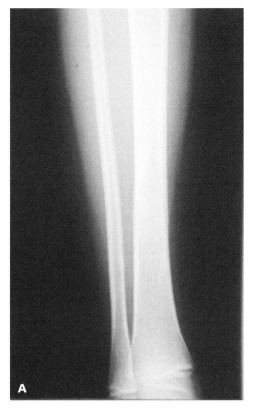
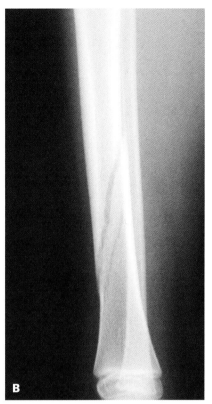
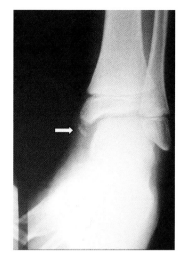

Figure 10-15 Ossification of the tip of the medial malleolus is common (arrow). One can often quickly establish that this is not a fracture in children who have sprained their ankles and have only lateral tenderness.

Figure 10-14 A spiral fracture of the tibia may be difficult to appreciate if only one radiographic view is obtained. These radiographs illustrate the importance of orthogonal radiographs when evaluating a child with the possibility of a fracture.

fixation. For medial malleolar fractures (Salter III), also be aware of subtle medial angulation of the fracture, which is indicative of displacement and an indication for surgery (Fig. 10-16). A technical point is to remember that the plafond of the tibia is arched, so both the AP and lateral images are needed to insure that the screws are not in the joint (Fig. 10-17).

In Salter I and II fractures more than 2 mm displacement is usually considered acceptable, and operative reduction is traditionally considered uncommonly needed. This approach has been recently questioned by one study, in which the rate of premature physeal closure was found to be 3.5 times higher (60% premature closure) in Salter I and II fractures if there was residual fracture displacement of more than 3 mm in postreduction films. The authors attributed this to interposed periosteum.[22] These fractures often occur in older children, in which a premature physeal closure may not have clinical relevance.

Interposed Periosteum in Physeal Fractures: Evildoer or Passive Hitchhiker?

In 2002, Gruber et al reported a histologic study in rats to examine the role of interposed perisoteum in proximal tibial physeal fractures.[23] If the physis was intentionally ablated, a physeal bar predictably resulted. If the physis was left intact, however, they found the physis was able to repair itself even in the presence of interposed periosteum. They concluded that "interposed periosteum seems to play a passive role in physeal fracture healing… (with) no histologic evidence of any osteogenic potential."

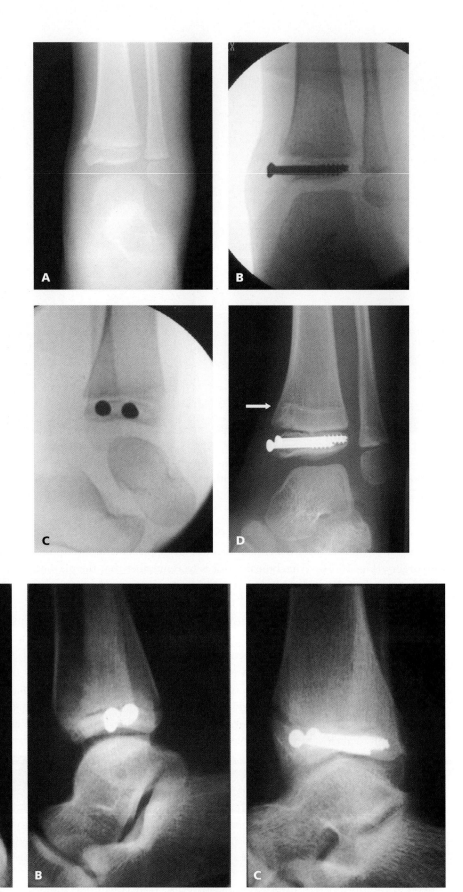

Figure 10-16 **A:** Displaced Salter IV fracture of the distal tibia in a 5-year-old child. Unlike diaphyseal or metaphyseal fractures that will remodel with growth, fractures with displacement of the joint or physis should be treated aggressively with anatomic reduction and fixation. **B, C:** AP and lateral imaging intraoperatively ensure both screws are not in the joint or the physis. **D:** Ten months following the injury a growth arrest line parallel to the physis confirms normal growth of the physis.

Figure 10-17 **A:** Fixation for a medial malleolar fracture appears to be in acceptable position on a mortise radiograph of the ankle. **B, C:** Lateral and oblique views demonstrate one screw is intra-articular. These views should have been obtained with intraoperative imaging to allow the screws to be replaced prior to leaving the operating room.

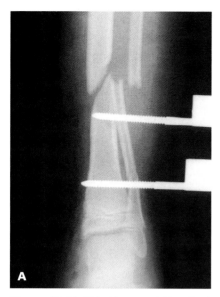 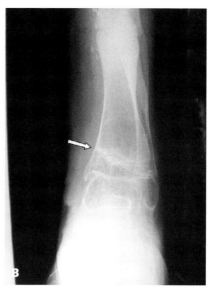 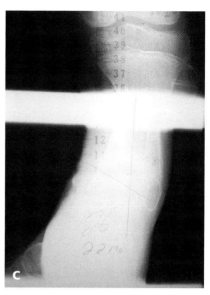

Figure 10-18 This 10-year-old boy had a grade 3 open tibia and fibula fracture with severe soft-tissue loss medially. **A:** The shear injury to the medial malleolus and physis were initially not appreciated. **B:** Thirteen months later, a growth arrest of the medial physis is evident by the angulation of the growth plate. The lack of a normal sized medial malleolus is appreciated in this radiograph as well. **C:** Twenty-two months later there is 26° of angulation.

SHEAR INJURY TO THE MEDIAL MALLEOLUS

Common mechanisms of this injury include road drag or lawn mower. The soft tissue and portion of the bone and physis about the medial malleolus are injured or removed in shear, usually in a high-energy, dirty setting. Customarily, care efforts are focused on the open injury, and the consequences of the physeal damage are not apparent until much later (Fig. 10-18). While it is unproven, covering the exposed physeal edge in an effort to prevent the formation of a peripheral boney bar may be worthwhile. We have used bone wax for this. Warning the family ahead of time and recognizing and addressing the growth disturbance early may improve outcome and minimize surgery.

SOFT TISSUE LOSS ABOUT ANKLE

As for shear injuries to the medial malleolus, this often occurs from road drag or lawn mower injuries. Skin grafts and flaps are often needed, but plastic surgeons warn us they are at risk of not "taking" due to motion about the ankle. An external fixator spanning the ankle, with pins in the calcaneus and metatarsals, allows wound care, promotes soft tissue healing of graft or flap, and prevents the development of ankle equinus (Fig. 10-19).

Staying Out of Trouble With Lawn Mower Injuries

The American Academy of Pediatrics has recommended that children younger than 12 years should not operate a walk-behind power mower.[24] Of the 69 children with a lawn mower amputations in a study by Loder,[25] 68 were 13 years of age or younger at the time of the injury. Simply following the American Academy of Pediatrics guidelines would have eliminated nearly all of those injuries. The treating physician needs to be aware of the potential for family psychosocial issues following these injuries where a family member may be considered "at fault."

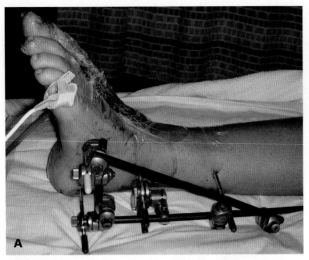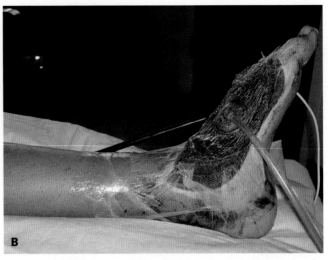

Figure 10-19 A pedestrian child was hit by a car and dragged, causing a distal tibia and fibular fracture, in addition to severe soft-tissue loss exposing bone and joint. **A:** An external fixator across the ankle helps maintain stability of the tibia fracture, prevents ankle equinus, and immobilizes the area of soft tissue injury to maximize chances of a future skin graft being successful. **B:** In this child a wound VAC was used to prepare the area of exposed bone and joints prior to skin grafting.

TRANSITIONAL FRACTURES

The distal tibial physis closes predominantly in a medial to lateral direction over about an 18 month period. Fractures through the partially opened lateral growth plate deserve mention because they are usually intra-articular, often require operative reduction, and have potential for being missed or under treated.

Over a 3-year period at Winnipeg Children's Hospital, of 26 patients with so-called Tillaux fractures, 9 could be diagnosed only by the oblique radiograph and 5 were initially missed.[26] A Tillaux fracture is an avulsion of the anterolateral corner of the distal tibial epiphysis by the anteroinferior tibiofibular ligament. These fractures are believed to occur secondary to external rotation of the ankle, so the maneuver for closed reduction is internal rotation. A triplane fracture has a more complex geometry with the fracture extending into the metaphysis. The fracture may be in three planes (hence the name), sagittal plane within the epiphysis and extending into the joint, the transverse plane along the open growth plate, and the frontal plane extending proximally into the metaphysis. The metaphyseal component of the fracture is surprisingly easy to miss at times and often best appreciated in the lateral view which demonstrates a posterior metaphyseal fragment. The fracture may be in one piece, or multiple pieces, but do not be distracted by the exact nature of the fracture pattern; it is of secondary importance.

Stay focused on the most important issue in these fractures—the joint surface. The amount of displacement and, more importantly, the amount of intra-articular step-off are notoriously difficult to assess on plain films, particularly when the child is in plaster. To stay out of trouble, consider a CT scan for a Tillaux or triplane fracture with *any* displacement seen on plain films (Fig. 10-20). Fractures which may appear minimally displaced on X-ray (1-2 mm) often are more displaced (>2 mm) on CT scan necessitating a change in treatment plan. For fractures of questionable displacement, the child may be placed in a long leg cast with internal rotation of the ankle, prior to the CT to evaluate the fracture after attempted closed reduction.

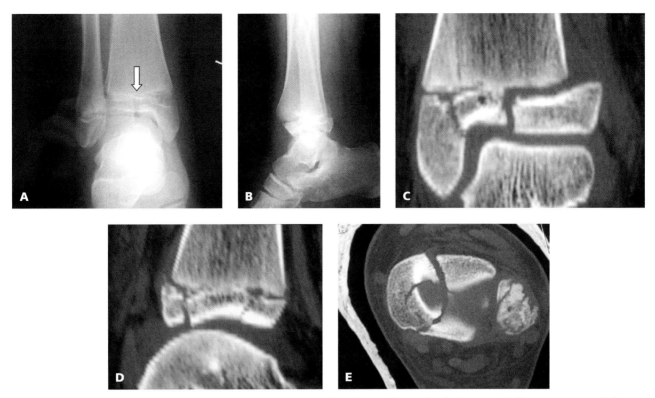

Figure 10-20 A: AP view of a triplane fracture. Note that on the plain radiographs the intra-articular component of the fracture (arrow) does not appear to be very displaced or have a step-off. **B:** Lateral view of fracture. **C-E:** CT further reveals extent of intra-articular step-off and comminution.

As this fragment of bone is intra-articular, operative treatment has been recommended for fragments with more than 2 mm of displacement, with series reporting an increased risk of poor results in such fractures. We think an important distinction should be made between joint step-off and fracture gap. Some surgeons will accept up to 5 mm of fracture gap in tri-plane fractures, and possibly even more in a Tillaux fracture that does not involve a significant amount of bone in a weight bearing region. However, no more than 2 mm of intra-articular step-off can be accepted, and if present, closed or open reduction using standard surgical principles is indicated. Cannulated screws are helpful in these fractures. Oftentimes, the posterior metaphyseal fragment can be reduced and fixed through an anterior incision.

One good thing about transitional fractures is there is no significant growth potential left in the growth plate, so in terms of treatment, the growth of the physis can be ignored. This is one of the only times you can put a screw across an open growth plate with a clean conscience. Beware that triplane fractures are associated with fibular fractures nearly 50% of the time, an ipsilateral tibial shaft fracture nearly 10% of times, and can even be associated with a proximal fibula fracture and syndesmotic injury (Maisonneuve equivalent).[27,28]

> **THE GURU SAYS...**
>
> The use of small joint scope and the arthroscopic ankle distractor may help with visualization of the articular reduction in some of these cases.
>
> KEVIN G. SHEA

ANKLE SPRAIN OR OCCULT FRACTURE: WHO CARES?

The differentiation of a nondisplaced Salter I fibula fractures from an ankle sprain in a child with an open physis may be difficult on physical examination, and initial radiographs in both conditions may be normal. In a fresh injury, the location of tenderness usually allows one to make the diagnosis with some confidence. If there is tenderness (and swelling) anterior to the distal fibula, along the anterior talofibular ligaments, assume there is a sprain. Fibular tenderness may be assessed by tapping with your finger on the posterior half of the distal fibula which is free of the anterior talofibular ligament. If there is boney tenderness, assume an occult Salter I fracture. The bottom line, however, is that either injury could be treated with functional bracing.

Foot

The apophysis at the base of the fifth metatarsal where the peroneus brevis attaches is frequently mistaken for a fracture by the unknowing. Remember that the normal apophysis is roughly parallel to the metatarsal, while a fracture tends to be roughly perpendicular to the metatarsal (Fig. 10-21). Jones fractures (metaphyseal-diaphyseal fractures of the fifth metatarsal) do occur in adolescent athletes. Unlike adult Jones fractures which are usually treated with intramedullary screw fixation in the athlete, pediatric and adolescent Jones fractures can heal well with closed treatment.

Although uncommon, Lisfranc injuries are often misdiagnosed and easily overlooked in children.[29] Fractures of the base of the second metatarsal is usually an indication of an associated tarsometatarsal joint injury. Remember the fourth metatarsal should line up with the medial cuboid and the second metatarsal with the lateral border of the medial cuneiform. In Lisfranc injuries in children, the proximal findings may be subtle, whereas the distal separation of the first and second metatarsals may be more obvious.

When a child's foot is run over by a car, there may be significant soft tissue injury, presumably from a combination of shear and compressive forces. Compartment syndrome is common in this instance, *even in the absence of fractures*. Anecdotal reports suggest compartment syndrome of the foot may be present even with relatively pain-free active motion of the toes, and neurologic or vascular symptoms are uncommon. I suggest the three-incision technique (incision over the second and fourth metatarsus and the medial border of the foot) to make certain all compartments are released.

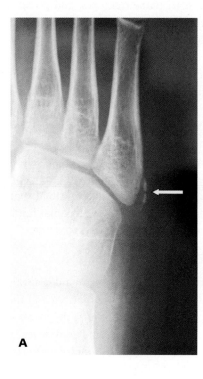 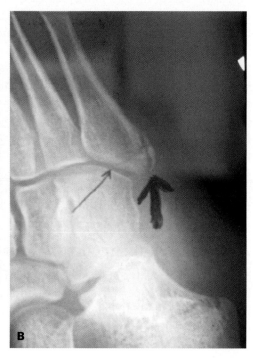

Figure 10-21 A: A normal apophysis of the base of the fifth metatarsal at the attachment of the peroneus brevis (arrow) in a 10-year-old girl. **B:** The thicker arrow points to the normal apophysis, which is roughly parallel to the metatarsal. The thinner arrow points toward a fracture, which is roughly perpendicular to metatarsal.

A   B

Puncture injuries of the foot, usually involving a nail, can lead to an infection with *Pseudomonas* being the most common organism. Beware that a septic joint or osteomyelitis can result from this injury as well. In phalangeal fractures, blood at the nail bed suggests an open fracture that should be treated accordingly.

A "stubbed" great toe with bleeding from the eponychium and a laceration proximal to the nail bed should alert physicians to the presence of a possible open fracture. These injuries can be easily missed, with delay in diagnosis leading to osteomyelitis and even growth arrest.[30]

Staying Out of Trouble With Trauma About the Knee, Tibia, and Foot

* In any traumatic knee lacking active extension, consider the possibility of a patella sleeve fracture and palpate for defect.
* Distal femoral fractures—use fixation for any displaced fractures.
  * Reduction is 90% traction and 10% manipulation.
  * Beware that intra-articular pins can lead to a septic knee.
* Make a concerted effort to look for a proximal tibial physeal fracture in children with high force injuries about the knee. It is frequently minimally displaced and easy to overlook.
  * Have high suspicion for arterial injury and compartment syndrome with proximal tibial physeal fractures.
* In length-stable open tibia fractures, flexible intramedullary nails may lead to quicker healing and leave the soft tissues more accessible for the plastic surgeons, than an external fixator.
* Plan for reduction and fixation of even minimally displaced medial malleolar fractures.
* For any fracture line extending into the tibial plafond on an AP or mortise radiograph, consider a triplane fracture and a obtain CT scan.
* A "stubbed" toe with bleeding about the proximal nail bed may be an open fracture.

SOURCES OF WISDOM

1. Grogan DP, Carey TP, Leffers D, et al. Avulsion fractures of the patella. *J Pediatr Orthop.* 1990;10(6):721-730.
2. Stanitski CL. Stress view radiographs of the skeletally immature knee: a different view. *J Pediatr Orthop.* 2004;24(3):342.
3. Thompson GH, Gesler JW. Proximal tibial epiphyseal fracture in an infant. *J Pediatr Orthop.* 1984;4:114-117.
4. Robert M, Moulies D, Longis B, et al. Traumatic epiphyseal separation of the lower end of the femur. *Rev Chirurgie Orthop.* 1988;74:69-78.
5. Eid AM, Hafez MA. Traumatic injuries of the distal femoral physis: retrospective study on 151 cases. *Injury.* 2002;33:251-255.
6. Riseborough EJ, Barrett IR, Shapiro F. Growth disturbances following distal femoral physeal fracture-separations. *J Bone Joint Surg Am.* 1983;65:885-893.
7. Hresko MT, Kasser JR. Physeal arrest about the knee associated with non-physeal fractures in the lower extremity. *J Bone Joint Surg Am.* 1989;71:698-703.
8. Graham JM, Gross RH. Distal femoral physeal problem fractures. *Clin Orthop Relat Res.* 1990;255:51-53.
9. Thomson JD, Stricker SJ, Williams MM. Fractures of the distal femoral epiphyseal plate. *J Pediatr Orthop.* 1995;15(4):474-478.
10. Janarv PM, Wikstrom B, Hirsch G. The influence of transphyseal drilling and tendon grafting on bone growth: an experimental study in the rabbit. *J Pediatr Orthop.* 1998;18(2):149-154.
11. Ashman CJ, Yu JS, Wolfman D. Satisfaction of search in osteoradiology. *Am J Roentgenology.* 2000;175:541-544.

12. Pace JL, McCulloch PC, Momoh EO, et al. Operatively treated type IV tibial tubercle apophyseal fractures. *J Pediatr Orthop.* 2013;33(8):791-796.

13. Davidson D, Letts M. Partial sleeve fractures of the tibia in children: an unusual fracture pattern. *J Pediatr Orthop.* 2002;22(1):36-40.

14. Pape JM, Goulet JA, Hensinger RN. Compartment syndrome complicating tibial tubercle avulsion. *Clin Orthop Relat Res.* 1993;295:201-204.

15. Wiss DA, Schilz JL, Zionts L. Type III fractures of the tibial tubercle in adolescents. *J Orthop Trauma.* 1991;5(4):475-479.

16. Fabricant PD, Yen YM, Kramer DE, et al. Fixation of traumatic chondral-only fragments of the knee in pediatric and adolescent athletes: a retrospective multicenter report. *Orthop J Sports Med.* 2018;6(2):2325967117753140.

17. Tuten HR, Keeler KA, Gabos PG, et al. Posttraumatic tibia valga in children. A long-term followup note. *J Bone Joint Surg Am.* 1999;81(6):799-810.

18. Brougham DI, Nicol RO. Valgus deformity after proximal tibial fractures in children. *J Bone Joint Surg Br.* 1987;69(3):482.

19. Robert M, Khouri N, Carlioz H, et al. Fractures of the proximal tibial metaphysis in children: review of a series of 25 cases. *J Pediatr Orthop.* 1987;7(4):444-449.

20. Yang JP, Letts RM. Isolated fractures of the tibia with intact fibula in children: a review of 95 patients. *J Pediatr Orthop.* 1997;17(3):347-351.

21. Caterini R, Farsetti P, Ippolito E. Long-term followup of physeal injury to the ankle. *Foot Ankle.* 1991;11(6):372-383.

22. Barmada A, Gaynor T, Mubarak SJ. Premature physeal closure following distal tibia physeal fractures: a new radiographic predictor. *J Pediatr Orthop.* 2003;23(6):733-739.

23. Gruber HE, Phieffer LS, Wattenbarger JM. Physeal fractures. Part II: fate of interposed periosteum in a physeal fracture. *J Pediatr Orthop.* 2002;22:710-716.

24. Smith GA. Committee on Injury and Poison Prevention. Technical report: lawn mower-related injuries to children. *Pediatrics.* 2001;107:E106.

25. Loder RT. Demographics of traumatic amputations in children: implications for prevention strategies. *J Bone Joint Surg Am.* 2004;86A:923-928.

26. Letts RM. The hidden adolescent ankle fracture. *J Pediatr Orthop.* 1982;2:161-164.

27. Rapariz JM, Ocete G, Gonzalez-Herranz P, et al. Distal tibial triplane fractures: long term follow up. *J Pediatr Orthop.* 1996;16:113-118.

28. Healy WA III, Starkweather KD, Meyer J, et al. Triplane fracture associated with a proximal third fibula fracture. *Am J Orthop.* 1996;25:449-451.

29. Hill JF, Heyworth BE, Lierhaus A, et al. Lisfranc injuries in children and adolescents. *J Pediatr Orthop B.* 2017;26(2):159-163.

30. Kensinger DR, Guille JT, Horn BD, et al. The stubbed great toe: importance of early recognition and treatment of open fractures of the distal phalanx. *J Pediatr Orthop.* 2001;21(1):31-34.

FOR FURTHER ENLIGHTENMENT

Cullen MC, Roy DR, Crawford AH, et al. Open fracture of the tibia in children. *J Bone Joint Surg Am.* 1996;78:1039-1047.

Kling TF Jr, Bright RW, Hensinger RN. Distal tibial physeal fractures in children that may require open reduction. *J Bone Joint Surg Am.* 1984;66:647-657.

Rapariz JM, Ocete G, Gonzalez-Herranz P, et al. Distal tibial triplane fractures: long-term follow-up. *J Pediatr Orthop.* 1996;16:113-118.

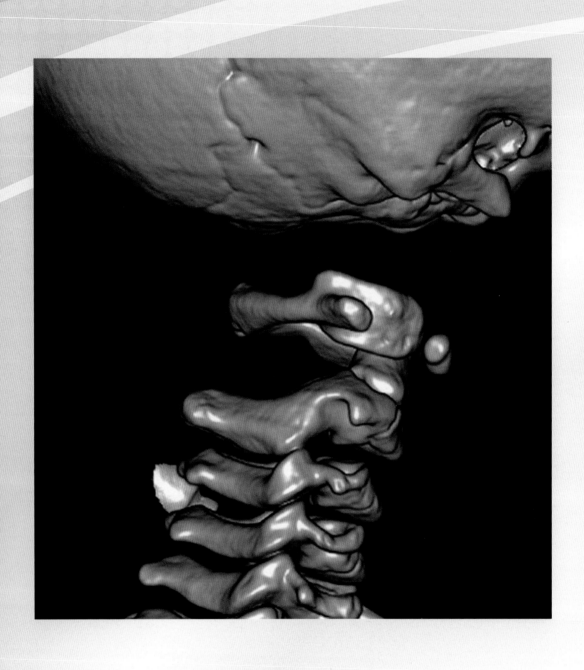

Chapter 11

Spine Trauma in Children

MICHAEL G. VITALE, MD, MPH and
RICHARD C. E. ANDERSON, MD

Gurus: Douglas L. Brockmeyer, MD and
Mark A. Erickson, MD, MMM

General Principles in Pediatric Spine Trauma

Significant pediatric spine trauma is fortunately rare but carries with it the possibility of significant trouble. Given the obvious challenges in obtaining a clear history and examination, and issues with imaging, diagnosis of these injuries can be difficult. Have a very high index for suspicion of a spine injury when presented with a child with multiple injuries or high-energy trauma.

It is helpful to understand a bit about the developmental anatomy and biomechanics of the growing spine as these injuries often follow specific patterns related to age and location.

Until around 8 or 9 years of age, the maturing spine is much more malleable resulting in specific injury patterns; after this age, the biomechanics approach those of adults, as do injury patterns.[1-3]

The main biomechanical difference between the pediatric and adult spine is that the developing spine is less ossified and more elastic. The child's spine is an able to undergo considerable movement between vertebral segments without damage, but at the cost of providing less protection to the underlying spinal cord.

For example, about half of all spine *injuries* in children involve the cervical spine, with the level of injury moving more caudal with progressive age. However, *fractures* of the cervical spine (as opposed to ligamentous injuries, subluxation, etc.) are less common until children are older than 13 years. To stay out of trouble, both fractures and ligamentous injuries must be ruled out prior to cervical spine clearance in young children. Similarly, thoracolumbar injuries are less common until adolescence.

It is also important to be aware that children very commonly sustain injuries at multiple levels of the spine (either contiguous or not), so it is important to carefully survey the entire spinal column in children. Don't be satisfied with the identification of a single abnormality; our job is to make sure the entire spine is clear. Finally, in younger children without an obvious history of high-energy trauma such as a fall or motor vehicle accident (MVA), it's important to rule out nonaccidental injury (child abuse) or pathological fracture.[4]

Given the plasticity of the child's spine, younger children can sustain pure ligamentous injuries without bony fracture. SCIWORA (spinal cord injury without radiographic abnormality) is a rare injury where there is subluxation or distraction of the spinal column, which then bounces back to its anatomical position "without radiographic abnormality."[5]

Strictly speaking, SCIWORA really means that there are no changes on MRI, but MRI in these cases often reveals disruption of the posterior ligaments and/or increased signal in the spinal cord. It is surprisingly common for SCIWORA to present up to 24 hours after the injury, so repeated neurological examinations are wise in a child with significant trauma, such as an MVA. Children with neurological injury in the cervical or thoracic spine can rapidly develop scoliosis (Fig. 11-1).

Evaluation of Children With Suspected Spine Injuries

The initial history and physical examination is critical. Learn as much detail as possible about the mechanism of injury, and search for signs of head injury or skin findings such as a lap belt sign across the abdomen. Remember that the disproportionately large head of young children will put them in a position of relative flexion/kyphosis if immobilized flat. The torso therefore needs to be bolstered if a cervical spine injury is suspected (Fig. 11-2). Similarly, a cervical collar can be

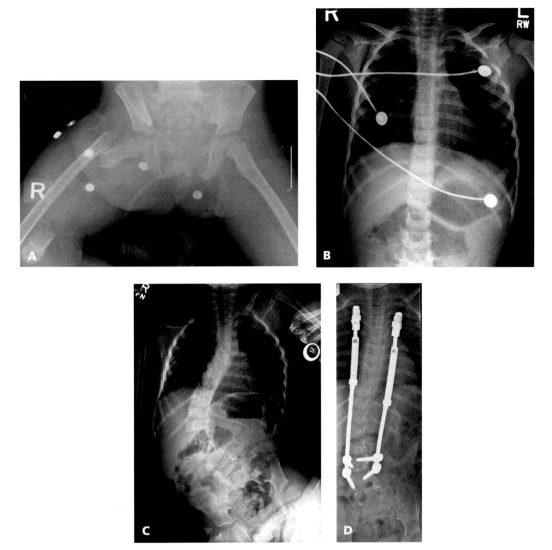

Figure 11-1 A 3-year-old boy presented after being struck by a car as a pedestrian. **A:** He had sustained multiple injuries, including head trauma, epidural hematoma, bilateral pneumothoraces with right lung contusion, multiple right rib fractures, ruptured bladder, pelvic fracture, and right femoral fracture. **B:** X-rays show no evidence spinal injury. Eight months later, the patient developed severe scoliosis **(C)**, which was treated with vertical expandable prosthetic titanium rib (VEPTR) **(D)**.

too large for young patients resulting in dangerous distraction forces. A history of loss of consciousness or facial or skull or even clavicle injury should raise concern about a possible cervical spine injury. In about 40% of children with cervical spine injuries, additional orthopaedic injuries are reported. Once any spine injury is noted, imaging and physical examination of the entire spine must carefully be assessed for other distant spine injuries, which are not uncommon. The isolated spine fracture should really be a diagnosis of exclusion.

If there is a potential spinal cord injury (SCI), document a thorough neurologic examination. Spinal shock results in loss of the bulbocavernosus reflex which almost always returns within 24 hours after injury. Complete injuries are defined by the absence of motor and sensory function below the level of SCI after the resolution of spinal shock. Sacral sparing, the presence of perianal sensation, rectal motor function, and/or great toe flexor function indicates a good prognosis for neurologic recovery.

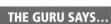 **THE GURU SAYS...**

Intubated, chemically paralyzed patients with head injuries in the pediatric intensive care unit (PICU) can have their hard cervical collars removed for periods of time in order to prevent pressure sores. As the patient wakes up, the collar goes back on until the neck is formally cleared.

DOUGLAS BROCKMEYER

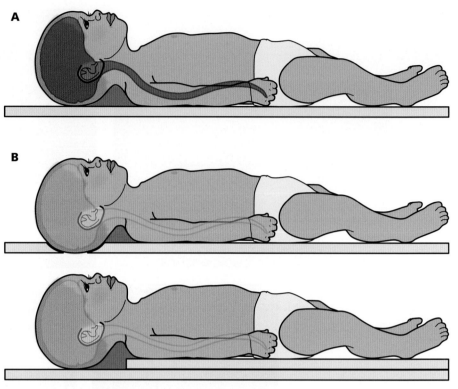

Figure 11-2 A: The relatively large head of the child forces the injured spine into flexion and can be a problem. **B:** Children need a modified backboard to hold their cervical spine in neutral.

Cervical spine X-rays are a part of most initial trauma evaluations. If these initial films are normal, but the child has neck pain, tenderness, about the spine, or concern of injury and is awake and cooperative, flexion/extension lateral cervical spine radiographs should be the next step. To stay out of trouble, clinicians should remember that ligamentous injury is more common than osseous injury in children and cannot be excluded based on normal bony anatomy demonstrated on static radiographs or CT scans. Don't be fooled by certain, classic false positives in children. These include retropharyngeal "swelling" due to crying and C2-3 pseudosubluxation (Fig. 11-3). Advanced imaging, including CT and MRI, is often necessary to better assess suspected spine injury in children. MRI has shown to be an effective method for clearing the cervical spine in obtunded children. As the sensitivity of MRI to detect edema associated with ligamentous injury is reduced after 48 hours from spinal column trauma, the study should be obtained within this time interval in order to be diagnostic.[6] So the bottom line is if in doubt, MRI the spine early.

While there is no consensus on which particular protocol is best, the use of defined protocols decreases the time needed to clear the cervical spine in children, reduces the number of missed injuries, and facilitates clearance by nonneurosurgical medical staff.[7-11] Figure 11-4 is a useful algorithm recently developed by a multidisciplinary group that stratifies by GCS rather than age or mechanism of injury.

THE GURU SAYS...

When clearing the pediatric cervical spine after trauma, a normal CT scan is extremely powerful. It is rare to need surgical stabilization if you have a normal cervical spine CT.

Douglas Brockmeyer

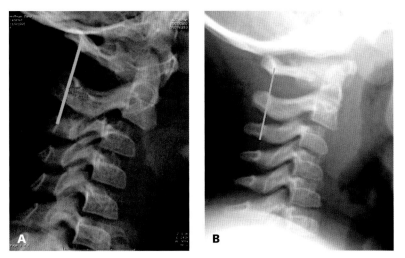

Figure 11-3 Pseudosubluxation of C2/C3. **A:** Pathological subluxation of C2/C3 with more than 1.5 mm step-off of the spinolaminar line (Swischuk line) drawn from spinolaminar point on C1 to C3. The spinolaminar point on C2 should be within 1.5 mm of the spinolaminar line. **B:** Pathological pseudosubluxation of C2/C3 with no significant stepoff at posterior line. Around 20% of children admitted for polytrauma will demonstrate this incidental finding, most commonly seen at C2/C3 and in children younger than 8 years. (Used with permission of the Children's Orthopaedic Center, Los Angeles.)

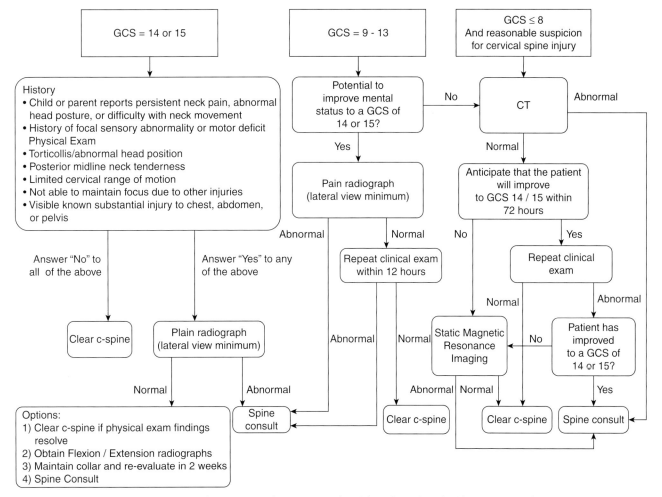

Figure 11-4 Pediatric cervical spine clearance working group algorithm. (Reprinted with permission from Herman MJ, Brown KO, Sponseller PD, et al. Pediatric cervical spine clearance: A Consensus Statement and Algorithm from the Pediatric Cervical Spine Clearance Working Group. *J Bone Joint Surg Am.* 2019;101(2):e1. Copyright © 2019 by The Journal of Bone and Joint Surgery, Incorporated.)

Traumatic Injuries of the Cervical Spine

ATLANTO-OCCIPITAL DISLOCATION

Atlanto-occipital dislocation (AOD) involves traumatic separation of the occiput from C1 and is an injury that occurs much more frequently in the pediatric population, due to the laxity of the ligamentous structures anchoring the occiput to the axial skeleton. Resulting from high-energy deceleration such as occurs in pedestrian MVAs, these injuries in children are often lethal. The dislocation usually severs the spinal cord at the foramen magnum, resulting in acute respiratory arrest[12] (Fig. 11-5).

To stay out of trouble, understand that these injuries may often not be appreciated on the initial presentation of the child to the trauma center. Some of these injuries reduce in the field or on transport to the trauma facility and then are not discovered until radiographs are done in a different position, especially traction. It is important to keep in mind that most survivors of AOD, including those with a severe initial presentation such a flaccid quadriplegia, have incomplete injuries and ultimately may have a good outcome. Radiographic findings on plain films may be subtle and AOD should be suspected in any child involved in a high-speed trauma, especially those presenting with cardiopulmonary instability and associated facial injuries. Maintain a high index of suspicion and obtain a thin-cut CT imaging from the occiput to at least C2 with sagittal and coronal reconstructions. The most accurate way to diagnose AOD is by measuring the condyle-C1 joint interval (CCI) on CT.[13] A CCI of greater than 4 mm in either the sagittal or coronal plane for one or both O-C1 joints is considered a positive finding (Fig. 11-6). AOD is exceedingly unstable so prompt external immobilization is critical. Stay out of trouble by remembering that cervical traction is contraindicated after AOD as it may result in additional cervicomedullary injury. Given that AOD is extremely unstable and there is a very real risk of further neurological injury with inadequate immobilization, internal fixation and fusion from O-C2 is typically performed.

C-1 INJURIES (JEFFERSON FRACTURE)

These injuries present some challenges in diagnosis. It is important to distinguish a Jefferson fracture (Fig. 11-7) from an unfused synchondrosis, which is generally

> **THE GURU SAYS...**
>
> AOD injuries require substantial forces to occur. Accordingly, beware of children presenting with severe head or facial injuries as they may also have an associated cervical spine injury like AOD.
>
> MARK ERICKSON

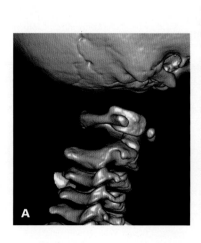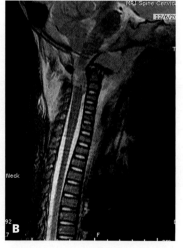

Figure 11-5 A: CT of a 1-year-old struck by a car demonstrating occiput-C1 dislocation. **B:** MRI demonstrates transection of the spinal cord. (Used with permission of the Children's Orthopaedic Center, Los Angeles.)

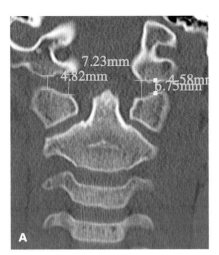
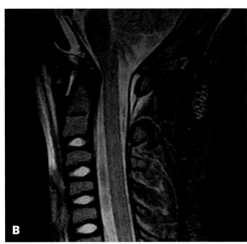
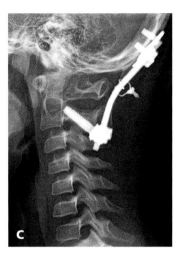

Figure 11-6 A: A 10-year-old boy pedestrian hit by a car presented with GCS 8 and imaging consistent with atlanto-occipital dislocation (AOD). **B:** Coronal CT demonstrates increased condylar-C1 interval (CCI) bilaterally and sagittal short-TI inversion recovery (STIR) MRI demonstrate ligamentous injury with clival hematoma. **C:** Postoperative lateral radiograph after occipital-C2 stabilization using rigid internal fixation and iliac crest structural allograft with cable.

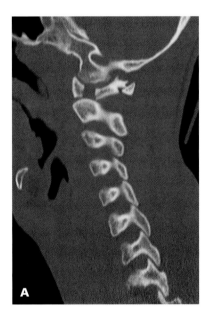
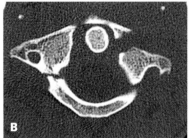
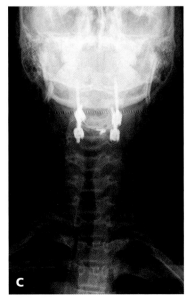
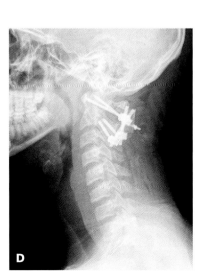

Figure 11-7 This 14-year-old boy had neck pain after colliding with a tree while snowboarding. **A, B:** Sagittal and axial CTs show multiple C1 fractures with displacement. MRI (not shown) demonstrated ligamentous injury. **C, D:** Postoperative AP and lateral radiographs after bilateral C1 lateral mass fixation, C2 pars screws, and iliac crest allograft with wire.

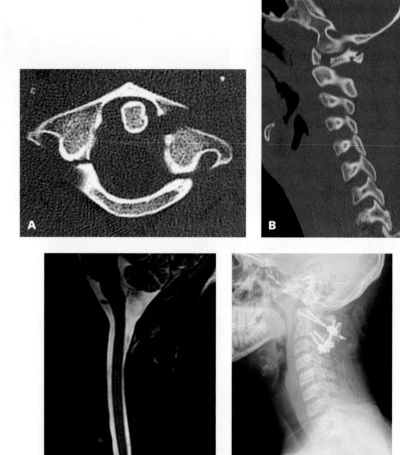

Figure 11-8 A 13-year-old boy brought in by EMS after head on collision playing football complaining of neck pain. Sagittal **(A)** and axial **(B)** CT scans demonstrate Jefferson fracture, and sagittal short-TI inversion recovery (STIR) MRI **(C)** shows ligamentous injury. **D:** Postoperative lateral radiograph after C1-C2 stabilization with rigid internal fixation and structural iliac crest allograft with cable.

not of any clinical significance. Alternatively, C1 fractures may occur through the synchondrosis and can be missed on plain radiographs. Atlas fractures may be accompanied by disruption of the transverse ligament, resulting in atlantoaxial instability. There is a high incidence of associated C2 fracture. CT imaging has led to an increased recognition of these fractures children[14] (Fig. 11-8). On odontoid view radiographs, transverse ligament disruption is suggested if the sum of the total overhang of the C1 lateral masses on C2 is 7 mm or more (the "rule of Spence"). Treatment of isolated Jefferson fractures with an intact transverse ligament is generally external immobilization in a rigid cervical collar, Minerva brace, or halo. If there is transverse ligament rupture and atlantoaxial instability, treatment should involve either halo immobilization or, rarely, C1-2 internal stabilization and fusion.

Translational Atlantoaxial (C1-2) Subluxation

Most of these injuries are nontraumatic in nature, associated with developmental disorders that result in either laxity of the transverse ligament or odontoid hypoplasia (i.e., Down syndrome, Klippel-Feil syndrome, juvenile rheumatoid arthritis, Morquio syndrome, skeletal dysplasias). Traumatic translational atlantoaxial subluxation can occur, but mortality is high C1/C2 instability is diagnosed by studying the atlanto-dens interval (ADI). The ADI in children has an upper limit of normal of 5 mm. If the ADI is greater than 5 mm on flexion/extension lateral radiographs in the setting of trauma, a C1/C2 fusion is recommended.

Atlantoaxial Rotatory Subluxation and Instability

Atlantoaxial rotatory subluxation and instability can also occur from traumatic and nontraumatic causes. Patients can present with mild rotatory subluxation or with a fixed position with no motion. Only 30% of these cases are traumatic in nature, usually from only minor trauma. When it comes to diagnosing C1-C2 rotatory subluxation, stay out of trouble by remembering that it is often best diagnosed with dynamic ("three-position") CT study[15,16] (Fig. 11-9).

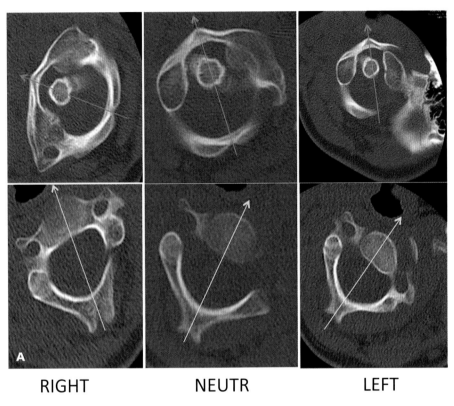

RIGHT   NEUTR   LEFT

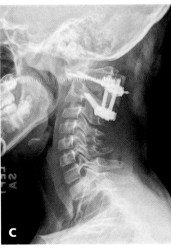

Figure 11-9 A 9-year-old girl had a fall while climbing tree (low height) and developed neck pain and head tilt. She was observed for 3 months by local physicians then referred for physical therapy without improvement. **A:** Three-position axial CT at 6 months demonstrates locked C1-C2 rotatory subluxation. **B, C:** AP and lateral radiographs after open reduction, fixation, and fusion with structural iliac crest allograft and wire.

ODONTOID FRACTURES

Odontoid fractures are generally related to translational C1-2 subluxation as a result of epiphysiolysis at the dentocentral synchondrosis, which is located slightly lower than the base of the dens within the rostral aspect of the C2 vertebral body, and is not fused until 8 to 11 years of age. This leads to a pattern similar to a type II odontoid fracture in adults. Many pediatric odontoid fractures will heal with reduction and halo vest immobilization. To stay out of trouble, be certain to get a satisfactory reduction, and document maintenance of reduction over the first 2 to 4 weeks. Most pediatric odontoid fractures will heal readily with immobilization, but they should be followed for at least a year. Some cases of os odontoideum are nonunions of early childhood odontoid fractures that either did not present at the time of injury or were missed.

HANGMAN'S (C2 PEDICLE) FRACTURE

Hangman's fractures are rare in the pediatric population. Treatment of C2 pedicle fractures is similar to that in adults. If the body of the atlas is not significantly displaced on C3, immobilization in a rigid collar should be adequate. If there is anterior displacement greater than 3 mm, external immobilization in a halo vest or Minerva cast is more appropriate. Surgical fusion is rarely required.

SUBAXIAL SPINE INJURIES

Subaxial cervical spine injuries can be divided into pure ligamentous injuries, anterior columns injuries, posterior column injuries, and combined anterior posterior injuries. Neck pain that persists for several weeks following trauma is unusual and should be investigated with radiological studies. White and Panjabi demonstrated that horizontal displacement of one vertebral body on another greater than 3.5 mm is consistent with significant ligamentous rupture in adults.[17] The pediatric spine exhibits greater physiologic movement in the horizontal plane than the adult spine. As such, displacement up to 4.5 mm at a given segmental level may be considered normal, and is termed pseudosubluxation, most commonly seen at C2-3 and C3-4.[2]

Most authors agree that a kyphotic angulation of more than 7° likely represents a significant ligamentous injury that may predispose the developing spine to further kyphosis and instability. CT scanning is helpful here. Patients with significant kyphotic deformities or unstable injuries (burst fracture with spinal cord compromise and fractures associated with significant ligamentous disruption) should be managed surgically (Fig. 11-10). Most osseous anterior column injuries in the subaxial cervical spine are stable fractures and heal in 4 to 6 weeks with conservative treatment. However, retropulsion of bone into the spinal canal can result in a neurological deficit warranting anterior cervical corpectomy and fusion with plating.

Osseous Posterior Column Injuries

Injuries to the bony elements of the posterior column of the subaxial cervical spine encompass several types of fractures, including those to the facets (including jumped and perched facets), lamina, pedicles, and spinous processes (clay shoveler's fracture). Isolated osseous posterior column injuries are rare in children and

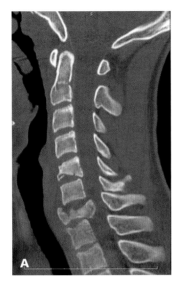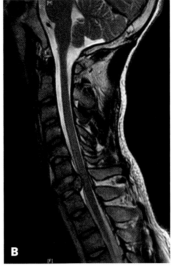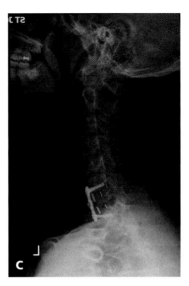

Figure 11-10 A 16-year-old-boy presented with neck pain and transient paresthesias after a snowboarding accident. Sagittal CT **(A)** and T2 MRI **(B)** demonstrate C7 burst fracture with canal compromise and anterior C5 body fracture. **C:** Postoperative lateral radiograph after C7 corpectomy with interbody cage and C6-T1 instrumentation. He was maintained in a hard collar for 6 weeks postoperatively with observation of the C5 fracture.

most often occur in combination with ligamentous injury. Unilateral and bilateral facet dislocations have been reported in some series to be the second most common injury to the pediatric subaxial cervical spine.[18]

Unilateral facet injury should be suspected when neck pain is accompanied by an isolated nerve root finding. Closed reduction in the alert awake patient may be attempted in a monitored setting but open reduction is often necessary. To stay out of trouble, obtain an MRI prior to reduction, to assess for a herniated intervertebral disk or impending spinal cord compression that may be exacerbated during reduction maneuvers. If malalignment of the facets can be corrected with closed reduction, the injury may heal itself over time with external immobilization only. In these instances, it is critical to take into account the amount of associated ligamentous injury and whether the anterior column is additionally involved. If conservative treatment is pursued, flexion-extension radiographs should be obtained 2 or 3 months after trauma to assess for maintenance of stability. Persistent neck pain despite appropriate reduction and external stabilization should raise the suspicion of significant concomitant ligamentous injury, warranting consideration of surgical fusion.

Combined Anterior and Posterior Column Injuries

Combined anterior and posterior column injuries involve disruption of all supporting structures (bone, ligaments, and soft tissues) of the subaxial cervical spine at one or more levels. Fracture-dislocation injuries fall into this category. Most children with combined anterior and posterior column injuries present following severe trauma with a high-energy mechanism. A large percentage of these patients have evidence of a neurological deficit from SCI. The main challenges of instrumented fusion in children compared with adults are (1) whether the anatomy of a given patient can accommodate the required instrumentation and withstand the stress applied by the construct, (2) a reduced amount of bone

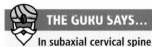
THE GURU SAYS...

In subaxial cervical spine trauma, both an anterior column injury and posterior column injury are necessary to create enough instability to require fusion.

DOUGLAS BROCKMEYER

surface for fusion to occur, and (3) the potential for alterations to spinal growth in young patients.

GENERAL SURGICAL PRINCIPLES IN CERVICAL SPINE TRAUMA

Positioning of the patient in the operating room is critical in children with cervical spine injuries. To stay out of trouble, remember that in the setting of cervical cord compression or an unstable cervical spine injury, fiberoptic nasotracheal intubation is usually the best approach in order to keep the cervical spine in neutral position. Somatosensory evoked potentials (SSEPs) and motor evoked potentials (MEPs) should be obtained both before and after positioning, as well as continued throughout the duration of the surgery.

Care must be taken during dissection of the pediatric spine. It is easy to get into trouble and inadvertently enter into the spinal canal through the midline cartilaginous tissue between nonfused laminae with monopolar electrocautery. Fusion of the laminae occurs postnatally, beginning in the lumbar spine, proceeding cranially, and is usually complete by 3 years of age. Nonfused laminae are most prevalent at the rostral and caudal ends of the spinal column, occurring at S1, L5, C1, C7, and T1, in order of decreasing frequency. In addition to careful dissection, discerning review of preoperative imaging can help prevent this error.

Traumatic Injuries of the Thoracic and Lumbar Spine

Thoracic and lumbar fractures are somewhat less common than cervical spine injuries in children and are most commonly the result of MVAs, falls, or other high-energy trauma. These injuries are generally described as they are in adults by the Denis classification, which includes compression (anterior wedge) fractures, burst fractures, flexion-distraction injuries (Chance fractures), and fracture-dislocations.

COMPRESSION FRACTURES

Compression fractures make up the most common fracture pattern, with loss of height of the anterior vertebra, classically from axial compression and/or flexion. Multiple vertebra are commonly involved. Neurological injury is rare, and pain is moderate so these fractures can present in a delayed manner. There is little reported about long-term outcomes of these injuries, but it is reasonable to treat patients with significant anterior wedging (especially over multiple levels) with a hyperextension thoracolumbar spinal orthosis (TLSO) in order to improve comfort, decrease activity, and perhaps stop the development of more kyphosis (Fig. 11-11). While radiographic follow-up on stable vertebral injuries in children is lacking, it appears that such injuries are generally not associated with long-term degenerative changes or disc disease.[19,20] Compression fractures can often be identified on lateral radiographs, but MRI is useful in better delineating the injury, ruling out other vertebral fractures which are common, and most importantly in identifying whether there is an associated posterior ligament injury.

BURST FRACTURES

Increased axial loads may cause vertebral burst fractures which involve both the anterior and middle columns. As opposed to compression fractures, burst fractures

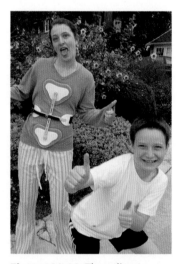

Figure 11-11 The editor's (D.L.S.) daughter demonstrates good patient acceptance of a hyperextension brace for a two-level lumbar compression fracture treated for 6 weeks. (Used with permission of the Children's Orthopaedic Center, Los Angeles.)

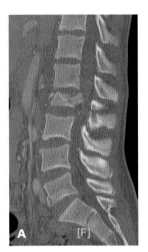 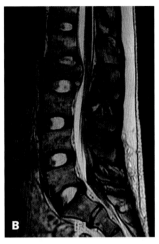 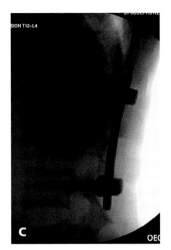 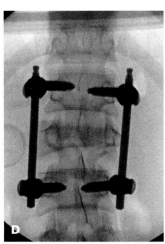

Figure 11-12 A 16-year-old girl jumped out of three-story window in a suicide attempt. Sagittal CT **(A)** and T2 MRI **(B)** demonstrate L2 burst fracture with three-column injury without significant canal compromise. Intraoperative AP **(C)** and lateral radiographs **(D)** after percutaneous L1-L3 instrumentation and stabilization.

more often result in retropulsion of bony fragments into the spinal canal, instability, and potential neurological compromise. Neurological compromise is more common in thoracic as compared with lumbar burst fractures.[21]

If the posterior ligamentous complex (PLC) is disrupted (which can be inferred from increased interspinous space in X-rays but best seen on MRI) it is likely the injury is actually a flexion-distraction injury. CT is helpful is assessing retropulsion and in quantifying the amount of kyphosis and loss of body height.

In children with no neurological symptoms and no evidence of instability (intact PLC), external immobilization in an extension TLSO for 8 to 12 weeks is appropriate for most patients. When the PLC is clearly disrupted, or in cases of neurological compromise, these fractures require decompression and surgical stabilization. Anterior, posterior, and (more recently) posterior percutaneous non-fusion techniques have been advocated for surgical treatment and the optimum approach in children remains controversial (Fig. 11-12). Dural leaks may occur as a result of tears sustained by fracture prompting some surgeons to prefer a percutaneous technique.[22]

FLEXION-DISTRACTION INJURIES (CHANCE FRACTURES)

Flexion-distraction injuries are often missed, even by spine surgeons.[23] These injuries classically result from forceful flexion of the lower thoracic spine over a lap seat belt without shoulder restraint and may leave a telltale sign on the abdomen (Fig. 11-13). On physical examination, there will be swelling and localized tenderness about the posterior elements that have failed in tension. If this is found on examination, get an MRI even in the setting of normal X-rays. X-rays do not always pick up interspinous ligament disruption. These injuries, which occur most commonly between T12-L2, involve all three and result in instability. To stay out of trouble, maintain a high index of suspicion for intra-abdominal injuries, which are commonly associated and often overshadowed by the spine injury. CT scanning is extremely useful to assess these injuries which can be underappreciated on plain X-rays. The classic finding on axial CT is the "empty facet" sign where distraction of the posterior elements interferes with the normal contact between inferior and superior facets so that only half of the facet at the injured level is captured on axial cuts (Fig. 11-14).

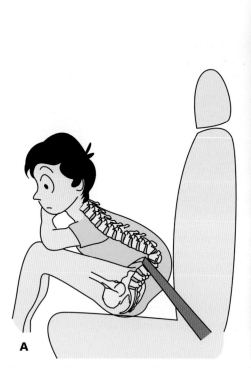
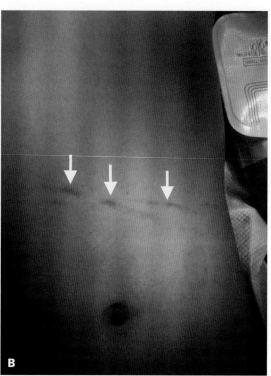

Figure 11-13 A: A lap belt used for a child can create a point of rotation about which the spine is flexed with an abrupt stop. This is a common mechanism for creating both intra-abdominal and flexion-distraction spinal injuries. **B:** A seatbelt sign may be subtle, as in this example of horizontal ecchymosis in the setting of a soft tissue L2–L3 chance fracture. In this case, the injury was missed on the initial radiology reading, and the clinical picture helped establish the diagnosis. Arrows demonstrate horizontal ecchymosis across the abdomen consistent with a seatbelt sign. (A: Reprinted with permission from Newton PO, Upasani VV. Thoracolumbar spine fractures. In: Waters PM, Skaggs DL, Flynn JM, eds. *Rockwood and Wilkins' Fractures in Children*. 9th ed. Philadelphia, PA: Wolters Kluwer; 2020:822-843. Figure 1.B: Used with permission of the Children's Orthopaedic Center, Los Angeles.)

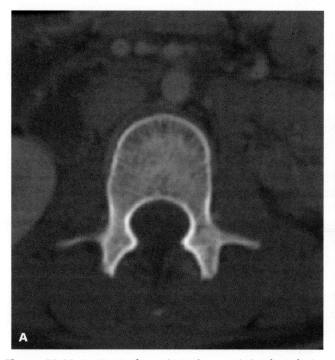
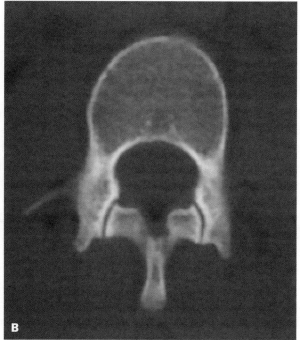

Figure 11-14 A: "Empty facet sign" characteristic of a soft tissue chance fracture. Normally, there would be both superior and inferior facets present in a transverse CT cut, but with separation of the posterior elements, only the superior facet is visualized. **B:** In contrast, this is an image of normal facet joints at an uninjured level in the same patient. (Used with permission of the Children's Orthopaedic Center, Los Angeles.)

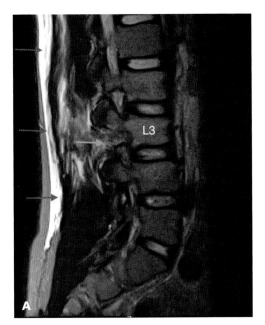
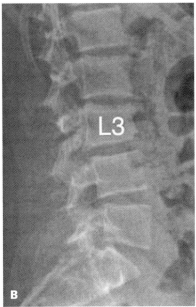
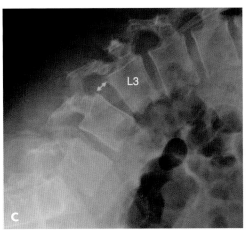

Figure 11-15 A: Classic MRI findings for a Chance fracture are disruption of the interspinous ligament (green arrow) and voluminous subcutaneous hematoma (red arrows), which is palpable as a boggy mass on fresh fractures. **B:** Unfortunately, this 14-year-old boy was treated conservatively. Standing X-rays 14 months later show some kyphosis. **C:** Flexion X-rays 14 months after the injury show gross instability. (Used with permission of the Children's Orthopaedic Center, Los Angeles.)

These horizontal fractures can be missed on the axial screening abdominal CT, so it is important to obtain multiplanar imaging when assessing Chance fractures. MRI imaging is essential to assess if there is an injury of the posterior ligaments, which render these injuries more unstable and less likely to heal without surgery (Fig. 11-15). In the uncommon purely boney Chance fracture (Fig. 11-16), as long as kyphosis can be corrected in a brace, the fracture can be treated conservatively. In the much more common Chance fracture with posterior ligamentous disruption, a posterior spinal fusion with instrumentation is the treatment of choice.[24]

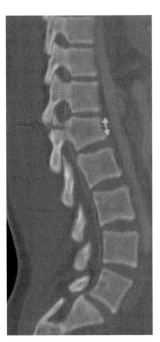

Figure 11-16 A pure bony Chance fracture with failure in tension through the posterior elements (red arrow) and compression across the vertebral body (green arrow). (Used with permission of the Children's Orthopaedic Center, Children's Hospital Los Angeles.)

FRACTURE-DISLOCATIONS

Among the most severe and unstable thoracolumbar fractures are fracture-dislocations, which result from more complex loading mechanisms. Nonaccidental injury has been associated with these injuries in very young children.[25]

Rates of neurological injury, including complete paraplegia, are high. While these injuries are often not radiographically subtle, at times the injury can self-reduce and X-rays can understate the extent of displacement that occurred. CT and MRI should be obtained to better define the injury and canal compromise, as well as to assess for very common associated injuries, including rib and pelvic fractures. These injuries generally require urgent operative decompression and stabilization to provide the best chance for neurological recovery, to prevent additional injury related to instability, and to allow more aggressive rehabilitation.

APOPHYSEAL RING OR GROWTH PLATE FRACTURES

Just like long bones, vertebrae have growth plates that are areas of weakness and subject to fracture. Growth plate fractures are often initially missed in kids, and misdiagnosed as a bulging disk (Fig. 11-17). Stay out of trouble by remembering that disk herniations in the immature skeleton are uncommon, and that an apophyseal ring fracture is best seen on CT.

> **THE GURU SAYS...**
>
> Thoracolumbar spine fracture-dislocations commonly result in complete spinal cord injuries. In this population, early stabilization of the spine is quite important to facilitate the necessary rehabilitation for SCI patients to achieve an optimal outcome.
>
> MARK ERICKSON

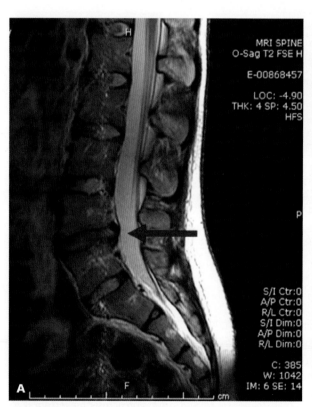
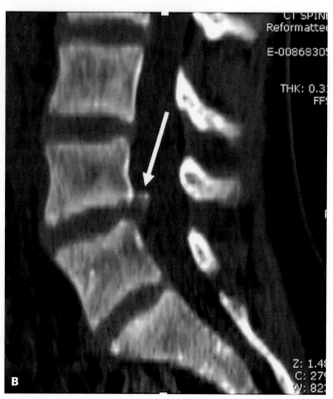

Figure 11-17 A 14-year-old girl felt a pop while kicking a soccer ball and had severe back pain. Months of steroid injections did nothing to relieve her pain. She was unable to walk or go to school. **A:** Arrow demonstrates L4 inferior end plate fracture on MRI. **B:** CT scan confirmed diagnosis of an end plate fracture. Surgical removal of the intracanal fragment adjacent to nerve roots relieved pain and the patient was able to return to soccer within a few weeks. Arrow more clearly demonstrates same injury on CT. (Used with permission of the Children's Orthopaedic Center, Los Angeles.)

Staying Out of Trouble With Spine Trauma in Children

✳ Remember that children's spines are different. Before about 10 years of age, children are more likely than older kids to sustain pure ligamentous injury and injuries to the upper cervical spine. Don't forget about SCIWORA, a uniquely pediatric injury.

✳ Injury level, pattern, and stability are directly influenced by the unique anatomic and biomechanical characteristics of the pediatric spinal column. The transition from an immature to mature spine, in biomechanical terms, occurs at roughly 8 or 9 years of age.

✳ The isolated pediatric spine injury should really be a diagnosis of exclusion given the high frequency of multiple spine injuries (contiguous and noncontiguous).

✳ Spinal column trauma is more likely to result in ligamentous injury rather than fractures in young children; the older the child, the more likely that a given injury involves a fracture.

✳ Most pediatric spine injuries can be treated with immobilization; however, surgical intervention is indicated for spinal column involving all three columns of the spine.

✳ Decompression of neural compression is a true surgical urgency, and children have a much higher chance of neurological recovery than adults.

✳ Distracting forces (e.g., traction) should be considered carefully in young children with cervical spine injuries given the high incidence of occipitocervical and atlantoaxial instability in this age group.

✳ Dynamic imaging and MRI, when appropriate, is of particular importance in the diagnosis of pediatric spinal column trauma given the high incidence of purely ligamentous injuries.

✳ MRI is often helpful in assessing the posterior ligamentous complex to determine the involvement of the posterior column which can affect treatment.

✳ Treatment of unstable injuries with rigid internal fixation and fusion often allows for a reduction in the duration and intensity of external immobilization.

SOURCES OF WISDOM

1. Bailey DK. The normal cervical spine in infants and children. *Radiology*. 1952;59(5):712-719.
2. Cattell HS, Filtzer DL. Pseudosubluxation and other normal variations in the cervical spine in children: a study of one hundred and sixty children. *J Bone Joint Surg Am*. 1965;47(7):1295-1309.
3. Fesmire FM, Luten RC. The pediatric cervical spine: developmental anatomy and clinical aspects. *J Emerg Med*. 1989;7:133-142.
4. Cirak B, Ziegfeld S, Knight VM, et al. Spinal injuries in children. *J Pediatr Surg*. 2004;39(4):607-612.
5. Pang D, Wilberger JE. Spinal cord injury without radiographic abnormalities in children. *J Neurosurg*. 1982;57(1):114-129.
6. Hadely MN. Management of pediatric cervical spine and spinal cord injuries. *Neurosurgery*. 2002;50(3 suppl):S85-S99.
7. Anderson RCE, Kan P, Vanaman M, et al. Utility of a cervical spine clearance protocol after trauma in children between 0 and 3 years of age. *J Neurosurg Pediatr*. 2010;5:292-296.
8. Anderson RCE, Scaife ER, Fenton SJ, et al. Cervical spine clearance after trauma children. *J Neurosurg*. 2006;105(5 suppl):361-364.
9. Brockmeyer DL, Ragel BT, Kestle JRW. The pediatric cervical spine instability study: a pilot study assessing the prognostic value of four imaging modalities in clearing the cervical spine for children with severe traumatic injuries. *Childs Nerv Syst*. 2012;28(5):699-705.

10. Frank JB, Lim CK, Flynn JM, Dormans JP. The efficacy of magnetic resonance imaging in pediatric cervical spine clearance. *Spine*. 2002;27(11):1176-1179.

11. Viccellio P, Simon H, Pressman BD. A prospective multicenter study of cervical spine injury in children. *Pediatrics*. 2001;108:E20.

12. Kaufman RA, Carroll CD, Buncher CR. Atlantooccipital junction: standards for measurement in normal children. *AJNR Am J Neuroradiol*. 1987;8:995-999.

13. Harris JH, Carson GC, Wagner LK, Kerr N. Radiologic diagnosis of traumatic occipitovertebral dislocation: 2. Comparison of three methods of detecting occipitovertebral relationships on lateral radiographs of supine subjects. *AJR Am J Radiol*. 1994;162:887-892.

14. Li Y, Glotzbecker MP, Hedequist D, Mahan ST. Pediatric spinal trauma. *Trauma*. 2011;14(1):82-96.

15. Lee V, Pang D. *Atlanto-axial rotatory fixation*. In: *Disorders of the Pediatric Spine*. New York, NY: Raven Press; 1995:531-553.

16. McGuire KJ, Silber J, Flynn JM, et al. Torticollis in children: can dynamic computed tomography help determine severity and treatment. *J Pediatr Orthop*. 2002;22(6):766-770.

17. White AA, Panjabi MM. *Clinical Biomechanics of the Spine*. Philadelphia, PA: JB Lippincott; 1990.

18. Ware ML, Auguste KI, Gupta N, et al. Traumatic injuries of the pediatric craniocervical junction. In: Brockmeyer D, ed. *Advanced Pediatric Craniocervical Surgery*. New York, NY: Thieme Medical Publishers; 2005:55-74.

19. Möller A, Maly P, Besjakov J, et al. A vertebral fracture in childhood is not a risk factor for disc degeneration but for Schmorl's nodes: a mean 40-year observational study. *Spine (Phila Pa 1976)*. 2007;32(22):2487-2492.

20. Möller A, Hasserius R, Besjakov J, et al. Vertebral fractures in late adolescence: a 27 to 47-year follow-up. *Eur Spine J*. 2006;15(8):1247-1254.

21. Vander Have KL, Caird MS, Gross S, et al. Burst fractures of the thoracic and lumbar spine in children and adolescents. *J Pediatr Orthop*. 2009;29(7):713-719.

22. Chou PH, Ma HL, Wang ST, et al. Fusion may not be a necessary procedure for surgically treated burst fractures of the thoracolumbar and lumbar spines: a follow-up of at least ten years. *J Bone Joint Surg Am*. 2014;96(20):1724-1731.

23. Andras LM, Skaggs KF, Badkoobehi H, et al. Chance fractures in the pediatric population are often misdiagnosed. *J Pediatr Orthop*. 2019;39:222-225.

24. Arkader A, Warner WC Jr, Tolo VT, et al. Pediatric Chance fractures: a multicenter perspective. *J Pediatr Orthop*. 2011;31:741-744.

25. Levin TL, Berdon WE, Cassell I, Blitman NM. Thoracolumbar fracture with listhesis—an uncommon manifestation of child abuse. *Pediatr Radiol*. 2003;33(5):305-310.

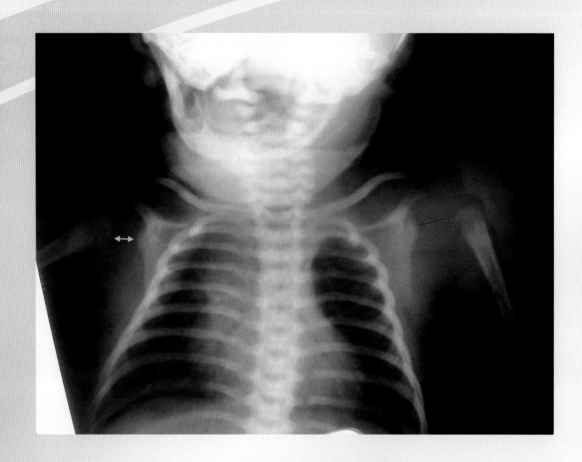

SPECIAL MALADIES AND CONCERNS

Chapter 12

Issues of the Newborn

DAVID L. SKAGGS, MD, MMM and JOHN M. (JACK) FLYNN, MD

Gurus: Paul D. Sponseller, MD and Jeffrey M. Bender, MD

Just as children are not merely little adults, newborns are not just little children. When you are called for a consult in the neonatal intensive care unit (NICU), remember that newborns and premature infants have their own unique physiology and pathology, hence the field of neonatology. While orthopaedic consults to the NICU or obstetrics are not too common, there are pearls and pitfalls worthy of discussion.

Infant's Arm Doesn't Move

One of the more common reasons for an orthopaedic consultation in the newborn nursery is for an infant who does not move an arm. The diagnoses that come quickly to mind are brachial plexus injury or fracture. However, infection is the most important diagnosis to make, as it can usually be treated successfully if recognized early, but may lead to permanent disability if the diagnosis is delayed (Fig. 12-1).

A newborn with a painful limb will demonstrate pseudoparalysis and not move the limb voluntarily. To the inexperienced, this may be misinterpreted as a true paralysis or brachial plexus injury. One approach to help differentiate pseudoparalysis from paralysis is to shake the arm; if you are being observed, perhaps explain what you are doing so you do not look like a calloused orthopod. If the child reacts to movement with pain, the diagnosis is likely fracture or infection. If there is no sign of pain, the diagnosis is likely neurologic injury. A potential pitfall of this approach is that an infant may have a fracture or infection *and* a brachial plexus injury, so a neurologic examination is essential even in the case of a known fracture or infection. One series reported that nearly 10% of newborns with a clavicle fracture also had a brachial plexus palsy.[1]

> ### THE GURU SAYS...
>
> The Moro reflex (allowing the head to gently extend) can help to distinguish a child with a fracture or infection from a child with a brachial plexus injury. A child with a fracture or infection will still move the arm somewhat while one with a brachial plexus palsy will not.
>
> PAUL D. SPONSELLER

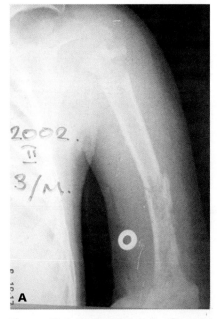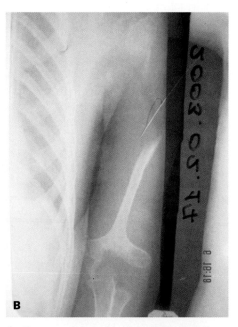

Figure 12-1 A: The diagnosis of neonatal infection was delayed in this child. An AP radiograph of the humerus at 3 months of age demonstrates significant osteomyelitis and subsequent fractures. **B:** Approximately 1 year later, there is an absence of most of the proximal humerus and severe changes of the distal humerus as well.

Infection

When dealing with the clinical diagnosis of infections in newborns, we enter into a different universe. In the first week of life, normal white blood cell count ranges between 9000 and 30,000 cells/mL. A total white cell count below 5000 cell/mL is generally considered to be suggestive of severe infection, although some overlap between infected and noninfected neonates occurs. Although over half of neonates with sepsis present with fever, hypothermia may be the leading sign of infection in 15% to 20% of infected neonates.

The diagnosis of osteoarticular infection may be suspected on clinical examination by a limb that appears painful when moved. In the absence of an obvious fracture on radiographs, an ultrasound should be performed which may demonstrate a septic shoulder or subperiosteal collection. Significant intra-articular pus may cause subluxation or dislocation of the joint (Fig. 12-2). A septic shoulder requires urgent surgical drainage if the newborn's condition permits. Adjacent osteomyelitis should be expected, as vessels cross the physis at this age. Of course, many of the principals here apply to the lower extremities as well. In particular, if there is a septic hip, the other hip should be closely investigated with ultrasound and/or aspiration (Fig. 12-3).

Most osteoarticular infections in this age group will be due to *Staphylococcus aureus*. That being said, given the high-risk nature of this population, Group B *Streptococcus*, *Escherichia coli*, *Kingella kingae*, *Candida* species, and other pathogens are seen much more commonly here than in older children. Obtaining cultures to help direct therapy is critical in successfully treating these infections (Fig. 12-4). There are some odd infections in the newborn, such as calcaneal osteomyelitis following a heel stick.[2]

> **THE GURU SAYS...**
>
> Although the erythrocyte sedimentation rate (ESR) is less reliable in newborns than in later age groups, elevated C-reactive protein (CRP) values have an approximately 60% positive predictive value for infection. More importantly, normal CRP values are very useful in ruling out infections with a negative predictive value exceeding 95%.
>
> JEFFREY BENDER

> **THE GURU SAYS...**
>
> Unfortunately, examinations in neonates can be exceedingly challenging. Many infants in NICUs are born prematurely and require significant medical interventions (lines, ventilators, etc.), which put them at high risk for invasive infections and make orthopaedic evaluations that much more difficult. It is of utmost importance to maintain appropriate infection prevention measures for these immunologically immature neonates. The most important thing we can all do to help is to adhere to strict hand hygiene practices whenever examining these infants.
>
> JEFFREY BENDER

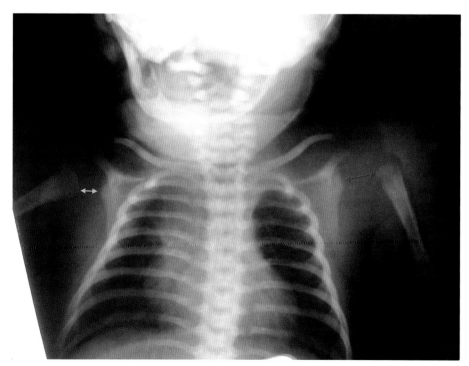

Figure 12-2 Note increased lateral translation of the proximal Humerus (red arrow) in routine chest X-ray, which helped diagnose a septic shoulder. Green arrow is the normal side.

THE GURU SAYS...

Check for finger movement to determine severity and prognosis. A high percentage of cases end up as malpractice suits against obstetricians. Do what you can early to defuse the situation. Make the referrals yourself so that patient falls into care of a knowledgeable orthopaedic surgeon. Many other (nonortho) specialists treating this condition do not have as much knowledge of natural history and of all treatment options.

PAUL D. SPONSELLER

THE GURU SAYS...

Slings for humeral fractures can be made with loop of stockinette (Fig. 12-7), or you can just fasten the sleeve of the garment to the chest with a safety pin. Another option for midshaft humerus fracture is to make functional above-elbow splint out of tongue depressors taped together.

PAUL D. SPONSELLER

THE GURU SAYS...

Pavlik is good for femur fractures in the first 3 months of life. However, in 3- to 6-month-old babies, I prefer a single-leg Gore-tex soft-cast spica for greater comfort. It is almost as easy to apply and is washable. The Pavlik does not rigidly immobilize the fracture. I have referenced an article that, while documenting the "success" of Pavlik for fractures, shows higher pain scores.[5]

PAUL D. SPONSELLER

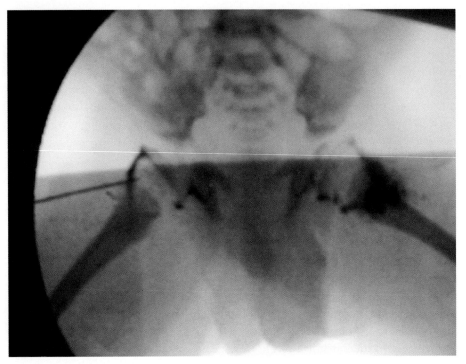

Figure 12-3 In newborns with a septic hip, the opposite hip should be evaluated very carefully for sepsis with aspiration and/or ultrasound.

Brachial Plexus Injury

There are many degrees of injury to the brachial plexus. In the most common type with upper plexus involvement, or Erb palsy, the characteristic appearance of waiter's tip—shoulder internal rotation, elbow extension, forearm pronation, and wrist flexion (Fig. 12-5)—aids in diagnosis. The surgeon should be aware that the phrenic nerve may be involved as well as a Horner syndrome (ptosis, miosis, and enophthalmos). Physical therapy should be started to maintain motion, as muscle imbalance may rapidly lead to contracture and joint incongruence.

Fractures

The big pitfall in fractures is a physeal fracture of the proximal humerus, or less commonly the distal humerus (Fig. 12-6). The humeral head and capitellum are not yet ossified, so the fracture is not easily appreciated on plain radiographs. On examination, there should be fullness, tenderness, and often warmth, similar to an infection. An ultrasound demonstrates the fracture. So the following clinical algorithm will help one make the diagnosis: arm hurts with movement, get a radiograph or ultrasound, depending on what is best at your institution. A radiograph will not show infection or some physeal fractures, so if the radiograph is negative, one must get an ultrasound. An ultrasound in the hands of an experienced user is probably the best study.[3]

Other fractures of the upper extremity and clavicle are more easily diagnosed on plain radiographs. Healing is very rapid, and outcome is benign with extensive remodeling the rule.[4] In the newborn, immobilization in generally needed for only 7 to 10 days (Fig. 12-8). For children with multiple fractures think about osteogenesis imperfecta, neonatal rickets, or neuromuscular disorders. Femur fractures in newborns are commonly treated in newborns with a Pavlik harness.

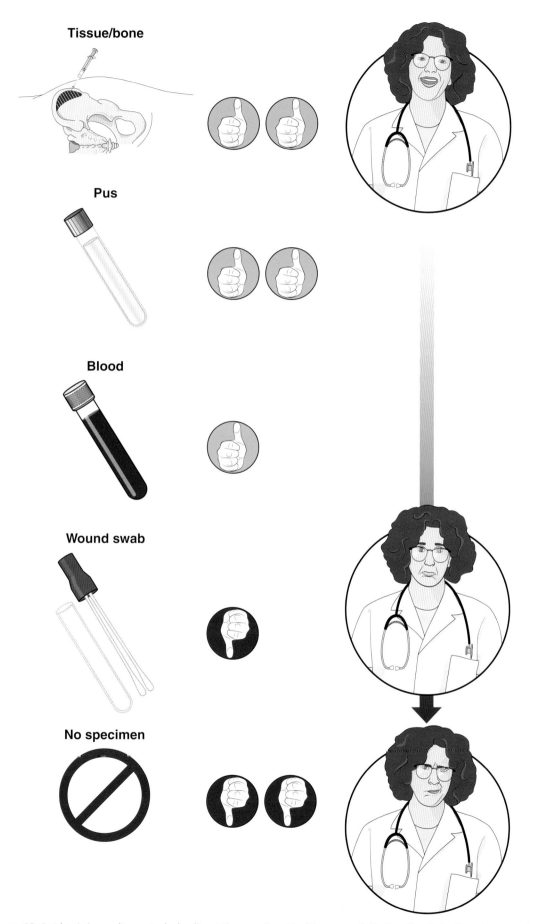

Figure 12-4 Obtaining cultures to help direct therapy is critical in successfully treating infections in neonates.

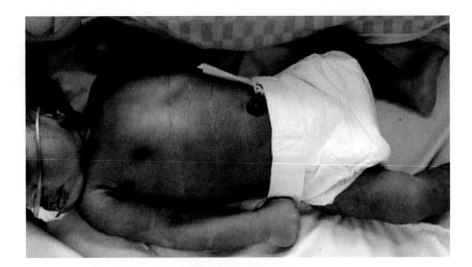

Figure 12-5 This infant with Erb palsy holds the right arm in the classic "waiter's tip" position of elbow extension, forearm pronation, and wrist flexion. (Used with permission of the Children's Orthopaedic Center, Los Angeles.)

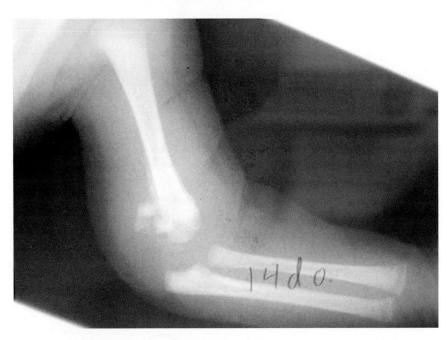

Figure 12-6 This transphyseal distal humerus fracture was sustained at birth. Note that this fracture may be difficult to identify on plain radiographs prior to the appearance of fracture callus.

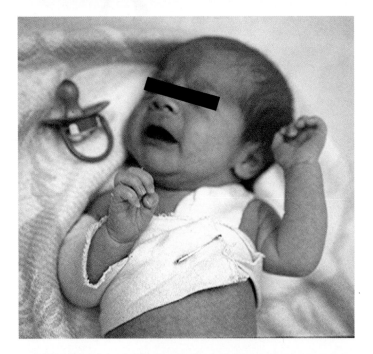

Figure 12-7 Standard slings and shoulder immobilizers do not fit the newborn with birth fractures of the upper extremity. This photo demonstrates one option of immobilization with cotton stockinette. The critical issue in treatment is to make certain a sling cannot migrate and obstruct the child's airway. A simpler option is to pin the shirtsleeve to the torso of the shirt.

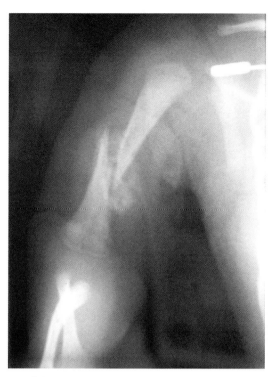

Figure 12-8 Fracture of the humerus sustained at birth demonstrates significant callus by the age of 14 days and was probably comfortable enough in 7 days to obviate the need for any immobilization.

Why Won't This Clavicle Fracture Heal?

Beware of the clavicle fracture that just doesn't look right or doesn't heal. Congenital pseudoarthrosis of the clavicle is a rare condition in which the medial and lateral ossification centers of the clavicle fail to unite (Fig. 12-9). Let the parents know it is not related to birth trauma. The patient is nontender, though a bump may be palpable, which can mislead one toward a diagnosis of fracture. The condition almost always occurs on the right side, and if it occurs on the left look for dextrocardia. The diagnosis is confirmed by lack of callous on subsequent radiographs. The natural history is most often benign,[6] though surgical treatment is likely to be successful if there is discomfort or if the almost ubiquitous bump is cosmetically concerning.[7]

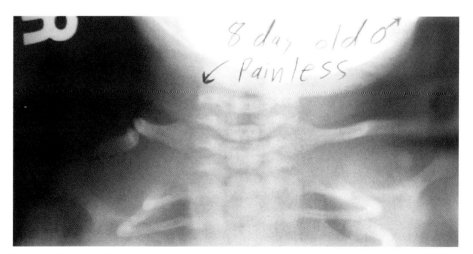

Figure 12-9 Pseudoarthrosis of the clavicle.

Hip Click

A consultation for a possibly dislocated hip is not emergent. Consider the child's overall health and other issues when deciding on timing and type of treatment. Pavlik harness application in the NICU can present challenges for caregivers and stress for parents. Beware that in the newborn a dislocated hip may not have decreased abduction. See Chapters 2 and 24 for further discussion.

Foot Problems

CLUBFOOT

Treatment of clubfoot is not emergent, but earlier manipulation and casting is probably best. Radiographs are of limited value in newborns but may be of assistance if the diagnosis is in question. A baby with a clubfoot has a higher likelihood of having developmental hip dysplasia,[8] so consider hip ultrasound and document your hip exam.

CALCANEOVALGUS FOOT AND POSTEROMEDIAL BOWING OF THE TIBIA

A calcaneovalgus foot looks a lot worse than it is. Both isolated calcaneovalgus of the foot and posteromedial bowing of the tibia generally resolve spontaneously. Gentle stretching of the foot by the parents may be helpful, though particularly severe cases may warrant a few stretching casts. Warn the parents that with

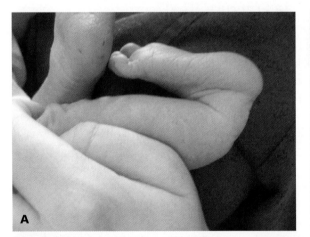
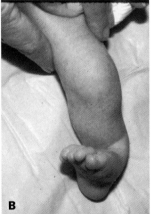
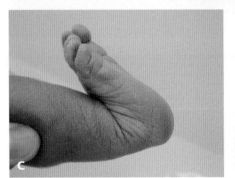
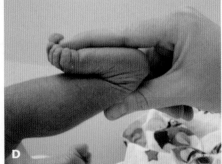

Figure 12-10 A, B: In posteromedial bowing of the tibia, the apex of the deformity is in the tibia. **C:** In calcaneovalgus foot, the apex is the joint. **D:** The dorsum of the foot can easily touch the anterior leg with out significant force or discomfort.

posteromedial bowing of the tibia, a 3- to 4-cm leg length discrepancy may result, and alert residents that a common test question highlights that leg length discrepancy is the most likely orthopaedic sequela.

Flexion Contractures

In newborns, flexion contractures of the knee, hip, and elbow are normal and resolve with time. For example, one study found the mean knee flexion contracture was 21° at birth, decreasing to 11° at 3 months and 3° at 6 months of age.[9] If these "normal" contractures are not present, suspect trouble. Full hip extension at birth is associated with hip dislocation.

Beware of the knee without a flexion contracture in a newborn. A fully extended knee may be a dislocated knee, whereas hyperextension of the knee is more common in a subluxed knee.

Early serial casting for congenital knee dislocation or subluxation is indicated, as earlier institution of casting decreases the likelihood of needing surgery.[10] Poor circulation of the foot is often noted after a cast has been applied to increase knee flexion, and the cast must be immediately removed. We have found soft fiberglass casting material to be convenient and effective in this setting.

> **THE GURU SAYS...**
> In a hyperextensible knee, a line drawn through the tibial shaft intersects the distal femoral epiphysis. In dislocated knee, the line falls anterior to the epiphysis (Figs. 12-11 and 12-12).
> PAUL D. SPONSELLER

> **THE GURU SAYS...**
> Casting is not often successful for true congenital dislocation of the knee. It can injure the physis.
> PAUL D. SPONSELLER

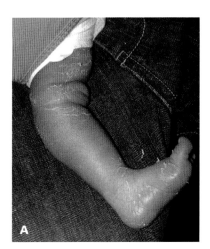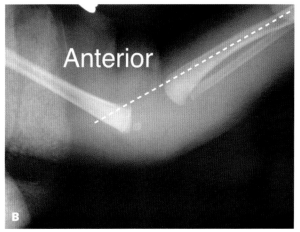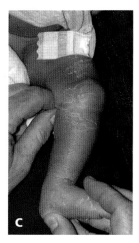

Figure 12-11 Congenitally subluxated (hyperextended) knee. **A:** Clinically, hyperextension is present. The clinical picture can be surprisingly confusing to the neophyte; some even suggesting the foot is on backward. **B:** Lateral X-ray shows a line down the tibia crosses the femur. **C:** This knee can be flexed past neutral at presentation. This signifies serial casting/manipulation/Pavlik harness is likely to be effective. (Courtesy of Kenneth J. Noonan, MD.)

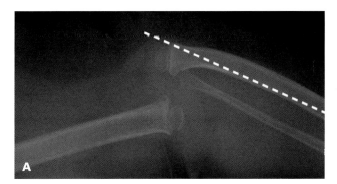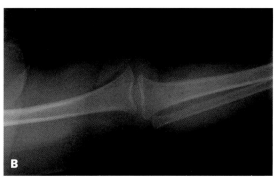

Figure 12-12 Congenitally dislocated knee. **A:** Lateral X-ray demonstrates that a line drawn along the tibial shaft does not intersect the femur. **B:** AP view alone can be confusing. (Used with permission of the Children's Orthopaedic Center Los Angeles.)

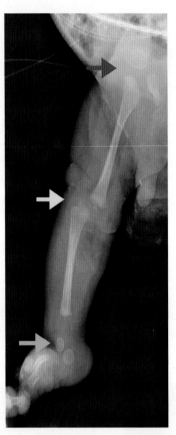

Figure 12-13 A congenitally dislocated knee is a sentinel finding that starts the search for associated orthopaedic conditions. This X-ray demonstrates a dislocated hip (*red arrow*), dislocated knee (*yellow arrow*), and vertical talus (*green arrow*) in a 2-month-old with Larsen syndrome. (Used with permission of the Children's Orthopaedic Center Los Angeles.)

Hip dislocations are present in up to 50% of children with congenital knee dislocations,[11] so all these children should have an ultrasound of the hips. Consider Larsen syndrome if both pathologies are present (Fig. 12-13). A Pavlik harness can be used to treat simultaneous hip and knee dislocations.[11]

Amniotic Band Syndrome

Although rare, an amniotic band can cause digital or limb ischemia in a newborn. Immediate removal of the band to prevent further damage to the digit or limb may be required.

Periosteal New Bone

Periosteal reaction may be seen in a variety of clinical scenarios in infants. Stay out of trouble by differentiating the normal from pathologic. Physiologic periosteal reaction of the newborn is a common finding in about 35% of infants aged 1 to 4 months. This is usually an incidental finding on radiographs obtained for other reasons. The periosteal reaction is thin, even, and symmetric, occurring along the femur, tibia, and humerus on both sides. Periosteal reaction is potentially abnormal if the child is premature or is younger than 1 month or older than 4 months. A thickness of greater than 2 mm of subperiosteal new bone is likely to be abnormal and should prompt further diagnostic evaluation.[12] It has also been shown that newborns receiving prostaglandin infusion[13] or on extracorporeal membrane

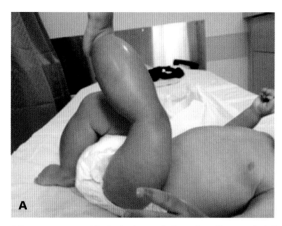
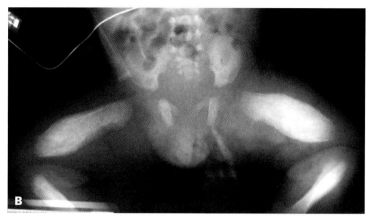

Figure 12-14 Clinical photo **(A)** and radiograph **(B)** of a patient with Caffey disease.

oxygenation (ECMO)[14] can have periosteal new bone formation. Pathologic causes of periosteal new bone formation in infants include Caffey disease (most commonly involving the mandible, ulna, and tibia) (Fig. 12-14), congenital syphilis, infection, malignancy, child abuse, and scurvy.

Staying Out of Trouble With Newborns

* If a limb is not moving voluntarily, consider fracture, nerve injury, and, most importantly, infection.

* An ultrasound of the shoulder may help differentiate infection from a transphyseal fracture.

* Traditional signs of infection such as temperature, serum white cell count, and ESR are less reliable in newborns than older children. CRP is best, but still imperfect.

* Significant flexion contractures of the knee, hip, and elbow are physiologic in the newborn and resolve spontaneously over the first year of life. An absence of knee or hip contractures is a red flag for a dislocation.

SOURCES OF WISDOM

1. McBride MT, Hennrikus WL, Shield WE II. Newborn clavicle fractures. *Orthopedics.* 1998;21(3):317-319.
2. Tural Kara T, Erat T, Ozdemir H, et al. Calcaneus osteomyelitis secondary to Guthrie test: case report. *Arch Argent Pediatr.* 2016;114(4):e260-263.
3. Eliahou R, Simanovsky N, Hiller N, Simanovsky N. Fracture-separation of the distal femoral epiphysis in a premature neonate. *J Ultrasound Med.* 2006;25(12):1603-1605.
4. Hsu TY, Hung FC, Lu YJ, et al. Neonatal clavicular fracture: clinical analysis of incidence, predisposing factors, diagnosis, and outcome. *Am J Perinatol.* 2002;19(1):17-21.
5. Podeszwa DA, Mooney JF, Cramer KE, Mendelow MJ. Comparison of Pavlik harness application and immediate spica casting for femur fractures in infants. *J Pediatr Orthop.* 2004;24:60-62.
6. Shalom A, Khermosh O, Weintraub S. The natural history of congenital pseudarthrosis of the clavicle. *J Bone Joint Surg Br.* 1994;76(5):846-847.
7. Grogan DP, Love SM, Guidera KJ, et al. Operative treatment of congenital pseudarthrosis of the clavicle. *J Pediatr Orthop.* 1991;11(2):176-180.
8. Perry DC, Tawfiq SM, Roche A, et al. The association between clubfoot and developmental dysplasia of the hip. *J Bone Joint Surg Br.* 2010;92(11):1586-1588.
9. Broughton NS, Wright J, Menelaus MB. Range of knee motion in normal neonates. *J Pediatr Orthop.* 1993;13(2):263-264.
10. Ferris B, Aichroth P. The treatment of congenital knee dislocation. A review of nineteen knees. *Clin Orthop Relat Res.* 1987;216:135-140.

11. Nogi J, MacEwen GD. Congenital dislocation of the knee. *J Pediatr Orthop*. 1982;2(5):509-513.
12. Kwon DS, Spevak MR, Fletcher K, et al. Physiologic subperiosteal new bone formation: prevalence, distribution, and thickness in neonates and infants. *AJR Am J Roentgenol*. 2002;179(4):985-988.
13. Velaphi S, Cilliers A, Beckh-Arnold E, et al. Cortical hyperostosis in an infant on prolonged prostaglandin infusion: case report and literature review. *J Perinatol*. 2004;24(4):263-265.
14. Kogutt MS, Lovretich JO. Periosteal reaction of the long bones associated with extracorporeal membrane oxygenation: cause and effect?. *Pediatr Radiol*. 1999;29(10):797-798.

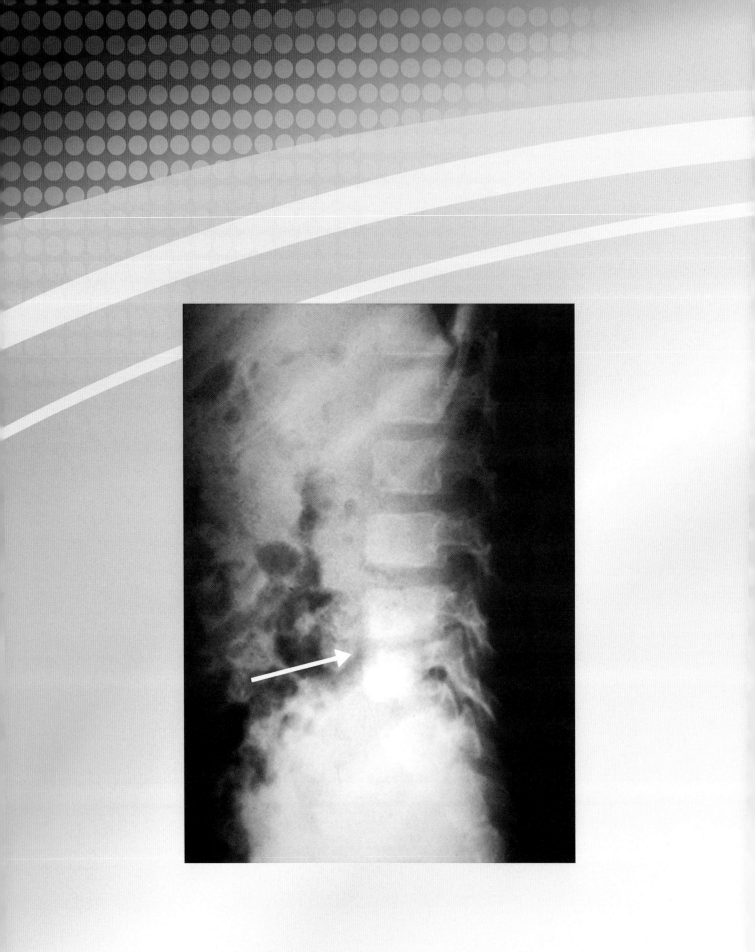

Chapter 13

The Limping Child

JOHN M. (JACK) FLYNN, MD, DAVID L. SKAGGS, MD, MMM, and MICHAEL G. VITALE, MD, MPH

Gurus: Haemish Crawford, FRACS and Nicholas D. Fletcher, MD

While many children presenting with a limp will have benign, self-limiting causes, the pediatric orthopaedic surgeon must keep their guard up to stay out of trouble and not miss something more serious. This is one of the most common reasons children are brought to our office, and the list of possible causes is long. Always take the parents' concern seriously. If a patient's mother says there is a limp, you should find it or prove her wrong. This is one of the areas where spending some time taking a good history is critical. Nail down the details regarding how long the limp has been there and the circumstances surrounding its first recognition.

Essential Questions When Evaluating a Limp[1]

* Is there pain?
* Is the child sick?
* Onset sudden or gradual?
* What type of limp?
* Can the problem be localized?
* Is the limp getting better, worse, or staying the same. Ones that are getting better can usually be watched with no further testing.

Reprinted with permission from Flynn JM, Widmann RF. The limping child: evaluation and diagnosis. *J Am Acad Orthop Surg*. 2001;9(2):89-98. Copyright © 2001 by American Academy of Orthopaedic Surgeons.

Get the child out into the hallway, and get him or her in shorts so you can see the whole lower limb. Do not hesitate to have the child walk or even run down the hallway. It's helpful to look at each segment (e.g., foot, ankle, knee, hip, torso) separately with each pass. Be patient as more subtle limps can become more obvious as the child becomes tired or forgets the doctor is watching.

During the tabletop exam, look at the whole limb (including the bottom of the feet). Look for subtle signs of muscle atrophy, swelling, or discoloration. When faced with the typically frustrating scenario of a limping toddler with normal x-rays and no helpful details in the history, search for the point of maximum tenderness (PMT). The PMT can sometimes be a little confusing. Thigh or knee pain (rubbing) is a clue to think of hip pathology. Remember, a toddler's fracture does not have to be in the tibia; it can be in the calcaneus or elsewhere (Fig. 13-1). Unless an obvious source reveals itself quickly (i.e., toddler fracture), range every joint (and that includes spine flexion/extension) (Fig. 13-2).

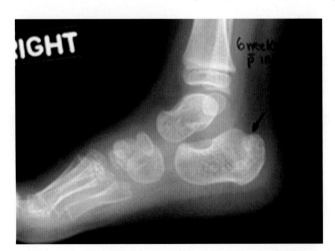

Figure 13-1 A "toddler's fracture" does not always have to be in the tibia. Children who jump down stairs or off playground equipment may sustain a fracture of the calcaneus that can be very difficult to see on initial radiographs. This calcaneus "toddler's fracture" revealed itself after 6 weeks in a short leg cast.

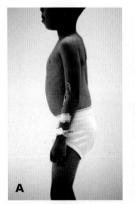
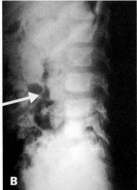

Figure 13-2 Diskitis presenting as a limp. **A:** This 6-year-old boy presented with a "limp" that was really an abnormal gait caused by his efforts to decrease motion in his lumbar spine. He walked with a very straight back and a slight crouch.
B: Lateral radiograph of the lumbosacral spine shows decreased disk height at L4-5 consistent with diskitis.

One way to think of the causes of limping is to consider the differential anatomically, from bottom to top: the ones on the top are often more serious (spinal cord tumor), more easily overlooked (diskitis), and are more difficult to localize on a physical exam since the structures are not as superficial (iliacus abscess).

Abnormal Gait

To recognize an abnormality, the orthopaedist needs to understand what normal should be for a given age. New walkers have a wide base gait, poor balance, and a tendency to toe walk, but none of these are "limps" (except maybe in the worried mind of a new parent). There are five unique limps, or abnormal gaits in children: antalgic, Trendelenburg, spastic, muscle weakness, and short limb gait. An antalgic limp does not have to come from the leg. It can come from the spine, pelvis, or sacroiliac joint. Sometimes you need to watch a longer stretch of walking or get the child to run in order to appreciate a subtler Trendelenburg gait. In a spastic gait, spasticity will affect the whole limb, so watch for the effects on multiple joints one at a time—floor to spine.

Look for signs of contracture (equinus, crouch gait due to hamstring contracture), or decreased motion and its effects (decreased knee motion is due to rectus spasticity, causing toe dragging). If suspicious of spasticity, always get the child to run. You may pick up subtle upper extremity posturing that clinches the diagnosis. A muscle weakness gait is seen in conditions such as Duchenne muscular dystrophy (DMD). To the uninitiated, this may not look like a "limp," just a "funny walk." It will be hard for the parent to describe, and it will come on gradually. You might see a lurch. Do a Gower test if there is any suspicion. Any loss of milestones is extremely concerning.

Short limb gait may be confusing. Leg length discrepancy (LLD) causes a limp when the difference gets to be 3% to 5%.[2,3] Remember that most kids with hemiplegia have a short limb on the affected side. Do not mistakenly blame LLD when it's the hemiplegia that's causing the limp

Imaging, Blood Work, and Other Diagnostic Tests

The presence or absence of pain, age, site of symptoms, and type of limp will help establish the differential diagnosis (Table 13-1). Make the pace and intensity of your workup (lots of tests immediately vs. watch and revisit) appropriate for the conditions on your differential diagnosis. Sometimes doing too much testing causes as much trouble as doing too little (e.g., you find some unrelated red herring on MRI that someone wants to biopsy and there is really nothing there. Or, you put a toddler under general anesthesia for an MRI that's not really needed). Good plain radiographs are always the starting point; they are quick, widely available, sensitive, and specific for many things on the differential diagnosis (Fig. 13-3). Oblique radiographs (especially of the foot) are valuable for seeing subtle abnormalities that might cause a limp. To stay out of trouble, keep in mind that plain radiographs may reveal no sign of early osteomyelitis. It can take 10 or more days for signs of infection to produce radiographic changes of the bone. Instead, the best early radiographic finding may be soft-tissue swelling. Comparison views may be helpful in seeing such subtle signs.

When dealing with a limping toddler in whom symptoms cannot be localized, consider plain radiographs of the entire lower extremity—hip to feet.

> **THE GURU SAYS...**
> While observing the gait, ask the child to walk on their toes and then heels. Ask them to sit on the floor and stand up. This gives you a quick assessment of neurologic status and muscle power.
> HAEMISH CRAWFORD

> **THE GURU SAYS...**
> Muscular dystrophy is often forgotten as a presenting cause of limp in modern medicine given the easier path to a genetically proven diagnosis, but this may continue to be one of the few conditions that you may be the first to diagnose. Always remember the Gower test in any boy with a new onset of a change in gait.
> NICHOLAS FLETCHER

TABLE 13-1 Differential Diagnosis of Antalgic Gait

Equinus Gait (Toe Walking)
Idiopathic thick ascending limb
Clubfoot
Cerebral palsy
Limb-length discrepancy

Trendelenburg Gait
Legg-Calve-Perthes disease
Developmental dysplasia of the hip
Slipped capital femoral epiphysis
Hemiplegic cerebral palsy

Circumduction Gait/Vaulting Gait
Limb-length discrepancy
Cerebral palsy
Any cause of ankle or knee stiffness

Steppage Gait
Cerebral palsy
Myelodysplasia
Charcot-Marie-Tooth disease
Friedreich ataxia

Reprinted with permission from Flynn JM, Widmann RF. The limping child: evaluation and diagnosis. *J Am Acad Orthop Surg.* 2001;9(2):89-98. Copyright © 2001 by American Academy of Orthopaedic Surgeons.

Technetium-99m bone scan can be a valuable tool when localization by history and physical, and plain radiographs have failed, but this is used less often these days given concerns about radiation.[4] Keep in mind that a cold on bone scan may indicate a particularly bad case of some of the osteomyelitis.[5] Remember, leukemia, which presents as musculoskeletal pain 25% of the time, may result

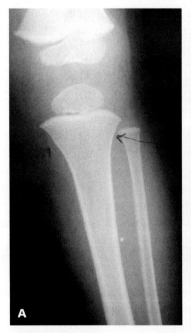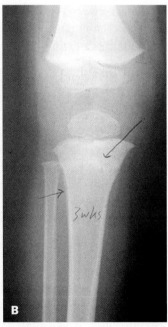

Figure 13-3 A subtle toddler's fracture. Although toddler's fractures are typically a nondisplaced spiral fracture of the tibial shaft, stay out of trouble by imaging the entire bone—or even the entire limb. Good-quality plain radiographs showing most of the lower limb will allow you to identify even very subtle changes suggesting a fracture. **A:** A very subtle cortical irregularity is seen in the proximal tibia. The child was placed in a long leg cast. **B:** Three weeks after injury, radiodense metaphyseal bone and periosteal new bone laterally is evident in this healing fracture.

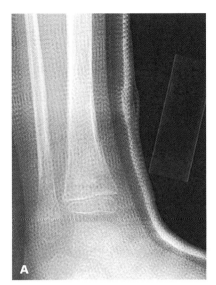
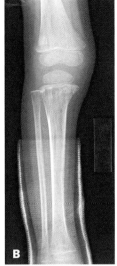
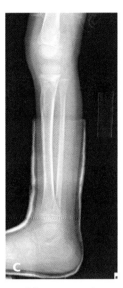

Figure 13-4 Leukemia presenting as a limp. This 3-year-old presented for a second opinion regarding persistent limping after an "ankle fracture" diagnosed at an outside hospital. **A:** An AP view of the ankle showed no clear sign of a fracture, but did show an irregular appearance to the bone. Fortunately for the child, the treating pediatric orthopaedist sent the child back for full-length AP and lateral of the tibia. AP **(B)** and lateral **(C)** radiographs of the entire tibia and distal femur show marked irregularities of the metaphyseal bone consistent with a systemic process. A rapid and aggressive workup quickly revealed that this child had leukemia.

in an increase, decrease, or no change in technetium-99m uptake[4] (Fig. 13-4). Metastatic neuroblastoma also presents in this age group (Fig. 13-5).

Ultrasound is the study of choice for rapid evaluation for a hip effusion in a child. Ultrasound can guide a successful aspiration, which has been shown to decrease the time to OR for septic hips by 50%.[6] However at some institutions, ultrasound is not readily available and one should not delay taking a child who has a story and exam suggestive of a septic hip to the OR. A CT scan can be valuable to diagnose a pelvic cause of a limp (Fig. 13-6). Although MRI should not be the first test chosen for the limping child, it is the best way to see processes in the bone marrow, joint, or cartilage. MRI can be valuable for finding malignancies and stress fractures once you have localized the area to look. MRI may be particularly valuable in identifying the cause of a limp that originates in the pelvis and spine, as a physical exam is limited in these areas (Fig. 13-7).

Laboratory tests are most valuable when the child presents with an acute, nontraumatic limp, especially if there are any constitutional symptoms, night pain, etc. White blood cell count (WBC) is the least helpful, as it is neither sensitive nor specific. WBC differential is helpful when leukemia is a consideration. ESR is too slow to rise to be helpful in the early phase of an acute process. If it is elevated above 50 in a limping child, there is a high likelihood of an infection; if it is over 100, osteomyelitis is likely. CRP rises within 6 hours of onset of an acute process and is a better measure than ESR.[7] Joint aspiration can be the most important test for septic arthritis evaluation. Because there is considerable overlap of WBC aspirates for different conditions, there is no magic number to definitively diagnose septic arthritis. From 50,000 to 80,000/mL is often used as a range above which the concern for septic arthritis becomes high.[8,9] The WBC differential, gram stain, and clinical picture are more important that the total WBC in the fluid (Table 13-2).

When dealing with the limping toddler (1-4 years old), do not be fooled by an immature gait. Fractures and infection usually top the list of most common causes

> **THE GURU SAYS...**
>
> Leukemia should always be considered in the differential for the limping child. A quarter of all leukemia cases will present with pain in an extremity. Laboratory analysis including a C-reactive protein (CRP), erythrocyte sedimentation rate (ESR), and complete blood count (CBC) with differential should be considered in children with a limp and fatigue, fevers, or systemic symptoms.
>
> NICHOLAS FLETCHER

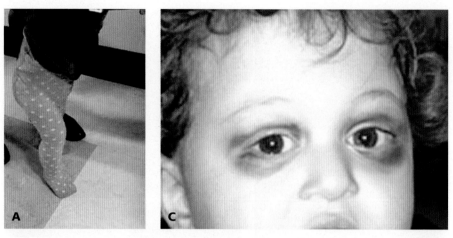

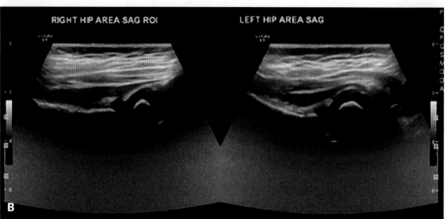

Figure 13-5 **A:** A 14-month-old had a fever and suddenly refused to bear weight. His ESR was 64 and CRP was 28. **B:** Ultrasound showed moderate effusion. He was taken to OR for irrigation and drainage of the hip with 2.5 mL turbid fluid. Cultures were negative but exam improved. **C:** Transaminases were noted to spike, and the patient developed bilateral periorbital ecchymosis—"raccoon eyes"—indicative of metastatic neuroblastoma, which was subsequently confirmed with biopsy.

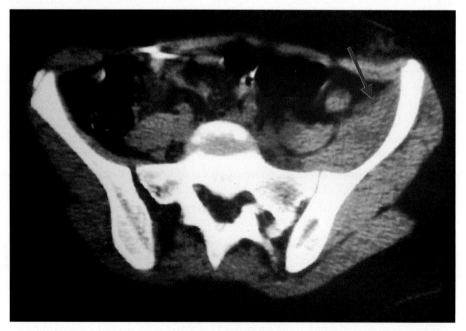

Figure 13-6 This child's mysterious limp, thought to be coming from his hip joint, was diagnosed as an abscess of the iliacus muscle, seen on this a CT scan cut.

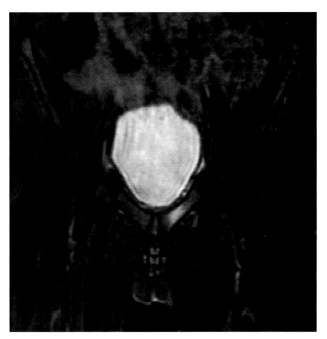

Figure 13-7 MRI of an 8-year-old girl with proximal femoral pain and a limp shows osteomyelitis of the superior pubic rami. She was afebrile and had only minor elevation of her ESR and CRP. A provisional diagnosis of hip septic arthritis or proximal femoral osteomyelitis was made, and IV antibiotics were started while she awaited the MRI.

of abnormal gait in this group. To stay out of trouble, you'll want to move quickly to nail down these diagnoses. For toe-walkers, get the pregnancy and birth history (was the child premature?).

Idiopathic toe walking should be bilateral; worry more when it's unilateral. However, bilateral is not always benign (DMD, diplegic cerebral palsy). Remember the Gower test in boys.

Children between ages 4 and 10 present a different scenario. Their gait is more mature and adult-like, so it is easier to recognize a true, pathologic limp. In this

> **THE GURU SAYS...**
>
> A fever plus a limping child equals osteomyelitis or septic arthritis until proved otherwise. Blood investigations and advanced imaging is mandatory. Do not hesitate to start IV antibiotics while still investigating the site of infection, as this will not alter subsequent cultures of the infected areas (Fig. 13-8).
>
> HAEMISH CRAWFORD

TABLE 13.2 Differential Diagnosis of Antalgic Gait

<4 y	4-10 y	>10 y
Toddler's fracture (tibia or foot)	Fracture (especially physeal)	Stress fracture (femur, tibia, foot, pars intra-articularis)
Osteomyelitis, septic arthritis, diskitis	Osteomyelitis, septic arthritis, diskitis	Osteomyelitis, septic arthritis, diskitis
Arthritis (juvenile rheumatoid arthritis, Lyme disease)	Legg-Calve-Perthes disease	Slipped capital femoral epiphysis
Discoid lateral meniscus	Transient synovitis	Osgood-Schlatter disease or Sinding-Larsen-Johansson syndrome
Foreign body in the foot	Osteochondritis dissecans (knee or ankle)	
Benign or malignant tumor	Discoid lateral meniscus	Osteochondritis dissecans (knee or ankle)
	Sever apophysitis	Chondromalacia patellae
	Accessory tarsal navicular	Arthritis (Lyme disease, gonococcal)
	Foreign body of the foot	Accessory tarsal navicular
	Arthritis (juvenile rheumatoid arthritis, Lyme disease)	Tarsal coalition
	Benign or malignant tumor	Benign or malignant tumor

Reprinted with permission from Flynn JM, Widmann RF. The limping child: evaluation and diagnosis. *J Am Acad Orthop Surg*. 2001;9(2):89-98. Copyright © 2001 by American Academy of Orthopaedic Surgeons.

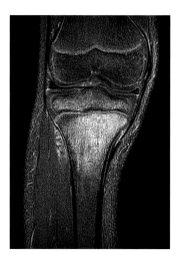

Figure 13-8 MRI of a 10-year-old boy with a painful proximal tibia with an antalgic gait and a mild fever. His CRP and ESR were also raised.

age group, infection is less likely to be the source of a limp compared to toddlers; injury (acute and overuse) and hip disorders (Perthes, transient synovitis) become very common causes. The diagnosis of DMD is often made at this age. One source of trouble is dismissing symptoms as "growing pains." Growing pains won't make you limp; instead, they are typically transient aching of the lower legs at night that is variable, is intermittent, and then resolves over time. More worrisome symptoms associated with leg aches include frequent night awakening, especially with pains referable to one side that causes limp or other functional problem during the day.

The school-aged child is old enough to provide a more useful description of their pain. A stress fracture of a tarsal is a frequently overlooked diagnosis that can cause limping.

Children 10 years of age and older can usually give an accurate history and help you localize the cause of the symptoms. Overuse and acute injury are important etiologies in this age group. You may not be able to localize the problem until after completing a good exam, or maybe not until you've done the correct diagnostic test. Examples include SCFE (slipped capital femoral epiphysis) that masquerades as knee or thigh pain, sacroiliac problems that seem to be the garden-variety low back pain, and stress fractures that cause vague regional symptoms.

Be careful when dealing with the teenage group. Teens can be very manipulative of any situation. Secondary gain rears its head in this age group. Teenagers can exaggerate symptoms to avoid something (e.g., gym class), or they can minimize symptoms so that they'll be permitted to participate (e.g., a high school basketball game) (Fig. 13-9). Back pain becomes more common in this age group and it's important to discern garden-variety muscular back pain from less frequent causes. History of antecedent overuse, chronicity, and relative mild symptoms support a diagnosis of muscular back pain. If a child really does not want to be bothered with a course of physical therapy, they are often telling you that their pain is mild and you can provide counsel to return if pain worsens.

This age group is also where we start to see rheumatologic issues. Pain in multiple joints, other autoimmune issues (e.g., eczema), and elevated markers are all things that should prompt evaluation by a pediatric rheumatologist.

> ### THE GURU SAYS...
> Remember that spinal disorders, especially discitis, are a common cause of a limp in the young child. Having the patient pick up a cell phone or toy placed on the floor can elicit the source of pain.
> NICHOLAS FLETCHER

> ### THE GURU SAYS...
> Do not forget to look at the spine and consider it as a cause of the limp! Spondylolisthesis, diskitis, disk prolapse, and intraspinal disease can all cause limping.
> HAEMISH CRAWFORD

> ### THE GURU SAYS...
> Every limping patient with one or more joints involved should be assessed for a generalized arthritic condition. Rheumatic fever is still common, so listening for a cardiac murmur will help make this diagnosis.
> HAEMISH CRAWFORD

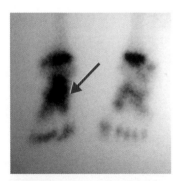

Figure 13-9 Bone scan was used to diagnose this stress fracture in an elite 13-year-old runner. Initial plain radiographs were normal. She did not want to see the doctor fearing her running would be restricted. A persistent limp led to a bone scan and the diagnosis of stress fracture.

Staying Out of Trouble With a Limping Child

* If a patient's parent says there is a limp, you should find it or prove them wrong.
* Do not allow the confines of the exam room cause you to miss something subtle like a balance problem or a limp that can only be seen with running.
* A toddler's fracture does not have to be the tibia; it can be the calcaneus, or elsewhere.
* Always perform a Gower test. This is easy *to do*, hard *to remember* to do.
* Oblique radiographs (especially of the foot) are valuable for seeing subtle abnormalities that might cause a limp.
* Leukemia, which presents as musculoskeletal pain 25% of time, may result in increased, decreased, or no change on bone scan.
* Idiopathic toe walking should be bilateral; worry more when it's unilateral. However, bilateral is not always benign (DMD, diplegic cerebral palsy).
* Growing pains shouldn't make you limp.

SOURCES OF WISDOM

1. Flynn JM, Widmann RF. The limping child: evaluation and diagnosis. *J Am Acad Orthop Surg.* 2001;9(2):89-98.
2. Song KM, Halliday SE, Little DG. The effect of limb-length discrepancy on gait. *J Bone Joint Surg Am.* 1997;79(11):1690-1698.
3. Kaufman KR, Miller LS, Sutherland DH. Gait asymmetry in patients with limb-length inequality. *J Pediatr Orthop.* 1996;16(2):144-150.
4. Aronson J, Garvin K, Seibert J, et al. Efficiency of the bone scan for occult limping toddlers. *J Pediatr Orthop.* 1992;12(1):38-44.
5. Pennington WT, Mott MP, Thometz JG, et al. Photopenic bone scan osteomyelitis: a clinical perspective. *J Pediatr Orthop.* 1999;19(6):695-698.
6. Zawin JK, Hoffer FA, Rand FF, Teele RL. Joint effusion in children with an irritable hip: US diagnosis and aspiration. *Radiology.* 1993;187(2):459-463.
7. Levine MJ, McGuire KJ, McGowan KL, Flynn JM. Assessment of the test characteristics of C-reactive protein for septic arthritis in children. *J Pediatr Orthop.* 2003;23(3):373-377.
8. Fink CW, Nelson JD. Septic arthritis and osteomyelitis in children. *Clin Rheum Dis.* 1986;12(2):423-435.
9. Morrissey RT. Bone and joint sepsis. In: Morrissey RT, Weinstein SL, eds. *Pediatric Orthopaedics.* Vol 1. 5th ed. Philadelphia, PA: Lippincott Williams & Wilkins; 2001:459.

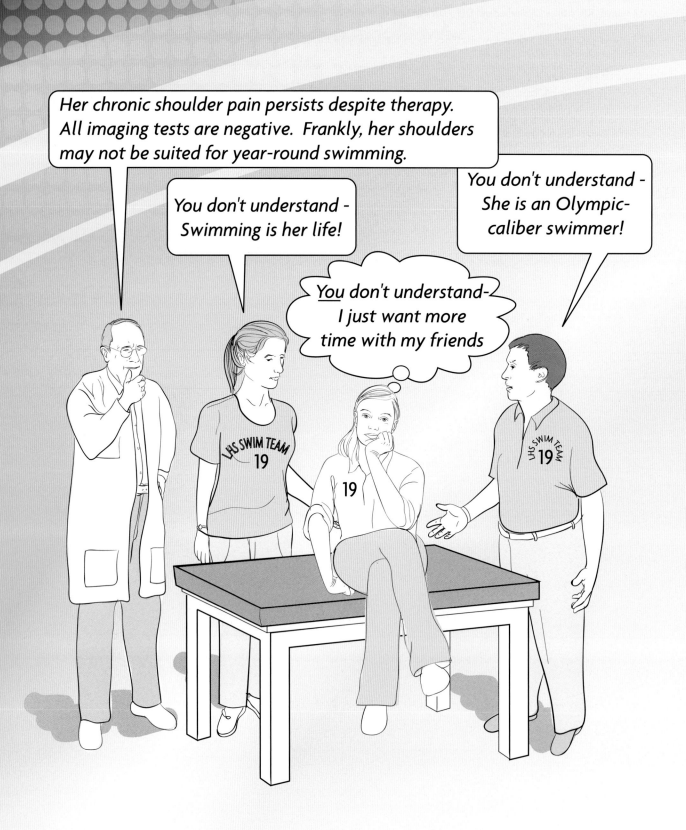

Chapter 14

The Pediatric Athlete

MININDER S. KOCHER, MD, MPH

Gurus: Theodore J. Ganley, MD and Michael T. Busch, MD

Pediatric Sports Medicine

Pediatric sports medicine is an emerging subspecialty that is a hot field! It is hot in orthopaedic surgery, with new subspecialty organizations such as PRISM (Pediatric Research in Sports Medicine) and study groups such as ROCK (osteochondritis dissecans), PLUTO (pediatric ACL), and JUPITER (patellofemoral instability). Pediatric sports medicine sessions are now regular occurrences in orthopaedic meetings, including AAOS, POSNA, AOSSM, IPOS, AAP, and AANA. Most children's hospitals have established sports medicine programs. Orthopaedic trainees interested in pediatric sports medicine are often pursuing dual fellowship training in both pediatric orthopaedics and sports medicine, or they are pursuing a single fellowship that has a large pediatric sports medicine component. A recent review of 14,636 pediatric sports medicine cases submitted by candidates for Part II certification by the American Board of Orthopedic Surgeons from 2004 to 2014 showed a large increase in the number of cases performed by dual pediatric and sports medicine fellows from 2.1% to 21.4% over a 10-year period.[1]

Pediatric sports medicine is also a hot field for patients and families. More than 30 million children and adolescents are participating in youth sports in the United States. With increased participation in competitive sports at a young age come increasing rates of injury. More than 3.5 million children 14 years old and younger receive treatment annually for youth sports injuries. Children 5 to 14 years old account for 40% of sports-related injuries in emergency rooms. Recent trend in youth sports includes professionalization, early sports specialization, and increasing rates of burnout and dropout. Youth sports has become a big business, estimated as a $17 billion market. Young athletes are specializing in a single sport year-round at early ages.[2,3] With increasing competition, pressure, and specialization come increasing rates of burnout. Almost 45% of children aged 6 to 12 played a team sport regularly in 2008, and now only 37% do. And 70% of adolescents are dropping out of sports by age 13. These children and adolescents leaving youth sports may forgo the health and psychosocial benefits of being physically active.

Trouble comes in many forms when caring for the young athlete. Although the conditions are not as grave as tumors, serious infections, and trauma, the acute and overuse injuries that affect the young, active child are very common. Sports medicine, like much of pediatric orthopaedics, is the treatment of low-energy trauma or repetitive microtrauma. Demographic evaluations now show that although the total number of children involved in organized sports decreases as the children get older, the intensity of the competition, and training for that competition, increases—and with it, many injuries.[4]

Sources of trouble caring for the pediatric athlete are both clinical and psychosocial. The orthopaedic surgeon will have frequent contact with the overzealous sports parents. Managing these interactions is a key to staying out of trouble. **NEWSFLASH! These families often have heavily invested both financially and psychosocially in their child's sports.** Often, the parents are living vicariously through the child's athletic accomplishments or projecting their athletic insecurities on the child (Fig. 14-1). Other times, parents are simply doing what they think is best for their children, and the whole family structure is focused around the children's sports activities. Parents may have dreams of their child becoming a professional athlete or getting an athletic scholarship to college, even though the odds of this are exceedingly unlikely. Or parents may simply want their child to excel in one dimension, be popular and respected, or get special consideration

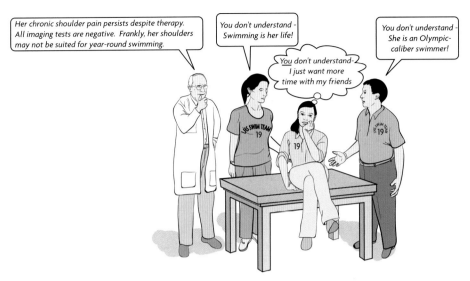

Figure 14-1 The overbearing sports parents.

for college admission. Just as treating any child with a medical condition, when treating the child athlete, you must consider the whole family. Beware the "crazy sports parents." These are parents, who have overly invested in the kid's sports: devastated at injury, pushing to get them back as soon as possible, and always telling you how great an athlete the child is. These crazy sports parents may require an approach that focuses on putting the injury in perspective and the long-term health of the child. And they may require a clinic visit that lasts longer than 15 minutes.

> ▶ **Red Flags for Crazy Sports Parents**
>
> - ▶ Parents talk more than the child.
> - ▶ Parents say "we got injured" or "our injury."
> - ▶ Parents are wearing the uniform or clothing of their child's sports team.
> - ▶ Parents who say that their child is "elite" or "being recruited" when their child is less than 14 years old.
> - ▶ Parents whose first question is "When can she get back to sports?"
> - ▶ Parents who can recite their child's sports statistics from memory.
> - ▶ Parents who have multiple videos of their child's sports on their phone.
> - ▶ Parents with radar guns to measure their pitch velocity.
> - ▶ Parents who tell you their child has a "high pain threshold."
> - ▶ Parents whose whole social life and family vacations are tied around youth sports tournaments.

Regardless, the young athlete themselves is often also very invested in their sport. Often their identity and peer group is tied to their sports. Their psychosocial functioning is closely associated with their identity as an athlete. When injured, they may lose this identity and experience psychosocial stress. They may become distraught or cry when you diagnose them with an anterior cruciate ligament (ACL) tear. As pediatric orthopaedic surgeons who have treated patients with osteosarcoma, cerebral palsy, myelodysplasia, or skeletal dysplasia, it can be hard for us to appreciate the impact that a sports injury can have on a young athlete and their family. Although it may seem minor compared to children with more severe conditions, we still must realize how real and devastating the news is to them. When giving bad sports injury news such as a torn ACL, it can often be helpful to pause and let the family digest the diagnosis and circle back to them in clinic to discuss treatment and outcome since they may be in "shock" from the initial diagnosis with poor retention of information thereafter. Sometimes, even scheduling another clinic visit later in the week can be helpful. Tell the family that you appreciate what bad news this is for them, but let them know that this is a common injury and emphasize the good prognosis in terms of return to sports. There will be time later in the treatment pathway to lay crepe with discussions of reinjury, graft failure, complications, and long-term arthritis.

Watch for the young athlete who is not coping well from their injury. Initially, many patients and families go through the Kubler-Ross stages of denial, anger, bargaining, depression, and acceptance. However, some patients may experience a true adjustment disorder or major depression that they are unable to cope with. Having had a handful of high-level youth athletes who committed suicide or attempted suicide at some point after their sports injuries, I think it is very important to be proactive and vigilant regarding depression. I let patients know that this injury can have a large psychosocial impact on them. I suggest they talk about how they are feeling, stay connected with their team, redirect their athleticism and training to physical therapy (PT), and focus on the goal of returning to sports. It can be helpful to talk to friends or teammates who have recovered from a similar injury. While it is normal to feel bummed out from being out of sports, if they are having difficulty coping or feeling depressed, then they should seek help. It can be hard to talk to their parents, or teammates, in the limited time we have in the clinic about these issues. We work closely with sports psychologists within our sports medicine program and sports psychologists in the community. Working with a "sports" psychologist has less of a stigma than working with other mental health professionals.

Also be alert for the child athlete who is looking to you or their injury to rescue them from overbearing athletic expectations. They may have played a sport for a long time, but now it is no longer fun or they are not as good as they were. An injury is a "safe" way to drop the sport. This is could be a swimmer with shoulder pain, a gymnast with back pain, or a dancer with patellofemoral pain. They may not be getting better with regular treatment and have negative imaging examinations. Be wary of a pain syndrome, such as chronic regional pain syndrome (CRPS). In fact, many cases of CRPS are diagnosed in the sports medicine clinic.[5] But sometimes these are patients trying to leave their sport. Telling them that they need a break from their sport or redirecting to another sport may come as a relief to the athlete and gradual acceptance by the parents. Unfortunately, the higher the level of the athlete, the more difficult such issues are to sort out.

Staying Out of Trouble as a Team Physician

Many sports medicine surgeons and physicians are team physicians. Being a team physician can be an incredible fun and rewarding experience. It can also be a source of stress, pressure, and time sink. I am a team physician for two local high schools, supervise coverage at the Boston Public Schools, am head team physician at a Division 3 college, am the orthopaedic consultant for a Division 1 college, and also cover a number of other events such as the Boston Ballet, the Boston Marathon, USA Track & Field, and the US Ski Team. Being on the sideline at a high school football game, the wings at a ballet performance, or the finish at a ski race allows you to appreciate the athlete in their native environment. It also gives

THE GURU SAYS...

It's important to have everyone treating these athletes—including nutritionists, NPs, PAs, medical and surgical specialists—understand warning signs such as the examination and outcome measures to collectively provide patients with the best referrals and overall clinical care.

THEODORE J. GANLEY

you a sense of the demands on the athlete and injury mechanisms. Working with athletic trainers at the high school or college level as a well-functioning team is essential. Respect the trainer's experience and judgment. Let them run out onto the field first and call you over when they need you. Don't assert your medical credentials as they often know the athlete better than you and may have seen more of a certain injury than you! **NEWSFLASH! Being a team physician takes time and energy. The commitment is commensurate with the level of sport.** Being a professional team physician sounds glamorous but can be completely time consuming and stressful. As pediatric orthopaedic surgeons, we have unique expertise as high school team physicians and in youth sports leagues. Also look for undercovered sports such as gymnastics, figure skating, running, and dance. These sports may greatly appreciate the attention and can become very devoted to your practice.

Being a capable team physician requires a knowledge base beyond pediatric orthopedics and sports surgery. **ORTHOPAEDICS 101: A good team physician has an understanding of concussion, heat-related illness, dehydration, the female athlete, infectious diseases, nutrition, the adaptive athlete, and sports psychology.** Look for this in your fellowship training. After training, look to acquire or maintain these skills through team physician courses or becoming involved in organizations such as ACSM and AMSSM.

Remember that youth sports has become a big industry. As a result, you will be faced with questions regarding nutritional supplements, performance enhancement, strength and conditioning training, and specialized equipment. Children don't need extra nutrients to perform athletically. Supplemental vitamins and minerals for the pediatric athletic are usually expensive and unnecessary. Performance-enhancing substances are a major source of trouble for young athletes.[6,7] Chances are very good that if you care for many young athletes, you care for a population that is taking a performance-enhancing substance.[6] It has been estimated that 10% to 20% of adolescent athletes (depending on the sport) use some kind of performance-enhancing substance. Although anabolic steroids are the most risky and have received the most attention, creatine, diuretics, amphetamines, and other stimulants can also be problematic.

Children and adolescents are at risk for heat injury and dehydration just as pro athletes are, maybe more so. Children are less efficient at regulating heat because they perspire less when they are hot. Children also make more metabolic heat per body mass than do adults. As a team doctor, you must be proactive in preventing heat injury. You can recommend and enforce a policy that includes mandatory periodic water drinking, cancellation or modification of practice in unsafe weather, and the discouragement of weight loss through water loss (e.g., wrestlers). Helmets should be removed when children are not in contact situations, so heat loss can occur through the head. Daily weights may be done before and after practice to monitor fluid loss.

Sometimes as a team doctor you have to speak up for young athletes who are put in dangerous situations due to limited budgets. You should also insist on proper fitting equipment that is in good repair. Sports equipment and playing fields should be age and size appropriate. Have discussions with the coaches and trainers regarding injury prevention and proper warm-up. Although coaches are loath to give up practice time, emphasizing performance benefits and keeping players on the field can be a convincing argument for warm-up. The medical team should practice simulated cervical spine injury protocols using a backboard and collar. Equipment to remove the facemask of helmets should be readily accessible. Protocols to access emergency medical services (EMS) should be reviewed.

THE GURU SAYS...
Injuries in these athletes can be at times underappreciated relative to those in collision sports. Remembering the exceptional focus and grit demonstrated by these young athletes during extended hours of training can help us to better detect, treat, and prevent overuse injuries.
THEODORE J. GANLEY

THE GURU SAYS...
Be aware that the principles of preventing heat injury and dehydration applies year-round rather than just during summer months.
THEODORE J. GANLEY

THE GURU SAYS...
During the warm-up time, coaches can address flexibility, strength, and neuromuscular training with programs such as "Ready, Set, Prevent" and the Micheli Center Prevention Program. They are both exercise and injury-prevention programs tailored to pediatric athletes and can be included in prepractice or team practice routines.
THEODORE J. GANLEY

Recent news headlines have exposed team physicians who have sexually assaulted young athletes. Being a team physician means that you are in a position of trust and a position of power. Respecting the moral and ethical obligations of this position is essential. Team physicians should not put themselves in a position where they could be compromised or accused of inappropriate behavior. Examining the athlete should be done with appropriate clothing and ideally with others observing.

THE GURU SAYS...

Most problems in youth sports are nonoperative and really a part of primary care. Most primary care physicians are particularly talented at taking thorough histories, understanding the big picture, and communicating with families.

MICHAEL T. BUSCH

THE GURU SAYS...

We encourage our sports practitioners to contact at least one pediatrician per day and text or call every orthopaedic surgeon who refers a patient. Our athletic trainers who work in the clinic are critical to keeping the lines of communication open with the physical therapists and trainers associated with their patients.

MICHAEL T. BUSCH

How to Build A Pediatric Sports Medicine Practice

1. You need credibility as both a pediatric orthopaedic surgeon and a sports medicine surgeon. This may mean dual fellowships in pediatric orthopaedics and sports medicine. If you do only a pediatric orthopaedic fellowship, then the local sports medicine surgeons may not respect you as a sports surgeon. Also, ABOS board certification (CSQ) in sports medicine may be required for sports privileges. If you do only a sports medicine fellowship, then the pediatric orthopaedic surgeons may not think you understand growth and the pediatric patient.

2. Sports medicine is more than sports injury surgery. Strive to understand the medical issues of the whole athlete: concussion, nutrition, psychology, cardiac issues, the adaptive athlete, female athlete triad, biomechanics, etc.

3. Work closely with medical sports medicine physicians, ideally in your practice. This is a synergistic relationship. Treat them with respect and understand their skills. There are conditions such as back pain, concussion, and patellofemoral dysfunction for which they may have a more effective therapeutic approach. They can also make your practice more surgically efficient by seeing acute injuries and if they need surgery, involving you. In addition, they may be proficient in ultrasound-guided office injections. Incorporation of medical sports medicine physicians, sports psychologists, athletic trainers, and sports nutritionists allows you to provide holistic sports medicine care. Patients and referring providers appreciate this and this may be a competitive advantage in your market.

4. The pediatricians can be your greatest allies. The pediatrician manages the pediatric and adolescent patient, often until they complete college in their early 20s. As such, they often control and recommend referrals. Pediatricians will appreciate your emphasis of pediatric sports medicine. They say, "The child is not a little adult." Your mantra should be, "The child athlete is not a little adult athlete!"

5. If your practice and/or hospital environment limits patients that you can see to 18 years old, you will be limited. This may skew your practice to nonoperative treatment. If you can treat college age patients, this allows you to see similar injuries as older adolescents, follow your high school athletes through college, become a college team physician, and skew toward operative cases. If the pediatricians are seeing the patients through college, you can make the practical case and business case to your hospital administrators. Remember, as an orthopaedic surgeon you are a large net revenue producer for the hospital and ancillary services.

6. Tip O'Neill said that "all politics are local." Similarly, develop strong local roots. Become a high school team physician. Coach your kids' sports and sponsor their team. Give talks to pediatricians, physical therapists, athletic trainers, and parents. Interface with youth sports organizations. The national and international talks that you give are important, but don't neglect your local connections. These build the bulk volume of your practice.

7. The number one complaint of referrers is lack of communication! This holds for pediatricians, primary care physicians, other orthopaedic surgeons, physical therapists, and athletic trainers. Get back to them. Your electronic medical record (EMR) may claim that it automatically sends notes to the referrer, but EMR has glitches, the person listed as the referrer may not actually be who referred the patient to you, and a computerized EMR note may be hard to wade through for the bottom line. Send them an email or a text. You will automatically become the most communicative and accessible orthopaedic surgeon they have ever encountered!

8. Physical therapists can also be your great allies. If possible, try to send patients to local therapists in their community. It is easier for them and it builds local relationships. Give talks to therapists. Appreciate their skills. Learn their language: neuromuscular facilitation, Graston, McConnell taping. After a surgery or an injury, they are often spending much more time with the patient than you are. If a therapist raises a concern about a patient, take it seriously. Soon the therapists will be recommending you to injured athletes and even to patients who are not improving under care of another provider. If a therapist refers a patient to you, refer them back to the therapist for nonoperative or postoperative treatment. It upsets a therapist who refers you a patient to then have that therapist referred to therapy within your system.

9. Look for underrepresented sports. Everyone wants to cover high school football and in some communities, there is fierce competition to be the team physician. Being a high school team physician does not guarantee that the injured athlete will be treated by you. In point of fact, the patient will be referred by their pediatrician or primary care physician. Figure skating, gymnastics, running clubs, and dance are often undercovered and thrilled to have a physician interested in their unique issues. They tend to be very vibrant communities that will be faithful to your practice.

> **THE GURU SAYS...**
>
> The average high school football team has one or less operative injuries per year. Being a team physician is a true dedication, and not a shortcut to a busy operative schedule.
>
> MICHAEL T. BUSCH

Sports Injuries

Many of the acute injuries that occur to the pediatric athlete are fractures covered elsewhere in this text. This section emphasizes the most commonly encountered pediatric athletic injuries, with the focus on staying out of trouble as you help these young athletes return to sports.

SHOULDER INJURIES

Typical shoulder injuries in young athletes include sternoclavicular (SC) joint injuries, clavicle fractures, acromioclavicular (AC) joint injury, glenohumeral instability, and little league shoulder.

Sternoclavicular Joint Injury

SC joint injuries, although still uncommon, are being seen with increased frequency. Posterior SC joint injuries are usually traumatic resulting from a direct blow to the medial clavicle.[8] There is deformity and pain at the SC joint. There may be hoarseness, difficulty swallowing, or vascular insult from posterior displacement of the medial clavicle toward the important mediastinal structures of the esophagus, trachea, and large vessels (Fig. 14-2A). Staying out of trouble with SC joint injuries includes not missing the diagnosis. These injuries are notoriously difficult to view on plain X-ray, including the serendipity view. Three-dimensional imaging (CT or MRI) is required to make the diagnosis and to characterize the injury (Fig. 14-2B). Although traditional teaching is that these injuries are usually medial clavicle physeal fractures since the medial clavicle physis closes late, a recent study showed that nearly half of these injuries in adolescents are true joint dislocations.[9] Treatment should be urgent and in the operating room with vascular/cardiac surgery backup. Rare cases have been reported of serious blood loss from reduction of a posterior SC joint dislocation. Stay out of trouble and inform your vascular surgeons. Don't do this case at the surgery center! Closed reduction has been described with abduction of the shoulder in the horizontal plane with a beanbag between the shoulder blades and percutaneous reduction with a towel clamp. Because closed or percutaneous reduction may redislocate or is often unsuccessful, I tend to operate on posterior SC joint dislocations. This involves open reduction, repairing the intra-articular disk if torn, repairing the periosteal

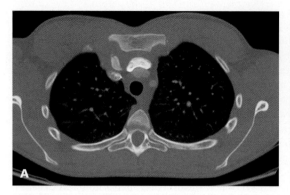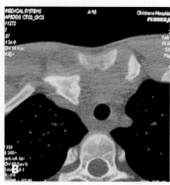

Figure 14-2 Axial **(A)** and sagittal **(B)** CT scans showing posterior displacement of the right SC joint with impingement on the mediastinal structures. Stay out of trouble by recognizing that this is an injury requiring urgent management. Posterior displacement can result in difficulty breathing, difficulty swallowing, or injury to the major mediastinal vessels.

THE GURU SAYS...

By contrast, posterior displaced fractures that do not compromise the airway or vessels can be allowed to heal and often remodel without surgery.

MICHAEL T. BUSCH

tube, and stabilizing the medial clavicle and sternum with heavy suture. Ligament reconstruction is not typically needed.

Anterior SC joint injuries are different than posterior SC joint. Although some are traumatic, many are atraumatic and associated with ligamentous laxity. Some cases are asymptomatic: they have a pop that is not painful, have full motion, and have full function. These can be observed. Cases that are symptomatic will require surgery: open reduction and ligamentous reconstruction. I usually use allograft gracilis tendon through drill holes in the medial clavicle and sternum weaved in a figure-of-8 fashion (Fig. 14-3). Stay out of trouble by drilling carefully in the mediastinum. Chucking up the drill so it can only extend a few millimeters from the tissue protector and connecting the drill holes with an angled curette saves some angst.

Clavicle Fracture

Clavicle fractures are common in sports. Special considerations in athletes include time to return to play and shoulder function. Open reduction internal fixation (ORIF) of displaced clavicle fractures has gained enthusiasm in adolescents extrapolating from treatment trends in adults (Fig. 14-4). However, recent studies have shown similar results in terms of function with nonoperative treatment. Children and younger adolescents have greater remodeling potential. Some sports

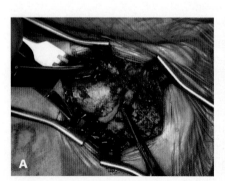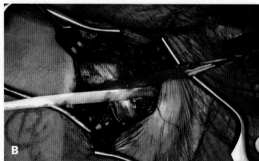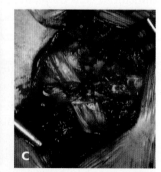

Figure 14-3 A: Open reduction of the SC joint, with forceps on the intra-articular disk. **B:** Allograft tendon weave through drill holes in the medial clavicle and sternum. **C:** Completed repair. Stay out of trouble by alerting your thoracic surgery colleagues that you will be operating on the SC joint and need thoracic backup. Don't be the cavalier surgeon who attempts this procedure at an outpatient surgery center!

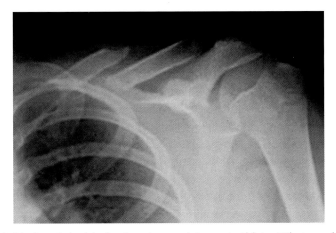

Figure 14-4 Displaced clavicle fracture in an adolescent athlete. What would you do? Stay out of trouble by not being dogmatic; not all displaced clavicle fractures in an adolescent need surgery and not all fractures can be managed nonoperatively. This is a great opportunity for shared decision-making with the family and patient.

parents may push surgical treatment for a sooner return to play. However, in contact sports this may be 6 to 12 weeks with surgery compared with 12 to 16 weeks with nonoperative treatment. Avoid trouble by adopting a shared decision-making approach erring toward nonoperative treatment.

Acromioclavicular Joint Injuries

Most AC joint injuries in children and adolescents are sprains without substantial displacement (types 1-3) that are treated nonoperatively. Even displaced AC joint injuries (types 4 and 5) in children and early adolescents may be treated nonoperatively. Unlike in adults, the ligaments are rarely disrupted. Instead, the periosteum remains attached to the intact ligaments, allowing excellent healing—sometimes so abundant that the callus is mistaken for a tumor (Fig. 14-5). Avoid trouble by simply watching these injuries recover in most children.

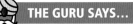

THE GURU SAYS...

The most definitive indications for surgery are open fracture, impending skin necrosis, and neurovascular compromise. The dominant shoulder in a late adolescent upper extremity athlete, with significant shortening or angulation, is probably a reasonable indication.

MICHAEL T. BUSCH

THE GURU SAYS...

Distal clavicle injures in youths are fractures until proved otherwise.

MICHAEL T. BUSCH

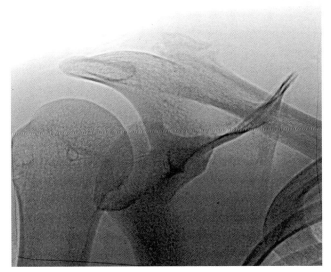

Figure 14-5 This distal clavicle physeal fracture had so much associated bony callus that it presented as a concern for a shoulder tumor. (Courtesy of C. Stanitski, MD.)

Glenohumeral Instability

Shoulder instability is seen frequently in adolescent athletes and can be classified as anterior instability, multidirectional instability (MDI), and posterior instability.[10] Anterior instability is usually traumatic and often results in anteroinferior capsulolabral disruption (Bankart lesion). The risk of recurrent dislocation is high in patients 18 years of age and younger, probably over 70%. Fixing the first-time dislocator versus fixing the recurrent dislocator is controversial. A one-size-fits-all approach does not work. I find an MRI helpful to delineate the extent of injury. In the acute setting, an MRI arthrogram is not necessary due to the arthrogram effect of the hemarthrosis. If there is a more extensive labral tear, ALPSA (anterior labral periosteal sleeve avulsion) lesion, HAGL (humeral avulsion of the glenohumeral ligament) lesion, or loose body, then surgery may be indicated initially. I find, however, that most patients can be managed nonoperatively and have surgery if they dislocate again. If the shoulder has dislocated two or three times, the patient and family usually appreciate that the shoulder is dysfunctional preoperatively. If you operate on a first-time dislocator, the shoulder was "normal" to the family before you operated. Stay out of trouble by adopting a shared decision-making process in these cases. Some families are risk averse and want to avoid surgery. Others are more averse to recurrent instability that may take the athlete out of sports and want to have it fixed initially. Also, the timing of the season may impact decision-making. A patient with a dislocated shoulder in the beginning or middle of the football season can often return to sports and have it fixed at the end of the season. I usually do an arthroscopic labral repair and capsulorrhaphy (Fig. 14-6). Open stabilization may be indicated for instability after prior arthroscopic surgery. However, open surgery has potential complications of subscapularis rupture or losing external rotation. Latarjet coracoid transfer has become very popular in adults and is being performed more frequently in adolescents. Indications for Latarjet include glenoid bone loss, large engaging Hill-Sachs lesion, and "off track" lesions. However, the Latarjet procedure is a larger operation than arthroscopic stabilization and has substantial risks such as nerve injury, nonunion, and stiffness.

MDI is very different from anterior instability. The direction of instability is usually posteriorly and inferiorly. The pathology is usually capsular laxity, not

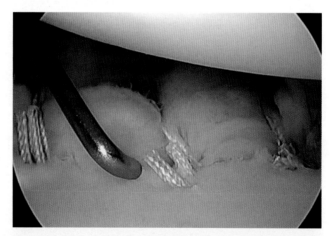

Figure 14-6 Arthroscopic anterior labral repair and capsulorrhaphy for recurrent anterior traumatic instability. Anteroinferior labral tear without glenoid bone loss is the most common pathology in recurrent anterior traumatic instability in adolescents. Stay out of trouble by not going overboard with shoulder instability treatment in the adolescent; Latarjet, remplissage, or allograft ligament reconstruction is rarely indicated.

a labral tear. The typical patient is a ligamentously lax adolescent female. Look for Ehlers-Danlos syndrome and refer to genetics if appropriate. Do a Beighton score. Staying out of trouble means the initial treatment should be PT. Identify shoulder therapists who like to work with these patients as both physical and mental therapist. The shoulder PT for MDI should address strengthening, scapular mechanics, scapular winging, shoulder posture, snapping scapula, and pain control. Beware of the voluntary dislocator with psychiatric overlay. Although I try to avoid surgery in MDI patients, some patients fail PT and have instability that impairs activities of daily living (ADLs). In these patients, shoulder stabilization can be performed by arthroscopic capsulorrhaphy or open capsular shift. I favor open inferior capsular shift in patients with Ehlers-Danlos syndrome or generalized ligamentous laxity as it reduces capsular volume to a greater extent than arthroscopic capsulorrhaphy.[11] Be careful of operating in overhead athletes with MDI such as swimmers, throwers, and gymnasts. If their symptoms are with sports but not ADLs, then they may have difficulty returning to sports because of loss of motion and they may be unhappy. If they are having difficulty with ADLs, then I think surgery is reasonable, and I tell them that return to sports is possible but not assured.

Little League Shoulder

Little league shoulder is widening of the proximal humeral physis from repetitive rotational stress. This is often a cause of chronic shoulder pain in younger pitchers, whereas internal impingement is often the cause of chronic shoulder pain in older adolescent pitchers. Interestingly, proximal humeral physeal changes and acquired increased humeral retroversion is an adaptive change in pitchers to allow for the increased external rotation of the throwing arm seen in adult pitchers. The diagnosis can be made from history, physical examination, and comparison X-rays showing increased widening of the involved arm (Fig. 14-7). The treatment is nonoperative with activity restriction, PT, and pitching mechanics. Stay out of trouble by giving the family a realistic expectation for return to throwing at 4 months instead of 3 to 6 weeks.[12] Emphasize PT and pitching mechanics to avoid recurrence. Try to find a biomotion lab that does pitching mechanics, physical therapists who like pitchers, and pitching coaches who understand pitching mechanics and injury.

ELBOW INJURIES

Medial Epicondyle Fracture

Medial epicondyle fractures can occur in throwing or upper extremity weight-bearing athletes such as gymnasts. In throwers, there may be an antecedent history of medial elbow pain before the acute fracture. Whereas there is controversy regarding operative versus nonoperative treatment of displaced medial epicondyle fractures in a typical pediatric patient, I would recommend surgical fixation for the high-demand elbow athlete such as a baseball or softball thrower, or a gymnast (Fig. 14-8). **ORTHOPAEDICS 101: The humeral origin of the UCL originates from the medial epicondyle, so the medial epicondyle must be important.** Acute fixation followed by early mobilization typically leads to good results. If treated nonoperatively, this can lead to symptomatic nonunion with pain, valgus instability, and ulnar neuropathy. Fixing an established medial epicondyle nonunion is challenging in terms of scar, protecting the ulnar nerve, and mobilizing the fragment back to its base.[13] Thus, staying out of trouble with this fracture in the athlete involves ORIF to avoid symptomatic nonunion.

> **THE GURU SAYS...**
> Attention to detail regarding a youth athlete's core strengthening, hip strengthening, lower extremity balance training, and scapular stabilizers will help ensure that their entire upper extremity has an appropriate, stable platform. Stay out of trouble by strengthening the entire kinetic chain and do not focus solely on the involved joint.
>
> THEODORE J. GANLEY

> **THE GURU SAYS...**
> While the average kid may tolerate some loss of motion and a very delayed union, many dedicated athletes and families don't.
>
> MICHAEL T. BUSCH

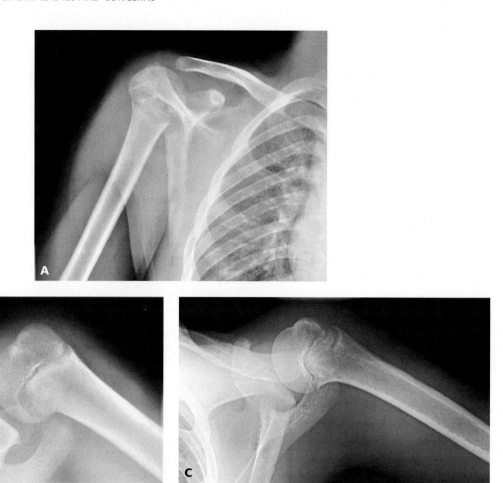

Figure 14-7 Humeral epiphysiolysis in a 13-year-old pitcher. Mom said that her son was so good that she had him pitching in three different leagues. **A, B:** Views of the right proximal humerus at presentation. He had significant shoulder pain. There is widening of the physis consistent with proximal humeral epiphysiolysis. **C:** This lateral image of the proximal humerus after 6 months of rest shows that the physeal appearance has returned to normal.

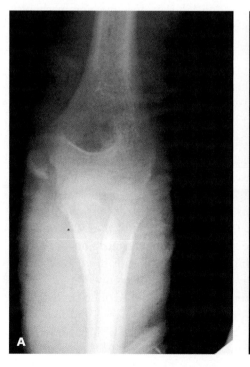
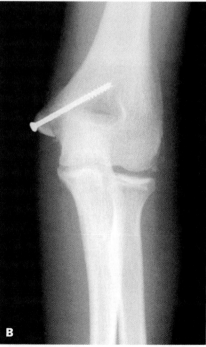

Figure 14-8 Medial epicondyle displaced fracture in adolescent athlete treated with ORIF (open reduction internal fixation). The management of displaced isolated medial epicondyle fractures is controversial—surgical versus nonsurgical. However, this indication is not. Medial epicondyle fractures associated with elbow dislocation or entrapped within the joint should be fixed!

Little League Elbow

Little league elbow describes injuries about the pediatric throwing elbow related to repetitive valgus loading.[14] These injuries include medial injuries from repetitive distraction (medial epicondyle apophysitis), lateral injuries from repetitive compression (OCD [osteochondritis dissecans] of the capitellum), and posterior injuries from repetitive shear (olecranon apophysitis).

Medial epicondyle apophysitis is characterized by medial elbow pain, tenderness at the medial epicondyle, and widening of the apophysis on X-ray. Treatment is nonoperative and similar to little league shoulder: stop throwing, PT, pitching mechanics. Staying out of trouble is setting reasonable expectations regarding returning to throwing, usually in 6 to 8 weeks. If the child throws through medial elbow pain, they can sustain a medial epicondyle avulsion fracture (see above). This warning usually gets the families' attention and facilitates compliance.

OCD of the Capitellum

Repetitive compressive loading of the capitellum can lead to OCD in throwers and gymnasts. OCD involves fragmentation of the subchondral bone with articular cartilage and can lead to instability and a loose fragment (Fig. 14-9). OCD can be suspected on X-rays and MRI is useful for staging the lesion. If detected early with intact articular cartilage, OCD can be treated nonoperatively with cessation of sports. Approximately 40% of lesions will heal in the elbow, which is lower than the knee (60%).[15] Lesions that do not heal can be treated with arthroscopic drilling. Later-stage lesions are treated with either fragment removal and microfracture or cartilage resurfacing with OATS (osteochondral autograft transfer system) plugs from the knee. This can be done through a direct anconeus splitting approach in hyperflexion. High-demand athletes such as pitchers and high-level gymnasts may have better results with OATS. Staying out of trouble in OCD of the capitellum means trying to detect the lesions early where treatment is simpler.

Ulnar Collateral Ligament Injury

Ulnar collateral ligament (UCL) injuries are being seen more frequently in older adolescent pitchers. Once the medial epicondyle apophysis fuses, the weak link becomes the UCL. UCL injuries are diagnosed by medial elbow pain, decreased pitch velocity or accuracy, and valgus instability on examination. MRI helps to confirm the attritional tearing of the UCL (Fig. 14-10). UCL reconstruction, "Tommy John" surgery, is one of the most recognizable surgeries to the lay public and has taken on almost mythical status. Because of the success of Tommy John surgery in returning high-profile MLB (Major League Baseball) pitchers back to sport, some families view this operation as a performance-enhancing surgery. In fact, I have had families demand Tommy John for their child with elbow pain but an intact UCL!

UCL reconstruction is a long recovery—often 9 to 12 months—until throwing, and the data suggest that many throwers do not get back to the same level, particularly adolescent throwers. This is important to discuss with young athletes and their families, as their expectations may come from selected success stories in professional athletes. Modern UCL surgery typically involves flexor-pronator split, ulnar nerve decompression but not transposition, and a docking technique with palmaris longus or gracilis tendon (Fig. 14-11).

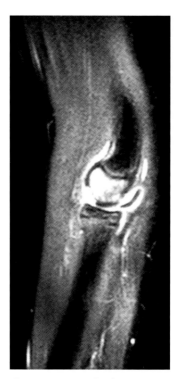

Figure 14-9 Sagittal MRI showing loose body associated with OCD of the capitellum. Should you do a simple procedure (scope, removal loose body, microfracture) or a complex procedure (OATS): the decision should be driven by patient factors (upper extremity athlete such as gymnast or baseball pitcher) and lesion factors (large lesions, poor underlying bone, cystic changes in the bone, uncontained lesions without a shoulder).

THE GURU SAYS...

Be sure the family understands that it takes at least 6 months for the graft to fully incorporate.

Michael T. Busch

THE GURU SAYS...

I periodically see referrals for acute UCL injuries, for instance, from an elbow dislocation. UCL reconstructions are almost exclusively indicated for chronic tissue fatigue injuries that do not have the biologic stimulus to heal. Not everyone understands that.

Michael T. Busch

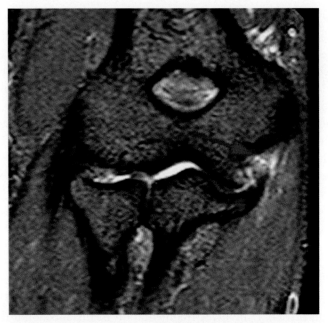

Figure 14-10 Coronal MRI showing ulnar collateral ligament tear.

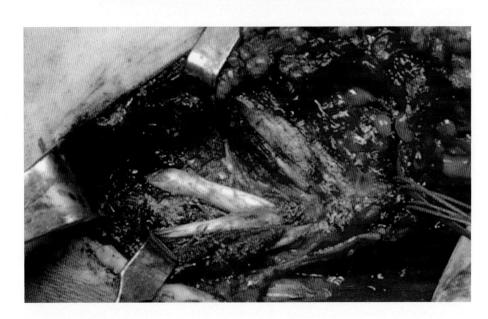

Figure 14-11 Ulnar collateral ligament (UCL) reconstruction with a docking technique. UCL reconstruction is a reliable operation to restore valgus stability and return to pitching. However, beware the crazy sports parents who demand Tommy John surgery for their child with a UCL sprain or medial epicondyle apophysitis!

WRIST INJURIES

Gymnast Wrist

Like little league shoulder in throwers, repetitive impact and weight-bearing on the hand and wrist in gymnasts can lead to pain and widening of the distal radial physis (gymnast wrist). However, unlike little league shoulder, gymnast wrist has a real risk of growth disturbance, resulting in shortening of the radius, overgrowth of the ulna, and ulnar-carpal impaction. The diagnosis is made in a patient with wrist pain, tenderness to palpation of the distal radius, and widening of the physis on comparison X-rays (Fig. 14-12). Gymnast wrist can be bilateral. In unclear cases, MRI can demonstrate widening of the physis and edema. Stopping the impact and loading on the wrist is key to treatment. This can result in resolution of pain, normalization of the widened physis, and avoidance of growth disturbance.[16] However, many gymnasts and gymnast families are extremely driven to

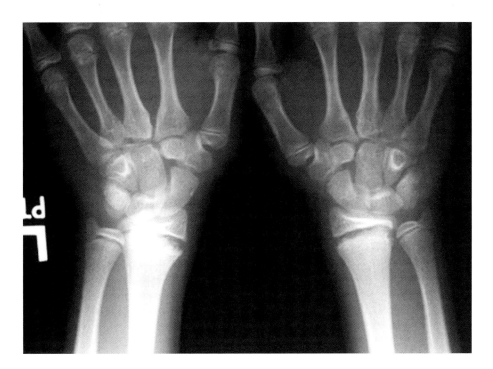

Figure 14-12 Gymnast wrist. Radiographs showing bilateral widening of the distal radius physis in a gymnast. Stay out of trouble by taking this seriously. Unlike little league shoulder, gymnast wrist can result in growth disturbance that can then lead to ulnar overgrowth, ulnocarpal impaction, and triangular fibrocartilage complex tears. So scare the patient and family. Keep them out of gymnastics until the pain resolves and the X-rays normalize, often 4 to 6 months. They will drive you crazy and level 10 gymnasts are not to be trusted, but the consequences of growth disturbance may end their gymnastics career!

compete and compliance can be challenging. Emphasize the avoidance of serious growth disturbance with resultant need for surgery. Cases with growth disturbance with ulnar-carpal impaction are usually treated with ulnar shortening and TFCC (triangular fibrocartilage complex) repair. Return to high-level gymnastics is unlikely.

HIP INJURIES

Labral Tears and Femoroacetabular Impingement

Labral tears are occurring and being diagnosed with increased frequency in adolescents. Labral tears often present as deep groin pain that can radiate around the hip and has been recalcitrant to PT for soft-tissue tendonitis or bursitis. On examination, patients will have pain with flexion and internal rotation. Labral injuries are particularly susceptible in certain athletes such as ice hockey players, field hockey athletes, and dancers. MRI arthrogram or plain MRI with radial sequences demonstrate the tear; however, MRI may show labral tears in asymptomatic patients, so it is important to correlate imaging with symptoms and physical examination findings. Ultrasound-guided injection about the hip (intra-articular, iliopsoas, trochanteric bursa) may be very helpful both therapeutically but also in identifying the etiology of hip pain. Stay out of trouble by identifying underlying structural abnormalities that may predispose to labral tearing such as femoroacetabular impingement (FAI) or acetabular dysplasia. Although many patients are referred with an MRI, make sure you get radiographs (standing AP pelvis, bilateral Dunn laterals, false profile) to understand the underlying structural abnormalities such as cam FAI (Fig. 14-13A), pincer FAI (Fig. 14-13B), and acetabular dysplasia (Fig. 14-13C).

Patients with labral tears should be given an initial trial of nonoperative treatment with PT and/or injections as many adolescent patients may be successfully treated nonoperatively.[17] Patients who fail nonoperative treatment may be candidates for arthroscopic surgery. This typically involves labral repair or refixation (Fig. 14-14). There may be articular cartilage injury such as full-thickness

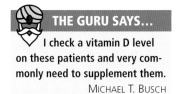

THE GURU SAYS...

I check a vitamin D level on these patients and very commonly need to supplement them.

MICHAEL T. BUSCH

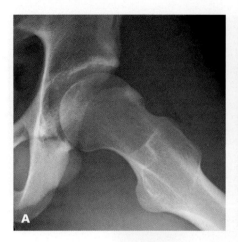
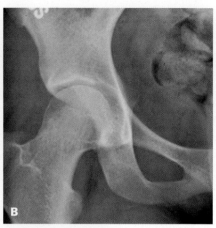
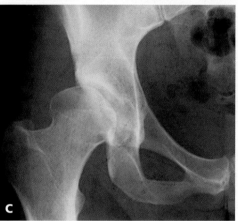

Figure 14-13 A: Cam femoroacetabular impingement (FAI). Dunn lateral radiograph demonstrating convex deformity at the femoral head-neck junction in an adolescent hockey player. **B:** Pincer FAI. AP radiograph of the right hip showing a positive crossover sign, indicating acetabular retroversion. **C:** Acetabular dysplasia. AP of right hip radiograph showing acetabular dysplasia. Stay out of trouble by recognizing the underlying structural issues associated with a labral tear. Don't be the hip arthroscopist who scopes a hip when a periacetabular osteotomy is needed for moderate to severe dysplasia! Also recognize that many adolescent athletes may have underlying FAI anatomy but their pain may be due to something else such as iliopsoas tendonitis or sports hernia!

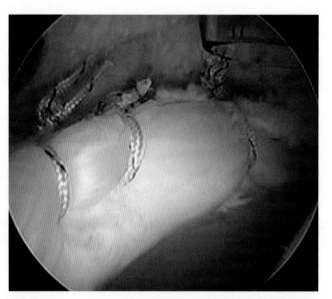

Figure 14-14 Hip arthroscopy with labral repair and refixation. Stay out of trouble by not being too zealous with the scope. Labral tears on MRI may be overread or may be an incidental finding when the patient's pain is from another diagnosis. Try nonoperative treatment (physical therapy, activity restriction, injections) as many patients with a labral tear may improve and not need surgery. A positive pain response to an intra-articular injection is a good sign that the patient may improve from arthroscopy.

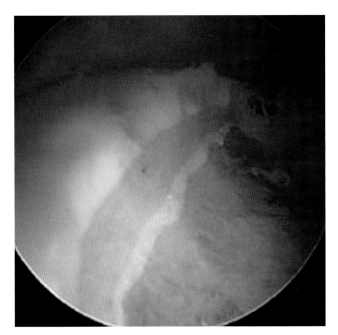

Figure 14-15 Hip arthroscopy with femoral osteochondroplasty for cam femoroacetabular impingement (FAI). Note the edge of the physis in an adolescent patient. Don't worry about growth issues in the adolescent with cam FAI. Most proximal femoral growth is over by this stage of development. Instead, think about the cause of cam FAI with respect to repetitive stress on the proximal femoral physis that leads to extra bone formation and distalization of the lateral physis.

chondral defects or chondral delamination, particularly in patients with cam FAI. Stay out of trouble by not just treating the labral tear, but also addressing the underlying structural issue.[18] This would be femoral osteochondroplasty for cam FAI (Fig. 14-15) and acetabular osteochondroplasty for pincer FAI. Ligamentously lax adolescent female athletes with borderline acetabular dysplasia can be particularly challenging. Avoid acetabular osteochondroplasty in these patients and capsular plication may be required for hip instability. Refer patients with moderate and severe dysplasia to your young adult hip colleagues for periacetabular osteotomy. These patients will not do well with arthroscopy alone.

Apophyseal Injuries About the Hip

Apophyseal injuries about the hip are common in skeletally immature adolescent injuries. Sports commonly associated with this injury are soccer, gymnastics, sprinting, hurdling, and jumping. These injuries include ASIS (anterior superior iliac spine) apophysitis or avulsion, AIIS (anterior inferior iliac spine) avulsion, iliac apophysitis, lesser trochanter apophyseal avulsion, and ischial tuberosity apophyseal avulsion. The vast majority of these injuries can be treated successfully nonoperatively with return to sports around 6 to 12 weeks. Stretching should be emphasized as many of these patients have structural tightness. Two apophyseal avulsion fractures that may be more complicated are AIIS avulsion and ischial tuberosity avulsion injuries. AIIS injuries can heal with deformity or bone that results in hip impingement (subspinous impingement) requiring arthroscopic decompression (Fig. 14-16). Ischial tuberosity avulsions can result in persistent pain or sciatic symptoms requiring fixation, particularly large fragments that are widely displaced (Fig. 14-17). Stay out of trouble by considering acute fixation of large, displaced ischial tuberosity fractures. Chronic fixation is challenging with retraction of the hamstrings and scar around the sciatic nerve.

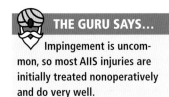

THE GURU SAYS...

Impingement is uncommon, so most AIIS injuries are initially treated nonoperatively and do very well.

MICHAEL T. BUSCH

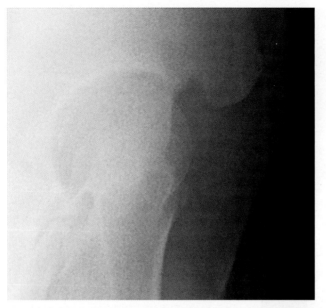

Figure 14-16 nterior inferior iliac spine (AIIS) apophyseal avulsion fracture that healed with subspinous impingement deformity. Not all AIIS avulsion fractures do well. Stay out of trouble by warning the family and following these patients over time for subspinous impingement.

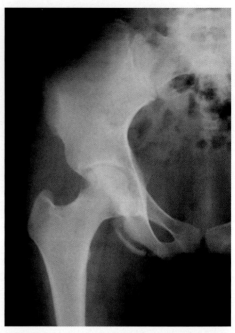

Figure 14-17 Ischial apophysis avulsion fracture can lead to sitting pain and sciatica. Stay out of trouble by warning these families also of subsequent problems. Consider fixing large fragments with wide displacement initially!

KNEE INJURIES

Tibial Spine Fracture

Tibial spine fractures were once thought to be the pediatric ACL injury equivalent injury in skeletally immature patients. Although ACL injuries in this age group are increasing in frequency, tibial spine fractures continue. **ORTHOPAEDICS 101: The mechanism of tibial spine fracture is an avulsion of the intercondylar eminence by the ACL. Thus, the ACL is not torn, but it may undergo plastic deformation at the time of injury.** Tibial spine fractures often present with a large hemarthrosis from the intra-articular fracture. There may be lack of extension from the bony block and ACL laxity from the discontinuity of the ACL-eminence structure. Diagnosis is usually by X-ray.

Closed reduction for displaced fractures (Meyers and McKeever type 2 or 3) can be attempted with aspiration of the knee and knee extension. However, this is usually not successful in type 2 fractures and I have never seen a truly type 3 fracture reduce. In addition, an entrapped intermeniscal ligament or anterior horn medial meniscus may prevent reduction (Fig. 14-18). Most type 2 or 3 fractures are thus treated with arthroscopic reduction and internal fixation. Internal fixation may be performed with epiphyseal cannulated screws (usually 4.0 mm diameter × 18 mm length) or suture fixation. Suture fixation is gaining popularity as this is biomechanically stronger and may allow for better reduction with tightening of the ACL (Fig. 14-19). I prefer suture fixation as it can be performed in smaller or comminuted fractures, it tightens the ACL, which may undergo plastic deformation, and there is no metal screw fixation for later hardware removal or interference with MRI.

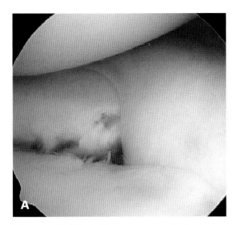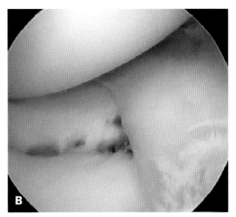

Figure 14-18 **A:** Entrapment of the intermeniscal ligament under the tibial spine fragment. **B:** Disentrapment of the intermeniscal ligament to its anatomic position above the fragment. Stay out of trouble by looking for meniscus entrapment. This may prevent anatomic reduction or may be a lateral source of pain. Extract it from the fracture site and retract it with a suture or a wire.

Stiffness is a common complication of tibial spine fractures. Stay out of trouble by early mobilization of the fracture. Knees should not be immobilized for more than 2 weeks after surgery. I aim for strong fixation so I can move the knee right away. If stiffness is identified, treat it early with aggressive PT and dynamic splinting.[19] If persistent at 3 months, arthroscopic lysis of adhesions followed by gentle manipulation under anesthesia is done.[20] Be careful to not fracture the distal femoral physis with aggressive manipulation[21] (Fig. 14-20).

The outcome is good for return to sports after tibial spine fractures usually at 4 months postoperatively. Because of the plastic deformation of the ACL or the athletic level of these patients to begin with, families should be warned about potential future ACL injury.

> **THE GURU SAYS...**
> Following an acute injury, timely and stable fixation as well as early mobilization can minimize the risk of stiffness. For patients presenting late with limited knee motion, having the patient regain knee motion prior to fixation can help prevent postoperative knee stiffness.
> THEODORE J. GANLEY

> **THE GURU SAYS...**
> Strongly agree that knees should not be immobilized for more than 2 weeks after surgery. Most epiphyseal fractures are healed by 3 weeks and hopefully the fixation is enough to compensate for early motion. It is easier to recover from nonunions than stiff knees.
> MICHAEL T. BUSCH

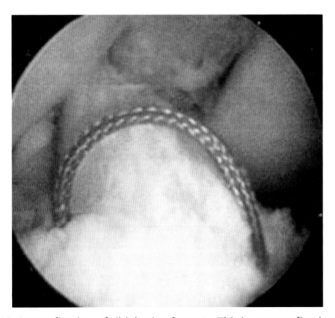

Figure 14-19 Suture fixation of tibial spine fracture. This is now my fixation of choice for tibial spine fractures as it can be performed for all fractures (even those with comminution or small bony fragments have higher biomechanical strength and do not require secondary surgery for screw removal).

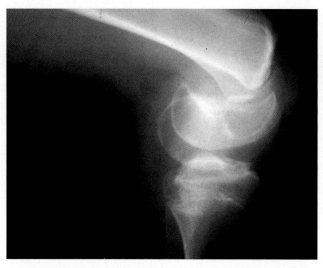

Figure 14-20 Distal femoral physeal fracture after manipulation for stiffness from tibial spine fracture. Stay out of trouble by doing a gentle manipulation after an arthroscopic lysis of adhesions. This is a bad complication that can lead to growth disturbance!

> **THE GURU SAYS...**
>
> Failure to diagnose can lead to young athletes returning to sports on unstable knees, with severe consequences. Educating trainers, coaches, and primary care physicians should be one of our focuses.
>
> MICHAEL T. BUSCH

> **THE GURU SAYS...**
>
> Stay out of trouble by recognizing and treating meniscal root tears and meniscocapsular separation ramp lesions to maintain circumferential hoop stress and cartilage viability.
>
> THEODORE J. GANLEY

ACL Injury

ACL injuries in children and adolescents have gained a lot of attention.[22-24] These injuries are being seen with increased frequency over the past decade or two. A traumatic hemarthrosis after a noncontact twisting injury or a contact injury with a pop should raise the suspicion of ACL tear. ACL insufficiency can also be seen congenitally either as isolated congenital absence of the cruciate ligaments or in association with other congenital conditions such as proximal focal femoral deficiency, fibular hemimelia, and tibial hemimelia. Physical examination may be difficult in a young child with a painful hemarthrosis because of guarding. MRI is useful to confirm the diagnosis and to look for associated injuries. **NEWSFLASH! Associated meniscal or chondral injuries occur in 50% of ACL tears in skeletally immature patients.**

Older treatment recommendations were for nonoperative treatment of ACL injuries in skeletally immature patients with a delay for surgery until skeletal maturity. This would involve PT, bracing, and keeping the patient out of cutting, pivoting, or contact sports. Although some partial ACL tears may do well without surgery, for complete ACL tears nonoperative treatment is problematic for two reasons. First, it is very challenging to keep these young athletes out of sports and activities. Sports commonly associated with this injury are soccer, gymnastics, sprinting, hurdling, and jumping. It may affect them and the family psychosocially. In addition, free play may result in cutting and pivoting. Secondly, these patients are at high risk for further meniscal or chondral injury. Recent studies have shown a much higher rate of meniscal or chondral injury with delay in treatment longer than 12 weeks.[25] These meniscal and chondral injuries have significance in terms of the long-term health of the knee. Stay out of trouble by having a shared decision-making process with the athlete and family, but emphasizing the risk and importance of further meniscal or chondral injury. Most pediatric ACL injuries should be treated with surgery.

Surgical treatment should respect the growth plates about the knee. The distal femoral and proximal tibial physes are the fastest growing growth plates in the body. An assessment of growth remaining is important when treating skeletally immature patients with ACL tears. Stay out of trouble by getting a hand film for bone age, estimating Tanner stage, and getting full-length AP hips to ankle X-rays for alignment and leg lengths prior to treatment. Surgical treatment options include physeal-sparing techniques, partial transphyseal techniques that go through the proximal tibial physis but avoid the distal femoral physis by going over the top or epiphyseal in the femur, and transphyseal techniques. In adolescent patients, transphyseal reconstruction is usually performed with anatomic positioning, fixation away from the growth plates (cortical fixation on the femur, interference screw or post/staple on the tibia), and soft-tissue autograft (hamstrings or quadriceps tendon). With more modern femoral tunnel drilling techniques such as anteromedial portal or outside-in, it is important to not go too obliquely across the distal femoral growth plate. In prepubescent patients, physeal-sparing techniques are recommended. These include intra-articular, extra-articular reconstruction with IT band and epiphyseal femoral and tibial tunnels.

> ### THE GURU SAYS...
> Those of us who have developed different all epiphyseal ACL reconstruction techniques owe a debt of gratitude to the wonderful creative mind and the original description of this technique by the late Dr. Allen Anderson.
>
> THEODORE J. GANLEY

The major concern about ACL reconstruction in skeletally immature patients is the risk of growth disturbance (leg length discrepancy and/or angular deformity). Cases of growth disturbance have been described with all techniques including transphyseal reconstruction and epiphyseal reconstruction (Fig. 14-21). Stay out of trouble by avoiding hardware across the growth plates, bone blocks across the growth plates, large tunnels, and aggressive dissection in the over the top position near the perichondrial ring.[26] Consider modifying your technique based on the amount of growth remaining with transphyseal techniques in adolescents and physeal-sparing techniques in prepubescents.

Return to sports after ACL reconstruction is evolving. Instead of time-based criteria such as 6 months, functional criteria are being emphasized, such as quadriceps and hamstring strength, balance, functional tests (hop tests), and neuromuscular control (drop landing tests). This has resulted in delaying return to sports to 9 months in most patients. Use of ACL braces after ACL reconstruction is controversial. ACL prevention programs should be emphasized to avoid reinjury to the operative knee and the higher risk of ACL tear in the contralateral knee. Skeletally immature patients should be followed up to the end of growth given the risk of growth issues and the higher risk of ACL graft tear than adult patients.

Meniscal Injury

Meniscal injuries are seen frequently in adolescents either as isolated injuries or in association with ACL tears. MRI, however, can overcall meniscal tears due to vascular and developmental changes in younger patients (Fig. 14-22). Stay out of trouble by reviewing the MRIs yourself and looking for meniscal signal change that extends to the articular surface of the meniscus. Compared to adults, treatment of meniscal tears in children and adolescents should emphasize meniscal preservation when possible.[27] The biomechanical function of the meniscus is important in terms of shock absorption, stress transmission, and stability of the knee. Total or near total meniscectomy results in early arthritis of the knee

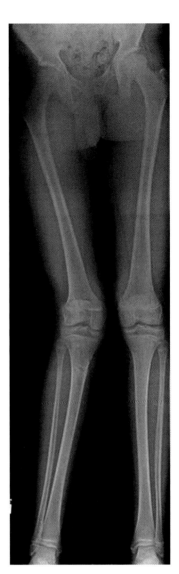

Figure 14-21 Growth disturbance after transphyseal anterior cruciate ligament reconstruction in a prepubescent patient. This may be rare, but when it happens the consequences are severe often requiring complex leg lengthening and angular correction surgery. Stay out of trouble by avoiding transphyseal surgery in prepubescent patients!

> ### THE GURU SAYS...
> I use a physeal-sparing technique for boys 12 years old and younger, and for girls 10 years and younger (skeletal ages). This typically translates to growth remaining of greater or less than 5 cm at the knee.
>
> MICHAEL T. BUSCH

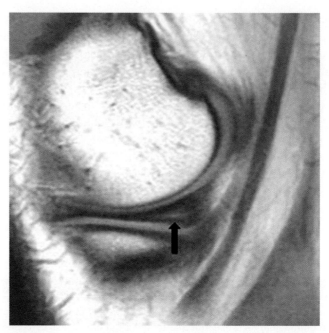

Figure 14-22 Normal meniscal signal change in a pediatric patient. Stay out of trouble by reviewing your own MRI scans and looking for signal change that extends to the articular surface of the meniscus and correlating with symptoms and physical examination.

THE GURU SAYS...

Overzealous repairs of the improbable can result in higher failure rates, which lead to disappointment, greater time lost from sports, reoperation, and potentially to articular damage.

MICHAEL T. BUSCH

THE GURU SAYS...

Counsel patients with an asymptomatic discoid meniscus to return to see you if they develop locking, catching, persistent swelling, or increasing pain that can signify a discoid meniscus tear. Treating acute tears can be significantly easier than treating chronic tears.

THEODORE J. GANLEY

THE GURU SAYS...

Like hip dysplasia, we recommend clinical follow-up every couple of years for the more severely involved. Also obtain alignment films to check for insidious onset of valgus.

MICHAEL T. BUSCH

within 10 years. Even partial meniscectomy can dramatically increase contact stress. **NEWSFLASH! Children and adolescents likely have increased vascularity and cellularity than the adult pattern of vascularity in the peripheral third of the meniscus only. Thus, meniscal repair can be successfully performed in children and adolescents in the middle third of the meniscus or in tear patterns such as radial tears or horizontal cleavage tears.** Stay out of trouble by not removing too much meniscus in the pediatric patient. Meniscal repair techniques include all-inside devices, inside-out sutures, and outside-in sutures. Be careful of penetrating too far with all-inside devices in the posterior horn of the medial and lateral meniscus in smaller children because of risk of injury to the popliteal neurovascular structures.

Discoid lateral meniscus is a unique pediatric condition. In young children, this may present as an otherwise asymptomatic popping knee or a lack of extension.[28] The diagnosis is confirmed by MRI (Fig. 14-23). Asymptomatic patients without tearing of the meniscus should be treated with observation, such as nonpainful occasional popping in a young child. Stay out of trouble—you can always make them worse with surgery instead of better! In the symptomatic discoid meniscus, surgery is indicated. This involves saucerization to a more normal shape and meniscal repair if unstable to probing after saucerization (Fig. 14-24). Stay out of trouble by looking for instability after saucerization both anteriorly and posteriorly. Repair is usually best done with inside-out sutures. Horizontal cleavage tears are common. These can be treated with meniscal repair with superior surface-inferior surface "sandwich" sutures. Warn the family that retear is not uncommon, approximately 20%, and may require further surgery. Avoid subtotal meniscectomy as this may lead to arthritis. When stuck with a pediatric patient after total or subtotal meniscectomy who is symptomatic and developing arthritic changes, consider meniscus transplantation. Physeal-sparing lateral meniscus transplantation techniques in skeletally immature patients have been described.[29]

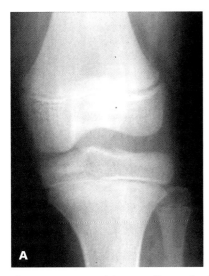
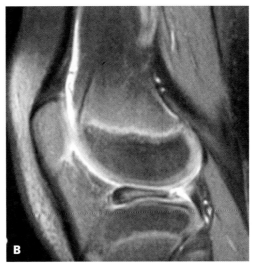

Figure 14-23 **A:** This AP radiograph of the knee in a girl with "clicking" shows widening of the lateral hemijoint. The orthopaedist suspected discoid meniscus. **B:** This sagittal MRI cut shows classic discoid meniscus with the bulk of the abnormal meniscus anterior.

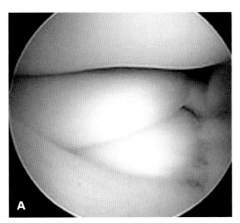
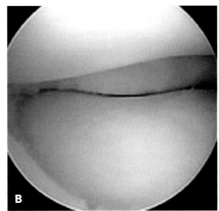

Figure 14-24 **A, B:** Saucerization of a discoid lateral meniscus. Stay out of trouble by going slowly with meniscus saucerization. You can always take more tissue but you can't put it back! Use multiple instruments that are angled (baskets, shavers, arthroscopic knives). After saucerization, probe the meniscus and move the knee. If the meniscus is unstable, it needs meniscal repair!

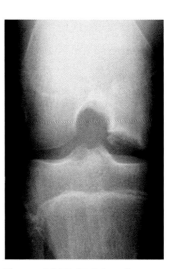

Figure 14-25 Notch radiograph showing osteochondritis dissecans (OCD) lesion of the medial femoral condyle. Stay out of trouble by ordering a notch radiograph in your standard knee series in children. You may miss the OCD lesion on AP and lateral views!

Osteochondritis Dissecans of the Knee

OCD of the knee is frequently encountered in the adolescent knee.[30,31] Early-stage lesions with intact cartilage may present as vague knee pain, often misdiagnosed as patellofemoral pain. Later stage lesions with instability have more obvious symptoms such as swelling, catching, and locking. Stay out of trouble by getting X-rays, particularly the notch view (Fig. 14-25), in patients with unilateral knee pain. Also get contralateral knee X-rays because OCD may be present in 25% to 33% of cases and treatment is simpler if it is caught in earlier stages. MRI is essential for staging OCD lesions and looking for size, chronicity, edema, articular cartilage fissuring, and instability (Fig. 14-26).

Early-stage lesions with intact articular cartilage (Hefti 1-2) can be treated nonoperatively. This involves activity restriction and PT for 3 or 4 months. Protected weight-bearing and unloader bracing may be useful adjuvants. MRI

THE GURU SAYS...

Educate your primary care colleagues that persistent knee pain in adolescents should not be ignored and that notch views are essential.

MICHAEL T. BUSCH

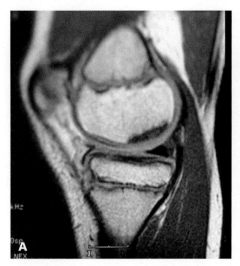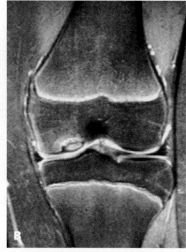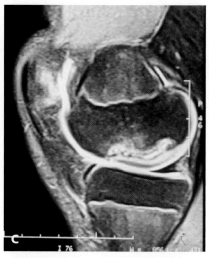

Figure 14-26 The good, the bad, and the ugly of osteochondritis dissecans lesions of the distal femur. Stay out of trouble by recognizing the difference. **A:** The good (probably will heal with immobilization). This sagittal image shows that the articular surface is completely intact. There is no effusion and the lesion is not marginated. **B:** The articular surface is intact but the lesion is marginated and the child is approaching skeletal maturity. Drill and pray. **C:** In this case the articular surface is disrupted and the lesion is partially detached. Major trouble—prepare the family for more than one operation.

can be repeated to assess progression toward healing. If the lesion is worsened or not improved, arthroscopic drilling is recommended (Fig. 14-27A). This can be done technically transarticular or retroarticular. Both techniques show high success rates. Stay out of trouble by avoiding drilling through the physis. Fissured (Hefti 3) or unstable lesions (Hefti 4-5) are treated surgically usually with fixation and drilling (Fig. 14-27B). Bone grafting may be required in some chronic lesions. Fragment fixation should be emphasized in young patients instead of fragment removal and chondral resurfacing given their higher healing ability and the preference of retaining their own articular cartilage. In cases that have failed prior fixation or those cases not amenable to fixation, excision with chondral

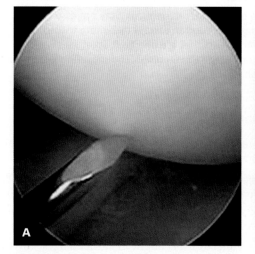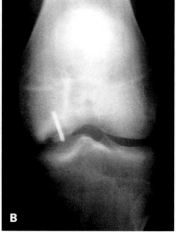

Figure 14-27 A: Transarticular drilling of osteochondritis dissecans (OCD). This can be done transarticular or retroarticular, but make sure you have adequately drilled the lesion to stimulate blood supply! **B:** OCD fixation with a variable pitch metallic screw. Whenever possible, try fixation of the OCD lesion before removal and chondral resurfacing. Keeping the patient's own cartilage is usually better than trying to stimulate cartilage growth or using allograft!

resurfacing may be necessary. Chondral resurfacing techniques include microfracture, OATS, osteoarticular allograft, ACI (autologous chondrocyte implantation) with sandwich technique, and MACI (matrix-induced autologous chondrocyte implantation).

Patellofemoral Instability

The peak incidence of patellofemoral instability is in adolescence. Try to develop a systematic approach to these patients. Determine if this is habitual dislocation in a pediatric orthopaedic–type patient or acquired dislocation in a sports medicine–type patient. Stay out of trouble by a thorough assessment of the multiple factors that can contribute to patellofemoral instability such as ligamentous laxity, genu valgum, femoral anteversion, external tibial torsion, pronation of the foot, trochlear dysplasia, and patellar alta.

I find it useful to obtain an MRI for the first-time patellar dislocator. If there is a loose body (20% of dislocators), surgery is recommended with fixation or excision of the loose body and medial patellofemoral ligament (MPFL) repair (Fig. 14-28). Stay out of trouble by identifying if there is a loose body. If there is no loose body (80% of dislocators), then nonoperative treatment is indicated including PT and patellofemoral bracing. Emphasize quadriceps and VMO (vastus medialis oblique) strengthening but also hip abductor strengthening and neuromuscular control. If the patient subsequently redislocates, then surgery is indicated.

Surgery should be individualized for each patient. If there is lateral retinaculum tightness with tilt short of neutral, then limited lateral release can be performed. Don't overdo the lateral release. If there are insufficient medial structures, then MPFL reconstruction is recommended. MPFL reconstruction has become a hot surgery. MPFL reconstruction has higher success rates to medial plication alone. A variety of MPFL techniques have been described using various grafts and fixation devices.[32] In the skeletally immature patient, the femoral origin of the MPFL is very close to the physis. Fluoroscopy should be used to place the MPFL just

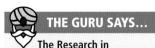

THE GURU SAYS...

The Research in Osteochondritis Dissecans of the Knee (ROCK) group established terminology that can help you accurately describe these lesions.

THEODORE J. GANLEY

THE GURU SAYS...

Limited lateral release is almost never an isolated procedure for instability. It is needed for fixed or the obligate dislocator, and relatively contraindicated for the hypermobile patient.

MICHAEL T. BUSCH

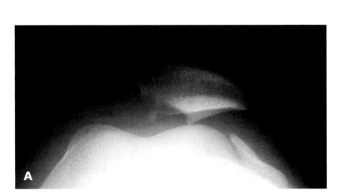
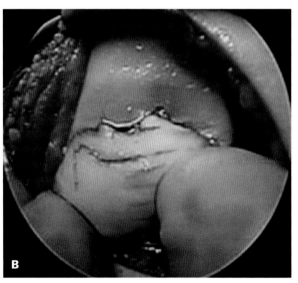

Figure 14-28 A: Patella dislocation with a fracture of the medial patellar facet. **B:** Surgical fixation of the fracture. Stay out of trouble by having a high index of suspicion of an osteoarticular fracture associated with traumatic patellofemoral dislocation. Sometimes the fragments can be very larger from the medial patellar facet or the lateral femoral condyle.

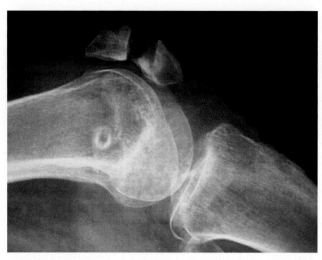

Figure 14-29 Patella fracture after medial patellofemoral ligament (MPFL) reconstruction with transverse patellar tunnel. Stay out of trouble by avoiding transverse tunnels across the patella for MPFL reconstruction. Consider anchor fixation, periosteal fixation, or biotenodesis.

THE GURU SAYS...

Unless the valgus is mild, fix the alignment first and do the patellar stabilization later. Realignment alone can fix some cases of instability. Stabilizing a patella with the knee in excessive valgus can result in an overcorrection when the alignment improves.

MICHAEL T. BUSCH

distal to the physis. The MPFL should be tensioned with the knee flexed so the patella engages the trochlear groove. Be careful of overtensioning the graft and medial subluxation. Be careful of transverse tunnels across the patella, which can lead to patella fracture (Fig. 14-29).

Additional procedures should be performed as indicated. In skeletally mature patients with an increased (>20 mm) TT-TG distance, anteromedialization tibial tubercle osteotomy can be performed. In skeletally immature patients with an increased TT-TG distance, Roux-Goldthwait lateral hemipatellar tendon transfer can be performed. Also consider guided growth in skeletally immature patients with associated genu valgum.

Checklist for Patellofemoral Instability

- Rotational alignment (femoral anteversion, external tibial torsion)
- Coronal alignment (genu valgum)
- Ligamentous laxity
- Trochlear dysplasia
- Patella alta
- Lateral retinacular tightness
- Medial retinacular/MPFL laxity/insufficiency
- Loose bodies
- Patella articular cartilage status
- TT-TG distance

Patellofemoral Pain

Patellofemoral pain is a "headache of the knee" for both the patient and the clinician. This is often an overuse complaint in an adolescent female athlete. Patellofemoral pain may be associated with patellofemoral maltracking with increased lateral tracking and tilt. Treatment is supportive and nonoperative. A good physical therapist is essential to work on lateral stretching, medial strengthening, proprioception, neuromuscular control, and coping. Bracing may or may not be beneficial.

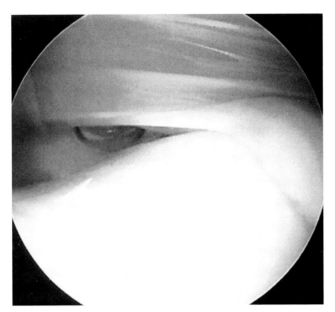

Figure 14-30 Staying out of trouble with plica means knowing which ones will benefit from surgical resection. Arthroscopic view of a plica that is substantial in size and notching the articular cartilage of the femoral condyle.

In patients who are not improving, look for alternative diagnoses such as plica, articular cartilage defect of the patella, or CRPS. CRPS must be considered in the differential diagnosis of anterior knee pain, either before or after surgery. The primary complaint is out of proportion to the inciting event. Early in the condition skin trophic changes are not present and imaging changes are also lacking. Also, don't forget to examine the hip. Hip issues such as slipped capital femoral epiphysis (SCFE) may present primarily with knee or distal thigh pain. Stay out of trouble by examining the hip and if the hip is painful with flexion-internal rotation, get hip X-rays.

Stay out of trouble by trying to avoid operating on patellofemoral pain. Surgery for patellofemoral pain (isolated lateral release, chondroplasty for chondromalacia, fat pad debridement) often fails and is frustrating to the patient and provider. If suspecting a plica, make sure it is symptomatic (Fig. 14-30). Ultrasound-guided injection can help confirm the diagnosis of a painful plica.

Popliteal Cysts

Popliteal (Baker) cysts may cause trouble through misdiagnosis or overtreatment. The vast majority of children who present with a popliteal mass will have a classic popliteal cyst, which requires no treatment other than observation. Although soft-tissue sarcomas are rare, they can occur in this area and should not be dismissed as a Baker cyst.[33] If the cyst is soft, in the classic location, and appears fluid-filled by transillumination, observation is warranted. If the cyst is in an unusual location or is firm or does not transilluminate, an ultrasound is a simple, relatively inexpensive, noninvasive way to confirm the diagnosis. If ultrasound does not show the classic fluid-filled cyst, MRI may be valuable to stay out of trouble. Another source of trouble with popliteal cysts is overtreatment. Families should be counseled that these cysts will generally resolve in children, but resolution may take several years. The popliteal cysts should not be routinely resected—observation is recommended as most will resolve or become smaller and asymptomatic.[34] After resection, scarring and soft-tissue problems can be significant, and neurovascular structures can be at risk with misguided surgery. Finally, the recurrence rate of these cysts can exceed 70%, which is discouraging to all involved.

THE GURU SAYS…

It's unfortunate that the same term is used for adults and children. In adults, cysts in the popliteal region typically arise from the posterior joint capsule and are usually related to intra-articular pathology. In children, these cysts arise from the semimembranosus bursa and are not related to the knee joint itself.

MICHAEL T. BUSCH

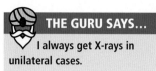
Osgood-Schlatter Syndrome

Osgood-Schlatter (OS) syndrome is commonplace. Patients point to pain over an enlarged tibial tubercle apophysis. X-rays may show enlargement, fragmentation, or an ossicle at the apophysis (Fig. 14-31). Although you may be tempted to forgo X-rays in a patient with classic OS symptoms, if there are any atypical symptoms such as night pain or rest pain, get X-rays because atypical lesions can present (Fig. 14-32). These patients are often jumping or kicking athletes. They are also frequently tight. Most children who present with OS have recently gone through a period of rapid growth and have significant quadriceps and hamstring contractures. If there is acute severe pain, often after chronic mild pain, consider a tibial tubercle apophyseal fracture.

Treatment is supportive. Stop the running and jumping. Ice the bump if painful. NSAIDs may be of benefit. PT is helpful to work on tightness. When they are nontender to palpation and do not have pain with resisted extension, they can gradually return to sports. This may take 3 to 6 weeks. A strap across the tendon may be of benefit for some patients. Another key to staying out of trouble with OS is to avoid casting. Although casting will give the knee a rest, it just leads to more atrophy and contracture at the quadriceps, thus aggravating the underlying cause and assuring recurrence upon return to sports. OGS often returns periodically. Teach the family how to manage it by modifying activity and working on baseline flexibility. Although it almost always resolves with skeletal maturity, there are patients who may remain symptomatic after skeletal maturity because of a painful ossicle. In these patients, ossicle excision with burring down the tubercle prominence can be helpful.

Sinding-Larsen-Johansson (SLJ) syndrome represents pain at the apophysis of the inferior pole of the patella. The pathophysiology is very similar to OS; most of these young athletes also have a quadriceps contracture and an overuse injury.

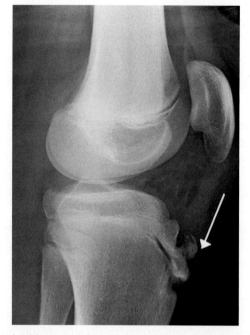

Figure 14-31 Osgood-Schlatter syndrome with widening and fragmentation of the proximal tibial apophysis. Although this can almost always be treated nonoperatively, stay out of trouble by warning families that sometimes pain can persist after skeletal maturity requiring fragment removal.

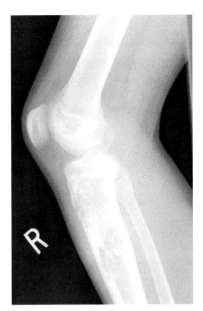

Figure 14-32 This 14-year-old boy presented with pain over his tibial tubercle. In many ways his symptoms were classic for Osgood-Schlatter syndrome. Fortunately, the orthopaedist obtained knee X-rays, which demonstrated a destructive process in the proximal tibia. The biopsy revealed osteosarcoma. (Courtesy of J. Dormans, MD.)

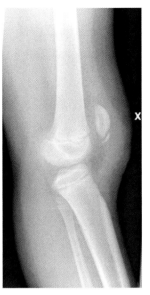

Figure 14-33 This lateral knee radiograph is of a 9-year-old girl who presented with anterior knee pain and swelling after a fall. She would not voluntarily extend her knee and could not hold it extended against gravity. The surgeon diagnosed a patellar sleeve fracture and rushed her to the OR. At surgery, her extensor mechanism was found to be intact. Final diagnosis was Sinding-Larsen-Johansson syndrome.

To stay out of trouble, it is important to clarify the difference between SLJ and a true patellar sleeve fracture. Just because a child will not do active extension does not mean that the extensor mechanism is disrupted (Fig. 14-33).

LEG, FOOT, AND ANKLE INJURIES

Stress Fractures

Although stress fractures are a rare cause of lower extremity pain in children, they must be on the differential diagnostic list when a young athlete presents with activity-related pain.[35] The tibia is one of the most common sites of stress fractures in children (Fig. 14-34). Tumors and infections share some presenting features with stress fractures; however, most stress fractures cause pain primarily with activity, while tumors and other conditions can cause pain at rest or during the night.

To stay out of trouble, do not perform a biopsy for a stress fracture: healing bone may have a histologic appearance that can be difficult to distinguish from malignant bone; furthermore, the biopsy can become a stress riser, leading to a complete fracture.

NEWSFLASH! Femoral neck stress fractures are very rare in children. Be sure to rule out more common causes, such as SCFE.[36] An MRI will help distinguish a femoral neck stress fracture from a very mild SCFE. More aggressive treatment is usually needed for adolescent femoral neck stress fractures, especially on the tension side. Completion of the fracture and displacement can lead to avascular necrosis.

Try to treat the whole patient and not just the stress fracture. Adolescents with stress fractures often have low bone density.[37] Identifying low bone density via DEX scan can have substantial implications in terms of improving bone health. Consider the female athlete triad, now known as relative energy deficiency syndrome, in the female athlete. Working in collaboration with a bone health clinician with these patients can be very beneficial.

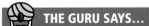

THE GURU SAYS...

When athletes return to sports after stress fractures, I prefer that in their first season back they start with one sport rather than returning to multiple sports at once. When returning to a single sport, it is preferred that they play for only one team and not multiple teams at once.

THEODORE J. GANLEY

THE GURU SAYS...

I always take a dietary history from all young athletes in whom I suspect demineralized bone, and I usually get a vitamin D level.

MICHAEL T. BUSCH

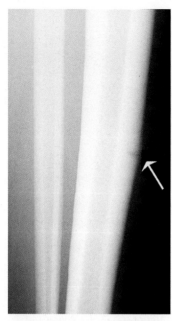

Figure 14-34 The "dreaded black line." This teenage runner was treated for bad shin splints that would not get better. Eventually she presented to the orthopaedist and was diagnosed with a tibial stress fracture. Although the two can be difficult to distinguish, this girl had very dramatic point tenderness localized to the anterior tibia, rather than diffuse medial tibial pain.

> **THE GURU SAYS...**
>
> The symptoms of antero-lateral impingement can mimic instability, so be sure that there are significant physical examination findings of laxity before undertaking a lateral ankle ligament reconstruction.
>
> MICHAEL T. BUSCH

> **THE GURU SAYS...**
>
> Beware of groove deepening in the skeletally immature patient, and I completely agree that transfer of the CFL is a very successful procedure.
>
> MICHAEL T. BUSCH

Leg Pain

Exertional compartment syndrome can cause recurrent lower extremity pain in runners. Compartment contents expand with exercise and cause pain, but rarely result in muscle necrosis. Pain typically develops after a specific duration of exercise. This pattern contrasts with the symptoms in a stress fracture, in which pain occurs early and intensifies with use. The most commonly involved compartment is the anterior compartment. The diagnosis is confirmed by compartment pressure testing at rest and after exercise.[38] To stay out of trouble, don't do a unilateral compartment release if there are *any* symptoms on the contralateral side (if you do, after the first release, the runner will feel much better and push her activity up to the point where she has symptoms on the opposite side).

> **THE GURU SAYS...**
>
> Posterior compartments have the highest failure rate, so a thorough release (particularly of the deep posterior compartment) and realistic expectations are important.
>
> MICHAEL T. BUSCH

Iliotibial band syndrome, a fairly common overuse problem, should be in the differential diagnosis of a runner with lower extremity pain. Look for a lower extremity malalignment, especially knee varus. To stay out of trouble, stick to rehabilitation and avoid surgical management. Release of the iliotibial band or bursa excision is rarely indicated and often does not give the kind of pain relief the young athlete expects.

Ankle Instability

Ankle sprains are perhaps the most common sports injury. Common in cutting and pivoting sports, an acute sprain can be treated supportively with RICE and return to sports usually within 1 to 3 weeks. However, more complex sprains may occur including medial deltoid ligament involvement or syndesmotic involvement. These sprains may take longer (3-6 weeks) to return to sports. In patients with lots of pain, swelling, or inability to weight bear, get X-rays to rule out fractures.

In patients with recurrent ankle instability, PT and bracing are recommended. In those who remain symptomatic or sustain recurrent sprains, ankle instability surgery can be performed. Anatomic procedures such as the modified Broström procedure have high success rates in adolescent patients.[39] This can be combined with ankle arthroscopy for anterolateral impingement in certain patients.

Peroneal Tendon Instability

Peroneal tendon instability may present similarly to recurrent ankle instability. Look for localization of the pain to the posterolateral ankle with subluxation of the tendons on resisted eversion or active eversion from an inverted position. Many of these patients have ligamentous laxity. If the popping is not painful or limiting, then simply observe. If painful and limiting, surgery can be beneficial. A variety of techniques have been described including groove deepening procedures and retinacular repair. I have had very good results with transferring the calcaneal fibular ligament (CFL) from deep to the tendons to superficial to the tendons.[40]

Osteochondral Lesions of the Talus

Osteochondral lesions of the talus can cause ankle pain, swelling, and mechanical symptoms in the adolescent athlete.[41] Medial lesions tend to be from recurrent loading and deeper. Lateral lesions may be more acute and tend to be shallower and more anterior. As with OCD, if these lesions are stable with articular cartilage, then they may heal with nonoperative treatment. However, if they do not heal or they are more advanced, then they may require surgery. Surgical treatment included drilling for stable lesions, fixation for unstable lesions, and excision with microfracture. Chondral resurfacing has been described as a salvage procedure but is infrequently required and is technically challenging in the ankle.

Os Trigonum

Look for os trigonum when encountering posterior ankle pain in a dancer. The os may be an extension of the posterior process of the talus, it may be a process that has fractured, or it may be an accessory bone. In plantarflexion athletes, such as ballet dancers, this may cause posterior ankle pain and impingement. A lateral X-ray of the ankle in demi-pointe demonstrates the pathology well to the dancer and her parents (Fig. 14-35). Look for other causes of posterior ankle pain such as Achilles tendonitis and initial treatment should be nonoperative. However, if PT fails, excision of the os can be beneficial. This can be done through either an arthroscopic or open approach. If the patient is having associated FHL tendonitis, then associated release of the FHL is beneficial.

Sever Disease

Sever apophysitis is a common cause of heel pain in young athletes. To stay out of trouble, be certain the diagnosis is correct. Good quality radiographs are recommended for heel pain (especially unilateral heel pain) to rule out bone cysts, acute fractures, and other conditions. Some evidence suggests that at least some cases may be calcaneal stress fractures.[42] Staying out of trouble also means understanding that the calcaneal apophysis in a school-age child usually has an "injured" appearance: sclerotic, fragmented, or cracked. Sometimes it is hard to convince parents that there is not an injury in this area. The essential elements of managing Sever apophysitis include relative rest from high-impact activities, stretching a tight gastrocsoleus muscle, and counseling the family about proper shoes.

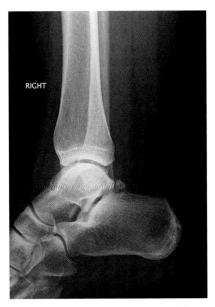

RIGHT

Figure 14-35 Os trigonum in an adolescent dancer. Consider this diagnosis in the adolescent ballet dancer with posterior ankle pain or impingement. A lateral ankle X-ray in demi-pointe makes the diagnosis obvious.

Many children with Sever apophysitis are running on hard surfaces in cleated shoes. A turf shoe, true running or silicone heel pad shoe often gives much relief. Recommend the same guidelines for return to play described above for Osgood-Schlatter—limping from Sever apophysitis gets the child pulled out of the game or practice.

Staying Out of Trouble With the Pediatric Athlete

General

* Managing interactions with sometimes overzealous sports parents is key.
* Be proactive and vigilant regarding depression and other psychological effects of a sports injury.
* Be wary of a pain syndrome.
* Team doctors can recommend and enforce a policy that includes mandatory periodic water drinking, and cancellation or modification of practice in unsafe weather, as well as discouraging weight loss through water loss.
* Sports medicine is more than sports injury surgery and involves understanding the medical issues of the whole athlete: concussion, nutrition, psychology, cardiac issues, the adaptive athlete, female athlete triad, biomechanics, etc.

Specific Sports Injuries

* SC joint injuries: Don't miss the diagnosis; seek 3D imaging.
* Clavicle fractures: Shard decision-making and err toward nonoperative treatment.
* AC joint injuries: Lean toward treating nonoperatively.
* Glenohumeral instability: Adopt a shared decision-making process.
* MDI: Start with PT.
* Little league shoulder: Set a realistic expectation for return to throwing at 4 months instead of 3 to 6 weeks.
* Medial epicondylar fracture: ORIF to avoid symptomatic nonunion.
* Little league elbow: Set reasonable expectations regarding returning to throwing, usually in 6 to 8 weeks.
* Osteochondritis dissecans of the capitellum: Detect the lesions early, so treatment is simpler.
* Gymnast wrist: Emphasize the avoidance of serious growth disturbance with resultant need for surgery.
* Hip labral tears: Identify and treat underlying structural abnormalities that may predispose to labral tearing.
* Hip apophyseal injuries: Consider acute fixation of large, displaced ischial tuberosity fractures.
* Tibial spine fracture: Early mobilization (by 2 weeks) to avoid stiffness.
* ACL injuries: Share decision-making process with the athlete and family, but emphasize the risk and importance of further meniscal or chondral injury.
* ACL reconstruction: Avoid hardware or bone blocks across the growth plates, large tunnels, and aggressive dissection in the over-the-top position near the perichondrial ring.

Staying Out of Trouble With the Pediatric Athlete *(continued)*

* Meniscal injuries: Review the MRIs yourself to look for meniscal signal change that extends to the articular surface of the meniscus.

* Meniscus repair: Do not remove too much meniscus.

* OCD of the knee: Order X-rays, particularly the notch view, in patients with unilateral knee pain.

* Patellofemoral instability: Thoroughly assess the multiple factors that can contribute to patellofemoral instability; identify if there is a loose body.

* Patellofemoral pain: If the hip is painful with flexion-internal rotation, get hip X-rays; try to avoid surgery.

* Osgood-Schlatter syndrome: Order X-rays to assess for atypical lesions.

* Sinding-Larsen-Johansson syndrome: Clarify the difference between SLJ and a true patellar sleeve fracture.

* Stress fracture: Do not perform a biopsy.

* Exertional compartment syndrome of the leg: Don't perform a unilateral compartment release if there are *any* symptoms on the contralateral side.

* Iliotibial band syndrome: Stick to rehabilitation and avoid surgical management.

SOURCES OF WISDOM

1. Obey MR, Lamplot J, Nielsen ED, et al. Pediatric sports medicine, a new subspeciality in orthopedics: an analysis of the surgical volume of candidates for the American Board of Orthopaedic Surgery. Part II. Certification exam over the past decade. *J Pediatr Orthop*. 2019;39(1):e71-e76.

2. Fabricant PD, Lakomkin N, Sugimoto D, et al. Youth sports specialization and musculoskeletal injury: a systematic review of the literature. *Phys Sports Med*. 2016;44(3):257-262.

3. LaPrade RF, Agel J, Baker J, et al. AOSSM early sport specialization consensus statement. *Orthop J Sports Med*. 2016;4(4):2325967116644241.

4. Metzl JD. Expectations of pediatric sport participation among pediatricians, patients, and parents. *Pediatr Clin North Am*. 2002;49(3):497-504.

5. Wilder RT, Berde CB, Wolohan M, et al. Reflex sympathetic dystrophy in children: clinical characteristics and follow-up of seventy patients. *J Bone Joint Surg Am*. 1992;74(6):910-919.

6. DesJardins M. Supplement use in the adolescent athlete. *Curr Sports Med Rep*. 2002;1(6):369-373.

7. Tokish JM, Kocher MS, Hawkins RJ. Ergogenic aids: a review of basic science, performance, side effects, and status in sports. *Am J Sports Med*. 2004;32(6):1543-1553.

8. Lee JT, Nasreddine AY, Black EM, et al. Posterior sternoclavicular joint injuries in skeletally immature patients. *J Pediatr Orthop*. 2014;34(4):369-375.

9. Bae DS, Kocher MS, Waters PM, et al. L. Chronic recurrent anterior sternoclavicular joint instability: results of surgical management. *J Pediatr Orthop*. 2006;26(1):71-74.

10. Heyworth BE, Kocher MS. Osteochondritis dissecans of the knee. *JBJS Rev*. 2015;3(7):pii: 01874474-201503070-00003.

11. Vavken P, Tepolt FA, Kocher MS. Open inferior capsular shift for multidirectional shoulder instability in adolescents with generalized ligamentous hyperlaxity or Ehlers-Danlos syndrome. *J Shoulder Elbow Surg*. 2016;25(6):907-912.

12. Heyworth BE, Kramer DE, Martin DJ, et al. Trends in the presentation, management, and outcomes of little league shoulder. *Am J Sports Med*. 2016;44(6):1431-1438.

13. Smith JT, McFeely ED, Bae DS, et al. Operative fixation of medial humeral epicondyle fracture nonunion in children. *J Pediatr Orthop*. 2010;30(7):644-648.

14. Klingele KE, Kocher MS. Little league elbow: valgus overload injury in the paediatric athlete. *Sports Med*. 2002;32(15):1005-1015.

15. Niu EL, Tepolt FA, Bae DS, et al. Nonoperative management of stable pediatric osteochondritis dissecans of the capitellum: predictors of treatment success. *J Shoulder Elbow Surg*. 2018;27(11):2030-2037.

16. DiFiori JP, Puffer JC, Mandelbaum BR, et al. Distal radial growth plate injury and positive ulnar variance in nonelite gymnasts. *Am J Sports Med*. 1997;25(6):763-768.

17. Pennock AT, Bomar JD, Johnson KP, et al. Nonoperative management of femoroacetabular impingement: a prospective study. *Am J Sports Med.* 2018;46(14):3415-3422.

18. Yen YM, Kocher MS. Clinical and radiographic diagnosis of femoroacetabular impingement. *J Pediatr Orthop.* 2013;33(suppl 1):S112-S120.

19. Pace JL, Nasreddine AY, Simoni M, et al. Dynamic splinting in children and adolescents with stiffness after knee surgery. *J Pediatr Orthop.* 2018;38(1):38-43.

20. Fabricant PD, Tepolt FA, Kocher MS. Range of motion improvement following surgical management of knee arthrofibrosis in children and adolescents. *J Pediatr Orthop.* 2018;38(9):e495-e500.

21. Vander Have KL, Ganley TJ, Kocher MS, et al. Arthrofibrosis after surgical fixation of tibial eminence fractures in children and adolescents. *Am J Sports Med.* 2010;38(2):298-301.

22. Ardern CL, Ekås GR, Grindem H, et al. Prevention, diagnosis and management of paediatric ACL injuries. *Br J Sports Med.* 2018;52(20):1297-1298.

23. DeFrancesco CJ, Storey EP, Shea KG, et al. Challenges in the management of anterior cruciate ligament ruptures in skeletally immature patients. *J Am Acad Orthop Surg.* 2018;26(3):e50-e61.

24. Fabricant PD, Kocher MS. Management of ACL injuries in children and adolescents. *J Bone Joint Surg Am.* 2015;99(7):600-612.

25. Vavken P, Tepolt FA, Kocher MS. Concurrent meniscal and chondral injuries in pediatric and adolescent patients undergoing ACL reconstruction. *J Pediatr Orthop.* 2018;38(2):105-109.

26. Kocher MS, Saxon HS, Hovis WD, et al. Management and complications of anterior cruciate ligament injuries in skeletally immature patients: survey of the Herodicus Society and the ACL Study Group. *J Pediatr Orthop.* 2002;22(4):452-457.

27. Kocher MS, Klingele K, Rassman SO. Meniscal disorders: normal, discoid, and cysts. *Orthop Clin North Am.* 2003;34(3):329-340.

28. Kocher MS, Logan CA, Kramer DE. Discoid lateral meniscus in children: diagnosis, management, and outcomes. *J Am Acad Orthop Surg.* 2017;25(11):736-743.

29. Kocher MS, Tepolt FA, Vavken P. Meniscus transplantation in skeletally immature patients. *J Pediatr Orthop B.* 2016;25(4):343-348.

30. Kocher MS, Tucker R, Ganley TJ, Flynn JM. Management of osteochondritis dissecans of the knee: current concepts review. *Am J Sports Med.* 2006;34(7):1181-1191.

31. Flynn JM, Kocher MS, Ganley TJ. Osteochondritis dissecans of the knee. *J Pediatr Orthop.* 2004;24(4):434-443.

32. Spang RC, Tepolt FA, Paschos NK, et al. Combined reconstruction of the medial patellofemoral ligament (MPFL) and medial quadriceps tendon-femoral ligament (MQTFL) for patellar instability in children and adolescents: surgical technique and outcomes. *J Pediatr Orthop.* 2019;39(1):e54-e61.

33. Oztekin HH. Popliteal glomangioma mimicking Baker's cyst in a 9-year-old child: an unusual location of a glomus tumor. *Arthroscopy.* 2003;19(7):E19-E23.

34. Van Rhijn LW, Jansen EJ, Pruijs HE. Long-term follow-up of conservatively treated popliteal cysts in children. *J Pediatr Orthop B.* 2000;9(1):62-64.

35. Coady CM, Micheli LJ. Stress fractures in the pediatric athlete. *Clin Sports Med.* 1997;16(2):225-238.

36. Wolfgang GL. Stress fracture of the femoral neck in a patient with open capital femoral epiphyses. *J Bone Joint Surg Am.* 1977;59(5):680-681.

37. Sonneville KR, Gordon CM, Kocher MS, et al. Vitamin D, calcium, and dairy intakes and stress fractures among female adolescents. *Arch Pediatr Adolesc Med.* 2012;166(7):595-600.

38. Beck JJ, Tepolt FA, Miller PE, et al. Surgical treatment of chronic exertional compartment syndrome in pediatric patients. *Am J Sports Med.* 2016;44(10):2644-2650.

39. Kocher MS, Fabricant PD, Nasreddine AY, et al. Efficacy of the modified Broström procedure for adolescent patients with chronic lateral ankle instability. *J Pediatr Orthop.* 2017;37(8):537-542.

40. Stenquist DS, Gonzalez TA, Tepolt FA, et al. Calcaneofibular ligament transfer for recurrent peroneal tendon subluxation in pediatric and young adult patients. *J Pediatr Orthop.* 2018;38(1):44-48.

41. Kramer DE, Glotzbecker MP, Shore BJ, et al. Results of surgical management of osteochondritis dissecans of the ankle in the pediatric and adolescent population. *J Pediatr Orthop.* 2015;35(7):725-733.

42. Ogden JA, Ganey TM, Hill JD, et al. Sever's injury: a stress fracture of the immature calcaneal metaphysis. *J Pediatr Orthop.* 2004;24(5):488-492.

43. Stanitski CL, Paletta GA Jr. Articular cartilage injury with acute patellar dislocation in adolescents: arthroscopic and radiographic correlation. *Am J Sports Med.* 1998;26(1):52-55.

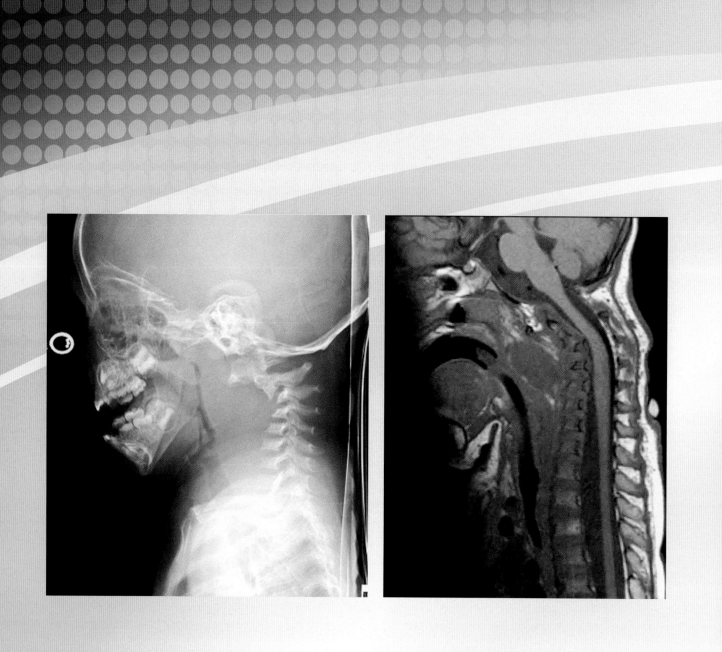

Chapter 15

Syndromes Important in Pediatric Orthopaedics

JOHN M. (JACK) FLYNN, MD, DAVID L. SKAGGS, MD, MMM, and MICHAEL G. VITALE, MD, MPH

Gurus: Paul D. Sponseller, MD and
William Mackenzie, MD, FRCSC, FACS

General Principles of Managing Children With Syndromes

Evaluating children with genetic syndromes is a part of being a pediatric orthopaedist. In fact, you may be the first to consider the diagnosis. Although any particular syndrome is rare, when taken together, the incidence of orthopaedic genetic abnormalities is about 5 in 1000.[1] The point is this: You are going to have to deal with syndromes on a regular basis in pediatric orthopaedics.

Just because the child looks like the parent does not mean that they both don't have a syndrome. Trust your gut instinct if a child looks "different" and consider a genetic consult. An astute pediatric orthopaedic surgeon can help entire families discover previously unrecognized genetic disorders.

When you encounter a congenital abnormality (e.g., congenital hand abnormality, clubfoot, hemivertebrae), ask yourself "Am I looking at a child with a syndrome?" Some syndromes are common enough to have their own multidisciplinary program (neurofibromatosis, for example). In such cases, these syndromes are easier to manage because there are a lot of interested experts who can lend a hand. Other syndromes are once-in-a-career rare. You may find that it is just you, a textbook, and perhaps an interested geneticist trying to do the job.

Even the brain of a pediatric orthopaedist has some limitations; remembering the name, orthopaedic manifestations, and associated systemic problems of every known syndrome that one might encounter will test those limitations. Therefore, to stay out of trouble, back up your pattern recognition skills with a good syndrome textbook,[2] as well as a computer in your clinic that has Internet access. With computer access, you can search for a syndrome by name or type OMIM into your favorite search engine to get the Online Mendelian Inheritance in Man website.

> **THE GURU SAYS...**
>
> It is not a failure to work with a geneticist to establish the diagnosis of a rare syndrome. The geneticist can also act as the family doctor for these families and be very helpful in patient management.
>
> WILLIAM MACKENZIE

> **THE GURU SAYS...**
>
> Remember to examine the entire child. The child should have shoes and socks off and be wearing shorts and a T-shirt. This can help you pick up many cutaneous and extremity findings.
>
> PAUL D. SPONSELLER

> **THE GURU SAYS...**
>
> Encourage parents to show off their knowledge of syndromes. Many are extremely knowledgeable, can teach you a lot, and will respect you for listening.
>
> PAUL D. SPONSELLER

Steps to the Diagnosis of a Syndrome[3]

1. Obtain history and physical, with more gentle interrogation on the family history than an orthopaedic surgeon would normally do.
2. Give the parents an informal examination, looking for syndromic features.
3. Find an excuse to leave the room, consult a text (or internet), and construct a mental list for a reevaluation.
4. Go back in the room and reexamine the child, looking for the specific features mentioned in the book.
5. Obtain appropriate radiographs or other confirming diagnostic testing.
6. Consult genetics.
7. Set follow-up visit to synthesize consultant's reports, all test results. Counsel family and construct orthopaedic treatment plan.

Always keep in mind that assigning a condition to a genetic cause is a loaded issue. It carries the possibility of blame assignment to one of the parents or to in-laws, with important implications for future offspring.

Don't get caught up in the mental exercise of assigning a name and lose sight of the true goal: providing timely treatment for the child's problems. Associated problems of other affected tissues and organ systems can be potential sources of trouble with syndromes. These other manifestations may suddenly become pertinent when the child is undergoing anesthesia for an orthopaedic procedure (Table 15-1). Guide parents to support groups so they are not alone.

TABLE 15-1 Trouble When Operating on a Child With a Syndrome

Syndrome	Potential Trouble
Down	Congenital heart disease, upper cervical spine instability, infections, hypothyroidism
Morquio	C1-C2 instability, myelopathy
Marfan	Mitral valve prolapse, aortic dilatation
Neurofibromatosis	Hypertension (renal artery stenosis or pheochromocytoma)
de Lange	GE reflux and swallowing disorders add risk to anesthesia; self-mutilating behavior
Proteus	Intubation can be difficult due to overgrowth of structures adjacent to trachea
Larsen	C-spine instability, airway problems, tracheomalacia
Freeman-Sheldon	Oral and laryngeal involvement complicates anesthesia
Nail-patella	Abnormal renal function
Familial dysautonomia	Autonomic dysfunction, decreased stress tolerance, decreased sensitivity to pain
Rubinstein-Taybi	Congenital heart defects, problems with neuromuscular blocking agents, keloids, and scarring problems
Turner	Cardiac abnormalities
Prader-Willi	Morbid obesity is anesthesia risk
Beckwith-Wiedemann	Huge tongue can complicate intubation, airway post-op
VACTERL/VATER	Congenital heart defects, renal abnormalities
Goldenhar	Difficult intubation, congenital heart defects
Hurler-Scheie	C-spine abnormalities
Beal	Cardiac abnormalities
Homocystinuria	Thromboembolism
Ehlers-Danlos	Cervical instability, abnormal wound healing
Klippel-Trénaunay	Hemorrhages and thromboembolism, cellulitis, wound healing
Osteogenesis imperfecta	Basilar impression, elevated intraoperative temperature, accidental fractures from tourniquets and positioning

Top 11 Syndromes of Importance in Pediatric Orthopaedics

DOWN SYNDROME

Down syndrome is thought to be the most common congenital malformation (1 in 660 live births), so there is a high likelihood that most orthopaedists will care for several patients with this condition. Staying out of trouble with Down syndrome means focusing on the child and not abnormal radiographs. Down syndrome patients can have all kinds of unusual physical examination and radiographic findings and yet function at a very high level. Focus on the problems that will hamper function or cause pain.

Beware of spine problems in Down syndrome, including cervical instability, scoliosis, and spondylolisthesis. When evaluating cervical spine instability, don't just look at C1-C2, look at occiput C1 as well (Fig. 15-1). A simplified and reasonable approach to cervical spine instability in Down syndrome is as follows:

- Asymptomatic instability with ADI less than 10 mm: No treatment
- Instability (ADI more than 10 mm) but no myelopathy: Check an MRI. If MRI shows cord impingement in flexion, then fuse. Increased signal in the cord is also a sign that there is abnormal motion and a relative indication for stabilization.
- Instability with myelopathy: Fuse.

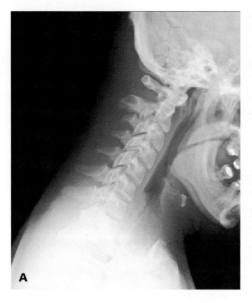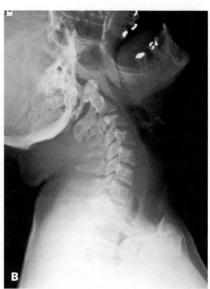

Figure 15-1 Be alert to the fact that the instability in the cervical spine of a child with Down syndrome can be at the occipitocervical junction, not just C1-C2. Note the relatively normal flexion film (**A**), but the movement of the occiput on C1 with extension (**B**).

> ### THE GURU SAYS...
>
> In children with osteogenesis imperfecta, look for skull-based abnormalities such as platybasia or basilar invagination, which may cause significant spinal cord compression.
>
> WILLIAM MACKENZIE

Don't recommend a fusion of C1-C2 just because the atlanto-dens interval is greater than 5 mm. Consider the risk and benefits carefully, because attempts at fusion are known to be associated with a very high complication rate.[4] In addition to instability, these children can also develop deformity in the subaxial spine related to spondylolysis and precocious osteoarthritis. Hip instability in Down syndrome, including complete hip dislocation, can develop late (Fig. 15-2).

The hip can look good initially, but go on to complete dislocation between the ages of 2 and 10 years. The acetabulum of the Down syndrome hip can have a normal radiographic appearance, which belies the real problem: extraordinary patholaxity of the soft tissues. Additionally, behavior is a major component of problems in Down syndrome hips. Children can be habitual hip dislocators, creating a challenge similar to managing multidirectional shoulder instability in an adolescent with generalized ligamentous laxity. In general, the surgical management of hip instability in Down syndrome is extremely difficult. If you plan surgery, do osteotomies on both sides of the joint—femoral and iliac—because you

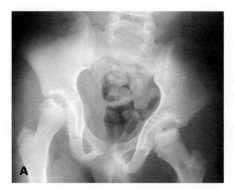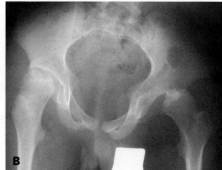

Figure 15-2 The hips in Down syndrome make their own rules. **A:** This boy presented at age 12 y with a few acute episodes of hip pain over the previous year, followed by refusal to bear weight for a few days, then a return to normal. The radiograph shows reduced, irregularly shaped femoral heads, and irregularly shaped acetabuli that seemed to provide good "coverage." **B:** He returned at age 15 y with a painful, fixed dislocation of the left hip, subluxation of the right hip, and shallow, dysplastic acetabuli. Could this trouble have been avoided? Can it now be successfully treated?

cannot rely on the soft tissues for stability. Long-term postoperative bracing may help to avoid redislocation. The complication rate of Down syndrome hip surgery can approach 50%.[5]

Be alert for slipped capital femoral epiphysis (SCFE) in a Down syndrome patient who develops an abnormal gait or complains of knee or thigh pain. Some authors have suggested that hypothyroidism may play a role.[6] It is well known that children with Down syndrome are more likely to get avascular necrosis (AVN) after an SCFE than otherwise normal children. A recent report showed AVN in five of eight patients.[7]

Most children with Down syndrome have hypermobile patellae. Given high rates of complications and recurrence of instability with surgical treatment, it is wise to restrict surgical treatment only to children who are symptomatic.

NEUROFIBROMATOSIS

There are two major types of neurofibromatosis: NF1 and NF2. Because the orthopaedic problems are confined to NF1, you should learn its diagnostic criteria (Fig. 15-3). Neurofibromatosis is relatively common (about 1 in 3000 infants), and many pediatric institutions have NF programs, so you are certain to see affected children. Be alert that NF can cause bone changes that are tumorlike in appearance (e.g., cysts or scalloping) and that neurofibromas can undergo malignant degeneration with an incidence of about 1%. Be alert for spinal manifestations of neurofibromatosis. The curves can be short and sharp, and there can be rib penciling and other findings (Fig. 15-4). Scoliosis and neurofibromatosis can start early and progress relentlessly. Bracing is usually ineffective. The enlarging neurofibroma can erode away at the pedicles (screw fixation can be difficult).

Fusion rates are lower in children with NF, and families should be counseled that more than one operation may be necessary. Dystrophic kyphosis is particularly dangerous (Fig. 15-6). This spinal deformity can lead to paralysis fairly rapidly. Historically, some have advocated for by both anterior and posterior fusion to increase fusion rates, but posterior-only operation has become more popular.[8-10]

> **THE GURU SAYS...**
>
> Surgical management of dystrophic spine deformity in neurofibromatosis can be very difficult due to the dural ectasia and erosion of the normal architecture. Be sure to get advanced imaging to assess for dural ectasia, rib intrusion into the canal, and plan fixation, which can be extremely challenging (Fig. 15-5).
>
> PAUL D. SPONSELLER

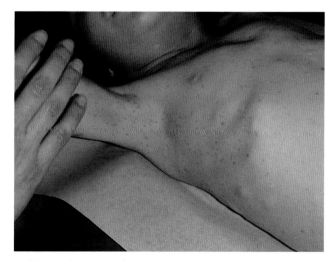

Figure 15-3 Axillary and inguinal freckling in neurofibromatosis. If there are freckles where the sun don't shine, it is neurofibromatosis until proven otherwise. Axillary or inguinal freckles can serve as a quick screen for neurofibromatosis. (Used with permission of the Children's Orthopaedic Center, Los Angeles.)

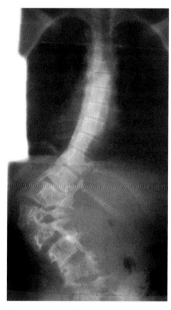

Figure 15-4 Scoliosis in a child with neurofibromatosis. Note the short, sharp curve that are classic in this NF spine trouble.

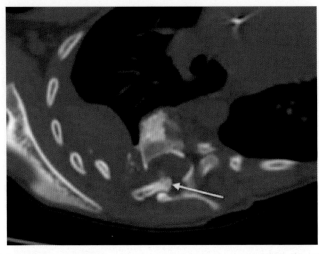

Figure 15-5 Advanced imaging can warn about the presence of rib penetration into the spinal canal in children with neurofibromatosis and keep you out of trouble in spine deformity correction.

> **THE GURU SAYS...**
>
> Don't forget the neck in NF-1. It is the least talked about but potentially most difficult to treat. When operating, fuse all dystrophic areas (Fig. 15-7).
>
> PAUL D. SPONSELLER

Erosion of the pedicles in the cervical spine can lead to cervical instability over time (Fig. 15-7). Be sure to monitor involved children closely.

Congenital pseudoarthrosis of the tibia is famous for the trouble that it causes. Perhaps the best testament to the trouble with congenital pseudoarthrosis is the fact that amputation was a common treatment (and still is for some cases).[11] It is important to remember that congenital pseudoarthrosis affects not just the tibia (Fig. 15-8) but can also affect the femur, clavicle, and either bone of the forearm. To stay out of trouble, don't do an osteotomy through bone affected by neurofibromatosis. Clamshell bracing may be the best protection in the very young. A comprehensive discussion of the risks and benefits of different treatment methods is beyond the scope of this book. Variable success has been reported with the Ilizarov device and Spatial Frame,[12] microvascular bone transfer,[13] and bypass grafting with preoperative bisphosphonates.[14] To stay out of trouble treating

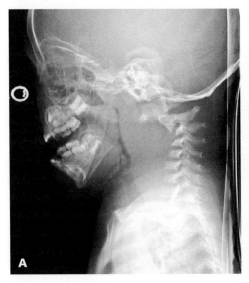
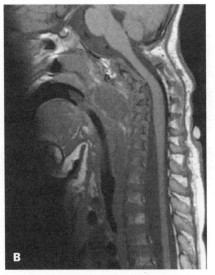

Figure 15-6 A: This 2-year-old boy with NF developed severe cervical kyphosis. **B:** An MRI showed a large neurofibroma anteriorly, with impingement on the cord in flexion. He was managed with anterior and posterior fusion with halo vest immobilization. (Courtesy of J. Dormans, MD.)

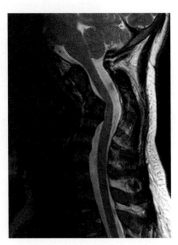

Figure 15-7 Subaxial cervical kyphosis resulting in cord compression and myelopathy in an 11-year-old with NF-1.

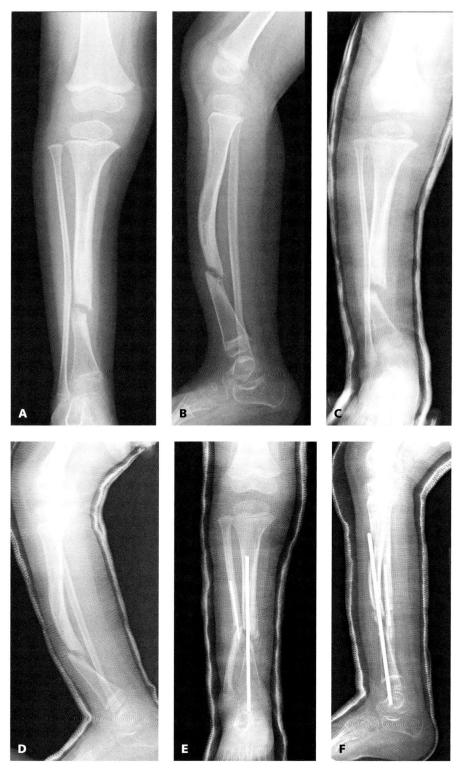

Figure 15-8 This 3-year-old with NF has a congenital pseudoarthrosis of the tibia that will be trouble for years to come. AP (**A**) and lateral (**B**) radiographs show a tibial pseudoarthrosis with an intact fibula. **C, D:** Prolonged casting had no effect. **E, F:** One year later, surgical management was begun. There was still no sign of healing, and the deformity had worsened. Many more procedures surely lie ahead. (Courtesy of R. Davidson, MD.)

congenital pseudoarthrosis of the tibia, prepare yourself and the family for multiple procedures and follow-up to maturity before success is declared. These cases may be best handled by the small group of surgeons who have done several.

ARTHROGRYPOSIS AND OTHER CONTRACTURAL SYNDROMES

Arthrogryposis is not a disease or diagnosis—it is a physical finding of rigid joint contractures. This category of syndromes includes dozens of distinctly different diseases including arthrogryposis multiplex congenita (AMC), Larsen syndrome, Freeman-Sheldon syndrome, and the pterygium syndromes. Children with AMC often present difficult multiple orthopaedic problems. To stay out of trouble, operate on joints early before adaptive changes secondary to the contractures make it difficult to get satisfactory results. Do osteotomies closer to the end of growth to avoid recurrence of deformity.

If you are consulted to see an infant with possible AMC, don't prescribe neonatal range of motion or other infant physical therapy until birth fractures have been ruled out. In general, warn the parents and the physical therapist against aggressive and forceful manipulation that may cause fractures.

Closed reduction of a hip dislocation in a child with AMC is rarely successful. Recent reports of open reduction, followed by only a brief period of postoperative spica casting, seem to be giving better results than in the past (when orthopaedic surgeons often would wait to see which children will walk and which would not).[15,16]

If a knee flexion contracture is greater than approximately 30°, soft tissue lengthening or release is recommended in the first year of life. Knee extension contractures can be treated at the same time as reduction of a dislocated hip, but knee flexion contractures should not: it is very hard to hold a hip reduced when you are casting and splinting the knees in extension. For an AMC clubfoot, casting alone is rarely successful. Avoid talectomy as an initial procedure.[17] Instead, stay out of trouble by using early multiple releases with a shortened period of postoperative casting.[18] In the upper extremities, it may be valuable to try to get one of two rigidly extended elbows to flex to 90°. Surgery on both elbows is not recommended.

LARSEN SYNDROME

If you are consulted to see an infant with dislocated knees, be alert to the fact that you may have encountered Larsen syndrome. These patients can have so many joint and spine problems that they can spend much of their childhood preparing for and recovering from orthopaedic surgery.

In Larsen syndrome, the anterior cruciate ligament (ACL) is often absent, and there may be patellar malalignment as well as dislocations of the radial head. If done early, manipulative treatment to reduce the knees may result in distal femoral fractures. Children with Larsen syndrome can have abnormal cervical spine segmentation. They develop kyphosis and myelopathy. Get a C-spine series before the first birthday.

Popliteal pterygium is a very difficult problem to manage (Fig. 15-9). To stay out of trouble, be alert that the popliteal artery will be deep, but the sciatic nerve can be very superficial[19] in the popliteal web and thus at risk for accidental surgical lengthening (not recommended). If full knee extension cannot be achieved by soft tissue surgery alone, consider shortening the femur.

THE MUCOPOLYSACCHARIDOSES

The mucopolysaccharidoses include a bewildering number of conditions. In this category of syndromes, the names change frequently and new ones are added

THE GURU SAYS...

Gradual correction of flexion contractors about the knee in syndromes like arthrogryposis often makes the surgeons appear brilliant in the short term but reoccurrence is extremely likely.
WILLIAM MACKENZIE

THE GURU SAYS...

In arthrogryposis, you can change the endpoints of the range of motion but not increase its total arc. Osteotomies take from one direction to give to another.
PAUL D. SPONSELLER

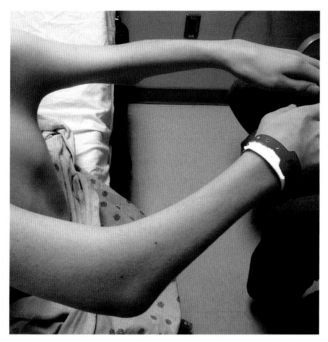

Figure 15-9 Arm pterygia with lack of flexion creases.

from time to time. Although each mucopolysaccharidosis (MPS) is rare, the entire group as a whole is not unusual. It can be difficult to establish the diagnosis on physical examination and radiographs in an infant. Be alert that children with Hurler syndrome can have odontoid hypoplasia and a spinal canal soft tissue mass. Children with Morquio syndrome are infamous for the trouble they cause the orthopaedist. Use braces after realignment osteotomies to protect their unstable knees. The cervical spine in Morquio is a major source of trouble.[20] C1-C2 instability can lead to death even in the first year of life. Be certain to get flexion/extension cervical spine films before any general anesthetic is contemplated for a child with Morquio syndrome.[21]

Newly available enzyme replacement medicines are now being used to treat several of the MPS with some early positive results, though it is unclear that this will positively affect the natural history of the orthopaedic manifestations of the disease.[22]

VACTERL/VATER

If your practice includes spinal disorders or hand and upper extremity surgery, you will certainly be consulted on children with VACTERL/VATER (acronyms to refer to congenital anomalies: *v*ertebral, *a*nal, *c*ardiac, *t*racheal, *e*sophageal, *r*enal, *limb/v*ertebral defects, imperforate *a*nus, *t*racheoesophageal fistula, *r*adial, and *r*enal dysphasia). These consults can come from the neonatal intensivist or general surgeon right after birth or the primary care doctor during the first year of life. As you manage the spine or hand problem, stay out of trouble by keeping in mind the high rate of congenital heart and renal abnormalities.

MARFAN SYNDROME

Marfan syndrome is a relatively common (1 in 10 000) autosomal dominant disorder. It can be difficult to make the diagnosis because the clinical manifestations can vary greatly (Fig. 15-10). If you are seeing a patient with long flat feet,

---

THE GURU SAYS...

Growth modulation can be highly effective in children with syndromes who have limb deformity. Be sure to evaluate remaining growth. In Morquio syndrome (MPS IV), there is little growth after age 10 years.

WILLIAM MACKENZIE

Dr. Skaggs Adds

An orthopaedic surgeon in California was sued for not diagnosing Hurler syndrome on a lateral spine X-ray. The parents reported they would not have had a second child with the disease had they been warned in time.

THE GURU SAYS...

In children with syndromes with severe spinal deformity, particularly in the sagittal plane, postoperative unexpected spinal cord injury can occur after extremity surgery. Consider the use of neuromonitoring on these patients.[22]

WILLIAM MACKENZIE

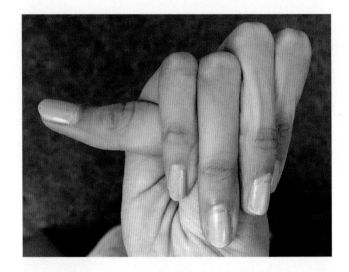

Figure 15-10 Steinberg's thumb sign is useful in the diagnosis of Marfan syndrome. (Used with permission of the Children's Orthopaedic Center, Los Angeles.)

THE GURU SAYS...

The recognition of Marfan syndrome can be lifesaving, since cardiovascular care is so successful.

PAUL D. SPONSELLER

THE GURU SAYS...

Failure of fixation is largely preventable in Marfan syndrome if you are aware of it and leave the case with good fixation at the end vertebrae.

PAUL D. SPONSELLER

THE GURU SAYS...

If a child looks like (s)he has Marfan syndrome with club-feet, think Loeys-Dietz syndrome (Fig. 15-12).

PAUL D. SPONSELLER

scoliosis, and ligamentous laxity, it is wise to get the geneticist, cardiologist, and perhaps the ophthalmologist involved if Marfan is suspected.

The management of scoliosis in children and adolescents with Marfan syndrome is also a source of trouble. The spinal deformity can follow the management guidelines of idiopathic scoliosis, but bracing is less successful.[24] The complications rate of spinal fusion is higher in children with Marfan syndrome.[25,26] Particular risks include pseudoarthrosis, progression outside the fusion levels, and instrumentation levels and progressive kyphosis at top or bottom of the instrumentation.[27]

Splenic rupture has recently been reported after spinal fusion in Marfan.[28] Stay out of trouble by getting a cardiology consult before any surgery is contemplated on children with Marfan syndrome. Some children may need cardiac surgery first.

Children with Marfan syndrome can have a severe pectus that crates a "double hit" for pulmonary function when accompanied by thoracic lordoscoliosis. Consider treatment of the pectus before spine surgery and involve general surgeon early in decision-making (Fig. 15-11).

Protrusion of the hip also occurs in Marfan syndrome. Howard Steel recommended closing the triradiate cartilage to halt protrusion before age 10 years.[29]

FAMILIAL DYSAUTONOMIA

Chances are you will encounter a child with familial dysautonomia, also known as Riley-Day syndrome, if your practice includes spinal deformity, particularly if there is a large Eastern European Jewish population in your area. In this ethnic group, the rate of Riley-Day syndrome is 1 in 3700. Stay out of trouble by understanding some special features of spinal deformity in this group. In a large percentage of cases, scoliosis starts early and progresses rapidly. Bracing is less effective in children with familial dysautonomia than in adolescent idiopathic scoliosis. Also, kyphosis is an important part of the deformity in many.[30] In correcting their spinal deformities, try to manage the problem without an anterior thoracic approach. Posterior osteotomies and pedicle screw fixation may allow you to stay out of the chest (Fig. 15-13). Be aware that the mortality after spine surgery is much higher in this group than in patients with idiopathic scoliosis. Some children die in childhood of pulmonary problems even without any thoracic surgery.

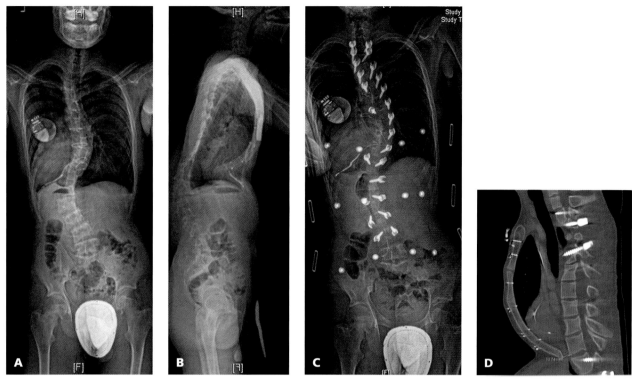

Figure 15-11 Fifteen-year-old boy with Marfan syndrome and severe pectus excavatum underwent aortic root replacement and insertion of an implantable defibrillator. **A, B:** Preoperative X-rays show frontal plane curve of 47/58 and 64°. Perhaps more important is the significant thoracolumbar kyphosis in the area of the sever pectus carinatum seen on the lateral radiograph (**B**). Attempts at surgical correction of the spinal deformity were aborted due to profound intraoperative hemodynamic instability resulting from compression of major blood vessels during corrective maneuver. Initial surgery was aborted, and staged correction was undertaken after pectus repair. **C, D:** Note the relationship between spine, pectus, and great vessels.

In Riley-Day syndrome, be alert that the insensitivity to pain in this syndrome can result in unrecognized or untreated fractures. If you see a child with Riley-Day syndrome and osteochondritis dissecans, the disease can behave more like a Charcot joint. The lesion can be refractory to typical osteochondritis dissecans management.

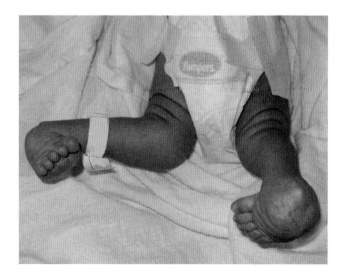

Figure 15-12 Infant with Loeys-Dietz syndrome with severe clubfoot, dislocated knees, and hip dysplasia.

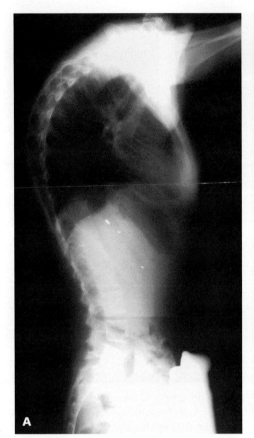
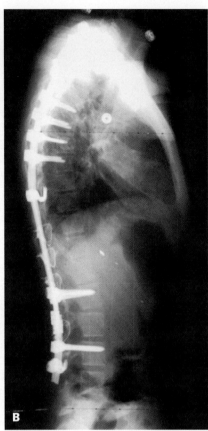

Figure 15-13 A: Kyphosis is often an important component of the spinal deformity in Riley-Day syndrome. **B:** This case was managed with a posterior instrumented fusion without anterior release.

PROTEUS SYNDROME

Proteus syndrome is characterized by overgrowth, manifesting as limb hypertrophy, macrodactyly, or other size incongruity. Although the bony overgrowth can be halted in macrodactyly, there is not a good solution for the overgrown soft tissue. Involved feet often require amputation or ray resection. To stay out of trouble with Proteus syndrome, exhaust nonoperative methods and counsel parents extensively before attempting any surgical management. Recurrences and complications are very common. In general, it is considered better to amputate rather than debulk in cases of macrodactyly.[31] Simple epiphysiodesis of the overgrown leg is usually better than limb lengthening, which can be fraught with complications. Angular deformities can recur rapidly after surgical correction.

KLIPPEL-TRÉNAUNAY-WEBER SYNDROME

Klippel-Trénaunay syndrome is manifest by limb hypertrophy with cutaneous nevi and varicosities. The current theory is that it is due to an abnormality of the walls of the veins of the extremities.

Simple resection of venous and lymphatic tissue is likely to result in recurrence. If you plan to operate, it may be wise to evaluate the full extent of the lesion with an MRI.

Children with Klippel-Trénaunay syndrome are prone to excessive bleeding during surgery, so it is essential to have blood and blood products available when contemplating surgery.

BECKWITH-WIEDEMANN SYNDROME

Consider Beckwith-Wiedemann syndrome if you are managing a large "cerebral palsy" (CP) patient with a leg-length inequality.[32] To stay out of trouble, keep in mind that there is a 10% incidence of abdominal tumors, especially Wilm tumor, associated with the hemihypertrophy. Involve your referring pediatrician or your institution's oncology team in surveillance for these abdominal tumors.

OTHER SYNDROMES THAT CAN LEAD TO TROUBLE

Russell-Silver Syndrome

Timing epiphysiodesis in children with Russell-Silver syndrome can be a source of trouble. In this syndrome, they can have very abnormal growth patterns, which can vary greatly between individuals.[32]

Turner Syndrome

In Turner syndrome, the administration of growth hormones can lead to rapid worsening of scoliosis. Stay out of trouble by working with your endocrinologist and following these children closely while they are on growth hormones.

Rett Syndrome

Rett syndrome is an X-linked disorder that can present to you in your CP clinic as a girl who seemed to be normal in her first year or two, but then progressively develops dementia, autism, ataxia, and repetitive hand motions. To stay out of trouble, don't ignore the scoliosis because you believe that Rett syndrome is lethal. In some cases of Rett syndrome, life expectancy is normal. Therefore, the spinal deformity should be managed with a full understanding of life expectancy and careful counseling of the family.[33] The spinal deformity is managed similarly to neuromuscular curves in children with CP, in whom segmental fixation and fusion to the pelvis gives the best results. The onset of scoliosis is usually before age 8 years, and rapid curve progression is usually detected early in the second decade. In Rett syndrome, sagittal deformity with excessive kyphosis can progress and necessitates close observation. Orthotic treatment does not alter the natural history of scoliosis or kyphosis. Indications for surgery are curve progression exceeding a 40° or 45° Cobb angle or curves that cause pain or loss of function.[34]

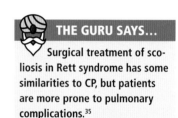

THE GURU SAYS...

Surgical treatment of scoliosis in Rett syndrome has some similarities to CP, but patients are more prone to pulmonary complications.[35]

PAUL D. SPONSELLER

Trouble With Bone Disease Syndromes

OSTEOGENESIS IMPERFECTA

Osteogenesis imperfecta (OI) represents a collection of conditions of greatly varying severity in which the fundamental problem is a defect of type 1 collagen. As such, it is easy to remember that these children have fragile bones, but don't forget about the ligamentous laxity, spinal deformities, hearing loss, easy bruisability, and other manifestations. One potential source of major trouble may occur at your first encounter. Fractures of infancy, and the mishandling of the diagnostic dilemma of child abuse versus OI, cause lots of trouble for families, doctors, and institutions[36-38] (Fig. 15-14). Diagnosis is easy when there is a family history of OI or other features of the syndrome (e.g., blue sclera, etc.) or when the history or injury constellation suggests abuse. Unfortunately, such history and examination features are absent. In very ambiguous cases, work up both child abuse and OI simultaneously and enlist all the help you can from Genetics and the appropriate authorities. To stay out of trouble, expect that anything you write or say regarding an infant's OI fracture may end up in a court of law.

Besides creating deformity, multiple fractures in OI can have some unexpected consequences. Be vigilant for growth arrests that are caused by multiple injuries

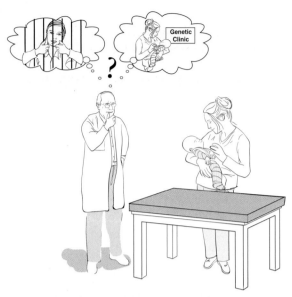

Figure 15-14 Child abuse versus osteogenesis imperfecta.

in the physeal region. Hypertropic callus can be mistaken for osteogenic sarcoma, leading to unnecessary amputation. Yet, osteogenic sarcoma can certainly occur in OI as it can in any child or adolescent.

Don't contribute to the fragile bone problem. Standard fracture immobilization protocols further decrease bone density and disuse atrophy. To avoid osteopenia, immobilize fractures only until symptoms resolve. In children with very high fracture rates, a "fracture kit," containing a series of splints for each upper and lower extremity limb segment, saves hospital visits and prolonged immobilization in full casts.

Sofield-type osteotomies have become the mainstay of treatment for the deformities associated with OI. Even in the best of hands, the complication rate can be high, particularly when nailing is performed in young patients[39,40] (Fig. 15-15). Migration of the nail has been a particularly common source of trouble.[41] When planning Sofield osteotomies, have every size of intramedullary device available and be prepared to modify devices as needed. The minimum internal diameter of the bone may be very hard to evaluate preoperatively.[42] Staging of multiple osteotomies in four different limbs may be necessary to avoid very high blood loss. Increasingly, Sofield osteotomies are being done through small percutaneous incisions.[43] Regarding timing after fracture, a Sofield osteotomy should either be done within a few days after fracture[44] or after complete fracture healing. If the osteotomy is done 1 to 3 weeks after fracture, the orthopaedic surgeon may encounter excessive bleeding from hyperemia of bone healing. Be prepared that there may be no true medullary cavity. Reaming is sometimes necessary. The child should be allowed to weight bear as soon as tolerated in casts or braces to maintain maximum bone strength.

Spinal deformities in OI are difficult to manage.[45] Pulmonary function deteriorates as curves reach 60°.[46] Corrective bracing can be difficult and detrimental. The children often cannot tolerate the brace because of the excessive sweating related to their condition. The corrective scoliosis brace can also deform the soft ribs of a child with OI. For surgical correction, it is important to plan an instrumentation strategy that involves multiple points of fixation. Preoperative halo

THE GURU SAYS...

When rodding the humerus in OI, be aware that the radial nerve can be entrapped in scar or callus from prior fractures.

PAUL D. SPONSELLER

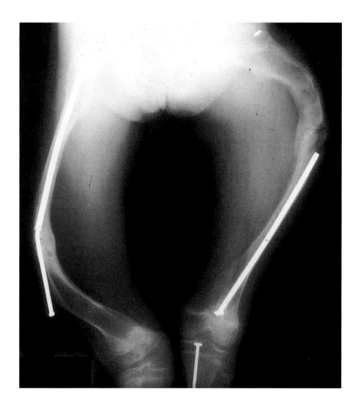

Figure 15-15 This single image illustrates the spectrum of trouble the orthopaedic surgeon may encounter when treating deformities and fractures in osteogenesis imperfecta. There has been separation of the Bailey-Dubow rod and subsequent removal in the left femur, causing refracture; in the right femur, there was bending of the Bailey-Dubow rod, with progressive deformities on both sides. Lack of follow-up made management even more difficult. (Courtesy of Michael Vitale, MD, MPH, Childrens Hospital New York-Presbyterian.)

gravity traction has been used with some success.[47] Iliac crest autograft is often insufficient, so the family should be consented for allograft. Postoperative immobilization is tolerated poorly.

RICKETS

Although classic nutritional rickets is seen less frequently than it was generations ago, you may occasionally be asked to correct deformities or manage problems of children with rickets, especially the forms related to an inherited metabolic disorder. To stay out of trouble with the correction of angular deformities, optimize the medical management first.[48,49] Work with the patient's pediatrician or with the endocrinologist to be sure that the child is getting the optimum doses of calcium and vitamin D (depending on the underlying metabolic problem). In most cases, slight overcorrection of the angular deformity is recommended to reduce the risk of recurrence. Finally, think of SCFE in children with renal osteodystrophy who present with hip, thigh, or knee pain. Consider prophylactic pinning of the unslipped opposite side because bilateral SCFE is very common in this population.

OSTEOPETROSIS

Osteopetrosis, a genetic defect in the osteoclast, compromises the ability of these cells to reabsorb bone, leading to very dense bone, fractures, and deformities. If you encounter a fracture in a child with osteopetrosis, be alert that these fractures can be slower to heal than you would normally expect. Corrective osteotomies for coxa vara and other deformities can be difficult to perform. Intramedullary fixation is difficult, as drills, saw blades, and other tools become very dull and can break during work on this extremely hard bone.[50] Be alert to the fact that children with osteopetrosis are also at increased risk of osteomyelitis (Fig. 15-16).

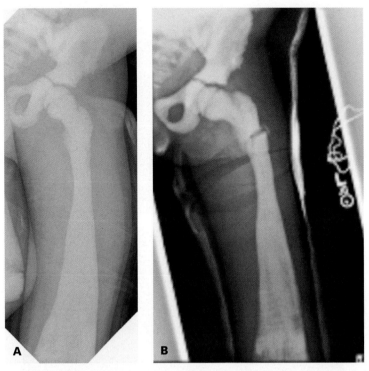

Figure 15-16 Treating fractures in osteopetrosis is trouble, particularly hip and proximal femur fractures. **A:** This nondisplaced subtrochanteric fracture was treated with cast immobilization alone. **B:** Four months later, after prolonged casting and wedging, the fracture still shows little sign of healing.

Staying Out of Trouble With Syndromes

General Principles

* Syndromes are unavoidable. Discover the syndrome before it finds you (and gets you in trouble).
* Back up your pattern recognition skills with a good syndrome textbook, as well as a computer in your clinic that has Internet access.
* Get a geneticist involved as early as possible.
* Don't forget other organ systems: cardiac, renal, etc.

Specific Syndromes

* Down syndrome: focus on the problems that hamper function or cause pain; look at the entire cervical spine, and don't do a fusion just because the ADI is increased.
* NF spinal deformity can lead to paralysis fairly rapidly.
* Arthrogryposis: rule out birth fractures before starting PT; do osteotomies closer to the end of growth to avoid recurrence.
* Larsen syndrome: cervical kyphosis and myelopathy can develop later in childhood.
* Morquio syndrome: C1-C2 instability can lead to death, even before the first birthday.

Staying Out of Trouble With Syndromes *(continued)*

✳ Marfan syndrome: get a cardiology consult before any surgery is contemplated.

✳ Klippel-Trenaunay-Weber: prone to excessive bleeding during surgery.

✳ Child abuse versus osteogenesis imperfecta: in very ambiguous cases, work up both child abuse and OI simultaneously, and enlist all the help you can from Genetics and the appropriate authorities.

SOURCES OF WISDOM

1. Van Regemorter N, Dodion J, Druart C, et al. Congenital malformations in 10,000 consecutive births in a university hospital: need for genetic counseling and prenatal diagnosis. *J Pediatr.* 1984;104:386-390.

2. Goldberg MJ. *The Dysmorphic Child: An Orthopedic Perspective.* New York, NY: Raven Press; 1987.

3. Rang M. Syndromology. In: Wenger DRM, ed. *The Art and Practice of Children's Orthopaedics.* New York, NY: Raven Press; 1993:752.

4. Dormans JP, Drummond DS, Sutton LN, et al. Occipitocervical arthrodesis in children: a new technique and analysis of results. *J Bone Joint Surg Am.* 1995;77:1234-1240.

5. Bennet GC, Rang M, Roye DP, et al. Dislocation of the hip in trisomy 21. *J Bone Joint Surg Br.* 1982;64:289-294.

6. Bosch P, Johnston CE, Karol L. Slipped capital femoral epiphysis in patients with Down syndrome. *J Pediatr Orthop.* 2004;24:271-277.

7. Dietz FR, Albanese SA, Katz DA, et al. Slipped capital femoral epiphysis in Down syndrome. *J Pediatr Orthop.* 2004;24:508-513.

8. Parisini P, Di Silvestre M, Greggi T, et al. Surgical correction of dystrophic spinal curves in neurofibromatosis: a review of 56 patients. *Spine.* 1999;24:2247-2253.

9. Halmai V, Doman I, de Jonge T, et al. Surgical treatment of spinal deformities associated with neurofibromatosis type 1: report of 12 cases. *J Neurosurg Spine.* 2002;97:310-316.

10. Hanna BG, Pill SG, Drummond DS. Irreducible thoracic spondyloptosis in a child with neurofibromatosis: a rationale for treatment. *Spine.* 2002;27:E342-E347.

11. Carney BT, Daniels CL. A retrospective review of congenital pseudarthrosis of the tibia. *Iowa Orthop J.* 2002;22:57-60.

12. Boero S, Catagni M, Donzelli O, et al. Congenital pseudarthrosis of the tibia associated with neurofibromatosis-1: treatment with Ilizarov's device. *J Pediatr Orthop.* 1997;17:675-684.

13. Gilbert A, Brockman R. Congenital pseudarthrosis of the tibia: long-term followup of 29 cases treated by microvascular bone transfer. *Clin Orthop.* 1995;314:37-44.

14. Strong ML, Wong-Chung J. Prophylactic bypass grafting of the prepseudarthrotic tibia in neurofibromatosis. *J Pediatr Orthop.* 1991;11:757-764.

15. Staheli LT, Chew DE, Elliott JS, et al. Management of hip dislocations in children with arthrogryposis. *J Pediatr Orthop.* 1987;7:681-685.

16. Akazawa H, Oda K, Mitani S, et al. Surgical management of hip dislocation in children with arthrogryposis multiplex congenita. *J Bone Joint Surg Br.* 1998;80:636-640.

17. Cassis N, Capdevila R. Talectomy for clubfoot in arthrogryposis. *J Pediatr Orthop.* 2000;20:652-655.

18. Niki H, Staheli LT, Mosca VS. Management of clubfoot deformity in amyoplasia. *J Pediatr Orthop.* 1997;17:803-807.

19. Oppenheim WL, Larson KR, McNabb MB, et al. Popliteal pterygium syndrome: an orthopaedic perspective. *J Pediatr Orthop.* 1990;10:58-64.

20. Stevens JM, Kendall BE, Crockard HA, et al. The odontoid process in Morquio-Brailsford's disease: the effects of occipitocervical fusion. *J Bone Joint Surg Br.* 1991;73:851-858.

21. Muenzer J. Early initiation of enzyme replacement therapy for the mucopolysaccharidoses. *Mol Genet Metab.* 2014;111(2):63-72.

22. Morgan KA, Rehman MA, Schwartz RE. Morquio's syndrome and its anaesthetic considerations. *Paediatr Anaesth.* 2002;12:641-644.

23. Pruszczynski B, Mackenzie WG, Rogers K, White KK. Spinal cord injury after extremity surgery in children with thoracic kyphosis. *Clin Orthop Relat Res.* 2015;473(10):3315-3320.

24. Sponseller PD, Bhimani M, Solacoff D, et al. Results of brace treatment of scoliosis in Marfan syndrome. *Spine.* 2000;25:2350-2354.

25. Jones KB, Erkula G, Sponseller PD, et al. Spine deformity correction in Marfan syndrome. *Spine.* 2002;27:2003-2012.

26. Lipton GE, Guille JT, Kumar SJ. Surgical treatment of scoliosis in Marfan syndrome: guidelines for a successful outcome. *J Pediatr Orthop.* 2002;22:302-307.

27. Sponseller PD, Sethi N, Cameron DE, et al. Infantile scoliosis in Marfan syndrome. *Spine.* 1997;22:509-516.

28. Christodoulou AG, Ploumis A, Terzidis IP, et al. Spleen rupture after surgery in Marfan syndrome scoliosis. *J Pediatr Orthop.* 2004;24:537-540.

29. Steel HH. Protrusio acetabuli: its occurrence in the completely expressed Marfan syndrome and its musculoskeletal component and a procedure to arrest the course of protrusion in the growing pelvis. *J Pediatr Orthop.* 1996;16:704-718.

30. Rubery PT, Spielman JH, Hester P, et al. Scoliosis in familial dysautonomia: operative treatment. *J Bone Joint Surg Am.* 1995;77:1362-1369.

31. Turra S, Santini S, Cagnoni G, et al. Gigantism of the foot: our experience in seven cases. *J Pediatr Orthop.* 1998;18:337-345.

32. Alman BA, Goldberg MJ. Syndromes of orthopaedic importance. In: Morrissy RT, Weinstein SL, eds. *Pediatric Orthopaedics.* Vol 1. 5th ed. Philadelphia, PA: Lippincott Williams & Wilkins; 2001:287-338.

33. Kerr AM, Webb P, Prescott RJ, et al. Results of surgery for scoliosis in Rett syndrome. *J Child Neurol.* 2003;18:703-708.

34. Huang TJ, Lubicky JP, Hammerberg KW. Scoliosis in Rett syndrome. *Orthop Rev.* 1994;23:931-937.

35. Cohen J, Klyce W, Kuchadkar SR, Kotian RN, Sponseller PD. Respiratory complications after posterior spinal fusion for neuromuscular scoliosis: children with Rett syndrome at greater risk than those with cerebral palsy. *Spine.* 2019;44:1396-1402.

36. Kruse RW, Harcke HT, Minch CM. Osteogenesis imperfecta (OI) may be mistaken for child abuse. *Pediatr Emerg Care.* 1997;13:244-245.

37. Blumenthal I. Osteogenesis imperfecta, non-accidental injury, and temporary brittle bone disease. *Arch Dis Child.* 1996;74:91.

38. Kocher MS, Kasser JR. Orthopaedic aspects of child abuse. *J Am Acad Orthop Surg.* 2000;8:10-20.

39. Zionts LE, Ebramzadeh E, Stott NS. Complications in the use of the Bailey-Dubow extensible nail. *Clin Orthop.* 1998;348:186-195.

40. Oznur A, Tokgozoglu AM, Alpaslan AM. Complications in the use of the Bailey-Dubow extensible nail. *Clin Orthop.* 1999;366:286-287.

41. Janus GJ, Vanpaemel LA, Engelbert RH, et al. Complications of the Bailey-Dubow elongating nail in osteogenesis imperfecta: 34 children with 110 nails. *J Pediatr Orthop B.* 1999;8:203-207.

42. Chotigavanichaya C, Jadhav A, Bernstein RM, et al. Rod diameter prediction in patients with osteogenesis imperfecta undergoing primary osteotomy. *J Pediatr Orthop.* 2001;21:515-518.

43. Li YH, Chow W, Leong JC. The Sofield-Millar operation in osteogenesis imperfecta: a modified technique. *J Bone Joint Surg Br.* 2000;82:11-16.

44. Panzica M, Garapati R, Zelle B, et al. Combination of femoral fracture treatment and corrective osteotomy in a child with osteogenesis imperfecta. *Arch Orthop Trauma Surg.* 2004;124:341-345.

45. Oppenheim WL. The spine in osteogenesis imperfecta: a review of treatment. *Connect Tissue Res.* 1995;31:S59-S63.

46. Widmann RF, Bitan FD, Laplaza FJ, et al. Spinal deformity, pulmonary compromise, and quality of life in osteogenesis imperfecta. *Spine.* 1999;24:1673-1678.

47. Janus GJ, Finidori G, Engelbert RH, et al. Operative treatment of severe scoliosis in osteogenesis imperfecta: results of 20 patients after halo traction and posterior spondylodesis with instrumentation. *Eur Spine J.* 2000;9:486-491.

48. Choi IH, Kim JK, Chung CY, et al. Deformity correction of knee and leg lengthening by Ilizarov method in hypophosphatemic rickets: outcomes and significance of serum phosphate level. *J Pediatr Orthop.* 2002;22:626-631.

49. Rubinovitch M, Said SE, Glorieux FH, et al. Principles and results of corrective lower limb osteotomies for patients with vitamin D-resistant hypophosphatemic rickets. *Clin Orthop.* 1988;237:264-270.

50. Armstrong DG, Newfield JT, Gillespie R. Orthopedic management of osteopetrosis: results of a survey and review of the literature. *J Pediatr Orthop.* 1999;19:122-132.

FOR FURTHER ENLIGHTENMENT

Akyol MU, Alden TD, Amartino H, et al.; MPS Consensus Programme Steering Committee; MPS Consensus Programme Co-Chairs. Recommendations for the management of MPS IVA: systematic evidence- and consensus-based guidance. *Orphanet J Rare Dis.* 2019;14(1):137.

Ando K, Kobayashi K, Ito K, Tsushima M, et al. Occipitocervical or C1–C2 fusion using allograft bone in pediatric patients with Down syndrome 8 years of age or younger. *J Pediatr Orthop B.* 2019;28:405-410.

Bernstein RM. Arthrogryposis and amyoplasia. *J Am Acad Orthop Surg.* 2002;10(6):417-424.

Doherty C, Stapleton M, Piechnik M, et al. Effect of enzyme replacement therapy on the growth of patients with Morquio A. *J Hum Genet*. 2019;64:625-635. doi:10.1038/s10038-019-0604-6.

Helenius IJ, Sponseller PD, Mackenzie W, et al. Outcomes of spinal fusion for cervical kyphosis in children with neurofibromatosis. *J Bone Joint Surg Am*. 2016;98(21):e95.

Kerr AM, Webb P, Prescott RJ, et al. Results of surgery for scoliosis in Rett syndrome. *J Child Neurol*. 2003;18:703-708.

MacCarrick G, Black JH 3rd, Bowdin S, et al. Loeys-Dietz syndrome: a primer for diagnosis and management. *Genet Med*. 2014;16(8):576-587.

Mikles M, Stanton RP. A review of Morquio syndrome. *Am J Orthop*. 1997;26(8):533-540.

Shaw ED, Beals RK. The hip joint in Down's syndrome: a study of its structure and associated disease. *Clin Orthop*. 1992;(278):101-107.

Stricker S. Musculoskeletal manifestations of Proteus syndrome: report of two cases with literature review. *J Pediatr Orthop*. 1992;12(5):667-674.

Van Regemorter N, Dodion J, Druart C, et al. Congenital malformations in 10,000 consecutive births in a university hospital: need for genetic counseling and prenatal diagnosis. *J Pediatr*. 1984;104:386-390.

Vitale MG, Guha A, Skaggs DL. Orthopaedic manifestations of neurofibromatosis in children: an update. *Clin Orthop Relat Res*. 2002;(401):107-118.

White KK, Bompadre V, Goldberg MJ, et al.; Skeletal Dysplasia Management Consortium. Best practices in peri-operative management of patients with skeletal dysplasias. *Am J Med Genet A*. 2017;173(10):2584-2595.

White KK, Jester A, Bache CE, Harmatz PR, et al. Orthopedic management of the extremities in patients with Morquio A syndrome. *J Child Orthop*. 2014;8(4):295-304.

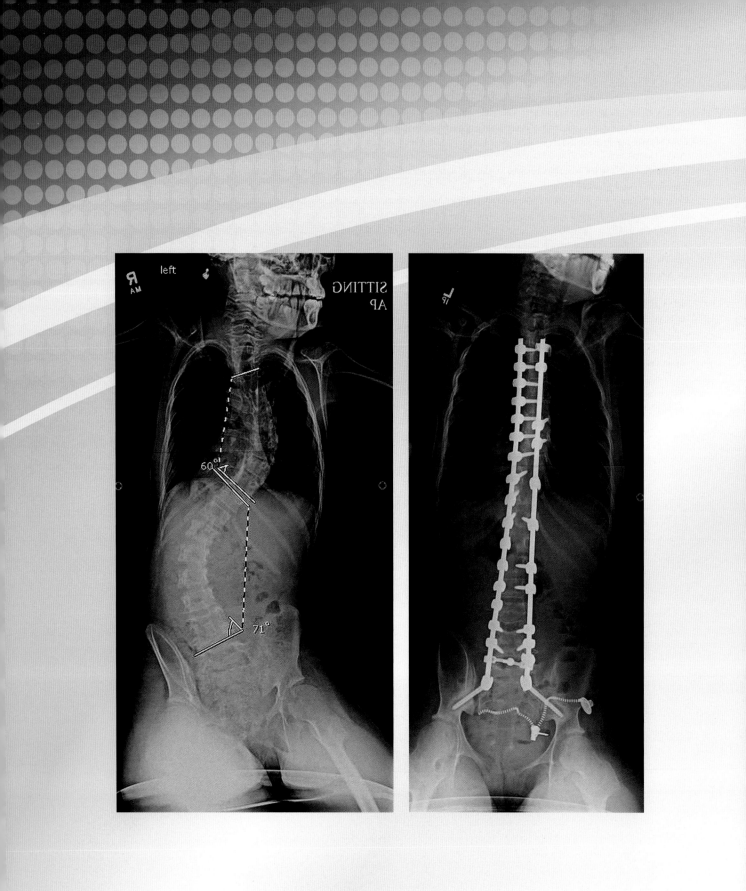

Chapter 16

Cerebral Palsy

ROBERT M. KAY, MD and JOHN M. (JACK) FLYNN, MD

Guru: Jon R. Davids, MD

General Considerations

Cerebral palsy (CP) results from damage to the immature brain, typically before age 2 years. Despite medical advances over the past several decades, the incidence of CP has not declined, and CP remains the most common motor disease of childhood. Currently, CP is estimated to affect 1 in every 300 to 400 children in the United States, with nearly 1 million affected individuals in the United States and 17 million worldwide. As a result of increased life expectancy in people with CP, there are now more affected adults with CP than children.

Historically, risk factors cited for CP have included premature birth, multiple gestation (e.g., twins, triplets, etc.), low birth weight, and need for oxygen following birth. In fact, the vast majority of children with CP do not have any known risk factors for having CP. Genetic causes of conditions presenting like CP are becoming increasingly recognized.

CP is now considered to be a group of disorders characterized by a static brain lesion which occurs before age 2 years. Although CP is typically thought of as a motor disorder, children with CP often have limitations in cognition, sensation, proprioception, and thermoregulation, and many affected individuals have pulmonary, gastrointestinal, genitourinary problems, and/or seizure disorders.

One of the important things to understand about people with CP is that they often have very different functional abilities in different domains. For example, some people with CP have severe motor involvement and are completely dependent for activities of daily living (ADLs) but have very good intellectual capacity, while others may have minimal motor limitation, but be severely cognitively impaired.

The brain lesion itself in CP is nonprogressive, though the peripheral manifestations (stiffness, contractures, and bone deformity) often progress with time. If there *does* seem to be progression of the neurologic problems in a child with CP, you should consult a neurologist, developmental pediatrician and/or geneticist to confirm the proper diagnosis, and whether or not other issues may have arisen (such as onset or progression hydrocephalus).

Classification

There are numerous ways to classify people with CP.[1] Some of the common classification methods include systems based on geographic distribution of the CP, type of motor involvement, and functional level. By sorting out and categorizing these children, you can stay out of trouble by expecting certain problems more frequently in particular groups.

GEOGRAPHIC CLASSIFICATION

Over time, the most common classification scheme has been based on geographic distribution of CP. This classification has categorized affected people as having hemiplegia (one side of the body involved), diplegia (both legs involved, with relative sparing of the arms), triplegia (both legs and one arm involved, with relative sparing of the other arm), quadriplegia (all four extremities involved), or tetraplegia (all four extremities plus bulbar involvement). Because there are gray areas in this classification scheme (e.g., essentially all children with "diplegia" have some degree of upper extremity involvement as well), health care providers in Europe often classify people as having unilateral or bilateral CP.

Because there are some useful distinctions when using a geographic classification of involvement (as discussed later), we believe there remains some value in such a classification of involvement for those with CP. Classifying the type of CP—diplegic, quadriplegic, hemiplegic, spastic, athetoid, etc.—can be difficult in some children but is helpful overall.

MOTOR INVOLVEMENT CLASSIFICATION

A common way to categorize those with CP is by the type of motor involvement they have. Those with spasticity (also sometimes referred to as having "spastic cerebral palsy") have increased tone and stiffness in the muscles with an exaggerated stretch reflex (and resultant increase in their reflexes, also known as "hyperreflexia"). Children with spastic CP are often the ones whom we can help most as orthopaedic surgeons. The opposite of spastic CP is "hypotonic" (low-tone) CP. These children have low tone and decreased stretch reflexes but have many of the same nonoperative needs (though fewer operative ones) than those with spastic CP.

Dystonia has become increasingly recognized as a significant problem in patients with CP. Dystonia is abnormal muscle tone in muscle(s), which typically results in repetitive posturing by the affected person. Although the particular muscles involved and the particular postures that result vary among affected individuals, the affected muscles and postures are very repetitive and consistent for a given person. For example, for one person, the dystonia may involve repetitive foot and ankle posturing into specific positions, while, in another, the posturing will affect different extremities and muscle groups. Dystonia often is not evident in young children but becomes more evident and problematic with time, particularly as children near and pass through adolescence.

Many children with CP have mixed patterns of CP that involve a combination of the aforementioned types of motor involvement. In young children, hypotonia of the trunk ("truncal hypotonia") is often seen in conjunction with spasticity of the extremities. Dystonia is often combined with spastic and/or hypotonic CP.

FUNCTIONAL CLASSIFICATION SYSTEMS

The most widely used classification system currently used is the Gross Motor Functional Classification System (GMFCS). The GMFCS has become the preferred classification system for communication among those treating children with CP.[1-3] There are five GMFCS levels. GMFCS I and II children both walk in the community without ambulatory aids, with the difference being that level I children do not use handrails while climbing stairs (level II children do) and GMFCS I children do well on all surfaces and level II children may have difficulty on uneven surfaces. Level III children are community ambulators with ambulatory aids (crutches or walkers). Level IV children do limited walking in therapy and/or other therapeutic settings (e.g., school, particularly with adaptive physical education). Level V children do not have head and neck control and are dependent for mobility; however, they may be placed upright in fully supportive standers.

Other classification systems are used, though less commonly by orthopaedic surgeons. These include the Manual Activity Classification System (MACS), which rates children on an ordinal rating system with five levels. The extremes include MACS I (a child who handles objects essentially without limitation) and MACS V children who do not handle objects. Similarly, the Communication Functional Classification System (CFCS) is a five-level system, with level I children easily and effectively sending and receiving messages in the majority of settings with the majority of people and level V children rarely effectively communicating with anyone.

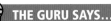 **THE GURU SAYS...**
All children with CP should receive a GMFCS and CFCS assessment. With this information, the provider will have insight into the degree of both motor and cognitive impairments. Parents are frequently offended if a provider presumes that the presence of significant motor impairment implies significant cognitive impairment.

JON DAVIDS

Evaluation

The first time a patient with CP comes into your office can seem overwhelming. Unlike the simple assessment of an otherwise-healthy child with a buckle fracture of the radius, adequately addressing the myriad issues common in children with CP can make this task seem insurmountable.

As with other complex processes, the key is to simplify by coming up with a problem list and a treatment plan to address these problems. You can sometimes even start the process before entering the patient's room. For instance, you may be able to observe how the child gets to the examining room. Do they walk or use a manual or power wheelchair? Who is with the child and how does the child interact with those accompanying them? If the child walks, take this opportunity as they walk to the room to observe their gait, since this may well be more representative than the "doctor's walk" the child will do for you after you have met and they know you are watching (and possibly considering bracing or surgery).

When addressing the child and family, ask about their main concerns. Many of the assumptions we may have as health care providers are very different from the priorities for the patient and family. Making sure to find out their needs—and making sure to do our best to meet those needs—is critical to patient and family satisfaction. **NEWSFLASH! Once the child is in the room, make sure to talk to them and not just those accompanying them. In addition to being humane and considerate, asking questions directly to the child will help you assess their cognitive abilities, including expressive and receptive language.**

Although the entire health care team caring for a child with CP should be working from a comprehensive history and physical examination, the orthopaedic surgeon should specifically be attuned to a few very important pieces of information. Birth history, including any problems during the pregnancy and delivery, is sought. Motor and cognitive milestones are assessed, and it is often helpful to ask the parent(s) how these milestones compared to their other children. Asking when they first noted that there was a problem is useful. You should ask about when the child demonstrated "handedness." **NEWSFLASH! Children should use both hands essentially symmetrically until at least 12 months old. A child who shows hand dominance before age 1 year has pathology affecting the non-dominant arm; commonly, this is due to hemiplegic (or unilateral) CP.**

Physical examination requires a thorough assessment of the entire child. Patience is key as the child is often anxious and/or fearful, either of which will typically increase spasticity and make examination more challenging. Tone is assessed in the trunk, spine, and extremities. Any dystonia should be noted. The child is asked to perform gross and fine motor tasks, as possible, based on both cognitive and motor function. All extremities are taken through a range of motion to assess for any contractures as well. Bilateral examination is critical for assessing symmetry. Subtle findings such as unilateral increased tone of the forearm pronators may be one of the only upper extremity findings in early hemiplegic (unilateral) CP. Watching the child handle objects while you are talking to him and the parents can be very telling.

There are several pitfalls to avoid while examining a child with CP. Hip abduction should be tested with the hips and knees extended. Patience is essential. If the examination is done hastily, the child's muscles will tense up and you will probably be testing spasticity more than you are testing the actual joint range of motion. When testing popliteal angles, the opposite hip must remain fully extended. It is a rookie error to allow the opposite hip to flex, which relaxes the hamstrings and leads to underestimation of the popliteal angle. Test ankle dorsiflexion with

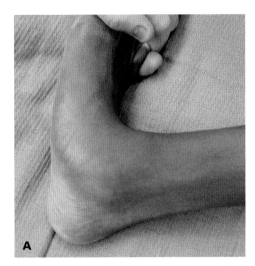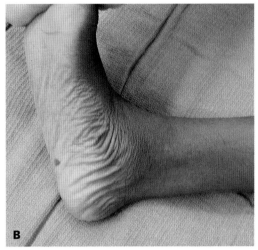

Figure 16-1 A: The incorrect way to check ankle dorsiflexion, because the examiner allowed the subtalar joint to go into eversion; this allows dorsiflexion to occur through the midfoot and may fool the examiner into thinking that there is suffi-cient ankle dorsiflexion. **B:** The correct technique, using hindfoot inversion, reveals that there actually is an ankle equinus contracture in this child. (Used with permission of the Children's Orthopaedic Center, Los Angeles.)

the knee flexed and extended (Silfverskiöld test), and be sure that the hindfoot is inverted, so that dorsiflexion through the midfoot does not fool you into over-estimating ankle dorsiflexion and underestimating the extent of the equinus con-tracture (Fig. 16-1). It is best to first check dorsiflexion with the hip and knee flexed, to get the child into a flexor pattern and increase static ankle dorsiflexion. For quadriplegic children with severe CP, if you get them in the sitting position to examine, the spine you will be able to evaluate how their spine is positioned when upright. Having the child lie on his side will allow you to check how flexible the spine is. True (rather than "postural") scoliosis is heralded by rotational defor-mity of the trunk. Postural curves, and or early nonstructural curves, will not have a fixed rotatory component.

Depending on upper extremity function, the child can be presented with objects to grasp, asked to transfer from hand to hand, and may be asked to do finger tapping, rapid alternating movements, and/or bimanual activities (donning and doffing socks or shoes, buttoning buttons, zipping up zippers, etc.). In younger children, simply observing them handling toys and/or other familiar objects may be all you can accomplish.

In addition to tone and range of motion assessment in the lower extremities, standing, transferring, and/or gait are assessed, depending on the child's functional level. Whenever possible, it is useful to see a child in and out of her leg braces. If the child needs handheld support or ambulatory aids, gait can be assessed with such assistance and/or aids.

Evaluating the gait of an ambulatory child with CP can be overwhelming to the less experienced. A systematic method for examining gait is needed. It is import-ant to observe the child's gait from both the front and the side to assess the vari-ous joints, body segments, and planes of motion. By taking a stepwise observation strategy with each walk down the hall, you can get a better sense of the problems.

Watch the child walk with and without braces, so you can assess the optimal brace for that particular child. Look at the shoes of a walking child to assess whether the toes are wearing out. This can be an indicator of foot clearance prob-lems, which can be seen with ankle equinus and/or a stiff knee in swing phase (which is often associated with rectus spasticity).

THE GURU SAYS...

When performing obser-vational gait analysis, I pay particular attention to consis-tency between strides, turning, stopping, and starting. Problems with these gait-related func-tions, as well as the presence of variable facial expressions and excessive movements of the fingers and toes while walking, suggest the presence of a more complex movement disorder.

JON DAVIDS

Of course, there is no specific diagnostic test to establish the diagnosis of CP. Many neurologists obtain a brain MRI, looking for characteristic abnormalities. Parents will sometimes ask the orthopaedist to order the brain MRI or to review it with them. The potential value of the MRI must be weighed against potential risks, including the need for sedation in young children. In most cases, the need for an MRI can be determined by the neurologist. One case in which an MRI should be ordered by the orthopaedist is in a child with hemiplegia and no risk factors or history that provides an adequate reason for the hemiplegia.

Depending on your comfort level, you may want to work together with the neurologist when diagnosing a child with CP, since the diagnosis of CP can carry profound implications. Many parental emotions and fears are attached to the words "cerebral palsy," so it is extremely important to contextualize this diagnosis. Many parents have a misconception that every child with CP is severely involved, such as those who are at GMFCS IV and V. You need to explain that children with CP have very different functional abilities, and that they typically gain motor milestones for many years (usually until at least 6-8 years old). Parents of a young child who already stands or walks, for instance, should be informed that such progress is expected to continue. Explain to the parents that although CP is not a progressive neurologic problem, the musculoskeletal manifestations of CP can change with time and growth. It is important to understand that some degree of gross motor functional deterioration does often occur in adolescence in children at GMFCS III, IV, and V levels, though conveying such information is not a good idea on the visit during which the diagnosis is first made. Such a conversation is better deferred until there is a closer bond between physician, patient, and family, and the child's prognosis becomes clearer.

Although a CP team approach is not available to all orthopaedists, one of the best ways to stay out of trouble is to work with other health care professionals knowledgeable about children with CP. If your institution has such specialists (pediatric neurologists, neurosurgeons, developmental paediatricians, physiatrists, and physical, occupational, and speech therapists), it is best to involve others whose assessments can help maximize outcomes and quality of life.

Other Diagnoses That Can Be Confused With CP

- Familial spasticity paraparesis
- Mitochondrial disease
- Leukodystrophy
- Congenital ataxia
- Brain or spinal cord tumors or infections
- Metabolic or chromosomal abnormalities with spasticity
- Rett syndrome

Surgery to Improve Walking

If you plan to do surgery on a child with CP, there are some important things to consider to stay out of trouble. Mercer Rang taught us that one of the keys to staying out of trouble when caring for children with CP is to avoid the "birthday syndrome," in which a different muscle group is released each year, leading to extensive multiple surgeries. Dr. Rang also taught us that regarding the outcomes of surgery in children with CP, "The decision is more important than the incision." Today, most orthopaedic surgeons know the importance of correcting problems at multiple levels simultaneously in children with CP, rather than leaving some deformities uncorrected. Single-event multilevel surgery (SEMLS), in which multilevel bone and soft-tissue surgeries are performed simultaneously to improve gait and function, has been the standard of care in these children for many years.

Typically, the best candidate for SEMLS surgery is a child who meets the following criteria: (1) they are aged 6 to 10 years, (2) their gross motor function has plateaued for at least 6 months, and (3) there are no nonsurgical ways to address the musculoskeletal problems interfering with gait and function. Evaluation using computerized gait analysis (CGA) facilitates this assessment, particularly in children with complex walking patterns.[4,5] In the absence of CGA, the child should be examined on at least a few occasions prior to surgery, and video taken from the front and side of the child walking can greatly enhance decision-making preoperatively. There are many readily available and inexpensive software apps available for mobile phones which allow the video to be slowed down and even freeze-framed and allow the user to measure joint angles as part of the gait assessment.

To stay out of trouble, make certain that the patient and family are committed to the postoperative therapy. A "great" surgery without quality therapy will yield disappointing results. After extensive surgery, the patients typically need quality physical therapy at least two to three times weekly for 2 to 3 months. If the patient and family are not able to commit to the therapy, surgery should be deferred until a time when they can make the commitment. **NEWSFLASH! Even under optimal circumstances, it generally takes a child 4 to 6 months to return to baseline functional status after SEMLS, and functional improvement often occurs for 2 years after surgery.** In a teenager with CP, return to functional baseline may take up to a year. These older and bigger children are slower to heal and have a much less favorable strength-to-weight ratio. You will do everyone a favor by being up front about these issues before surgery.

Overlengthening of tendons can be a major source of trouble. Though most commonly thought of as a problem at the level of the ankle, overlengthening can be problematic at other levels as well. Overlengthening at the hip (especially if combined with obturator neurectomy) can lead to hip hyperabduction. Overlengthening of the hamstrings often leads to recurvatum and/or a stiff knee gait. Overlengthened heel cords result in calcaneal crouch.

Children with dystonia present significant challenges to the surgeon. Soft-tissue procedures, such as tendon lengthenings and transfers, have unpredictable results in children with dystonia and should be avoided whenever possible. Well-planned bone surgery can be of benefit in children with dystonia.

Casts can cause significant problems in children with CP, and their use is minimized when possible. When casts are used, the surgeon should exercise great care in cast application. Foam padding has been shown to be a low-cost way to decrease skin complications following lower extremity postoperative casting in children with CP.[6]

To keep children with CP comfortable after surgery, diazepam is used routinely to help with the muscle spasms. Narcotics may be helpful at first but are not as valuable as the antispasticity medicines perioperatively.

Specific Challenges by Anatomic Area

SPINE DEFORMITY

Spine deformity is one of the most common complaints of patients and families in children with CP. The rate of significant scoliosis is directly related to GMFCS level, with very low rates (similar to the overall population) in GMFCS I and II children, and significant scoliosis in the majority of GMFCS V children.

Early on, there is typically not a fixed deformity. In children whose deformity is due to trunk weakness and lack of postural control, the spine will be noted to curve when the child is upright but to be straight when the child is supine or lying on his side. Lying the child on his side will mitigate the effects of gravity on the spine and allow an easy assessment of whether there is a fixed spinal deformity.

When there is a fixed spinal deformity, there will be thoracic and/or lumbar "humps" due to the rotational component of the deformity. The development of a rotatory deformity is the typical indication for spine radiographs. The radiographic technique should be consistent from visit to visit (e.g., sitting or supine) to allow for accurate assessment of any deformity progression. Sitting X-rays have the benefit of assessing the spinal deformity when the child is upright during daily activities. It will uniformly look worse than a supine film. The supine film has the advantage of eliminating the effects of gravity and is a more accurate reflection of fixed deformity.

Treatment

Bracing

Bracing (with a thoracolumbosacral orthosis or TLSO) is commonly used in children with CP and spinal deformity. It is important to recognize that a TLSO has not been proven to significantly change the natural history of spinal deformity in children with CP. However, use of a TLSO can enhance the quality of life of the child and family, by facilitating sitting (especially when out of the wheelchair). By facilitating sitting, the TLSO can often free up the child's hands for use.

When a TLSO is used in a child with CP, it differs from that used with idiopathic scoliosis. The TLSO for a child with CP should be a softer, "flex foam" type of TLSO to allow for appropriate postural support. Children with CP rarely tolerate a rigid TLSO, and such rigid bracing can lead to pressure sores, particularly in those with limited ability to communicate.

Occasionally, for children with significant scoliosis and in whom the patient and family have decided against surgery, the spine deformity can be addressed with a custom molded back for the wheelchair. Though this does nothing to correct the deformity, it can facilitate positioning, and the custom mold essentially braces the child when she is in her wheelchair.

Surgery

The decision for spine fusion surgery is a big decision for the patient and family. These are large surgeries with a significantly higher risk profile than for idiopathic scoliosis. However, there is a high level of patient and caregiver satisfaction after successful spine fusion in these patients. Jain et al. have recently reported significant improvement in quality of life in children with CP following spine fusion in patients with CP.[7] It is important to assure that the family is ready for a journey that can include many setbacks—prolonged hospital stay, wound infection, changes to the seating system (ordering new a wheelchair for child with a new shape can take many months in some areas). It is wise not to book surgery the first time the curve magnitude crosses 50°. Instead, share the risks and benefits, then send the family away thinking, and perhaps getting any necessary preoperative medical consults. See them back in 4 to 6 months and make a plan. Be careful not to go more than about 6 to 9 months—the deformities can progress rapidly when the curve is more than 60° and the spine is collapsing in these children with softer vertebrae.

Waiting until curves get much larger (and stiffer) often results in longer, more complicated surgeries, greater blood loss, longer hospital stays, and a larger residual curve.

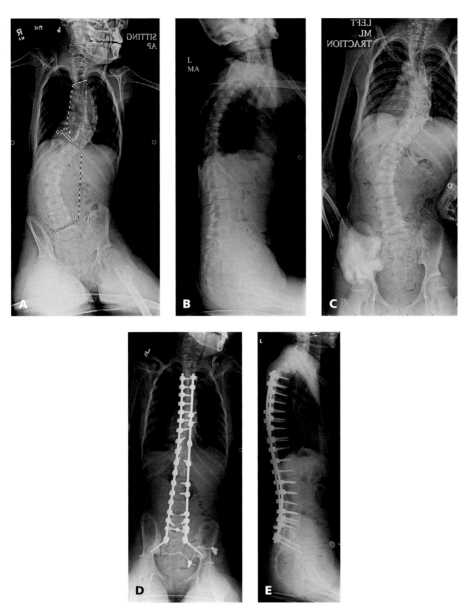

Figure 16-2 Spine deformity correction in CP.

Spine fusions are typically very long (upper T-spine to pelvis) for children with CP spine deformities (Fig. 16-2). Fusion to the pelvis is controversial. If the pelvis can be spared, complications such as pelvic pain, implant loosening, and surgical site infection are lower. Competent therapists note that seating is much easier if the child is not "a single cement block," as they say; having a jog of motion at the lumbosacral junction permits more comfortable seating. However, it is imperative that the technical execution for fusion to L5 be excellent. The pelvis at L5 must be leveled with intraoperative traction before the start of surgery. L3, L4, and L5 must have bilateral pedicle screw fixation, and each must be leveled. In general, the best deformities for fusion to L5 are the more flexible curves with a more cephalad apex. Unfortunately, if the fusion to L5 at the initial surgery does not level the three end vertebrae and revision surgery is required, the surgical times can be long and the blood loss similar to a primary long fusion to the pelvis.[8] So, to stay out of trouble, choose candidates for fusion to L5 wisely, and level those three lower vertebrae with bilateral screws. If you can, you are doing the child a favor for the rest of their sitting life. If it is not possible due to curve rigidity, magnitude, or caudal apex, then fuse to the pelvis.

Because of the traditional high rates of infection following posterior spinal fusion in this patient population, there have been recent trends toward more aggressive preoperative preparation, use of broad-spectrum antibiotics perioperatively, intraoperative wound lavage, and the use of impermeable dressings postoperatively (to avoid fecal contamination of the wound in these patients, who often lack bowel control). Such measures have markedly diminished the infection rate in this population.

HIP DISPLACEMENT

Hip subluxation is very common in children with CP. Previous studies have been all over the map as far as the risk of subluxation, ranging from less than 10% to more than 70%. Traditionally, the risk for hip subluxation was stratified by the geographic distribution of a child's CP, with low risk in those with hemiplegia, moderate in diplegia, and high in quadriplegia.

The GMFCS classification is the best way to stratify the risk of hip subluxation in CP. Soo et al. reported hip subluxation in 35% of their cohort of children with CP and a linear relationship between the risk of hip subluxation in children with CP, including a 0% risk in their GMFCS I patients and 90% in their GMFCS V children.[9] Previous authors have also shown that increased hip displacement is associated with a lower quality of life in children with CP.[10]

Since hip subluxation can only be detected definitively with radiographic evaluation, it is imperative that all children with CP undergo radiographic hip screening. **NEWSFLASH! There are different guidelines worldwide, but there is consensus that *all* children with CP need hip screening, typically beginning by age 2 to 3 years.** The frequency of screening thereafter varies depending on GMFCS level, previous radiographs (i.e., presence of subluxation and/or progressive hip migration), and physical examination. The frequency of screening X-rays should be greatest in children with the most severe involvement (GMFCS IV and V) and least frequent in those with mild involvement (GMFCS I and II). One group of highly functional children (GMFCS I or II) who have significant risk of later hip subluxation or dislocation are Winters and Gage type IV hemiplegics (who walk with a flexed, internally rotated hip, and flexed knee).[11] Remember that a screening hip radiograph can look relatively normal in a child with CP but can progress to complete dislocation (Fig. 16-3).

It is not unusual for the parent of a school-age child with CP to present to the orthopaedist's office complaining that the child has hip pain. To stay out of trouble, understand that there are many different things that cause pain besides

Figure 16-3 A: A screening X-ray in this patient with CP (GMFCS IV) at age 4 y shows well-reduced hips and good acetabular morphology.
B: Unfortunately, he did not undergo routine hip screening, and at age 17 y, he had windswept hips with a dislocated, misshapen, painful, and unreconstructible right hip. (Used with permission of the Children's Orthopaedic Center, Los Angeles.)

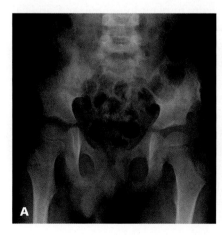
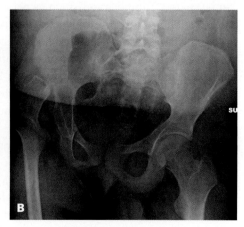

the hip joint itself. Even with a radiograph that shows some hip subluxation, be certain that there is not an abdominal source for the pain. Reflux, constipation, hernias, and other conditions can mimic the pain of spastic hip disease. Also, spastic hip adductors may be the real source of pain in a younger child. It is very unlikely to have actual joint pain in a younger child, even with severe subluxation.

On physical examination, there are three main findings to look for that are suggestive of hip subluxation and/or dislocation. The first is the Galeazzi sign, in which the hips are adducted and flexed to 90°; a positive Galeazzi (knee heights are different) is suggestive of asymmetric hip subluxation and/or dislocation. The second is the degree of hip abduction (typically tested in extension). Asymmetry between the hips, loss of abduction since the previous visit, and/or abduction <20° in extension are suggestive of the possibility of hip subluxation. Finally, posterior prominence of the femoral head is typically assessed with the hips and knees flexed to 90° as the examiner axially loads the knees (pushing posteriorly on the knees) and palpates for the femoral heads in the buttocks.

Beware of anterior hip dislocations. Although they make up <5% of hip sub-luxations and dislocations in children with CP, they can be more difficult to diagnose.[12] To stay out of trouble, understand that the radiographs in children with an anterior hip dislocation often shows little, if any, lateral hip displacement. These children do not have the classic hip flexion adduction posture. Instead, they are usually in figure 4 (or "frog") position with the hips extended, abducted, and externally rotated. If you feel an anterior prominence in the groin and see this figure 4 position, the diagnosis is an anterior dislocation. Though uncommon, some children with significant posterior subluxation will not show lateral translation either, and advanced imaging may be needed to assess their anatomy (Fig. 16-4).

Treatment

Nonoperative

For a child with a hip "at risk" for progressive subluxation and/or dislocation, hip adductor stretching (in therapy and/or at home) and nighttime hip adduction stretching with a hip abduction pillow or hip abduction orthosis (HAO) are commonly used. Botulinum toxin injection into the hip adductors may be considered, though this typically lasts only for 3 to 5 months following injection. These various nonoperative methods do not avoid the need for surgery but may delay the time until surgery is needed.[13]

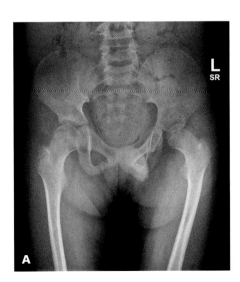

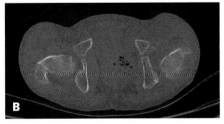

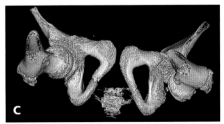

Figure 16-4 A 15-year-old boy with CP (GMFCS IV) had a positive Galeazzi sign and prominence of his femoral head posteriorly on physical examination. **A:** Plain radiographs (showed some widening of the medial clear space and mild lateral uncovering). **B, C:** CT scans showed significant posterior subluxation of the left femoral head with posterior acetabular dysplasia. (Used with permission of the Children's Orthopaedic Center, Los Angeles.)

THE GURU SAYS...

Early soft-tissue surgery about the hips reliably improves hip range of motion, facilitating perineal hygiene, which is appreciated by caregivers. This surgery is also useful as a "dry run" in anticipation of the much larger hip reconstruction surgery, giving the physicians on the care team an opportunity to learn more about how a child with severe CP tolerates surgery and recovery, and giving parents better insight into what is involved before, during, and following orthopaedic surgery.

JON DAVIDS

Surgery

Hip surgery is typically considered for hips with migration percentage above 40% and progressive displacement. The iliopsoas can be a significant element of the pathophysiology in spastic hip disease. In very young children (<3-4 years old), soft-tissue lengthenings of the adductors and often the psoas can be considered. The long-term results of these procedures in avoiding bone surgery are very low in most series, but such soft-tissue procedures may be used as a temporizing measure in order to delay the need for bone surgery in these patients. Don't forget about a child's medical comorbidities because many children with hip subluxation or dislocation are GMFCS IV or V and often have significant medical comorbidities.

As with many of the surgeries in children with CP, one of the major challenges after hip surgery in these children is tone management. Many children get significant spasms after surgery, particularly soft-tissue surgery, and most of the acute postoperative pain is due to spasms and responds better to tone management than to narcotic administration.

Bone surgery for hip subluxation or dislocation is common in these children. Typically, the migration percentage exceeds 40% to 50% when they come to surgery. When possible, it is best to avoid bone surgery in children younger than 5 years of age because of the high risk of recurrent hip displacement. Traditionally, the bone surgeries in these children were comprehensive ("global") surgeries, which included soft-tissue lengthenings (adductors ± psoas), varus derotational osteotomy (VDRO), open hip reduction, and pelvic osteotomy. When a VDRO is done, it is important to do an adequate adductor lengthening, since a varus osteotomy results is an adduction osteotomy (it increases hip adduction and decreases hip abduction); failure to do an adequate adductor lengthening when doing a VDRO exacerbates a hip adduction contracture (Fig. 16-5). These global

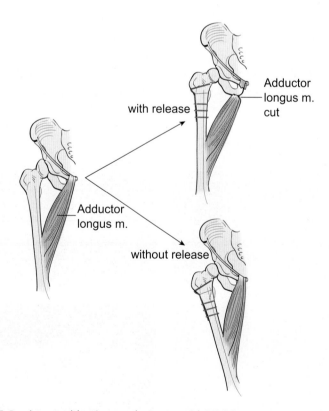

Figure 16-5 Persistent adduction made worse with VDRO.

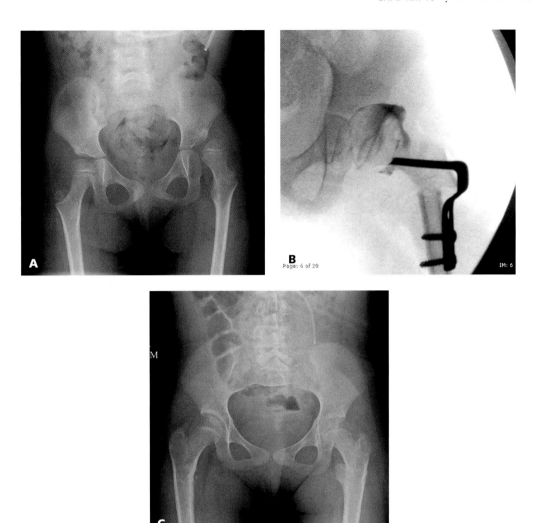

Figure 16-6 **A:** X-rays of a dislocated hip in a 6-year-old child with CP (GMFCS IV). **B:** Intraoperative arthrogram (prior to placement of the final two screws) shows good acetabular morphology and no significant medial dye pool; as a result, neither an open reduction nor a pelvic osteotomy was performed. **C:** Six-year follow-up X-rays (following hardware removal) with good acetabular morphology. (Used with permission of the Children's Orthopaedic Center, Los Angeles.)

surgeries typically have good results,[14] though most recent series using an "a la carte" approach, with routine use of the soft-tissue lengthenings and VDRO and selective use of the open reduction and/or pelvic osteotomy, show similar results.[15] Use of an "a la carte" approach results in significantly shorter operative times, lower blood loss, and less need for blood transfusion. Use of a hip arthrogram is very helpful in determining the need for the addition of an open reduction and/ or pelvic osteotomy when using the "a la carte" approach (Fig. 16-6). Since the psoas is lengthened as part of the VDRO (assuming the VDRO results in removal of the lesser trochanter, with attendant release of the psoas off the less trochanter), a separate psoas lengthening is not typically needed when a VDRO is performed.

One of the big questions is when to do bilateral surgery for hip subluxation in a child with CP who has unilateral hip subluxation or dislocation. In the vast majority of bilaterally involved children less than 10 years old, bilateral surgery is recommended by most experts. This allows for maintenance of symmetry and allows for some shortening of the femurs (usually 1.5-2 cm) at the time of surgery (which helps decrease the risk of recurrent muscle contracture and hip displacement). Unilateral VDRO surgery universally results in a significantly short leg on the operated side, and this limb length discrepancy (LLD) is not only visually unacceptable to many families but can interfere with seating, standing, and walking.

Anterior hip subluxation or dislocation rarely requires operative intervention. If surgery is contemplated, a CT scan of the pelvis can be very helpful to assess proximal femoral and acetabular anatomy. With anterior displacement, the anterior acetabulum may be deficient. A reshaping acetabular osteotomy (such as a Pemberton or a Dega osteotomy in those with open triradiates, or a PAO if the triradiates are closed) to enhance anterior coverage can be useful in this population.

There are many reasons that children with CP have a high complication rate after hip reconstruction. Low bone density, unfavorable biomechanics, abnormal tone, poor muscle control, limited cognition, and associated medical problems (particularly pulmonary and GI) can combine to make the postoperative period difficult. Be certain that the family knows the goals and risks of the surgery.

For painful hips with long-standing dislocations that are no longer able to be reconstructed, salvage surgery may be performed. The most common salvage procedures include proximal femoral resection (so-called Castle procedure), proximal femoral valgus (Schanz) osteotomy, proximal femoral Schanz osteotomy in combination with a Girdlestone procedure (McHale procedure), and prosthetic arthroplasty. Girdlestone procedures should not be performed in this patient population, due to poor results (including pain and stiffness), and arthroplasty has poor results in nonambulators in our experience.

The remaining procedures have similar benefits of pain relief (typically in about 80% of patients).[17] For patients and families who want the child to be able to do some standing with weight bearing on the operative limb, a McHale typically gives good pain relief while maintaining the ability to weight bear. The Castle procedure (proximal femoral resection at approximately the level of the lesser trochanter) can provide good pain relief but does not allow the child to weight bear on the operative leg and results in a short and "floppy" leg. Since windswept hips are common in those with chronic unilateral hip dislocation undergoing a salvage procedure, a VDRO (with internal rotation) is often indicated on the contralateral side to align the lower extremities better with the pelvis, which facilitates sitting, including positioning in the wheelchair. Regardless of which type of salvage procedure is undertaken, excellent pain relief often takes several months. Heterotopic ossification is also very common after proximal femoral resection, and we routinely provide a single dose of low-dose radiation on postoperative day 1. Because of proximal femoral remodeling, the proximal screws often become prominent and painful in the years following the McHale procedure, and hardware removal is commonly indicated (Fig. 16-7).

KNEE PATHOLOGY

Knee Contractures and Crouch Gait

As a result of hamstring spasticity and quadriceps weakness, many children with CP develop progressive knee contractures. Extension contractures are very rare and usually are seen in children after near-drowning hypoxic events.

For early hamstring contractures, conservative management with stretching is useful, and this can be augmented with the use of knee immobilizers at bedtime. If the contracture progresses, botulinum toxin injection can be considered.

Knee flexion during gait is typically referred to as crouch gait. As with any walking problem, it is important to assess what is happening at different levels

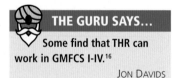

THE GURU SAYS...

Whenever possible, aggressive tone management, with intrathecal baclofen pump or selective dorsal rhizotomy, should be considered prior to performing palliative surgery for painful hip dysplasia in teenagers with CP. Occasionally, significant tone reduction results in adequate pain relief, obviating the need for the palliative hip surgery. Effective tone management facilitates postoperative pain management and recovery/rehabilitation following palliative hip surgery.

JON DAVIDS

THE GURU SAYS...

Some find that THR can work in GMFCS I-IV.[16]

JON DAVIDS

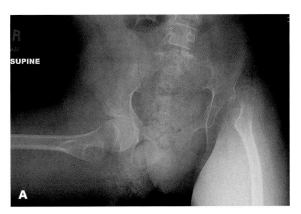
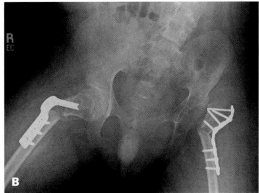
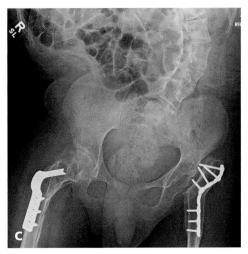

Figure 16-7 A: A 15-year-old boy presented with severe windswept hip deformity, left hip pain, and difficulty sitting. **B:** Postoperative X-rays after right VDRO and left McHale procedures. His pain resolved and sitting ability was markedly improved. **C:** X-rays 5 y postoperatively show remodeling of the proximal femur with hardware prominence and impingement, which caused significant pain. Hardware removal resulted in pain resolution.

when a child walks. Crouch gait is no exception. There are three main types of crouch gait, and, in all three, the hips and knees are flexed. The difference between these conditions is the ankle position: in calcaneal crouch, the ankle is dorsiflexed excessively; in apparent equinus, the ankle is neutral; and, in jump gait, there is ankle equinus.[18]

When surgery is contemplated, it is important to determine the extent of hamstring tightness and whether or not there is an associated knee flexion contracture. Hamstring lengthening can be considered if the popliteal angle exceeds 40° to 50° and the knees are excessively flexed during gait. **NEWSFLASH! Hamstring lengthening (HSL) surgery can worsen anterior pelvic tilt, and caution should be exercised for someone who already has anterior pelvic tilt in whom you are considering HSL.** A CGA can help assess anterior pelvic tilt preoperatively and can also be used to assess dynamic hamstring length. If the hamstrings are not short based on this hamstring length modeling on CGA, then HSL is not typically indicated. If HSL surgery is performed, a popliteal angle should *not* be checked intraoperatively, in order to minimize the risk of postoperative peroneal neuropraxia.

For a child with a significant knee flexion contracture (>10°) who is older than 10 years, bone surgery is typically needed to adequately address the knee contracture. Such bone surgery can include either guided growth (with distal femoral anterior hemiepiphysiodesis, DFAH) or distal femoral extension osteotomy (DFEO).

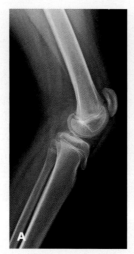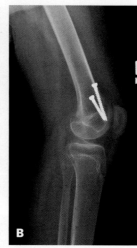

Figure 16-8 A: Patella alta and open physes in a 12½-year-old girl with CP (GMFCS III) and crouch gait prior to undergoing distal femoral anterior hemiepiphysiodesis and patella tendon advancement. **B:** Appropriate position of the screws (crossing the anterior third of the physis and the improved position of the patella). Patella baja does not appear to be problematic in these patients, and sufficient tensioning of the extensor mechanism is paramount. (Used with permission of the Children's Orthopaedic Center, Los Angeles.)

Whenever possible, DFAH is preferred over DFEO since DFAH is a much smaller, less morbid procedure, and allows immediate weight bearing. When DFEO is necessary, it should always be combined with a patellar tendon advancement (PTA), since the combination of DFEO with PTA has much better results than an isolated DFEO.[19] PTA may be performed concomitantly with DFAH in the case of significant patella alta and an incompetent extensor mechanism (Fig. 16-8).

Stiff Knee Gait

> **THE GURU SAYS...**
>
> Some believe that rectus femoris lengthening may be as effective as DFRT.[20]
>
> JON DAVIDS

Stiff knee gait is common in children with CP and can result in difficulties with foot clearance and tripping. If the stiff knee gait is interfering with function, then distal rectus femoris transfer (DRFT) can be considered. This surgery can help by improving the arc of motion of the knee from stance to swing phase and by making peak knee flexion occur earlier in the gait cycle.

The following indications must all be met for a child to be a good candidate for DRFT:

- Stiff knee in swing: This is best evidenced on CGA.
- Overactive rectus femoris muscle in swing phase: As seen with dynamic electromyography during CGA. In the absence of CGA, a positive Duncan-Ely (prone rectus) test can be used as a proxy for rectus spasticity.[21]
- GMFCS I or II: Previous work has shown poor results in GMFCS III and IV children.[22]

Knee Pain

Knee pain is an underappreciated problem in children with CP. Part of this results from difficulties in communication. These children often have many risk factors for patellofemoral pain, including weak quadriceps, tight hamstrings, patella alta, femoral anteversion, external tibial torsion, pes valgus, and other issues. Previous research indicated a 21% incidence of knee pain in a prospective study of 121 children presenting to a gait lab for routine testing.[23]

Most treatment of knee pain is conservative. Simple accommodations, such as sitting with the knees less flexed for part of the day, may be sufficient for some children. Hamstring stretching and quadriceps strengthening exercises are often useful, and knee immobilizers may also be used to stretch the hamstrings. Surgery is rarely performed solely for knee pain, though surgeries which improve knee extension in stance, decrease knee contractures, and address femoral anteversion, external tibial torsion, and/or valgus foot deformities likely decrease the prevalence and severity of knee pain in those with CP.

FOOT AND ANKLE PATHOLOGY

Equinus Contractures

Equinus refers to the position of the foot in plantarflexion. This can be the result of a contracture of the plantarflexors or simply due to dynamic positioning in equinus. When assessing someone with equinus, it is imperative to determine whether or not there is a true contracture. The Silfverskiöld test should be performed, to assess the amount of dorsiflexion with the knee both flexed and extended. One of the pearls when checking for ankle dorsiflexion is to first flex the child's hip and knee, in order to get the child into a flexor pattern in the leg being examined. Once the child's hip and knee are flexed, the plantarflexor tone is relieved and the ankle can be dorsiflexed more easily. After this is checked, then the knee is slowly extended to complete the Silfverskiöld test. If the ankle is initially examined with the hip and knee extended, the child's extensor pattern will result in increased tone in the plantarflexors and you will measure less dorsiflexion (and might be fooled into thinking there is a contracture). Regardless of how hard you push, you almost never can achieve as much dorsiflexion as an older and heavier child gets during gait, as his body weight overcomes the resistance in the plantarflexors.

If the ankle is only tight with the knee extended, then the gastrocnemius is tight but the soleus is not; but if the ankle is also tight with the knee in flexion, then the soleus is also tight. The gastrocnemius is a two-joint muscle (since it crosses the knee and ankle joints) and tends to be tight in CP, whereas the single-joint soleus is rarely tight.

When present, a fixed equinus contracture requires intervention to gain range of motion, which can include a range of treatments such as a stretching program, daytime and/or nighttime bracing, casting, and/or surgery. For dynamic equinus, appropriate daytime bracing is typically all that is needed, though botulinum toxin injection may be considered in some cases.

It is far better for heel cords to be too tight, rather than too loose. If the Achilles tendon is loose, the child typically stands and walks with excessive ankle dorsiflexion (the calcaneal crouch noted above), and there are no good treatments to reliably fix the problem. The natural history of children with CP is a progressive increase in dorsiflexion of the ankle and potential crouch, as the child grows toward adolescence,[5] and surgical intervention for the gastrocsoleus complex should be minimized. Even without surgery, children can progress from equinus to calcaneal crouch gait.[24]

If surgery is needed for a tight calf, gastrocnemius recession is the preferred surgery in the vast majority of patients. Achilles tendon surgery should be avoided in all but the most severe cases of equinus contracture since such surgery weakens the calf musculature much more than does a gastrocnemius recession and results in a much greater risk of overlengthening and calcaneal gait.[25]

For children with long-standing equinus contractures, the toe flexors are also often tight. When the ankle is brought to neutral at surgery (after equinus correction), toe flexor tightness with clawing of the toes may be present. If so, the toe flexors should be lengthened (just above the medial malleolus) at the same time.

Pes Varus

Varus foot deformities are much more frequent in those with unilateral (hemiplegic) CP than with bilateral (diplegic or quadriplegic) CP. The main problems with varus foot deformity in CP are the following: (1) less of the foot is contacting the ground during standing and walking, so the child does not have an adequate base of support; (2) varus often results in in-toeing, further compromising the child's base of support; and (3) brace fitting is difficult, frequently resulting in areas of high pressure and pain.

The anterior tibialis contributes to pes varus much more frequently than traditionally thought, and muscle contributors to the varus foot in CP include the posterior tibialis in about one-third of patients, the anterior tibialis in another third, and both the anterior and posterior tibialis in the remaining third.[26]

The only way to definitely determine which muscle(s) is contributing to the varus foot is with dynamic electromyography (EMG) during gait, though many people do not have access to a gait lab with such technology. In the absence of such access, the confusion test can be very helpful to evaluate the anterior tibialis. Since most children with CP do not have good selective motor control, the confusion test relies on a mass action pattern by the patient. The child is asked to actively flex the hip while seated; as he does so, the anterior tibialis contracts and dorsiflexes the ankle. If the foot supinates during this maneuver (a "positive" confusion test), the anterior tibialis is a likely contributor to varus foot deformity in this patient.

A varus foot can typically be controlled sufficiently for months or years in a well-made brace. Surgery can sometimes be completely avoided in these patients, but even if it cannot, the brace can temporize the situation until the child is older and ready for surgery. In order for a brace to control a varus foot well, it should have a wraparound component which can capture the hindfoot well and maintain a more neutral subtalar position. Such a wraparound hindfoot component also maximizes the surface area of contact between the brace and foot, thus minimizing contact forces and the risk of pressure areas and skin breakdown.

If surgery is needed, the dynamic EMG from a gait lab is very helpful. In the absence of such information, a reasonable option is to perform combined surgery for the anterior tibialis (with a split anterior tibial tendon transfer [SPLATT]) and posterior tibialis (with either a lengthening or split transfer). This combination has a high probability of success with a low risk of significant overcorrection. Another option is to do the confusion test preoperatively to assess whether there appears to be anterior tibialis contribution to the varus foot and to proceed as above when the anterior tibialis is involved ("positive" confusion test) and to do surgery to the posterior tibialis (but not the anterior tibialis) when the confusion test is "negative." When performing a SPLATT, it is best to transfer to the peroneus tertius (if available) and the peroneus brevis otherwise. Such tendon-to-tendon transfers allow better tensioning of the transfer and avoid the problems of buttons on the plantar foot (which are often used in SPLATT transfers to bone in these children; Fig. 16-9).

THE GURU SAYS...

Varus deformity of the foot associated with significant equinus during stance phase of gait suggests that the tibialis posterior is the primary cause of the varus and should be the target of surgery. Varus deformity associated with minimal equinus during the stance phase of gait suggests that the tibialis anterior is the primary cause of the varus and should be the target of surgery.

JON DAVIDS

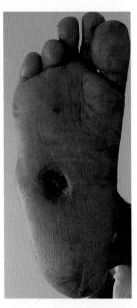

Figure 16-9 Pressure sore on the plantar foot following split anterior tibial tendon transfer to the cuboid, using a felt and button on the plantar foot; doing a tendon-to-tendon split anterior tibial tendon transfer avoids this potential complication and also allows better tensioning of the transfer. (Used with permission of the Children's Orthopaedic Center, Los Angeles.)

For fixed varus deformities, a calcaneal osteotomy is necessary in conjunction with the soft-tissue procedures noted above. Most commonly, a Dwyer (lateral closing wedge) osteotomy of the calcaneus is the procedure of choice, though some surgeons perform a lateral calcaneal slide.

Pes Valgus

Valgus foot deformity is more common in bilaterally involved children than in those with unilateral CP. For most with valgus foot deformity, there is still a stable base of support, though bracewear may be a problem, particularly due to pressure over the medial midfoot. Bracing suffices as treatment for most valgus feet. A significant midfoot break makes bracing more difficult and surgery more likely. **NEWSFLASH! One of the important things to remember to stay out of trouble is that sometimes a child who appears to have a valgus foot may actually have a valgus ankle.** Make sure to check the ankle alignment on physical examination. In a normally aligned ankle, the lateral malleolus is distal to the medial malleolus. If this is not the case, then the apparent foot valgus is likely due to ankle valgus instead. If there is any question about whether ankle valgus is present, get an AP ankle X-ray (preferably standing) to rule out ankle valgus (Fig. 16-10).

If surgery is needed for a valgus foot deformity, calcaneal osteotomy is typically necessary. This can be via a medial calcaneal slide or a calcaneal lengthening osteotomy. Anecdotally, it seems that a calcaneal lengthening osteotomy may have an increased risk of later overcorrection into hindfoot varus in children with CP, since a peroneus brevis lengthening is routinely performed as part of this surgery.

If a significant midfoot break is present, then medial column surgery is needed at the time of the lateral column lengthening surgery. For GMFCS I and II children, medial reefing of the talonavicular joint and possibly the posterior tibial

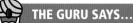

THE GURU SAYS...

The varus foot may also have fixed skeletal deformity of the midfoot and forefoot. Adduction deformity is best treated with lateral column shortening, when the deformity is small by cuboid closing wedge osteotomy, when the deformity is large by calcaneocuboid shortening arthrodesis. Significant forefoot supination deformity is best corrected by opening wedge plantarflexion osteotomy of the medial column (medial cuneiform or proximal first metatarsal). Significant forefoot cavus deformity is best treated by closing wedge dorsiflexion osteotomy of the medial column (medial cuneiform or proximal first metatarsal).

JON DAVIDS

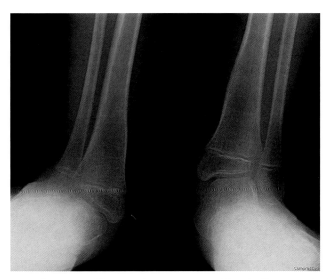

Figure 16-10 Standing AP ankle X-ray in an 11-year-old male (GMFCS IV) with bilateral valgus-appearing feet. The X-ray shows that the valgus emanates from the right ankle and the left foot. This is a case where valgus foot correction is the correct surgery for the left foot, whereas valgus ankle correction is needed on the right. (Used with permission of the Children's Orthopaedic Center, Los Angeles.)

Figure 16-11 A: Preoperative AP foot X-ray in a child with CP (GMFCS III) and midfoot breaks prior to bilateral medial calcaneal sliding osteotomies and talonavicular fusions. She was unable to tolerate bracing due to pain and skin problems. **B:** Two-year postoperative AP X-ray showing improved alignment. (Used with permission of the Children's Orthopaedic Center, Los Angeles.)

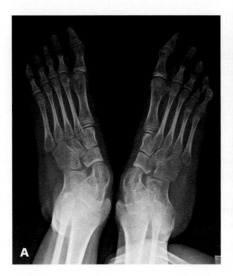
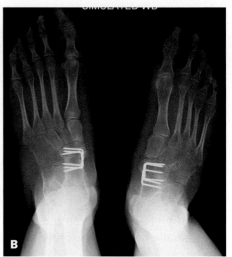

tendon is often helpful in the presence of a significant midfoot break. While this may not completely correct the midfoot break in these children with CP, it is beneficial and maintains hindfoot motion. For severe midfoot breaks in more limited ambulators and obligate brace users, a talonavicular fusion at the time of calcaneal lengthening osteotomy provides excellent stability, correction, and durability (Fig. 16-11).

Always remember that forefoot supination often occurs concomitantly with hindfoot valgus. Make sure to assess this at surgery when correcting these feet. A plantarflexion osteotomy (e.g., a medial cuneiform plantarflexion osteotomy) may be needed at the same surgery to address the supination.

If there is ankle valgus (rather than foot valgus), then surgery can be directed toward the ankle deformity via guided growth using medial malleolar screw placement or distal tibial and fibular osteotomies.

Hallux Valgus

Hallux valgus is most common in children with bilateral involvement, particularly those with valgus feet. For many cases of hallux valgus, a toe strap added to the brace suffices to control the toe position.

In children in whom the hallux valgus worsens, surgery may need to be considered. The main indications for consideration of surgery include underlapping of the great toe under the second toe, progressive pain (typically over the medial aspect of the first metatarsal head), and/or the inability to tolerate braces. If surgery is undertaken, preservation of range of motion at the first metatarsophalangeal joint (MTPJ) with standard hallux valgus reconstruction techniques is preferred for GMFCS I and II children, although their risk of recurrence is more than for typically developing children. For obligate bracewearers and nonambulators, first MTPJ fusion is indicated.

Dorsal Bunion

Dorsal bunions are more common in more involved (GMFCS III-V) children but may also occur in GMFCS I and II children, particularly those with varus feet. The dorsal bunion results in significant dorsal prominence of the first metatarsal head, which often causes pain and difficulty with shoewear and/or bracewear (Fig. 16-12).

THE GURU SAYS...

Great toe MTP arthrodesis is well tolerated in children with CP at all GMFCS levels. Proper sagittal plane alignment is essential for a good result. Inadequate dorsiflexion blocks third rocker in GMFCS I level patients (few GMFCS II or III patients achieve third rocker in stance phase). Excessive dorsiflexion results in interphalangeal (IP) joint flexion and dorsal prominence, which may be painful and compromise shoewear.

JON DAVIDS

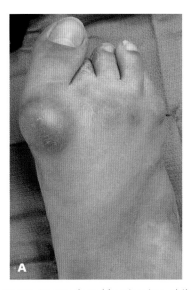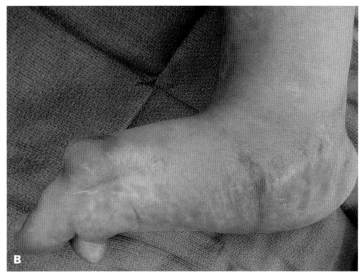

Figure 16-12 Severe dorsal bunion in a child which interfered with shoe and bracewear.

The tibialis anterior typically pulls the first metatarsal dorsally, in combination with overpull of the great toe plantarly by the flexor hallucis longus (FHL). The child ends up with pressure over the first metatarsal head and the plantar aspect of the tip of the great toe.

Soft (elastic-type) straps over the dorsum of the metatarsal heads can be affixed to the braces to minimize the symptoms when braced in many children. Sometimes bracewear must be abandoned due to pain. In some children, the only way to alleviate symptoms is to have them wear very soft shoewear (such as slippers) or no shoes whatsoever.

If surgery is needed, preoperative determination should be made regarding the rigidity of the deformity. For flexible dorsal bunions, soft-tissue surgery suffices. In such cases, anterior tibialis surgery (lengthening or split transfer), combined with a transfer of the FHL to the plantar aspect of the first metatarsal head, is the procedure of choice. If this is not sufficient for complete correction, then a plantarflexion osteotomy of the first ray may also be needed.[4]

For rigid deformities, weakening of the overpull of the anterior tibialis (via lengthening or SPLATT) is combined with fusion of the first MTPJ. A plantarflexion osteotomy of the first ray may also be needed.

IN-TOEING AND OUT-TOEING

In-toeing and out-toeing are not unique problems for children with CP. Unlike typically developing children, however, in-toeing and out-toeing can cause significant functional limitations in children with CP due to their limitations in balance, strength, and coordination. Based on Newton's third law—"For every action, there is an equal and opposite reaction"—when we walk, the ground pushes back against our feet as we push against the ground. The "ground reaction force" is abnormally positioned when we intoe or outtoe, and this results in lever arm dysfunction and inefficient gait (and can negatively impact the function of someone with a neuromuscular condition, including CP).[27]

The main causes of in-toeing in children with CP include femoral anteversion, tibial torsion, and varus foot deformity.[28] In one-third of all children with CP who intoe, there are multiple causes present within the same extremity, and the number rises to 50% for those with hemiplegia and intoe.[28]

The main causes of out-toeing in CP include external hip rotation during gait, femoral retroversion, external tibial torsion, and pes valgus. Many of these children also have multiple causes. For a child who is in-toeing or out-toeing, the physical examination should include the following:

- Internal and external hip rotation (in the prone position, whenever possible)
- Thigh-foot angle (TFA)
- Assessment of the foot (for varus or valgus)
- Gait assessment

When assessing hip internal and external rotation, any significant difference (>20°-30°) between internal and external rotation of a given hip is a potential cause for concern. For TFA (with a normal measure about 10° external), measures at least 15° external or 0 or more degrees internal are potentially problematic.

When assessing gait, the in-toeing and out-toeing are contextualized in relation to the child's overall gait and how it impacts her function. The observer should look at the child's foot progression angle (FPA) as an overall indicator of in-toeing or out-toeing. The observer should look at the knee progression angle (KPA) as an indicator of where the knee is relative to the direction in which the child is walking, with an internal KPA being an indicator of a cause of in-toeing above the knee (likely internal hip rotation due to femoral anteversion and/or internal pelvic rotation). An external KPA would indicate the opposite (external hip rotation, femoral retroversion, and/or external pelvic rotation). The observer should then compare the FPA and the KPA. If these are different (for instance, if the foot is more internally rotated than the knee), then there is a problem below the knee. If the foot is more internal than the knee, the common causes are internal tibial torsion and/or a varus foot. If the foot is more external than the knee, the common causes are external tibial torsion and/or a valgus foot.

Treatment

There are no nonoperative interventions that correct tibial or femoral torsion. Temporizing measures with various straps and/or twister cables can be used to decrease in-toeing or out-toeing until a time when surgery is performed.

If surgery is performed for long bone torsion, the affected bone(s) are addressed with derotational osteotomies. For the femur, good results can be obtained with proximal or distal osteotomies. Proximal osteotomies are necessary if there is concomitant coxa valga and hip subluxation. Correction for femoral osteotomies should be 1.5 to 2:1 of the abnormal hip rotation seen on gait (e.g., 30°-40° of correction if the hip is internally rotated 20° during gait), with the goal of having at least 20° more external than internal hip rotation at the end of surgery.[4] For tibial derotation, the osteotomy is done distally, to minimize the risk of neurovascular compromise. Only the tibia needs to be cut, unless more than about 50° of correction is needed, in which case, a fibular osteotomy may be performed.

The tibial correction should be 1:1, with the goal of a neutral thigh foot angle at the end of surgery.[4] Since children with CP tend to develop more external tibial torsion as they progress to adolescence,[5] the goal for surgery should be a neutral TFA, rather than the "normal" 10° of external TFA.

THE GURU SAYS...

Gait deviations due to abnormal transverse plane alignment of the femur and tibia are a consequence skeletal lever arm deficiency, which places muscles at a biomechanical disadvantage and compromises their ability to generate a moment. In my experience the magnitude of the skeletal malalignment is not linearly related to the magnitude of the gait deviation. From this perspective, surgical correction may be dosed to restore normal transverse plane alignment, which restores the lever arm available to the muscles and corrects the associated gait deviations.

Jon Davids

THE GURU SAYS...

In my experience, tibia torsion corrections of greater than 30° may require concomitant osteotomy of the fibula.

Jon Davids

Staying Out of Trouble With Cerebral Palsy

General Principles

* Children use both hands essentially equally in infancy. Hand dominance before 1 year is abnormal and is due to hemiplegia until proven otherwise.

* Patience during physical examination is crucial. If the examination is done hastily, the child's muscles will tense and you will be testing spasticity more than the actual joint range of motion. Serial examinations in the child help confirm the true degree of contractures and gait deviations.

* Surgery should rarely be recommended during an initial orthopaedic consultation with a patient and family, due to the complexity of these patients and the variability of their examination over time. An exception is a child referred for surgical consultation due to dislocated hip(s), severe scoliosis, or severe, long-standing gait deviations.

* The ideal candidate when considering for SEMLS surgery fulfills the following three criteria:
  * Age 6 to 10 years
  * Has plateaued with regard to motor function for at least 6 months
  * Has issues that cannot be adequately addressed nonoperatively

* Making certain that the patient and family are committed to the postoperative therapy is critical. A "great" surgery without quality therapy will yield less than stellar results. If the patient and family are not committed to the postoperative therapy, surgery should be deferred until a time when they can make the commitment.

* Warn families about the impact of multiple surgeries on older children. Rehabbing after SEMLS is more difficult in children older than 10 years of age.

* Be wary of doing soft-tissue procedures, such as tendon transfers or lengthenings, in children with dystonia. The results in this population are very unpredictable.

* Overaggressive lengthening results in poor outcomes at any level (hip, knee, or ankle) of the lower extremity and should be avoided.

Hip

* GMFCS level is the most accurate predictor of hip subluxation.

* *All* patients with CP need to undergo hip screening, typically beginning by age 2 or 3 years.

* The frequency of hip surveillance should be related to GMFCS level, degree (if any) of previous hip subluxation, and rate of progression of hip displacement.

* Hip displacement is often silent, so do not rely on physical examination alone. Radiographs are needed.

* Delay hip reconstruction in the very young, if possible: there is a much higher rate of failure if hip reconstruction is done in children younger than 5 years.

* A VDRO is an *adduction* osteotomy (the patient will lose abduction). It is important to do a satisfactory adductor lengthening prior to performing a VDRO, to avoid exacerbating a hip adduction contracture.

(continued)

Staying Out of Trouble With Cerebral Palsy (continued)

* Iliopsoas lengthening or release in nonambulators is often needed (either via soft-tissue lengthening or resection of the lesser trochanter during VDRO) for success in the surgical management of spastic hip disease.

* Be alert: the radiographs in children with an anterior hip dislocation often do not show any significant displacement.

Spine

* Work closely with family members to help them understand the effects of neuromuscular scoliosis on their child's function and health.

* Bracing with a TLSO has not been proven to stop curve progression but can improve sitting; it seems to slow progression in some children who tolerate high brace time use each day.

* Surgical management of neuromuscular scoliosis is a big undertaking, with significant risks, but can significantly enhance patient and family quality of life. Try not to book surgery at the time of the first discussion.

* Preoperative evaluation in this patient population typically involves both cardiac and pulmonary consultation and optimization.

* Preoperative GI consultation (and sometimes even G-tube placement) does not appear to enhance outcomes following spine fusion in these patients.

Knee

* Knee pain is common in CP, up to 21% of ambulatory children presenting to a gait lab.

* Hamstring overlengthening is a significant problem and can result in knee hyperextension and/or a stiff knee in swing.

* Distal rectus femoris transfer should only be considered in GMFCS I and II children.

Foot

* In the management of equinus, the most common source of trouble is overlengthening of the heel cord. A little equinus is much better than any calcaneus, especially in older children.

* Varus feet are not just due to overpull of the posterior tibial tendon. Typically, the anterior tibial tendon is causative in one-third of patients, the posterior tibial tendon in another third, and the combination of both the anterior and posterior tibial tendon in the remaining third.

In-toeing and Out-toeing

* In-toeing and out-toeing result in lever arm dysfunction but only cause functional issues in children with CP due to their difficulties with balance, strength, and coordination.

* When assessing in-toeing or out-toeing, look at both the FPA and the knee progression angle (KPA). If the KPA is abnormal, there is a problem above the knee (trunk, pelvis, and/or hip/femur). If the KPA and FPA are not equal, then there is a problem below the knee (typically tibial and/or foot deformity).

* Common causes of in-toeing include internal pelvic rotation, internal hip rotation, internal tibial torsion, and/or a varus foot.

* Common reasons for out-toeing include external pelvic rotation, external hip rotation, and/or a valgus foot.

SOURCES OF WISDOM

1. Rethlefsen SA, Ryan DD, Kay RM. Classification systems in cerebral palsy. *Orthop Clin North Am.* 2010;41(4):457-467.
2. Alriksson-Schmidt A, Nordmark E, Czuba T, Westbom L. Stability of the Gross Motor Function Classification System in children and adolescents with cerebral palsy: a retrospective cohort registry study. *Dev Med Child Neurol.* 2017;59(6):641-646.
3. Wood E, Rosenbaum P. The gross motor function classification system for cerebral palsy: a study of reliability and stability over time. *Dev Med Child Neurol.* 2000;42(5):292-296.
4. Kay RM. Lower-extremity surgery in children with cerebral palsy. In: Skaggs DL, Kocher MS, eds. *Master Techniques in Orthopaedic Surgery: Pediatrics.* 2nd ed.. Philadelphia, PA: Wolters Kluwer; 2016:149-192.
5. Rethlefsen SA, Blumstein G, Kay RM, Dorey F, Wren TA. Prevalence of specific gait abnormalities in children with cerebral palsy revisited: influence of age, prior surgery, and Gross Motor Function Classification System level. *Dev Med Child Neurol.* 2017;59(1):79-88.
6. Murgai RR, Compton E, Patel AR, et al. Foam padding in postoperative lower extremity casting: an inexpensive way to protect patients. *J Pediatr Orthop.* 2018;38(8):e470-e474.
7. Jain A, Sullivan BT, Shah SA, et al. Caregiver perceptions and health-related quality-of-life changes in cerebral palsy patients after spinal arthrodesis. *Spine.* 2018;43(15):1052-1056.
8. Nielsen E, Andras LM, Bellaire L, et al. Don't you wish you had fused to the pelvis the first time: a comparison of reoperation rate and correction of pelvic obliquity. *Spine.* 2019;44:E465-E469.
9. Soo B, Howard JJ, Boyd RN, et al. Hip displacement in cerebral palsy. *J Bone Joint Surg Am.* 2006;88(1):121-129.
10. Jung NH, Pereira B, Nehring I, et al. Does hip displacement influence health-related quality of life in children with cerebral palsy? *Dev Neurorehabil.* 2014;17(6):420-425.
11. Winters TF Jr, Gage JR, Hicks R. Gait patterns in spastic hemiplegia in children and young adults. *J Bone Joint Surg Am.* 1987;69(3):437-441.
12. Selva G, Miller F, Dabney KW. Anterior hip dislocation in children with cerebral palsy. *J Pediatr Orthop.* 1998;18(1):54-61.
13. Graham HK, Boyd R, Carlin JB, et al. Does botulinum toxin a combined with bracing prevent hip displacement in children with cerebral palsy and "hips at risk"? A randomized, controlled trial. *J Bone Joint Surg Am.* 2008;90(1):23-33.
14. McNerney NP, Mubarak SJ, Wenger DR. One-stage correction of the dysplastic hip in cerebral palsy with the San Diego acetabuloplasty: results and complications in 104 hips. *J Pediatr Orthop.* 2000;20(1):93-103.
15. Huh K, Rethlefsen SA, Wren TA, Kay RM. Surgical management of hip subluxation and dislocation in children with cerebral palsy: isolated VDRO or combined surgery? *J Pediatr Orthop.* 2011;31(8):858-863.
16. Houdek MT, Watts CD, Wyles CC, et al. Total hip arthroplasty in patients with cerebral palsy: a cohort study matched to patients with osteoarthritis. *J Bone Joint Surg Am.* 2017;99(6):488-493.
17. Chan P, Hsu A, Godfrey J, et al. Outcomes of salvage hip surgery in children with cerebral palsy. *J Pediatr Orthop B.* 2019;28(4):314-319.
18. Rodda JM, Graham HK, Carson L, et al. Sagittal gait patterns in spastic diplegia. *J Bone Joint Surg Br.* 2004;86(2):251-258.
19. Novacheck TF, Stout JL, Gage JR, Schwartz MH. Distal femoral extension osteotomy and patellar tendon advancement to treat persistent crouch gait in cerebral palsy: surgical technique. *J Bone Joint Surg Am.* 2009;91(suppl 2):271-286.
20. Ellington MD, Scott AC, Linton J, et al. Rectus femoris transfer versus rectus intramuscular lengthening for the treatment of stiff knee gait in children with cerebral palsy. *J Pediatr Orthop.* 2018;38(4):e213-e218.
21. Kay RM, Rethlefsen SA, Kelly JP, Wren TA. Predictive value of the Duncan-Ely test in distal rectus femoris transfer. *J Pediatr Orthop.* 2004;24(1):59-62.
22. Sousa TC, Nazareth A, Rethlefsen SA, et al. Rectus femoris transfer surgery worsens crouch gait in children with cerebral palsy at GMFCS levels III and IV. *J Pediatr Orthop.* 2019;39:466-471.
23. Rethlefsen SA, Nguyen DT, Wren TA, et al. Knee pain and patellofemoral symptoms in patients with cerebral palsy. *J Pediatr Orthop.* 2015;35(5):519-522.
24. Huh K, Rethlefsen SA, Wren TA, Kay RM. Development of calcaneal gait without prior triceps surae lengthening: an examination of predictive factors. *J Pediatr Orthop.* 2010;30(3):240-243.
25. Borton DC, Walker K, Pirpiris M, et al. Isolated calf lengthening in cerebral palsy: outcome analysis of risk factors. *J Bone Joint Surg Br.* 2001;83(3):364-370.
26. Michlitsch MG, Rethlefsen SA, Kay RM. The contributions of anterior and posterior tibialis dysfunction to varus foot deformity in patients with cerebral palsy. *J Bone Joint Surg Am.* 2006;88(8):1764-1768.
27. Rethlefsen SA, Kay RM. Transverse plane gait problems in children with cerebral palsy. *J Pediatr Orthop.* 2013;33(4):422-430.
28. Rethlefsen SA, Healy BS, Wren TA, et al. Causes of in-toeing gait in children with cerebral palsy. *J Bone Joint Surg Am.* 2006;88(10):2175-2180.

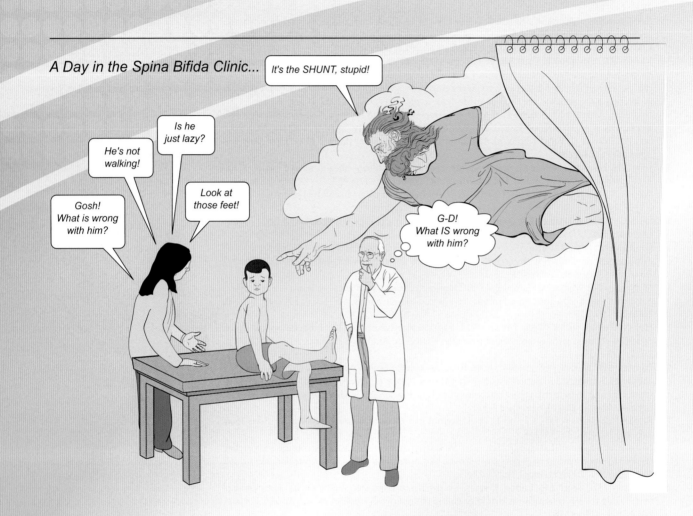

Chapter 17

Other Neuromuscular Conditions and Spina Bifida

KENNETH J. NOONAN, MD, MHCDS

Guru: Robert M. Kay, MD

Tips for Recognizing Neuromuscular Conditions

The array of diagnosable neuromuscular conditions presenting in children is interesting but sometimes intimidating. Most of this information is generally toward the periphery of most orthopaedic surgeons' knowledge. Stay out of trouble by knowing a few common threads in these conditions that can help you identify a child with a potential neuromuscular condition. Also, don't be afraid to ask parents what syndrome their child has and ask them to enlighten you. Parents like doctors who are not know-it-alls but are willing to learn from them.

A common scenario occurs when parents bring a child to an orthopaedic surgeon because the child walks funny, falls down, wants to be carried when walking far, or some other seemingly innocuous complaint. Ninety-nine percent of the time, it is age appropriate, but this chapter may help with the other 1%. Delay in diagnosis can have serious implications. In addition to delaying treatment of the child's condition, it can also result in transmitting the same disease to younger siblings; as an example, before Duchenne muscular dystrophy (DMD) is diagnosed, 20% of families already have conceived a second child. Do not hesitate to examine the parents (subtle cavovarus feet, café au lait spots, etc.) and ask for a family history. Many parents have unrecognized subtle forms of the same disease as their child. This aids in diagnosis of the child.

> ### ▶ Red Flags That a Child May Have a Neuromuscular Disorder
>
> ▶ "Floppiness" as an infant, inability to sit independently
> ▶ Delayed crawling
> ▶ Delayed walking (consider up to 18 months for achievement of independent ambulation "normal"—one must often clarify to the parents that this means the child walks without the child holding on to anything)
> ▶ Complains of tiring easily when walking
> ▶ Tripping or falling if new-onset or worsening gait
> ▶ Difficulty navigating stairs
> ▶ No complaints of pain
> ▶ Hypotonia or hypertonia (though this seems to be overdiagnosed these days)
> ▶ Changing or progressive deformity of feet (Fig. 17-1)
> ▶ Involvement is symmetrical (except for hemiplegia; if asymmetrical, think spine pathology)

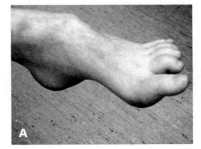 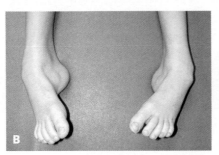 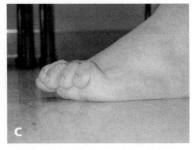

Figure 17-1 A: This child with a cavus foot has an underlying neuromuscular disorder. In children with unilateral foot deformity, consider spinal pathology as more likely; with bilateral foot deformity, consider underlying neuromuscular disease is more common. **B:** A child with bilateral cavovarus feet with Charcot-Marie-Tooth disease. **C:** Claw toes are also an indication of an underlying neuromuscular disease.

General Principles of Treatment

Do not become focused on one body part as many neuromuscular conditions have multiple orthopaedic implications. For example, a child with Charcot-Marie-Tooth (CMT) disease may present to you with a foot deformity, but do not forget there is an increased risk of scoliosis[1] and hip dysplasia.[2,3] This raises an important point even for pediatric orthopaedic surgeons who feel comfortable seeing children with neuromuscular conditions. Each condition has its own unique pitfalls, and it is probably worthwhile to quickly review literature on a child's condition prior to instituting treatment. For example, children with various muscular dystrophies have widely variable prognoses. Know the natural history and expected function of the condition prior to planning surgery as many of these children may never be expected to walk, or even live very long, which may influence whether surgery is indicated. If a muscle biopsy is required, biopsy the weak muscle—i.e., the deltoid, for shoulder girdle weakness.

> **THE GURU SAYS...**
>
> You should check with the pathologist before doing a muscle biopsy to confirm what type of specimen she wants. Placing muscle clamps on the muscle before taking the biopsy, and leaving them in place, is often preferred by pathologists since it allows the muscle to be at its resting length and maintain its structural properties and architecture while it is examined microscopically.
>
> ROBERT KAY

> **THE GURU SAYS...**
>
> As the field of medicine continues to advance rapidly, the natural history of neuromuscular diseases can be dramatically changed by new treatments. Spinal muscular atrophy (SMA) is a recent example of a disease whose prognosis has been dramatically improved by medical advances, which has also changed the orthopaedic treatment paradigm in patients with SMA.
>
> ROBERT KAY

> ### Latex Allergy: Not Just in Spina Bifida
>
> Many children with a variety of neuromuscular disorders (including cerebral palsy) have had multiple exposures to latex (ventriculoperitoneal shunt, catheterization, previous surgeries, etc.) and may be considered at risk for latex allergy and intraoperative anaphylaxis.[4]

> **THE GURU SAYS...**
>
> It's a good idea to always have a latex-free environment in both the office and operating room settings to avoid any potential latex reactions.
>
> ROBERT KAY

Fractures

Children with neuromuscular disease and decreased ambulation are at an increased risk for osteopenic fractures. In an insensate area, fractures are often not appreciated at the time of injury and present late as a swollen, red, and warm limb that is often mistaken for infection by the inexperienced. To make things even more confusing, the child may present with a fever and abnormal laboratory studies. This scenario unfortunately occurs in children who have severe communication challenges (Figs. 17-2 to 17-4).

Fracture care in these children is quite different than in otherwise normal, active children. First, mobilization should begin as early as possible. If a child with progressive weakness and increasing difficulty in walking (e.g., 11-year-old boy with Duchenne muscular dystrophy) is in a long leg cast that prevents walking for 6 weeks, the child may lose so much muscle strength that he *never* walks independently again. You do not want to contribute to that. Second, immobilize for as little a time period as possible. Immobilization leads to localized osteopenia. These children already have some degree of osteopenia to begin with; following immobilization, fractures at other areas in the limb are quite possible. One of the editors (D.L.S.) assumed care of a spina bifida patient who spent 11 months in lower extremity casts for multiple fractures at different locations. Third, these children often have abnormal sensation; soft-tissue problems from cast sores are more likely to occur, and less likely to be recognized, than in the general population.

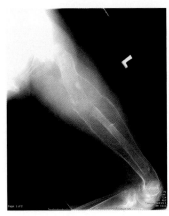

Figure 17-2 Radiograph of a femur of a nonambulator with cerebral palsy who has sustained multiple femur fractures. The clinical and radiographic appearance of this fracture may be confused with infection.

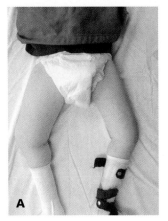 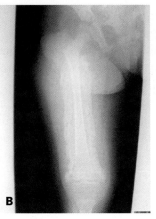 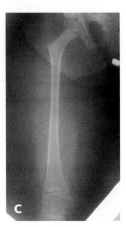

Figure 17-3 A: This boy with thoracic-level spina bifida presented with a chief complaint of (painless) leg swelling. The leg was warm to touch. **B:** Radiographs demonstrate copious new bone formation. **C:** To make matters even more confusing, when children with spina bifida fracture through the growth plate, there may be *no* callus formation. Clinically, this young girl with thoracic-level spina bifida had motion through the Salter I fracture of the distal femur.

We have found less-rigid immobilization is a useful technique for fracture care in nonambulatory children with neuromuscular conditions. This can be accomplished with semirigid fiberglass and/or significant padding, such as polyurethane foam. This decreases osteopenia secondary to immobilization, lessens the chance of a secondary fracture at the edge of a rigid cast, and decreases skin problems from poorly sensate soft tissues rubbing against the edge of a hard cast. The good news in this situation is that there's often rapid and overwhelming callus formation and the child's demands usually do not require anatomic reduction.

Pearls to Help Diagnosis Other Disease-Specific Conditions

- If there is no weight bearing on the upper extremities in the prone position and no head/neck extension by 3 months, think cerebral palsy.
- For new-onset lower extremity weakness and falling, think familial diplegia (also called hereditary spastic paraparesis; HSP).
- In a child with unilateral cavovarus feet, order a spine MRI scan for spinal dysraphism.
- In a child with bilateral cavovarus feet, look at the hands; if there is intrinsic muscle weakness (Fig. 17-5), think hereditary sensory motor neuropathy (CMT). Look at the parent's feet, if they have same foot deformity...bingo.
- If the child shakes your hand, then can't relax the grip, think myotonic dystrophy.
- If the primary complaint is an abnormality in gait, think Friedreich's ataxia.
- Tongue fasciculations = spinal muscular atrophy.
- Dermatomyositis: acute onset of weakness and a malar rash.

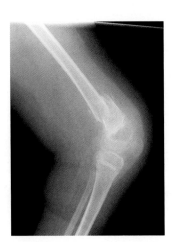

Figure 17-4 Nonambulators with osteopenia frequently have fractures of the distal femoral metaphysis. Have a high index of suspicion when children who were in a hip spica cast for hip surgery present with increasing pain shortly after the spica cast was removed.

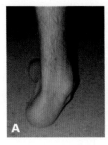 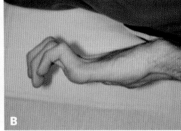

Figure 17-5 This young man with severe Charcot-Marie-Tooth disease has bilateral cavovarus feet (**A**) with clawing of his fingers (**B**). (Used with the permission of the University of Wisconsin Division of Pediatric Orthopaedics.)

THE GURU SAYS...

More tips for diagnosis:

- HSP can be difficult to differentiate from CP. Some potential helpful indicators include normal milestones at an early age, significant progression of the spasticity, lack of any upper extremity involvement, normal cognition, and—at times—other affected family members.
- Most children presenting to the orthopaedist's office with cavus (or cavovarus) foot deformity have one of the hereditary motor sensory neuropathies (HMSNs), most commonly CMT. There can be significant difference in the severity of the deformity in the two feet in CMT.
- Although the great bulk of foot deformities in CMT have a varus component, valgus deformities may also be seen in CMT (particularly in CMT type 2).

ROBERT KAY

Duchenne Muscular Dystrophy

Duchenne is the most common of the muscular dystrophies, and many other types of muscular dystrophy are less severe. The level of creatine phosphokinase (CPK) may be 20 to 200 times normal in children with DMD but can be elevated for patients with other forms of muscular dystrophy as well as many other types of muscle disease. The CPK may be elevated by birth in normal children, but should return to normal quickly. DMD is not that rare, occurring in 1 in 3500 births, so there is a good chance most orthopaedic surgeons will encounter a new patient at some point in their career. While DMD is X-linked and thus occurs only in boys, it can occur in a child with Turner syndrome (XO), and other forms of muscular dystrophies can occur in girls. Rarely, girls can prevent with a DMD phenotype in the setting of the Lyon hypothesis, in which there is inactivation of one of the two X chromosomes. Mental retardation may be present; just because a boy has mental retardation doesn't mean he doesn't have muscular dystrophy. Perhaps the greatest way to stay out of trouble in DMD is to make it a practice to do Gower's test on all 3- to 6-year-old boys with gait abnormalities other than torsion (see Fig. 2-1 in Chapter 2).

THE GURU SAYS...

Dystrophin abnormalities in the brain often lead to cognitive delays and behavioral problems in boys with DMD.

ROBERT KAY

Clues That a 3- to 6-Year-Old Boy May Have Duchenne Muscular Dystrophy

- Normal birth history
- Progressively worsening gait and function, new-onset toe walking
- Ankle equinus
- Waddling gait secondary to weak hip abductors
- Hyperlordosis and anterior pelvic tilt secondary to weak hip extensors
- Hyperextension of knee during standing phase
    - Partially in reaction to ankle equinus
    - Partially to augment weak quadriceps
- Pseudohypertrophy of calves—on palpation a hard, "rubbery" feeling (Fig. 17-6)

THE GURU SAYS...

While pseudohypertrophy of the calves is classic and is seen in the vast majority of children with DMD, 10% to 15% do not have pseudohypertrophy.

ROBERT KAY

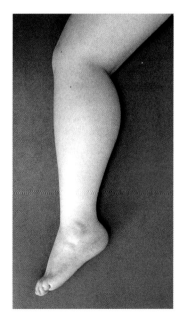

Figure 17-6 Pseudohypertrophy of the calf in the setting of weakness suggests Duchenne muscular dystrophy.

In a 1986 survey in England, the diagnosis of DMD was missed in every case referred to an orthopaedic surgeon (37 patients). Including visits to other specialists, there was a mean delay of diagnosis of 2 years. The authors of the original survey believe this delay has not changed since then and recommend that a serum CPK should be carried out in all boys presenting with nonspecific neuromuscular complaints.[5,6]

TREATMENT

In contrast to the past, there is now something that can be done for these children to prolong strength. Steroids are now routinely used in the treatment of children with DMD. Steroid treatment has been shown to significantly increase muscle strength, performance, and cardiac and pulmonary function, as well as slowing the progression of weakness and the development of scoliosis. Steroids are not tolerated by all patients, and complications include weight gain, change in appearance, behavioral changes, abnormal hair growth, osteoporosis, and the development of cataracts after several years of treatment. Gene therapies (such as eteplirsen) hold promise in the treatment of DMD, though the massive size of the dystrophin gene makes such gene therapy very challenging. Refer children with DMD to a neurologist with experience in the pharmacologic treatment of DMD, preferably one who heads a muscular dystrophy clinic.

Minimize periods of immobility; once children are in a wheelchair for 3 to 6 months, they are unlikely to ever walk again. In general, minimize surgery. For most children, a percutaneous tendo Achilles lengthening (TAL) and possibly a posterior tibial tendon release or transfer is all that is ever needed aside from possible spine surgery. Remember that the inability to dorsiflex the ankle past neutral is actually a good thing as it tends to augment the weakened quadriceps and assist knee extension in stance phase. Thus, do not be too aggressive in treating mild equinus in the ambulatory child, as this may be protective against knee flexion contractures. After a child is nonambulatory, foot surgery is unlikely to improve quality of life and is performed only for comfort.

Scoliosis

Scoliosis usually becomes progressive after cessation of walking. Use of steroids may delay the development and slow the progression of scoliosis.[7] As the disease progressively weakens the cardiac and pulmonary systems with time, stay out of trouble by performing a spinal fusion early, at 20° to 30° of scoliosis, before cardiopulmonary deterioration becomes severe. There is an estimated 4% loss of forced vital capacity (FVC) for every 10° of spinal curvature.[8] Some have suggested that an FVC of 35% is the minimum for safe spinal fusion, though with approval and support from the pulmonologist, cardiologist, and anesthesiologist; children with even worse pulmonary function undergo surgery safely and successfully. Make certain the family understands that although there is a realistic possibility of death, especially in children with small FVCs, the more likely outcome is the child needing a tracheotomy (which means a loss of verbal communication), as well as the possible need for permanent mechanical ventilation. It is also wise to discuss preoperatively with parents and the patient that if there is a loss of spinal cord function during the surgery, it will be wise to leave implants in place to maintain sitting balance. The indications to fuse to the pelvis have been debated. In our experience, and that of others, fuse to the pelvis during the primary surgery.[9] We believe the risk of fusing to the pelvis during primary surgery is much less than extending the fusion down to the pelvis years later following further cardiopulmonary decline.

THE GURU SAYS...

Psychological challenges are common in both boys with DMD and in other family members. Do not hesitate to consider referral to mental health professionals.

ROBERT KAY

THE GURU SAYS...

The early use of ankle-foot orthoses (AFOs) at nighttime can often significantly slow the progression of ankle equinus and obviate the need for heel cord lengthening.

ROBERT KAY

THE GURU SAYS...

The child and his family should be aware that scoliosis is extremely common and that fusion will be needed in most children after they become nonambulatory.

ROBERT KAY

Arthrogryposis

Arthrogryposis simply means "curved joint" and is heralded by stiffness, yet while the term seems rudimentary there over 150 specific disorders which can have features of arthrogryposis. Clinically, the phenotype can vary from mildly stiff fingers (distal arthrogryposis) to total body stiffness; there are common clinical characteristics including a history of deceased intrauterine movement. Children with the most common type, amyoplasia, are generally of normal intelligence or high intelligence (in the author's experience) and the majority will be able to ambulate. The joints (including bones, cartilage, muscle units, ligaments, and skin) have never had the necessary movement in utero for normal development and will never have normal motion. This is important for the surgeon and family to understand. Long-term physical therapy may be of little use and may be psychologically counterproductive when significant effort leads to little if any gains. The goal of treatment is *not* to create normal motion of joints, as this is a setup for failure. The goal is to align the extremities and joints to maximize the ability to stand, ambulate, and sit.

The care of each child with arthrogryposis is *highly* individualized, and the goal is to improve function, not cosmesis. Clubfeet are common in arthrogryposis and should be treated if only to get shoes on those children who will never walk. They should be initially managed with Ponseti manipulation and casting and improvement in foot position can be gained; yet there is a risk of cast sores as these feet are much stiffer. Many feet will need some surgery at a year of age to obtain full correction. Postoperatively the feet need to be braced with an AFO as recurrence is common. Knee contractures can be particularly difficult to manage, and the family and the provider have to determine if the knees should be in a sitting position or a standing position. Treatment options can include benign neglect, guided growth to gain knee extension (Fig. 17-7), distal femoral extension osteotomy in mature patients to gain knee extension, and, in some cases, knee disarticulation and prosthetic fitting have gotten children to walk. **ORTHOPAEDICS 101: When considering periarticular osteotomy or guided growth to improve joint position, remember that the total amount of joint motion will not improve.** The walking of a 16-year-old patient with knee flexion contracture of 35° (and a range from 35° to 85°) could potentially be improved with a distal femoral extension

> **THE GURU SAYS...**
>
> The ongoing involvement of physical and occupational therapists is key for these children and their families. The therapists are instrumental in assuring the child's needs are met, including assistance with obtaining appropriate durable medical equipment (DME) to facilitate activities of daily living (ADLs) and home and community access (including powered mobility).
>
> ROBERT KAY

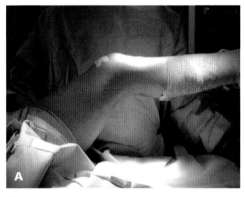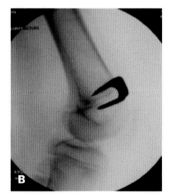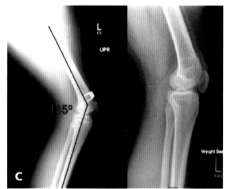

Figure 17-7 Knee flexion contractures can be difficult to treat in arthrogryposis. This child with 40° knee flexion contracture (**A**) underwent anterior hemiepiphysiodesis (**B**). **C:** At maturity, she lacks about 5° of full extension. In the author's opinion, this is a good method for 20° to 30° knee flexion contractures. It's critical that the patient has good knee flexion prior to the procedure. (Used with the permission of the University of Wisconsin Division of Pediatric Orthopaedics.)

osteotomy; yet if they only have 50° of knee motion, they won't be able to flex their knee more than 50° when sitting. This person may be best left alone. Hip contractures (Fig. 17-8) and hip dislocations are common in arthrogryposis, and patients with bilateral dislocations may be best left untreated. Unilateral hip dislocations should be treated if the child is relatively mildly affected in the other joints and who will likely be a good walker.

A newborn with severe flexion contractures of the hips can be helped with physical therapy and soft-tissue releases to get the legs down. Moderate residual hip flexion contractures can be accommodated for in gait by increasing lumbar lordosis or use of a shoe lift for functional leg length discrepancy (LLD). Similar to the knee, proximal femoral extension osteotomy should only be considered if the hip has enough flexion to make sitting possible in the new position. Scoliosis in arthrogryposis may require posterior spine fusion with instrumentation; the commonly cited goal of a level pelvis with fusion to the pelvis may not be appropriate for all patients as limited hip flexion can lead to relatively fixed infrapelvic obliquity that could make sitting difficult if the spine is fused straight to the pelvis. In these cases, some residual scoliosis in the spine below the fusion results in a little extra motion at L5-S1 and L4-L5 may make life easier for the child even if there is some residual deformity. *Scoliosis treatment is about balance, not perfect correction in all cases.*

Spina Bifida

First off, do not be confused by terminology. Spina bifida occulta, a lack of complete formation of the posterior arch (usually of L5 is present in about 10% of the population), is *not* what most orthopaedists would call spina bifida (which by convention has some neurologic involvement) (Fig. 17-9). By definition, spina

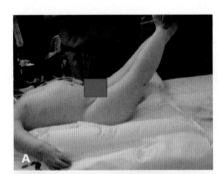
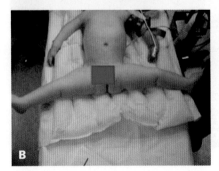
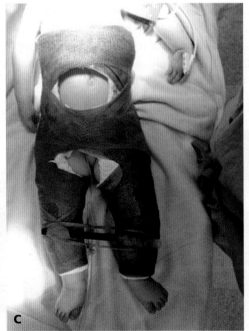
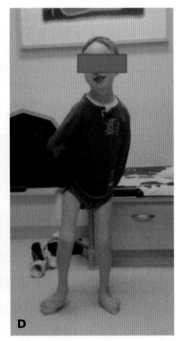

Figure 17-8 A, B: This 11-month-old boy with arthrogryposis had bilateral hip contractures. **C:** To improve his ambulatory potential, he underwent hip flexor release and spica cast in extension and adduction. **D:** He has been able to stand and walk as his childhood progresses. (Used with the permission of the University of Wisconsin Division of Pediatric Orthopaedics.)

bifida occulta is a normal variant, and some have correlated an increased incidence of spondylolisthesis with spina bifida occulta.

In true spina bifida (or myelomeningocele), it is important to remember that although the most obvious abnormality is at the end of the spine—the whole central nervous system (CNS) can be affected with hydrocephalus, Chiari malformation, or syrinx as part of spina bifida.

It's the Shunt, Stupid!!!

Any time a child with spina bifida has a problem without an obvious solution, think, "It's the shunt, stupid!"
- Shunt malfunction leads to hydrocephalus and is quite common. This may happen multiple times during childhood.
- The shunt can be evaluated by CT of brain, cerebrospinal fluid (CSF) pressure, and/or neurosurgical consultation.
- Symptoms may range from subtle behavior changes or difficulty concentrating, to subtle gait changes, to progressive scoliosis, to permanent brain damage.

LEVEL OF INVOLVEMENT

The child's function, and to some extent orthopaedic problems, is largely determined by the level of motor involvement, defined as the lowest level with 4/5 strength or better. The can-can dance can help one determine levels (Fig. 17-10). Document the level of involvement at every clinic visit to help recognize deterioration of function and, if needed, begin a search for the underlying cause such as tethered cord or shunt malfunction.

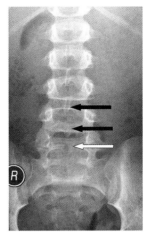

Figure 17-9 Spina bifida occulta. Spinous processes of L3 and L4 are visible (black arrows). An absent spinous process at L5 (white arrow) is consistent with spina bifida occulta in an otherwise-normal child.

THE GURU SAYS...

If there is any question about shunt malfunction, refer to the patient's neurosurgical team for prompt evaluation.

ROBERT KAY

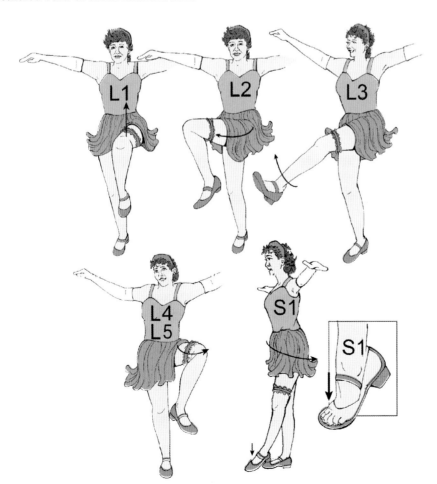

Figure 17-10 Can-can dance: spina bifida levels for everyone. Need 4/5 strength to make the level. These may not be exact, but they are easy to remember, easy to do, and makes it easy to notice when something is changing. *L1*, hip flexion (iliacus, psoas, sartorius); *L2*, hip adduction (hip adductors); *L3*, knee extension (quadriceps); *L4*, knee flexion (medial hamstrings); *L5*, hip abduction (tensor fascia lata, gluteus medius, gluteus minimus); *S1*, hip extension and ankle plantar flexion (gluteus maximus, gastrocnemius, soleus).

AMBULATION

It has been taught that if the medial hamstring muscles are grade 4/5 or better, the child has the potential to stand and do some walking with appropriate orthosis and assistive devices. Walkers are most often L4 (grade 4/5 hamstring) or better, though even many children with low-lumbar and sacral lesions will not be long-term walkers. In one study looking at patients between 10 and 30 years of age, half of those with sacral lesions are not community ambulators.[10]

There is a misconception that the disease is static and the level of function in childhood should be expected in adulthood. While the congenital lesion may not change, deterioration in ambulation can be expected for a variety of factors, including CNS problems (shunting and tethering) and increased obesity outstripping poor muscle strength.

While outcome varies by center and population, Rancho Los Amigos Medical Center reviewed 35 patients with sacral level lesions who were initially community ambulators. At an average age of 29 years, they found a decline in the ability to walk in 11 of 35 patients (31%), and more than 50% had osteomyelitis.[11] Keep out of trouble by sharing with families early on that deterioration in ambulation is an expected part of the disease and not necessarily anyone's fault. Adding to this challenge is the fact that there are few if any multidisciplinary clinics for adults with spina bifida as there are at every children's hospital. Orthopaedic surgeons who practice adult medicine are rarely interested in seeing these patients. Adults are especially at risk for delay in diagnosis and spotty medical care.

Hip and knee contractures are common and best prevented by positioning and range-of-motion exercises. For overall mobility, the importance of weight control cannot be overstressed to parents—*before* it becomes a problem. Up to one-third of children with spina bifida are latex sensitive, thus treat all children with this condition as if they are latex sensitive. There are no definitive tests to prove they are not, and the stakes of anaphylaxis are too high to risk when prevention is so simple.[4]

SPINE

If a spinal deformity is progressing rapidly, it may be secondary to underlying or changing CNS pathology (syrinx, Arnold-Chiari type II, tethered cord, shunt malfunction). Investigate with an MRI of the entire spine and neurosurgical assessment of shunt function. Scoliosis greater than 45° is very uncommon in L5 and sacral level patients, and, if present, is usually due to underlying CNS pathology (see Fig. 17-8). Beware that congenital scoliosis is also frequently present; go with traditional treatment such as early fusion of a unilateral bar opposite a hemivertebrae, as applicable.

When a severe lumbar kyphosis, or gibbus is present, the aorta and vena cava are too short to allow full correction of the deformity, thus vertebral bodies are removed to shorten the spine. There are anecdotes of acute vascular insufficiency leading to loss of legs following an overly aggressive correction. Consider an arterial line with blood pressure monitoring in the lower extremities or pulse oximetry when planning significant corrections of a sharp kyphosis.

A "tethered cord" is almost universally present on MRI in children with spina bifida. One should only consider surgical release of a tethered cord in the setting of signs and symptoms (new-onset lumbar, sacral or buttock pain, lower extremity

---

THE GURU SAYS...

As in many neuromuscular conditions, deterioration in adolescence is common due to an unfavorable change in the adolescent's strength-to-weight ratio.

ROBERT KAY

loss of function, or spasticity) or in accordance with surgical scoliosis correction that will significantly lengthen the spine. Beneficial effects of surgical release of a tethered cord are often underwhelming. Detethering has variable outcomes and can lead to neurologic worsening in many areas.[12]

Staying Out of Trouble During Spine Surgery With Myelomeningocele

* Make sure to consult other specialties prior to surgery.

* Consider having a plastic surgeon see the patient preoperatively to plan flaps and to help close—the tissue is almost always compromised from the original spinal closure.

* Assess shunt function preoperatively as per your neurosurgeon's routine. If the shunt is not functioning and CNS drainage through the spine is abruptly stopped intraoperatively, the child can die within minutes.

* Prior to spine surgery, consider urology consultation for the Malone antegrade colonic enema (MACE) procedure to help manage bowel continence by creating a stoma into the large intestine. Fusing in a position of excessive lordosis may make it impossible for females to self-catheterize.

* These children are likely to need spine imaging in the future (MRI); titanium instrumentation may be preferable.

* Pedicle screws are often essential when laminae are absent, but beware that the pedicle anatomy may be quite distorted. Pedicles may be facing almost straight lateral.

* Pelvic obliquity may lead to decubitus ulcers over an insensate pelvis—correct this aggressively.

* If the soft tissue appears to be too damaged to cover any instrumentation, spinal rods can be placed directly into vertebral bodies in cases of kyphosis (Fig. 17-11).

* Prevent incontinence from wound soiling. Ioban dressing with benzoin applied in the OR between the incision and anus is helpful (Fig. 17-12).

HIPS

Dislocated hips do not influence walking ability. A comprehensive study of ambulatory children with L3- and L4-level spina bifida who underwent surgical hip reduction found that benefits were marginal at best, and patients with failed operations had worse function than those who were not operated on.[13] A frequent and unfortunate outcome of attempts to reduce a dislocated hip in spina bifida is a stiff hip, which may interfere with positioning and transfers. In our experience, we tend to leave bilaterally dislocated hips alone. A unilateral dislocated hip could be considered for reduction if the patient has L5 level or sacral level of function.

KNEES

Stay out of trouble by telling the parents to expect knee (and hip) contractures to develop over time. Physical therapy and sleeping in a well-fitting knee orthosis

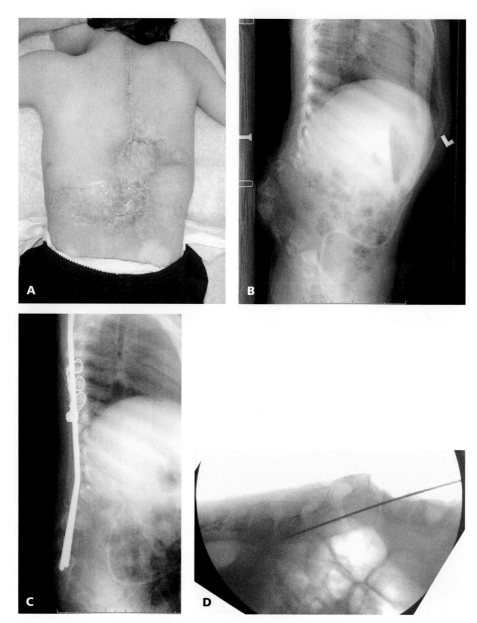

Figure 17-11 A: Child with thoracic-level spina bifida with skin graft directly adherent to bone over the progressive kyphotic gibbus with frequent ulceration. Plastic surgical consultation concluded that there were no means of providing soft-tissue coverage for traditional posterior spinal instrumentation. **B:** Preoperative lateral supine radiograph demonstrates rigid nature of kyphosis. **C:** Surgery was performed with no incision distal to L3, by placing the rods directly into the vertebral bodies of L-4-S1. **D:** Intraoperative imaging with preliminary Kirschner wires assists in correct placement of rods.

may help. A straight off-the-shelf knee immobilizer may lead to sores in a child with a knee flexion contracture. As many children with spina bifida have weak quadriceps to begin with, the addition of knee flexion contractures makes walking even more difficult. The use of ground reaction AFOs helps prevent knee flexion contractures, as well as help compensate for quadriceps weakness. Patients with fixed knee flexion contractures may actually have difficulty walking with ground reaction AFOs if the orthosis does not accommodate the deformity. If the knee

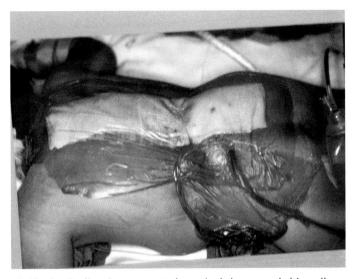

Figure 17-12 Placing iodine-impregnated surgical drape and skin adherent between the perineum and wound helps keep the wound from becoming soiled. Children with spina bifida have a much higher incidence of gram-negative and mixed floral infections, possibly due to wound contamination from incontinence.

lacks 20° of extension, the AFOs may need to have 10° to 20° of dorsiflexion. Children with absent or very weak quadriceps strength may benefit from knee-ankle-foot orthoses (KAFOs) to assist in standing, transfers, and ambulation. This is one of the few remaining indications for bracing above the knee in contemporary pediatric orthopaedics.

FEET

Stay out of trouble by remembering that the goal of orthopaedic care in spina bifida feet is a braceable, supple, plantigrade foot. Fusions are generally contraindicated, as a stiff, insensate foot is a setup for ulcers. Foot sores must be dealt with quickly and aggressively, often starting with total contact casting. An infected ulcer in a child with spina bifida can lead to osteomyelitis and amputation if not cared for appropriately. Educate parents to inspect feet every day and to seek medical care at the first signs of more than transient redness or ulcers. Adjustment of a pressure spot on an orthosis may prevent a frank ulcer when redness is identified early.

All children with clubfeet can be helped with Ponseti casting. Although complete correction is uncommon, moderate correction can help stretch out the soft tissues and make closure from surgery easier (Fig. 17-13). When performing clubfoot surgery, resect 1 to 2 cm of all tendons to help minimize recurrence and minimize future surgeries. Although this sounds extreme, a flexible, braceable foot is far superior to a rigid deformed foot prone to ulcers. Even in children with thoracic level involvement, in which the muscles to the foot are not normally innervated, the muscle tendon units can act as deforming forces.

THE GURU SAYS...

External tibial torsion may have significant negative effects on the knee. Not only does external tibial torsion result in lever arm dysfunction (and exacerbate the child's tendency to crouch), but it also introduces a valgus moment at the knee and may lead to meniscal damage.
ROBERT KAY

THE GURU SAYS...

Ironically, the highest functioning walkers (sacral-level spina bifida) have the greatest frequency of severe foot ulcers due to long distance walking on insensate feet.
ROBERT KAY

THE GURU SAYS...

Be aware of the development of ankle valgus over time in children with spina bifida. This deformity is not present at birth but often develops as the children grow and can contribute to bracewear problems and pressure sores.
ROBERT KAY

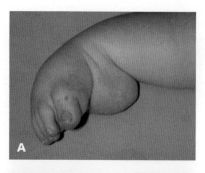

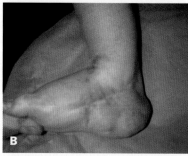

Figure 17-13 This child with spina bifida had severe bilateral clubfeet (**A**) and underwent 2 months of Ponseti casting prior to posterior medial release (**B**). The family was told she will require AFOs throughout her childhood to prevent recurrence. (Used with the permission of the University of Wisconsin Division of Pediatric Orthopaedics.)

Staying Out of Trouble With Other Neuromuscular Conditions and Spina Bifida

* Do a Gower's test on a young boy who seems to tire easily, falls, or is "doing worse."

* Think of the possibility of neuromuscular disease when parents report that falling or tiring when walking is worsening.

* Treat all children with spina bifida as if they are latex allergic.

* For almost any problem in spina bifida that does not have an obvious cause, your first thought should be "It's the *shunt*, stupid!"

SOURCES OF WISDOM

1. Walker JL, Nelson KR, Stevens DB, et al. Spinal deformity in Charcot-Marie-Tooth disease. *Spine*. 1994;19(9):1044-1047.
2. Kumar SJ, Marks HG, Bowen JR, et al. Hip dysplasia associated with Charcot-Marie-Tooth disease in the older child and adolescent. *J Pediatr Orthop*. 1985;5(5):511-514.
3. Pailthorpe CA, Benson MK. Hip dysplasia in hereditary motor and sensory neuropathies. *J Bone Joint Surg Br*. 1992;74(4):538-540.
4. Dormans JP, Templeton JJ, Edmonds C, et al. Intraoperative anaphylaxis due to exposure to latex (natural rubber) in children. *J Bone Joint Surg Am*. 1994;76(11):1688-1691.
5. Read L, Galasko CS. Delay in diagnosing Duchenne muscular dystrophy in orthopaedic clinics. *J Bone Joint Surg Br*. 1986;68(3):481-482.
6. Marshall PD, Galasko CS. No improvement in delay in diagnosis of Duchenne muscular dystrophy. *Lancet*. 1995;345(8949):590-591.
7. Alman BA, Raza SN, Biggar WD. Steroid treatment and the development of scoliosis in males with Duchenne muscular dystrophy. *J Bone Joint Surg Am*. 2004;86(3):519-524.
8. Kurz LT, Mubarak SJ, Schultz P, et al. Correlation of scoliosis and pulmonary function in Duchenne muscular dystrophy. *J Pediatr Orthop*. 1983;3(3):347-353.
9. Alman BA, Kim HK. Pelvic obliquity after fusion of the spine in Duchenne muscular dystrophy. *J Bone Joint Surg Br*. 1999;81(5):821-824.

10. De Souza LJ, Carroll N. Ambulation of the braced myelomeningocele patient. *J Bone Joint Surg Am*. 1976;58(8):1112-1118.

11. Brinker MR, Rosenfeld SR, Feiwell E, et al. Myelomeningocele at the sacral level. Long-term outcomes in adults. *J Bone Joint Surg Am*. 1994;76(9):1293-1300.

12. Cochrane DD, Rassekh SR, Thiessen PN. Functional deterioration following placode untethering in myelomeningocele. *Pediatr Neurosurg*. 1998;28(2):57-62.

13. Alman BA, Bhandari M, Wright JG. Function of dislocated hips in children with lower level spina bifida. *J Bone Joint Surg Br*. 1996;78(2):294-298.

FOR FURTHER ENLIGHTENMENT

Sarwak JF, Lubicky JP, eds. *Caring for the Child with Spina Bifida*. Rosemont, IL: American Academy of Orthopaedic Surgeons; 2004.

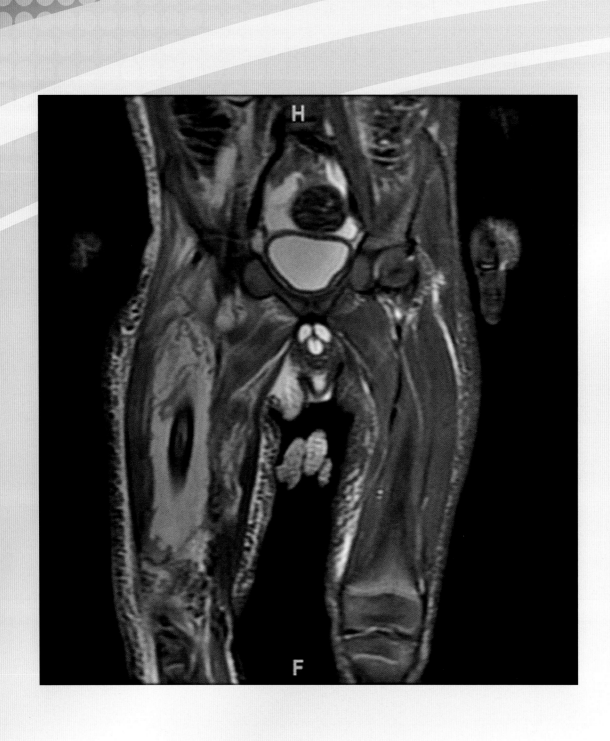

Chapter 18

Orthopaedic Infections

MICHAEL G. VITALE, MD, MPH

Gurus: Jonathan Schoenecker, MD, PhD and
Alexandre Arkader, MD

General Considerations

Osteomyelitis, pyomyositis, and septic arthritis were huge sources of trouble for our orthopaedic ancestors—and their patients. Today, with vastly superior imaging and antibiotics, most orthopaedic infections can be located, identified, and treated in a timely fashion with rare residual sequelae. To stay out of trouble, it is important to recognize several trends over the last couple of decades. Pyomyositis is now the most common musculoskeletal infection, although pyomyositis, osteomyelitis, and septic arthritis occur more commonly together than alone. Bacteria have developed virulence factors and resistance, and we must be vigilant for signs that what seems like a localized musculoskeletal infection is about to "metastasize" and become a life-threatening systemic multiorgan disease (Fig. 18-1). We know a lot more about the acute-phase response (APR) to infection which usually functions efficiently to control infection and allow repair (Fig. 18-2) but can sometimes be "hijacked" by bacterial mechanisms resulting in tissue damage, out-of-control spread of infection and even death (Fig. 18-3).

It is much more likely that the orthopaedist will see a child very early after the start of a bone or joint infection. This can make diagnosis very difficult, because inflammatory markers such as C-reactive protein (CRP) or erythrocyte sedimentation rate (ESR) may initially be normal or only slightly elevated. Inflammatory markers are not the only tests that may be normal initially. An aspiration may not yield any pus early after infection, and radiographs may well be normal also. Repeat the labs if there is any question as the trend can tell a lot about the severity or disease and prognosis (Fig. 18-4).

At the same time, in the modern era, while cases of isolated infections do occur, infections that lead to death or disability are metastatic, involving multiple tissues (e.g., bone, muscle, and joint) with systemic spreading (e.g., lung). Opposed to single isolated infections, the acute phase response to multifocal infections is more exuberant, correlating with the amount of tissue infected and the duration of the infection leading to morbidity and mortality from systemic inflammatory response syndrome and thrombosis. While some have previously argued that knee-jerk

> **THE GURU SAYS...**
>
> Pyomyositis can affect multiple muscle groups, and most frequently affects the musculature of the hip. In recent years, pyomyositis has been reported with greater frequency in large part due to the increased use of MRI in cases of pediatric musculoskeletal infection. A prospective study found that in children consulted for an acutely irritable hip, cases of pyomyositis outnumbered cases of septic arthritis at a rate of 2:1. As such, proper identification of pyomyositis (rather than septic arthritis) allows patients to be treated without the need for joint debridement.
>
> JONATHAN SCHOENECKER

> **THE GURU SAYS...**
>
> Musculoskeletal tissue injury evokes a cascade of carefully regulated pathways that are collectively known as the APR. The two principle roles of the APR are survival and tissue repair. Although most bacteria are trapped and killed by the APR, certain bacteria have developed mechanisms to "hijack" and utilize the APR to their advantage to support dissemination and evade the host immune response. As a result, these bacteria flock to injured tissue and the regulated and coordinated nature of the APR is lost, leading to potentially fatal systemic inflammatory response syndrome and thrombosis.
>
> JONATHAN SCHOENECKER

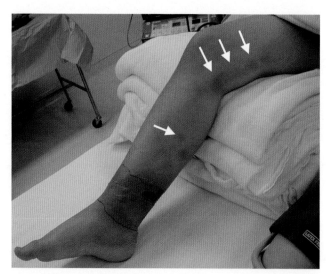

Figure 18-1 At the initial consultation for "cellulitis," the area of erythema was marked with a pen so any spreading could be noted. Hours later, rapidly ascending erythema, along with fever and high C-reactive protein, was highly suggestive of necrotizing fasciitis, which is a surgical emergency. (Used with permission of the Children's Orthopaedic Center, Los Angeles.)

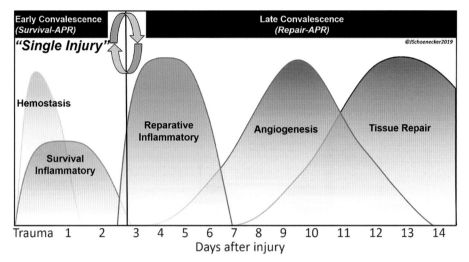

Figure 18-2 The acute-phase response (APR). The body's response to infection or any other injury includes the acute-phase response, which has two phases. The first is survival, which utilizes coagulation and inflammation to achieve hemostasis and prevents or eliminates infection. The second phase, recovery, attempts to recreate functional anatomy by eliminating scar and abscess tissue. It includes angiogenesis to revascularize structures and repair of damaged tissues. (With permission of Jonathan Schoenecker, MD.)

antibiotic administration may blunt the initial picture, current thinking is that early antibiotic administration rarely affects culture results. Holding antibiotics to wait for a culture result can lead to progression of the infection and complications.

As a general rule, be sure to get a medical specialist to help in the management of infants and younger children and in those who show any signs of systemic toxicity.

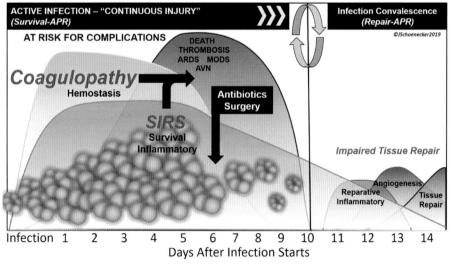

Figure 18-3 Acute-phase response (APR) to infection. In infection as in other injuries, the acute-phase response is critical but can also lead to complications. Excessive coagulation and inflammatory response can lead to thrombotic complications, organ failure, AVN, and even death. Inadequate acute-phase response will not eliminate the infectious threat to survival. An overexuberant acute-phase response can lead to significant tissue damage and even death. Some bacteria have mechanisms to hijack the normal acute-phase response. Antibiotics and surgery are often necessary to end the injury and help the body fight infection and enable convalescence and repair. ARDS, acute respiratory distress syndrome; AVN, avascular necrosis; MODS, multiple organ dysfunction syndrome; SIRS, systemic inflammatory response syndrome. (With permission of Jonathan Schoenecker, MD.)

THE GURU SAYS...

Trauma often precedes infection, making diagnosis of new-onset pain difficult. When trauma leads to acute hematogenous osteomyelitis (AHO), pain worsens over time. If there is any question, have the patient come back in 24 to 48 hours for a repeat examination and repeat labs. Statistically, the differential diagnosis of a limping child includes, in order from most to least common, trauma, infection, and neoplasm. Sometimes unwitnessed trauma may mimic the usual signs and symptoms of an infectious process. Adding labs and imaging is the next step in diagnosis.

ALEXANDRE ARKADER

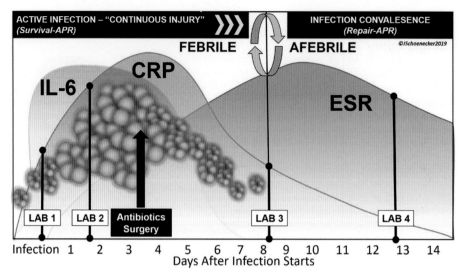

Figure 18-4 Acute-phase response (APR) markers and infection. Levels of acute-phase reactants change dramatically and predictably following the onset of infection and tissue injury. While IL-6 and procalcitonin peak earliest, C-reactive protein (CRP) is the most useful widely used marker. The extent and duration of an acute-phase response is dependent upon the severity of a tissue injury. CRP can rapidly spike to values greater than 100, indicating risk for overwhelming systemic infection and warranting aggressive emergent treatment. CRP drops more rapidly than erythrocyte sedimentation rate (ESR) heralding the entrance into the reparative phase of healing. IL, interleukin. (With permission of Jonathan Schoenecker, MD.)

Osteomyelitis

On first presentation of a child with osteomyelitis, there is often a trauma history. This may lead the orthopaedist down the path of looking for occult fractures, sprains, etc., delaying diagnosis. To stay out of trouble, recognize that if it is an injury, with each passing day, the area looks and feels better; in an infection, with each passing day, it looks and feels worse.

Be aware that children with neuromuscular conditions, especially spina bifida but also cerebral palsy and others, can present with a fracture and have a picture that mimics infection.

Although pain is a key feature, children may not complain of pain. Instead, they may limp or not walk or not move the body part. Don't forget about referred pain: pain from the back and the psoas area can refer to the hip, and pain that originates in the hip can refer to the distal thigh or knee region. Be sure to get a history of recent infections. A particularly important example is chicken pox: the virus lowers immunity and the skin lesions can be infected. In these cases, the bacterial pathogen is usually *Streptococcus* but can be *Staphylococcus*.[1]

To stay out of trouble, be alert to how unbelievably unreliable WBCs can be as a marker of infection.[2] WBC is often normal, although a left shift may be a clue that there is an infection. It is also essential to keep in mind that leukemia may be in the differential diagnosis. If this is a possibility, you will want your primary care doctors or infection consultants to look at a manual differential/smear to rule out leukemia. ESR rises slowly and is unreliable in the early presentation of bone and joint infections. It is also unreliable in the neonate or children with sickle cell disease. CRP can rise after trauma, giving you a false-positive result. It is also usually elevated in otitis media and other childhood infections, so like other markers, specificity is poor.

> **THE GURU SAYS...**
>
> Measures of inflammation such as CRP are useful in the early diagnosis of infection (within 4-6 hours), such that higher CRP levels are associated with increasing disease severity and more severe outcomes, including a longer length of stay in the hospital. If a treatment is effective, the CRP and other acute-phase reactants should begin to return to normal levels, with an expected spike associated with any surgical intervention. If values are not returning to normal, this indicates that further intervention is likely necessary.
>
> JONATHAN SCHOENECKER

Blood cultures are good, but the best way to isolate an organism is by aspirating the suspected site of osteomyelitis. When aspirating a potential site of osteomyelitis, do it under conscious sedation with careful localization. A common mistake in aspirating osteomyelitis is to be in the diaphyseal region, too far from the physis. One clue is that if it is hard to penetrate the bone, you are probably in the diaphysis. Use a C-arm if necessary. Localizing the point of maximum tenderness can be very valuable. Most osteomyelitis is in the metaphysis very near the physis. Interventional radiology can be helpful to localize a collection and obtain cultures but is not truly therapeutic with regard to decompressing and sterilizing a larger collection. If there is a large subperiosteal collection, it's usually better to do an operative irrigation and debridement.

Although imaging is often essential in managing pediatric orthopaedic infections, radiographs can fool you by lagging behind the actual clinical activity. You may encounter imaging that is normal after the disease has started or imaging that looks worse despite rapid clinical resolution (Fig. 18-5). It is well

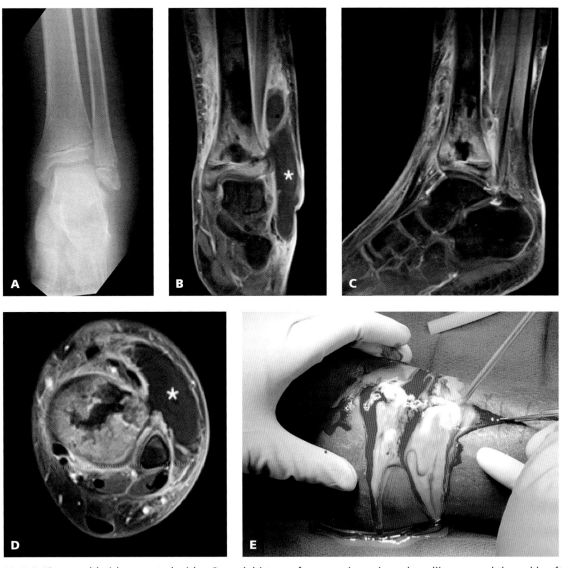

Figure 18-5 A 12-year-old girl presented with a 3-week history of progressive pain and swelling around the ankle after a minor trauma. She was overall healthy, with no constitutional symptoms except for report of a low-grade fever. **A:** AP radiograph of the ankle did not demonstrate any obvious bone involvement but showed some minor swelling in the lateral aspect of the ankle. **B–D:** MRI T1 images demonstrated significant tibia and fibula marrow changes, extension into the epiphysis, cortical disruption, and a very large abscess around the anterior lateral aspect of the ankle (*). **E:** Intraoperative image shows a large purulent abscess being evacuated right after skin incision is made. (Used with permission from CHOP Orthopedics, Philadelphia, PA.)

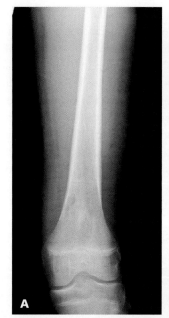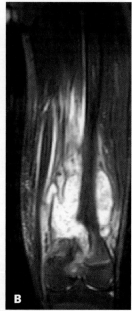

Figure 18-6 This 13-year-old boy presented for a consultation for limb-sparing surgery because the initial treating orthopaedist thought he had an osteosarcoma based on the plain radiographs (**A**) and MRI (**B**). Fortunately, Gram stain and culture were performed at the time of biopsy. Intraoperative culture grew methicillin-resistant *Staphylococcus aureus* (MRSA). The lesson: Culture every biopsy, and biopsy every infection. (Courtesy of J. Dormans, MD.)

> **THE GURU SAYS...**
>
> Chondroblastoma can resemble subacute osteomyelitis. They both present as a well-defined eccentric lytic lesion within the epiphysis adjacent to an open growth plate. Chondroblastoma may have a sharp sclerotic margin and intralesional calcifications, neither seen in osteomyelitis. MRI demonstrates significant edema surrounding the lesion, while osteomyelitis tends to have little or no edema.
>
> ALEXANDRE ARKADER

> **THE GURU SAYS...**
>
> By definition, acute osteomyelitis is a clinically managed disease—that is, usually successfully treated with antibiotics. The indications for surgical intervention include large subperiosteal abscess, joint involvement, or lack of clinical improvement with appropriate antibiotics.
>
> ALEXANDRE ARKADER

known that changes in the bone take more than a week to show up on plain radiographs after the start of AHO. To stay out of trouble, look for soft-tissue swelling as an early radiographic sign. For comparison, position both limbs symmetrically and ask for a soft tissue technique. Bone scan with pinhole views have been used in the past but have been largely replaced by MRI (Fig. 18-6). MRI can be incredibly helpful for localizing disease especially in contiguous areas.

In addition to diagnosis, the treatment of AHO can be a significant source of trouble. In the past, while IV antibiotics were generally used until inflammatory markers settle, most centers are finding oral antibiotics to be equally effective and there has been a trend for less IV antibiotic use. Today, most hospitals that would admit a child with AHO have infectious disease specialists on staff. Ask these experts, or the child's primary care doctor, to help you define the best antibiotic and antibiotic course. Remember that some antibiotics can cause side effects, such as neutropenia and kidney and liver toxicity. You or one of the primary doctors should be following a WBC.

The indications for irrigation and debridement of a potential site of osteomyelitis are not absolute though signs of systemic inflammatory syndrome or thrombosis would warrant emergent surgical treatment. Many orthopaedists use the failure to show clinical improvement after 24 to 36 hours of antibiotics as the main reason to do an irrigation and debridement. Others recommend doing an irrigation and debridement if the CRP is rising, if a significant volume of pus is aspirated, or if there are disruptive changes on radiographs. Extended follow-up may be warranted for young children with osteomyelitis. Because the infection in infants and young children occurs so close to the growth plate, there is a risk for growth arrest, and these kids should be followed for 6 to 12 months after resolution of symptoms with radiographs.

Conditions That Mimic Infection

- Leukemia: Remember that 15% of children with leukemia present with musculoskeletal complaints. Metastatic neuroblastoma is age related and often has multiple sites of involvement
- Metastatic neuroblastoma
- Langerhans cell histiocytosis
- Ewing sarcoma
- Sickle cell disease
- Infarct
- Gaucher disease

Septic Arthritis

Septic arthritis is a major source of trouble, especially in the hip, where it is a surgical emergency. Surgical irrigation and debridement is also recommended for most other joints, although there is some literature to support the efficacy of repeat aspirations and antibiotics for joints other than the hip.

To stay out of trouble, keep the differential diagnosis of a swollen joint in your head. You should consider Lyme arthritis in endemic areas as well as various rheumatologic conditions. The experienced examiner will note that in both Lyme arthritis and nonbacterial arthritis, there may be a large effusion but no significant short arc tenderness.[3] Juvenile rheumatoid arthritis (JRA) can appear suddenly and mimic septic arthritis. Some children with JRA or Lyme arthritis will have a synovial WBC greater than 100,000. Keep gonococcal arthritis in your differential. You won't see gonococcal arthritis exclusively in sexually active teens; sadly, you may encounter the infection in a younger child who has been sexually abused. As the organism responsible for gonococcal arthritis is notoriously difficult to grow in culture, be sure to obtain proper cultures for the differential diagnosis.

With imaging, there are several sources of trouble in septic arthritis. Widening of a hip joint space is a very unreliable sign of septic arthritis of the hip (Fig. 18-9). Such widening may be affected by positioning and is more common in infants. If you do see a true widened hip joint space, it means that there is substantial pressure on the joint. This is not usually present early in the process. Also keep in mind that ultrasonography itself cannot absolutely distinguish transient synovitis, pyomyositis from septic arthritis of the hip.[5] If a patient with a septic joint has had over 4 days of pain, there is a high chance of contiguous osteomyelitis, so an MRI of the area should be considered prior to surgery, but only if the patient is not in danger of being septic and the MRI can be performed in an urgent fashion.

In terms of treatment, stay on top of the changing bacterial pathogens responsible for septic arthritis in children. H flu is now nearly eliminated as a common pathogen, but the incidence of positive *Kingella kingae* cultures is rising.[6] It may be that *Kingella* has been present for a long time but is so difficult to isolate by culture that we are just isolating it more frequently now. To culture *Kingella*, use a blood culture bottle to help with your bacterial isolation.[7]

Special Scenarios

TRANSIENT SYNOVITIS VERSUS SEPTIC ARTHRITIS

Transient synovitis is the most common cause of hip pain in school-age children, while septic arthritis of the hip is a rare but potentially crippling disaster if unrecognized. Rapidly telling the difference between transient synovitis and septic arthritis is an essential skill to stay out of trouble in pediatric orthopaedics.[8] In septic arthritis, children are usually sick with a fever and are getting worse by the hour. In septic arthritis, they usually won't bear weight on the affected hip. You will usually find pain with simple log rolling of the hip. The CRP may be elevated, but the ESR may not, in the first 24 hours after the infection.[9]

You should aspirate any suspicious hip, and do an irrigation and debridement on any hip with bacteria or elevated WBC on Gram stain in the aspiration fluid. Remember a negative Gram stain does not mean that the patient doesn't have a septic hip, and we must follow the clinical picture and markers carefully and closely to stay out of trouble.

Make irrigation and debridement of the septic hip one of your most important pediatric orthopaedic emergencies. The timeliness of treatment is just as important as compartment syndrome and probably more important than a rapid irrigation and debridement of an open fracture.

Be alert to the many conditions that can mimic classic pediatric hip septic arthritis[10] (Fig. 18-7). Osteomyelitis of the pelvis and septic arthritis of the sacroiliac (SI) joint certainly fall into this category. Such patients are usually older children and teens, whereas septic arthritis of the hip is usually seen in younger children. Pelvic osteomyelitis usually has protean manifestations much like spinal infections. The flexion abduction external rotation test (FABER) can be very helpful to stress the SI joint and localize the problem to this area. Palpation over the SI joint or compression of the iliac wings can also be provocative for pain in the SI region. SI joint infection can usually be treated with antibiotics alone. An abscess of any of the muscles around the hip can also present looking just like septic arthritis of the hip.[11] Depending on the duration and how extensive, these hips are

> ### THE GURU SAYS...
>
> Toxic synovitis usually presents with lower CRP, so if there is a suspicion for septic arthritis and CRP is elevated, infection is more likely. One exception is neonates, who tend not to develop elevated inflammatory markers.
>
> ALEXANDRE ARKADER

> ### THE GURU SAYS...
>
> Despite multiple recent studies indicating that pre-treatment with antibiotics does not change the yield of local tissue aspiration, conventional treatment has been to hold antibiotics prior to aspiration. Importantly, I recommend that, no matter what, antibiotics should not be held to obtain cultures if the child is experiencing an exuberant APR that puts them at risk for morbidity and mortality (CRP > 150 mg/L and platelets < 200).
>
> JONATHAN SCHOENECKER

> ### *Intra-Articular Metaphysis*
>
> In these joints, osteomyelitis can break directly into the joint:
> - Hip
> - Proximal humerus
> - Proximal radius
> - Distal lateral tibia

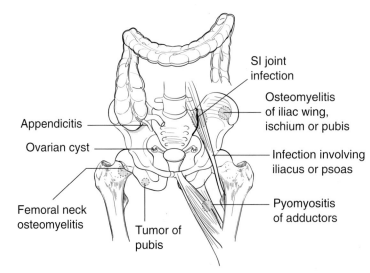

Figure 18-7 The various conditions that can mimic classic pediatric hip septic arthritis. SI, sacroiliac.

usually not so painful with general rotation at 90° but are worse with extension. After the pus has been dissected around the hip capsule, these children present much more like classic septic arthritis of the hips. Sometimes you can find tenderness over the brim of the pelvis. A quick way to distinguish psoas abscess from a septic hip is an ultrasound, which can often detect swelling of the psoas. An MRI may be also helpful to distinguish these two conditions.[12] Also, don't forget non-orthopaedic conditions like appendicitis, gynecologic conditions, or even hernias that can mimic some of the signs and symptoms of hip joint septic arthritis.

The hallmark of differentiating rheumatoid arthritis (RA) from septic arthritis is noting that, in RA, there is a joint effusion that is out of proportion to the symptoms. The patients can usually range their knee to 90° of flexion and remain ambulatory. The experienced examiner will detect a different feel to the synovial thickening in JRA as opposed to septic arthritis.

Once you have determined that the child has septic arthritis and not transient synovitis, it is important to adhere to certain surgical principles and techniques to stay out of trouble. Septic hips in young children are most often drained anteriorly to avoid disrupting the posterior blood supply to the femoral epiphysis. It is critical to do a definitive capsulotomy. Be sure that the joint is aggressively irrigated and that there is no purulent collection left behind. Some have recommended decompression of the femoral neck if there is associated osteomyelitis that has not decompressed itself into the joint. Most surgeons place a drain around the femoral neck, secure the drain carefully, and rest the child in bed for at least a day or so to keep the drain in and to allow the hip to quiet down.

For most cases of septic arthritis of the hip, our infectious disease colleagues recommend 4 weeks of antibiotics, following the clinical course and CRP closely.[13] Beware when the CRP does not rapidly normalize in the first week after surgery! You must ask yourself whether there is another collection of fluid, whether the fluid reaccumulated, or if you have the right diagnosis. Is it possible that you may have missed osteomyelitis of the femoral neck (Fig. 18-8)? In this clinical scenario, it is best to get an MRI to determine why the child has not had the expected clinical improvement. Finally, follow these children for a couple of years afterward to be certain that there is not AVN or any proximal femoral growth disturbance (Fig. 18-9).

THE GURU SAYS...

One current controversy in the treatment of hip infections is the need for drilling proximal femur osteomyelitis. Due to concern for avascular necrosis (AVN), traditional teaching has been that drilling of proximal femoral osteomyelitis is necessary to relieve pressure and reduce bacterial burden. However, animal studies have suggested that drilling of osteomyelitis and curettage may only cause damage to the bone, destroying intramedullary blood supply and serving to more widely inoculate the area with bacteria. Additionally, drilling of the femoral neck and proximal femur further weakens the bone, which is already at risk for fracture due to infection. Furthermore, improvement in antibiotics likely obviates the need for bony debridement, and antibiotic administration does not reduce culture yields even if debridement is felt to be necessary in the future. For these reasons, I no longer drill all proximal femoral osteomyelitis.

JONATHAN SCHOENECKER

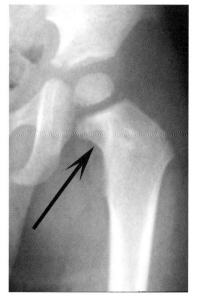

Figure 18-8 An associated femoral neck osteomyelitis, as shown in this AP hip radiograph (arrow), delays improvement after an irrigation and debridement of the hip.

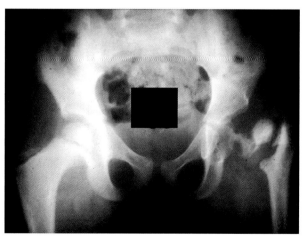

Figure 18-9 The disastrous consequences of missing a septic arthritis of the hip.

DISCITIS AND SPINAL OSTEOMYELITIS

Discitis and spinal osteomyelitis is really an infection, although the older literature called it inflammation and questioned the role for antibiotics. The infection is believed to start in the bone adjacent to the vertebral end plate. It often takes longer to present and diagnose than other pediatric musculoskeletal infections, so CRP and sedimentation rate are often quite high. Cultures, obtained rarely, are usually negative. To stay out of trouble, recognize that many children with such spinal infections will not have back pain. Younger children may refuse to walk or just present with lethargy. There may also be abdominal pain in the school-age child, although teenagers typically have true low-back pain. Children with these spinal infections often won't complain of back pain, but it can usually be elicited on examination. Classically, the children will walk bent over with their hands on their thighs in the worse cases. Knowing all the presentations is important so that the doctor recognizes them as signs of possible discitis. This should then lead to a proper examination, which will elicit physical findings of discitis: rigidity and lack of motion in the involved segments as well as tenderness on percussion.

To stay out of trouble, recognize that radiographs and bone scan may be negative in the first couple of weeks. An MRI is very helpful in early spinal infections (Fig. 18-10). Fight the urge to biopsy these children immediately. The cost and morbidity of biopsy can be high and the yield is so low that empirical treatment with antibiotics (be sure to cover *Staphylococcus*) is the standard of care. The indications for biopsy are soft but include a worsening clinical picture despite antibiotics.

It is wise to observe the child on inpatient intravenous antibiotics for a few days to be sure that there is no sign of an epidural abscess. An epidural abscess is rare but is certainly an emergency. An epidural abscess will present with worsening neurologic signs and should be drained immediately.

NEONATAL INFECTIONS

Neonatal osteomyelitis or septic arthritis should be considered in the first 2 months after birth, especially if the child is premature. The clinical scenario is much different in this group. To stay out of trouble, recognize that the lack of a mature immune system means that many of the inflammatory responses we count on as indirect evidence of infection will be absent. Routine lab tests are not even helpful in many cases. Most important, to stay out of trouble, look for more than one site of infection, especially in the NICU baby with invasive monitoring. Premature and term neonates present differently for these infections. Multiple sites of infection occur in 70% or more of cases in preterm infants, and there is a wide spectrum of organisms. For these neonates, you will definitely need a pediatrician or infectious disease specialist to help you with management.

Beware of potential postinfectious growth arrest. All infants with bone and joint infections should be followed for at least a year and probably longer after treatment.[14]

SICKLE CELL DISEASE

In sickle cell disease, osteomyelitis is often in the diaphysis, not the metaphysis (Fig. 18-11). The biggest source of trouble here is separating an infarct from an infection. In many ways, these two problems can have a very similar presentation. Both have pain and swelling, and the ESR may be falsely low because of the hematologic nature of the tests and the abnormal red blood cells. On the radiograph, you can see a periosteal reaction for both, and there can be edema on MRI in both conditions. If the picture is suggestion of an infection, it is important to get blood cultures and aspirate the site. Sequential radionuclide bone marrow and bone scans have also been shown to be helpful but are rarely used these days.

THE GURU SAYS...

Until recently methicillin-resistant *Staphylococcus aureus* (MRSA) was thought to be more virulent, more invasive, and lead to longer hospital stay, more surgeries, higher complication rate—including deep vein thrombosis (DVT) and septic emboli—and higher mortality than methicillin-susceptible *Staphylococcus aureus* (MSSA). However, both Panton-Valentine leukocidin (PVL)-positive MSSA and some strains of *Streptococcus* have the ability to elicit worse APR and systemic effects than MRSA. MSSA has now picked up many of the virulence factors, so don't be lulled into a false sense of security.

ALEXANDRE ARKADER

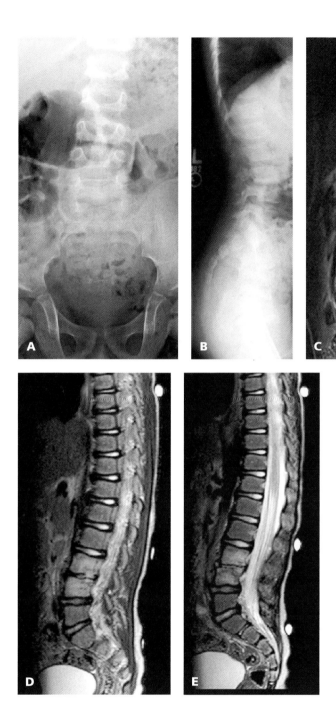

Figure 18-10 Discitis. This 4-year-old boy presented with fever, back pain, and an elevated C-reactive protein (CRP). AP (**A**) and lateral (**B**) radiographs showed narrowing of the L3-4 disc space. **C:** An MRI at presentation showed loss of normal fluid signal in the disc on T2 images and a small posterior collection. He was given the diagnosis of discitis/vertebral osteomyelitis, treated with IV antibiotics, and experienced rapid resolution of his symptoms. By 2 wk after presentation, his CRP had normalized. One month later, the infectious disease team ordered a routine follow-up MRI, despite the fact that he was completely asymptomatic and had normal lab tests. **D, E:** They called orthopaedics, alarmed that the MRI had "dramatically worsened, with loss of disc space and involvement of the entire anterior L3 and L4 vertebral bodies." They were wondering whether a biopsy should be performed. Fortunately, the orthopaedist had treated many such cases and recognized that this is the typical evolution of MRI appearance over time. The child was observed, and months later continued to have no symptoms or elevation in inflammatory markers.

It is important to cover both *Staphylococcus* and *Salmonella* until the cultures are positive. *Kingella* has probably been around for a long time. It is difficult to culture and is killed by most of the commonly used antibiotics. It may have accounted for many of the negative-culture septic arthritis cases that responded to antibiotics in the past.

THE GURU SAYS...

The microorganism profile of musculoskeletal infections has a strong regional/geographical bias. Anyone involved in the care of children with musculoskeletal infections should be aware of their regional "culprits." Specific management recommendations are not "one size fits all."

ALEXANDRE ARKADER

THE GURU SAYS...

While *Salmonella* species is the "classic" pathogen seen in osteomyelitis in children with sickle cell disease, *S. aureus* is still the most common pathogen seen in this patient population.

ALEXANDRE ARKADER

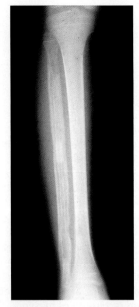

Figure 18-11 This AP radiograph was taken several weeks after a child with sickle cell disease showed signs of osteomyelitis of the fibula. Note the extent of diaphyseal involvement. Biopsy of the diaphysis can be more difficult; general anesthesia with fluoroscopic image localization is helpful. (Courtesy of J. Dormans, MD.)

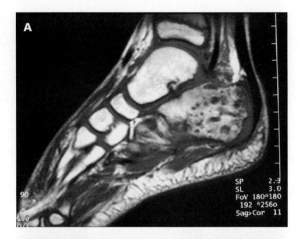

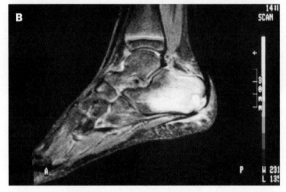

Figure 18-12 T1 (**A**) and T2 (**B**) images of the foot of a child who stepped on a nail. There is osteomyelitis of the calcaneus.

Miscellaneous Orthopaedic Infection Trouble

CHRONIC RECURRENT MULTIFOCAL OSTEOMYELITIS

Chronic recurrent multifocal osteomyelitis (CRMO) can be a difficult condition to manage. The cultures are almost always negative, so a biopsy of the tissue is not recommended, unless malignancy is in the differential diagnosis. It is important to follow the patients to maturity, because deformities can develop.[15] Growth arrest has also been described.[16]

FOOT PUNCTURE WOUNDS

Foot puncture wounds also present some problems[17] (Fig. 18-12). *Staphylococcus* is the most common cause of the soft-tissue infection. True osteomyelitis or foot septic arthritis develops in only a very small percentage of puncture wound cases. *Pseudomonas* infection occurs when the puncture goes through the sole of a shoe or when the child is in dirty water, such as a lake. *Pseudomonas* loves cartilage, so infections in cartilage should be sought out. Initial care involves a tetanus shot, limited superficial debridement, and antistaphylococcal antibiotics. If the infection develops in a bone or joint, you must perform an irrigation and debridement in order to truly irrigate the infection, especially if it is *Pseudomonas*. Broad-spectrum antibiotics are needed. Getting help from your infectious disease team is valuable in this scenario.

> **THE GURU SAYS...**
>
> CRMO is a diagnosis of exclusion. Total body MRI screening has become more popular to rule out other sites of disease. Diagnosis is based on histology findings.
>
> ALEXANDRE ARKADER

> **THE GURU SAYS...**
>
> Treating musculoskeletal infections is a team game. It is very important to keep lines of communication open with ER docs, pediatricians, infectious disease team, radiologists, and interventional radiologists.
>
> ALEXANDRE ARKADER

Staying Out of Trouble With Orthopaedic Infections

٭ Worry about kids with out-of-control acute-phase reactants as these kids often have metastatic disease and can deteriorate quickly.

Osteomyelitis

٭ Fever plus tenderness over a bone is AHO until proven otherwise.

٭ Be sure to get a pediatrician to help in the management of infants and younger children so that you don't miss other site infections that may be disastrous (such as meningitis).

٭ A common mistake in aspirating osteomyelitis is to be in the diaphyseal region, too far from the physis.

٭ MRI is an important part of the modern day evaluation of suspected osteomyelitis.

Septic Arthritis

٭ The hallmark of differentiating Lyme arthritis or RA from septic arthritis is noting that in the former, there is a joint effusion that is out of proportion to the symptoms.

٭ Remember: the patient doesn't have to be a sexually active teen to have gonococcus arthritis.

٭ Irrigation and debridement of the septic hip is more of an emergency than washing out an open fracture, though take the time to thoroughly evaluate the patient. MRI can identify pyomyositis that does not need surgery or septic joints that have associated noncontiguous sites of infection which need attention, so don't rush the diagnosis!

٭ When draining a septic hip, take out a small sample of the capsule with its synovium. This ensures adequate decompression and gives tissue for culture.

٭ These children need to be followed radiographically to rule out AVN.

Other Infection Issues

٭ Discitis: MRI is useful to rule out an epidural abscess or other "mimickers" of spinal infection but will often remain "bright" for a significant time after resolution of symptoms. Biopsy is rarely necessary.

٭ Neonatal infection: look for more than one site of infection, especially in the NICU baby with invasive monitoring.

SOURCES OF WISDOM

1. Konyves A, Deo SD, Murray JR, et al. Septic arthritis of the elbow after chickenpox. *J Pediatr Orthop B*. 2004;13(2):114-117.

2. Yamanaka L, Herbert ME. Myth: an elevated leukocyte count distinguishes septic arthritis from less serious causes of hip pain. *West J Med*. 2001;175(4):275-276.

3. Willis AA, Widmann RF, Flynn JM, et al. Lyme arthritis presenting as acute septic arthritis in children. *J Pediatr Orthop*. 2003;23(1):114-118.

4. Cruz AI Jr, Anari JB, Ramirez JM, et al. Distinguishing pediatric Lyme arthritis of the hip from transient synovitis and acute bacterial septic arthritis: a systematic review and meta-analysis. *Cureus*. 2018;10(1):e2112.

5. Gordon JE, Huang M, Dobbs M, et al. Causes of false-negative ultrasound scans in the diagnosis of septic arthritis of the hip in children. *J Pediatr Orthop*. 2002;22(3):312-316.

6. Gene A, Garcia-Garcia JJ, Sala P, et al. Enhanced culture detection of *Kingella kingae*, a pathogen of increasing clinical importance in pediatrics. *Pediatr Infect Dis J*. 2004;23(9):886-888.

7. Lejbkowicz F, Cohn L, Hashman N, et al. Recovery of *Kingella kingae* from blood and synovial fluid of two pediatric patients by using the BacT/Alert system. *J Clin Microbiol*. 1999;37(3):878.

8. Kocher MS, Mandiga R, Zurakowski D, et al. Validation of a clinical prediction rule for the differentiation between septic arthritis and transient synovitis of the hip in children. *J Bone Joint Surg Am*. 2004;86-A(8):1629-1635.

9. Levine MJ, McGuire KJ, McGowan KL, et al. Assessment of the test characteristics of C-reactive protein for septic arthritis in children. *J Pediatr Orthop*. 2003;23(3):373-377.

10. Wong-Chung J, Bagali M, Kaneker S. Physical signs in pyomyositis presenting as a painful hip in children: a case report and review of the literature. *J Pediatr Orthop B*. 2004;13(3):211-213.

11. Song J, Letts M, Monson R. Differentiation of psoas muscle abscess from septic arthritis of the hip in children. *Clin Orthop Relat Res*. 2001;(391):258-265.

12. Song KS, Lee SM. Peripelvic infections mimicking septic arthritis of the hip in children: treatment with needle aspiration. *J Pediatr Orthop B*. 2003;12(5):354-356.

13. Kim HK, Alman B, Cole WG. A shortened course of parenteral antibiotic therapy in the management of acute septic arthritis of the hip. *J Pediatr Orthop*. 2000;20(1):44-47.

14. Peters W, Irving J, Letts M. Long-term effects of neonatal bone and joint infection on adjacent growth plates. *J Pediatr Orthop*. 1992;12(6):806-810.

15. Duffy CM, Lam PY, Ditchfield M, et al. Chronic recurrent multifocal osteomyelitis: review of orthopaedic complications at maturity. *J Pediatr Orthop*. 2002;22(4):501-505.

16. Piddo C, Reed MH, Black GB. Premature epiphyseal fusion and degenerative arthritis in chronic recurrent multifocal osteomyelitis. *Skeletal Radiol*. 2000;29(2):94-96.

17. Eidelman M, Bialik V, Miller Y, et al. Plantar puncture wounds in children: analysis of 80 hospitalized patients and late sequelae. *Isr Med Assoc J*. 2003;5(4):268-271.

FOR FURTHER ENLIGHTENMENT

Al-Mayahi M, Cian A, Lipsky BA, et al. Administration of antibiotic agents before intraoperative sampling in orthopedic infections alters culture results. *J Infect*. 2015;71(5):518-525.

Benvenuti M, An T, Amaro E, et al. Double-edged sword: musculoskeletal infection provoked acute phase response in children. *Orthop Clin North Am*. 2017;48:181-197.

Benvenuti MA, An TJ, Mignemi ME, et al. A clinical prediction algorithm to stratify pediatric musculoskeletal infection by severity. *J Pediatr Orthop*. 2019;9(3):153-157.

Benvenuti MA, An TJ, Mignemi ME, et al. Effects of antibiotic timing on culture results and clinical outcomes in pediatric musculoskeletal infection. *J Pediatr Orthop*. 2019;39(3):158-162.

Bouchoucha S, Benghachame F, Trifa M, et al. Deep venous thrombosis associated with acute hematogenous osteomyelitis in children. *Orthop Traumatol Surg Res*. 2010;96:890-893.

Cunningham R, Cockayne A, Humphreys H. Clinical and molecular aspects of the pathogenesis of *Staphylococcus aureus* bone and joint infections. *J Med Microbiol*. 1996;44:157-164.

Dodwell ER. Osteomyelitis and septic arthritis in children: current concepts. *Curr Opin Pediatr*. 2013;25:58-63.

Harel L, Prais D, Bar-On E, et al. Dexamethasone therapy for septic arthritis in children: results of a randomized double-blind placebo-controlled study. *J Pediatr Orthop*. 2011;31:211-215.

Mignemi ME, Menge TJ, Cole HA, et al. Epidemiology, diagnosis, and treatment of pericapsular pyomyositis of the hip in children. *J Pediatr Orthop*. 2014;34:316-325.

Peltola H, Paakkonen M, Kallio P, Kallio MJT. Prospective, randomized trial of 10 days versus 30 days of antimicrobial treatment, including a short-term course of parenteral therapy, for childhood septic arthritis. *Clin Infect Dis*. 2009;48:1201-1210.

Riise ØR, Kirkhus E, Handeland KS, et al. Childhood osteomyelitis-incidence and differentiation from other acute onset musculoskeletal features in a population-based study. *BMC Pediatr*. 2008;8:45.

Schlapbach LJ, Straney L, Alexandre J, et al. Mortality related to invasive infections, sepsis, and septic shock in critically ill children in Australia and New Zealand, 2002–13: a multicentre retrospective cohort study. *Lancet Infect Dis*. 2015;15:46-54.

Section J, Gibbons SD, Barton T, et al. Microbiological culture methods for pediatric musculoskeletal infection: a guideline for optimal use. *J Bone Joint Surg Am*. 2015;97:441-449.

Zhorne DJ, Altobelli ME, Cruz AT. Impact of antibiotic pretreatment on bone biopsy yield for children with acute hematogenous osteomyelitis. *Hosp Pediatr*. 2015;5:337-341.

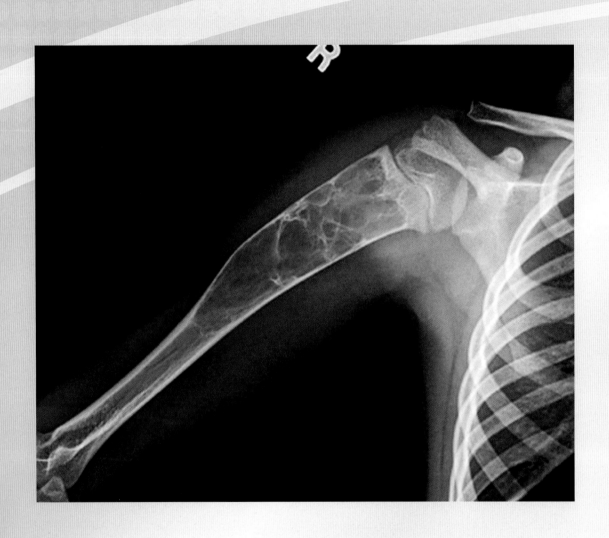

Chapter 19

Tumors

ALEXANDRE ARKADER, MD and JOHN M. (JACK) FLYNN, MD

Guru: Kristy L. Weber, MD

General Considerations

Rule number 1 of medicine is "Do no harm," and rule number 1 of orthopaedic oncology should be "Be aware of the zebras." While bone and soft tissue tumors are rare conditions, in particular in children, they will find you regardless of what your subspecialty interest may be. The incidence of cancer in the United States for 2018 was around 1.7 million. There were approximately 3500 new cases of bone and soft tissue malignant tumors, corresponding to 0.2% of the total, and only 25% of these were in patients younger than 20 years.[1] So you may ask yourself, why do I need to know about something so uncommon? Because orthopaedic surgeons are usually the first line of defense after pediatricians and primary care physicians for evaluation of these lesions. Furthermore, benign conditions are at least 10 times as common as malignancies. Therefore, in order to stay out of trouble, one should be comfortable diagnosing and managing the most common benign conditions, but at the same time comfortably recognize the "imitators", the "no touch" lesions and malignancies, avoiding burning bridges and impacting prognosis in a negative way. While the goal of this chapter is not to provide detailed comprehensive management of musculoskeletal tumors, we will review the basic principles and highlight areas of "caution" when evaluating one of these lesions.

Making the Diagnosis

HISTORY AND PHYSICAL EXAMINATION

Play the detective: obtaining a complete history is important and may provide clues for appropriate differential diagnosis. The main things to inquiry about are family history of systemic conditions, lesions, or tumors; past medical history, including presence of diagnosis such as metabolic diseases, previous infections, etc.; environmental factors exposure; prodromal symptoms such as pain, fever, or others; history of repetitive or acute trauma.

> **THE GURU SAYS...**
>
> Whereas typical pain from overuse or activity-related trauma can be treated symptomatically without initial imaging, these atypical pain symptoms require further workup starting with an X-ray.
>
> KRISTY L. WEBER

> ### Typical Scenarios of How a Bone or Soft Tissue Tumor May Present
>
> - **Incidental:** When a patient is getting an imaging examination for an unrelated condition, or acute trauma and a lesion is noted.
> - **Pain:** Pain is the most common presenting symptom. While some tumors have a characteristic pain pattern, such as osteoid osteoma, with pain at night alleviated with nonsteroidal anti-inflammatory drugs (NSAIDs), most lesions don't display a typical pattern.
>   **ORTHOPAEDICS 101: Classic "red-flag" symptoms that should raise awareness of treating physician are pain that wakes children from sound sleep, pain resistant to regular analgesics, and pain that has no relationship with the type of physical activity exerted throughout the day.**
> - **Limp:** Abnormal gait or limp can be the only presenting sign of a tumor. This is particularly true for younger children, who often will adapt or modify their gait pattern, rather than complain of discomfort. Limp without a witnessed trauma should be met with high level of suspicion.
> - **Mass:** This is one of the most objective signs of a tumor, but imitators such as infection, heterotopic ossification, and others may present in a similar fashion. In the case of soft tissue masses, the ability to move the mass from deep planes can help differentiate deep seated, large and adherent malignant lesions from the more superficial, small, and benign ones. Size also matters, as soft tissue lesions larger than 5 cm are very suspicious for a malignancy, especially if seated deep to the fascia. Transillumination of superficial masses is an easy and quick way to diagnose cystic lesions such as ganglion or popliteal cysts. Nothing is more telling about a palpable mass than its behavior.

- **Painless mass:** While painless masses are more often benign in nature, the absence of pain does not eliminate a possible malignant diagnosis. The classic example is synovial sarcoma, which can be present for years prior to causing any discomfort or rapidly growing.

    ORTHOPAEDICS 101: Synovial sarcomas are tumors that can be stable in size for quite a while before demonstrating their aggressive nature, with rapid growth pattern. They are the most common soft tissue tumor of the foot and between ages 20 and 40 years.

Understanding the behavior of a lesion is a key factor in determining its aggressiveness and urgency in which referral or treatment is needed. While it may be difficult to make that determination at first encounter, there are a few questions that can help you get there. These include the length of symptoms or presence of a palpable mass and its rate of growth, changes, or associated symptoms. In general, lesions that have been latent (stable in size) for several months or years are more likely to be slow growing and benign, while lesions that grow in a rapid and continuous fashion indicate an active process that is more suspicious for malignancy.

It is imperative that while examining a patient with a bone or soft tissue mass, the entire extremity is examined for the presence of enlarged nodes, skin changes, altered range of motion (due to mass effect or pain), and changes in neurovascular status. Skin changes, for example, can suggest a systemic condition or a nontumor diagnosis, such as a vascular malformation, or a syndromic diagnosis such as neurofibromatosis or McCune Albright (Fig. 19-1).

IMAGING

Radiographs are the single most useful imaging modality for diagnosis of bone lesions; it should be seen as the stethoscope of the orthopaedist. MRI is the gold standard for soft tissue lesions and is also very helpful for bone lesions.

The indications for CT are limited due to the concern of ionizing radiation, but it is still the best tool to identify osteoid osteomas and helpful to rule out pathologic fractures, as well as a preoperative planning tool for certain lesion associated with angular deformities such as fibrous dysplasia (Fig. 19-2) or unicameral bone cyst (UBC), by 3D reconstruction of models.

THE GURU SAYS...

Masses in general are more benign in nature, but sarcomas are almost always painless.
KRISTY L. WEBER

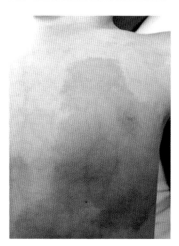

Figure 19-1 This is an 8-year-old boy with a diagnosis of McCune Albright syndrome. Note the large café-au-lait spot over the left chest and abdominal area. (Used with permission of CHOP Orthopedics, Philadelphia, PA.)

THE GURU SAYS...

MRI with/without gadolinium contrast is recommended for indeterminate bone lesions as it can differentiate solid from cystic lesions, determine the extent of marrow involvement, and delineate the boundaries between a soft tissue mass and surrounding neurovascular or bony structures.
KRISTY L. WEBER

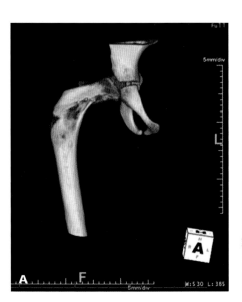
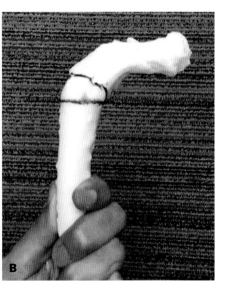

Figure 19-2 A: Right proximal femur 3D CT Recon of a child with fibrous dysplasia and shepherd's crook deformity. **B:** 3D-printed model of the deformity for preoperative planning. (Used with permission of CHOP Orthopedics, Philadelphia, PA.)

TABLE 19-1 Stepwise Approach to Radiographs

1. Tumor location	• What bone • Where in the bone • Central versus eccentric
2. Tumor effect on bone	• Margins • Type of lesion • Matrix
3. Bone reaction	• Cortical changes • Periosteum
4. Associated findings	• Pathologic fracture • Soft tissue mass • Interval progression • Multiple or second lesion

TABLE 19-2 Key Differential Radiographic Findings to Stay Out of Trouble

Benign Tumors	Malignant Tumors
Well-defined	Permeative
Continuous periosteal reaction	Destructive
Bone remodeling	Cortical breakthrough (with exceptions[b])
Solitary lesion (with exceptions[a])	Disorganized periosteal reaction
No soft tissue mass	Multiple lesions (with exceptions[a])
	Soft tissue mass

[a]Multiple osteochondromas, fibrous dysplasia, enchondromatosis.
[b]Benign lesions: nonossifying fibroma, aneurysmal bone cyst.

Radiograph assessment should be approached in a stepwise manner to facilitate generating a differential diagnosis (Table 19-1) and therefore staying out of trouble (Table 19-2).

Tumor Location

Most tumors have a predilection for the metaphyseal regions of long bones, especially during the growing years. In general, a short differential list can be generated based on location alone, for example, lesions in the posterior elements of the spine are usually benign (e.g., aneurysmal bone cyst, osteoid osteoma, and osteoblastoma), epiphyseal lesions differential is usually limited to chondroblastoma, Brodie abscess, or giant cell tumor. While common central lesions include UBC and enchondroma, eccentric lesion examples include aneurysmal bone cyst and nonossifying fibroma. **NEWSFLASH! In the metaphysis "anything can be anything," as this is the most common area for development of bone lesions.**

Effect on Bone

Rapidly growing and aggressive lesions will permeate the bone in a way that it is difficult to determine lesion boundaries. These lesions can at time lead to complete bone destruction and pathologic fractures.

Bone Reaction

If the lesion is not aggressive or if it has been present for a long time, the bone is able to adapt and "protect" itself, producing organized periosteal reactions, cortical thickening, expansion, etc. On the other hand, very slow growing benign lesions such as UBC or fibrous dysplasia can overtime lead to cortical thinning, with minimal bone response (Fig. 19-3).

Associated Findings

There are several red flag signs of a malignant or aggressive lesion, and those need to be readily recognized. They include but are not limited to cortical destruction, soft tissue mass, satellite lesions, etc. **ORTHOPAEDICS 101: Be attentive to the possibility of axial tumors, these lesions are often very difficult to visualize on radiographs, and low threshold for advanced imaging is recommended** (Fig. 19-4).

BIOPSY

While most pediatric orthopaedists will not routinely treat tumors, it is almost certain that they will encounter these lesions in their practice at some point. The key to staying out of trouble is to understand which lesions should and shouldn't

THE GURU SAYS...

The presence of a sclerotic rim or border around a lesion suggests that the bone had time to wall off the lesion, indicating its benign nature.

KRISTY L. WEBER

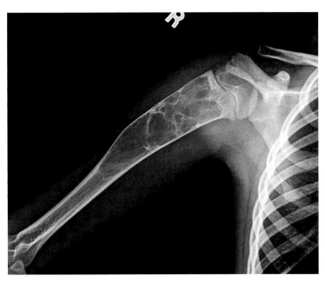

Figure 19-3 Radiographs of right proximal humerus in a 7-year-old boy, demonstrating a well-defined, lytic lesion in the meta-diaphysis. There is mild expansion and septation; there is no soft tissue mass, cortical disruption, or periosteal reaction. The lesion was consistent with an aneurysmal bone cyst. (Used with permission of CHOP Orthopedics, Philadelphia, PA.)

be biopsied by a generalist and how to safely and efficiently perform a biopsy. The Musculoskeletal Tumor Society (MSTS) has reported on the hazards of a poorly performed biopsy in two different occasions.[2] The inability to perform an adequate biopsy can lead to worse outcome, need for further procedures, and otherwise unnecessary amputations.

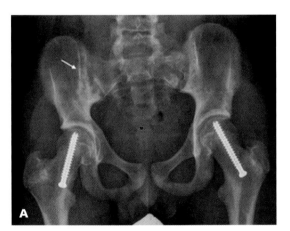

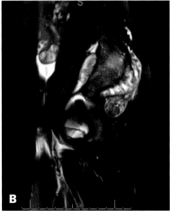

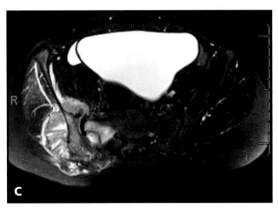

Figure 19-4 A: AP pelvis radiograph of a 12-year-old boy with a history of bilateral valgus slips, complaining of pain in the right hip. The arrow points to an area of increased sclerosis at the sacroiliac (SI) joint region. Sagittal (**B**) and axial (**C**) T2-weighted MRI demonstrates a bone forming lesion with an associated large soft tissue mass, expanding into the sciatic notch, sacroiliac, and sacral involvement of this osteosarcoma. (Used with permission of CHOP Orthopedics, Philadelphia, PA.)

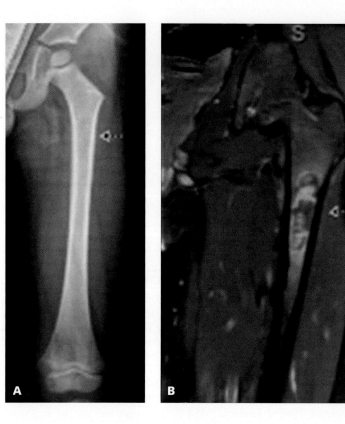

Figure 19-5 A: AP femur radiograph of a 3-year-old boy who presented with a limp. Note the subtle, but well-defined lytic lesion in the proximal metaphysis and diaphysis. **B:** T1-weighted coronal MRI demonstrates intramedullary marrow involvement and no soft tissue mass. The final diagnosis was Ewing sarcoma. (Used with permission of CHOP Orthopedics, Philadelphia, PA.)

After a patient with a bone or soft tissue lesion is evaluated in clinic, the treating physician needs to make sure that all necessary imaging studies are adequately completed and a differential diagnosis is formulated. The next step is to determine the urgency in which the biopsy/diagnosis needs to be made: the next 24 hours, the next few days, or the next few weeks. If there is a concern of a malignant or aggressive process, adequate referral to a tertiary center may be preferred over performing a biopsy.

While open incisional biopsy has been the standard of care for decades, most tertiary centers have moved toward image-guided needle biopsies in conjunction with interventional radiology. Percutaneous methods of biopsy, core needle in particular, are safe, less invasive, and less costly and avoid several risks associated to open biopsies such as infection, need for biopsy tract resection, pathologic fractures, etc. and have been shown to provide similar accuracy of diagnosis.[3] If an infectious process is in the differential diagnosis, culture and sensitivity should be sent at time of biopsy. **ORTHOPAEDICS 101: "Biopsy every culture and culture every biopsy" is a principle that should be followed, as several neoplastic processes may present in a very similar fashion as an infection. Ewing sarcoma, in particular, can resemble a low-grade infectious process on imaging and clinical presentation, including elevated inflammatory markers (Fig. 19-5).**

Benign Bone Tumors That Every Orthopaedist Should Know

UNICAMERAL BONE CYST

Unicameral bone cyst (UBC) is one of the most common lesions seen and treated by pediatric orthopaedists. Most cases are diagnosed at the time of a pathologic fracture and with few exceptions, such as displaced, or hip fractures, they should initially be treated conservatively (Fig. 19-6).

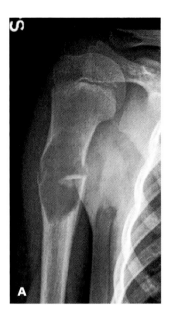
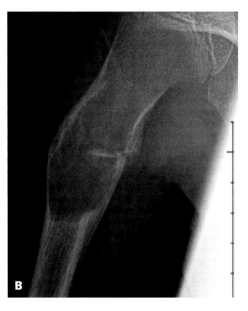

Figure 19-6 **A:** AP radiographs of a 6-year-old girl who presented with a pathologic fracture through a presumed unicameral bone cyst. **B:** After 4 wk, the fracture is healed but the cyst persists. (Used with permission of CHOP Orthopedics, Philadelphia, PA.)

Both the etiology and natural history of UBCs are poorly understood, and the ideal treatment is debatable with most modalities presenting high recurrence rate (~25%).[4] The best way to staying out of trouble with UBCs is to avoid under- and/or overtreating it. Lesions in weight-bearing bones, especially around the hip, may need to be aggressively treated to avoid the complications of a pathologic fracture; active lesions in very young children can lead to physeal arrest and growth compromise; therefore, those lesions may also require further imaging and active treatment (Fig. 19-7).[5]

For small latent lesions (further away from physis), particularly in the upper extremity, the approach should be conservative. There is no clear "best treatment" for UBCs; the most successful techniques recommend some combination

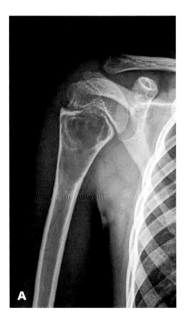
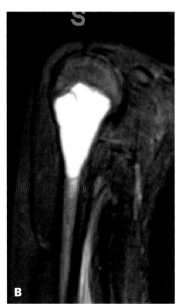
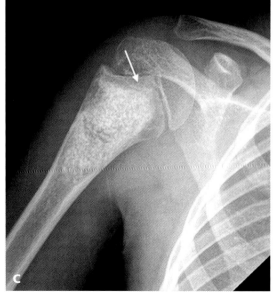

Figure 19-7 **A:** AP radiograph of the proximal humerus of a 6-year-old boy demonstrating a well-defined lytic lesion in the metaphysis with cortical thinning, consistent with a unicameral bone cyst. **B:** On MRI, there is physeal abutment but no crossing. **C:** About 1 y postoperatively, the patient has a well-healed cyst with normal physeal growth (arrow). (Used with permission of CHOP Orthopedics, Philadelphia, PA.)

of mechanical disruption of the cyst, with decompression to allow reestablishing normal blood/marrow flow to the affected area, followed by bone grafting. **NEWSFLASH! For active UBCs, close to the adjacent physis, preoperative MRI may be useful to ensure that there is no pretreatment physeal disruption.**

ANEURYSMAL BONE CYST

An important concept to understand regarding aneurysmal bone cysts (ABCs) is that these lesions may be secondary to other benign and/or malignant lesions, so the correct diagnosis is essential. The neoplastic basis in primary ABC was proven by demonstrating translocation on chromosome 17 leading to recurrent USP6 fusion oncogene under the regulatory influence of a CDH11 promoter. This does not seem to occur in secondary lesions.[6]

While most lesions can be biopsied at time of definitive treatment, if there are concerns of a potential associated lesion or malignancy (e.g., telangiectatic osteosarcoma), biopsy should be done prior to any surgical intervention and potential contamination of surrounding tissues.

ABCs may cause significant intraoperative bleeding. While this is usually a result of the tumor content, rather than tumor neovascularization, some ABCs can be hypervascular and benefit from preoperative embolization (Fig. 19-8).

It is advisable to review the preoperative imaging studies with a radiologist or IR team to determine whether preoperative selective embolization would be beneficial. While thorough curettage and bone grafting is still the standard of care for most ABCs, serial embolization or sclerotherapy is an alternative for recurrent or large lesions, especially around the pelvis or spine, where surgical morbidity may be significant. It can be used as the main treatment or as an adjuvant (Fig. 19-9).

NONOSSIFYING FIBROMA

Undoubtedly, nonossifying fibroma (NOF) is the most common lesion seen in children, with an estimated prevalence of 20%. NOFs are also referred as fibrous cortical defects (lesions usually <4 cm) or cortical desmoids. Most NOFs are incidentally found and can be left alone; they are the "intoers" of the orthopaedic oncologists, the exceptions being large lesions (>50% of the bone involved) in weight-bearing bones (Fig. 19-10), that can predispose to pathologic fractures or chronic pain (usually due to stress reaction or insufficiency fracture; Fig. 19-11). When treatment is warranted, curettage and bone grafting is sufficient to strengthen the bone and lead to lesional healing; at times, internal fixation is needed. Most NOFs should gradually heal/ossify by skeletal maturity; most lesions should be left alone.

THE GURU SAYS...

As parents are often extremely anxious when an NOF is noted incidentally after trauma, it is important to discuss the natural history and benign nature of the lesion. These "birthmarks" on the bone should not require any imaging other than plain X-rays.

KRISTY L. WEBER

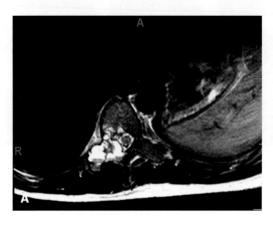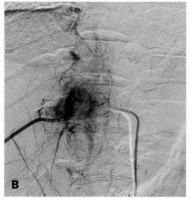

Figure 19-8 Aneurysmal bone cyst of the spine. **A:** MRI T2 axial demonstrates a right-sided expansile lesion involving the pedicle of T9 with expansion into the spinal canal. **B:** This patient underwent a preoperative angiogram and embolization. (Used with permission of CHOP Orthopedics, Philadelphia, PA.)

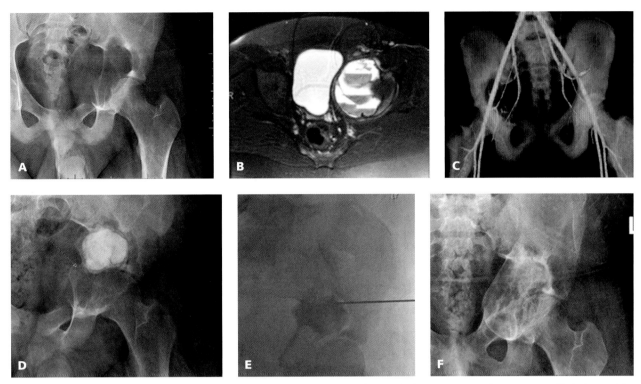

Figure 19-9 This is a 15-year-old boy with left hip pain. **A:** The AP radiograph demonstrates a large, expansile lesion arising in the supra-acetabular region of the left hip. **B:** Axial MRI demonstrates the classic fluid-fluid levels and significant pelvic expansion. **C:** Preoperative CT angiogram did not demonstrate increased blood supply to the region, and embolization was not performed. After curettage and bone grafting, there was a persistent area of aneurysmal bone cyst (ABC) medially (**D**) that was approached with embolization using doxycycline (**E**). **F:** At 1 y after embolization, the lesion is completely healed. (Used with permission of CHOP Orthopedics, Philadelphia, PA.)

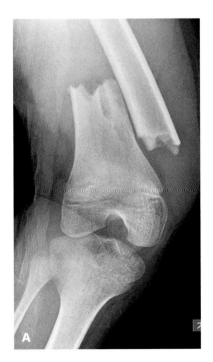
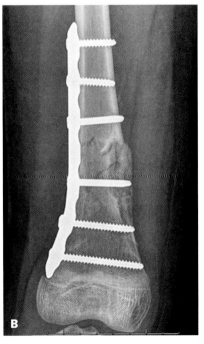

Figure 19-10 Pathologic fracture of the femur in an otherwise healthy 12-year-old boy. **A:** Note the medially cortical-based lesion with sclerotic border consistent with a large nonossifying fibroma. **B:** The fracture was approached with open reduction internal fixation (ORIF) through a lateral approach. (Used with permission of CHOP Orthopedics, Philadelphia, PA.)

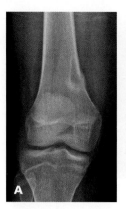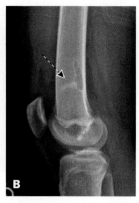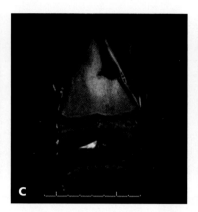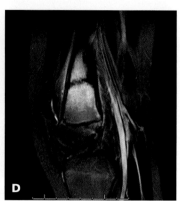

Figure 19-11 A 15-year-old female varsity runner presented complaining of thigh pain with activities. AP (**A**) and lateral (**B**) radiographs demonstrate a cortically based, lytic lesion with sharp sclerotic border, consistent with a nonossifying fibroma (NOF) and new bone formation with a sclerotic stress fracture across (arrow). **C, D:** MRIs better demonstrate surrounding edema and the "dreaded" black line diagnostic of the stress fracture. (Used with permission of CHOP Orthopedics, Philadelphia, PA.)

OSTEOCHONDROMA

Considered the most common benign bone tumor in children, osteochondromas usually present as a painless "bump." Some patients may complain of pain after a minor trauma, repetitive discomfort with activities, "locking" sensation, or deformity. The most common locations are the shoulder and knee due to the rapid growth nature of the adjacent physis (Fig. 19-12).

Osteochondromas are tumors of "growth years"; therefore, as long as the child is growing, the lesion is expected to grow as well. While most lesions will grow in proportion to skeletal growth, lesions closer to the adjacent physis are considered active and grow faster. The risk of malignant degeneration of an isolated osteochondroma is overinflated in some of the available literature and is likely less than 0.5%. Malignant degeneration is expected to occur only after skeletal maturity, presenting with new growth of a stable lesion and/or new associated symptoms such as pain.

Most malignant degenerations are to low-grade chondrosarcomas with a great prognosis.

Avoid overtreating an osteochondroma; the simple "trade" of a bump for a scar may not be worth it for the child. The complication rate with surgical resection may be as high as 12%, not justifying excision of asymptomatic lesions.[7] The indications for excision of osteochondroma should include chronic pain, impingement on musculotendinous structures, neurovascular symptoms, block to motion, or angular deformities.

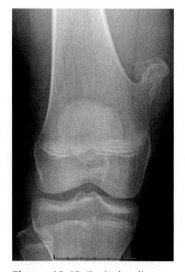

Figure 19-12 Typical radiographic appearance of a sessile osteochondroma of the distal femur. Note the continuity of the cortex with the outline of the lesion and continuity of the medullary canal into the lesion. (Used with permission of CHOP Orthopedics, Philadelphia, PA.)

> **THE GURU SAYS...**
>
> In general, operative excision should be reserved for pedunculated lesions rather than sessile lesions. The sessile lesions are generally not symptomatic and do not impinge on neurovascular structures. Removing them would often involve removal of a large portion of cortex, putting the child at risk for pathologic fracture.
>
> KRISTY L. WEBER

Always obtain adequate preoperative advanced imaging (e.g., MRI) for osteochondromas that are in proximity to neurovascular structures, even in the absence of symptoms of entrapment (Fig. 19-13). **NEWSFLASH! Multiple hereditary exostosis (MHE) is a "different animal" and should be routinely followed during growth years due to the increased risk of angular deformities (Fig. 19-14), decreased ROM, and malignant degeneration.**

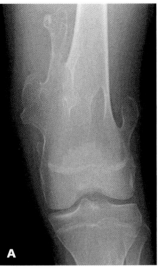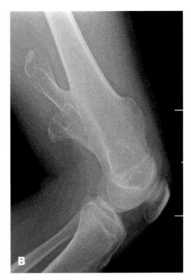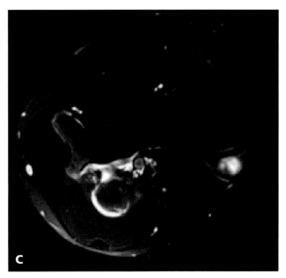

Figure 19-13 AP (**A**) and lateral (**B**) radiographs of a 15-year-old boy with multiple hereditary exostosis and knee pain. There is significant involvement of the distal femur with several osteochondromas around the meta-diaphysis. **C:** Axial MRI demonstrates the vascular bundle wrapping around the base of the lesion (arrow). (Used with permission of CHOP Orthopedics, Philadelphia, PA.)

OSTEOID OSTEOMA

Osteoid osteomas are benign bone tumors that have "read the book" and present with a classic history of localized pain, often intense, at times waking the child up from sound sleep, and rapidly responsive to NSAIDs or aspirin. Some of the challenges in making the diagnosis include the "not so typical" presentation especially

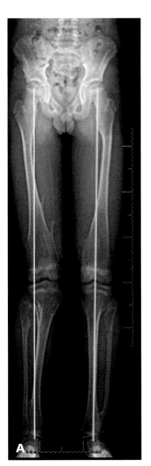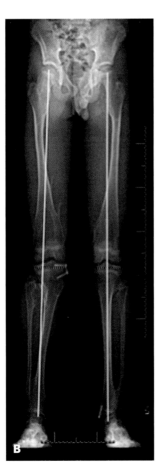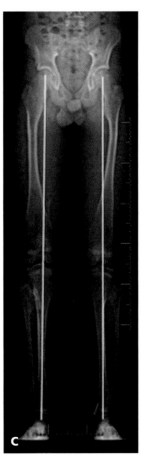

Figure 19-14 A: AP hip-to-ankle EOS imaging of a 13-year-old boy with multiple hereditary exostoses and right knee valgus deformity. The patient underwent hemiepiphysiodesis with plates and screws (**B**) and presented with normalization of his mechanical axis after hardware removal (**C**). (Used with permission of CHOP Orthopedics, Philadelphia, PA.)

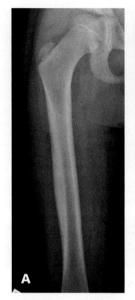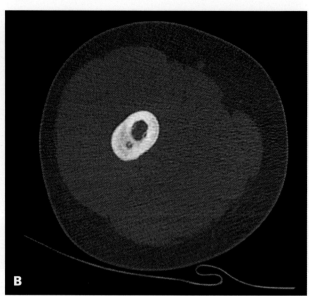

Figure 19-15 A: AP radiograph of the proximal femur of a 13-year-old boy presenting with intermittent pain and recurrent night pain at the right thigh. There is cortical thickening of the femoral shaft with continuous new bone formation and a questionable lucency in the lateral aspect of the femur (arrow). **B:** Axial CT scan clearly demonstrates the osteoid osteoma nidus within the femoral cortex. (Used with permission of CHOP Orthopedics, Philadelphia, PA.)

> **THE GURU SAYS...**
>
> The differential diagnosis of an osteoid osteoma includes a stress fracture or reaction, osteomyelitis or, less likely, Ewing sarcoma. A CT scan should identify the typical nidus.
>
> KRISTY L. WEBER

> **THE GURU SAYS...**
>
> For an osteolytic lesion in the skeletal of a growing child, LCH can almost always be in the radiographic differential.
>
> KRISTY L. WEBER

> **THE GURU SAYS...**
>
> Per the classic article by Yasko et al.,[9] injection of steroids into an LCH solitary lesion will induce resolution and avoid any need for surgical treatment.
>
> KRISTY L. WEBER

in young children, or secondary signs, such as atypical scoliosis associated with pain. Furthermore, these lesions are small (<1 cm) and can be missed on radiographs. Secondary focal periosteal new bone formation around the lesion may lead to the diagnosis. MRI often fails to define the lesional nidus due to significant surrounding bone edema; therefore, CT is the gold standard[8] (Fig. 19-15). In some instances, bone scanning may be required to localize small lesions, especially in the spine.

The current standard of care for the treatment of osteoid osteoma is image- (CT-) guided ablation. While radiofrequency ablation (RFA) has been used most often, other techniques, such as microwave ablation, have been recently used for areas such as the spine, where scattered heat may pose risk to nerves. The overall success of ablation is over 90%. Surgery is only indicated in select cases with close proximity to neurologic structures, or for recurrent lesions (RFA also used with success on recurrent lesions) that are readily visible on plain films (Fig. 19-16). **NEWSFLASH! In cases in which there is a high suspicion of osteoid osteoma, but X-rays and MRI aren't conclusive, make sure to order a fine cut (1-2 mm) CT, as some lesions can be missed even with a CT if the cuts are too wide.**

LANGERHANS CELL HISTIOCYTOSIS

While the treatment of these lesions may be limited to making the diagnosis, Langerhans cell histiocytosis (LCH) is referred to as the "great imitator" due to a rather nonspecific clinical and imaging presentation. While most lesions are diagnosed early in the second decade and primarily involve the musculoskeletal system, LCH can less commonly involve the skin and viscera and present as a disseminated multisystemic and life-threatening condition.

Spinal lesions will often present as a "vertebra plana" with symmetric or asymmetric vertebral body collapse (Fig. 19-17). Most lesions involve the anterior elements alone, but posterior elements extension may occur. MRI is recommended to rule out soft tissue expansion or intracanal involvement.

All suspected lesions should undergo biopsy. Besides formulating the definitive diagnosis, biopsy incites an inflammatory or reactive bone response that often stimulates lesional healing and resolution of solitary lesions.

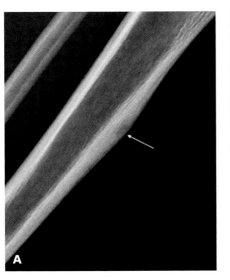

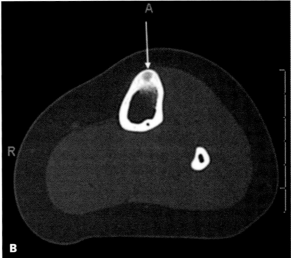

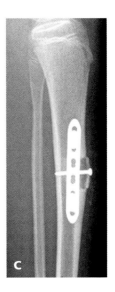

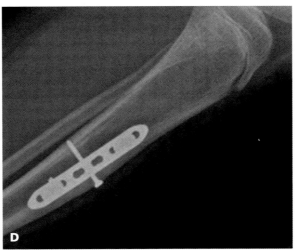

Figure 19-16 A: Osteoid osteoma nidus is visualized in the lateral radiograph of this 15-year-old boy. **B:** Axial CT confirms the anterior placed nidus within the tibial cortex (arrow). **C:** The patient failed to improve after radiofrequency ablation and underwent an en bloc resection with allografting. **D:** Two years later, he had complete healing and no pain or signs of recurrence. (Used with permission of CHOP Orthopedics, Philadelphia, PA.)

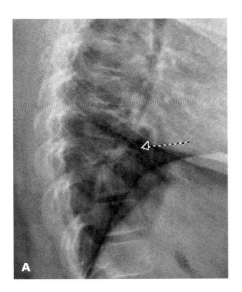

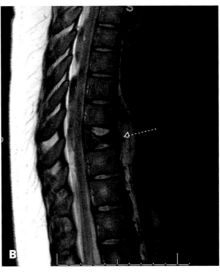

Figure 19-17 T11 vertebra plana from Langerhans cell histiocytosis (LCH) visualized on lateral radiographs (**A**) and sagittal MRI (**B**). Note the absence of soft tissue mass or canal involvement. (Used with permission of CHOP Orthopedics, Philadelphia, PA.)

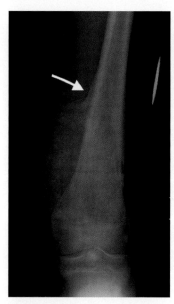

Figure 19-18 Classic appearance of a distal femur osteosarcoma. There is an ill-defined mixed lesion with large soft tissue mass, disorganized periosteal reaction, and Codman triangle (arrow). (Used with permission of CHOP Orthopedics, Philadelphia, PA.)

Determining whether this is a solitary lesion is essential to guide the treatment. Skeletal survey is the modality of choice, as a bone scan can miss these lesions. The skull is one of the most common sites of bone disease. While solitary bone lesions can be observed, multisystem or polyostotic disease is treated with chemotherapy utilizing "heavy anti-inflammatory" medication including prednisone, methotrexate, or vinblastine. **ORTHOPAEDICS 101: While vertebra plana is characteristic of LCH, it is not exclusive or pathognomonic of LCH, and in a recent study, almost 50% of vertebra plana had other etiologies, such as CRMO, leukemia, and Ewing sarcoma.**

How to Stay Out of Trouble With Malignancies

OSTEOSARCOMA

Osteosarcoma is the most common primary bone malignancy and is more often seen in the second decade, around the knee and shoulder. Knee pain is the most common presentation, and as this is a very common complaint in teenagers, it is important to keep a healthy level of suspicion and have a low threshold level to obtain radiographs of the involved area if there are atypical pain symptoms.

The WHO divides osteosarcoma in eight subtypes, most (90%) being the "conventional" osteoblastic type presenting as a metaphyseal, mixed destructive lesion associated with a soft tissue mass and disorganized periosteal reaction (Fig. 19-18).

Juxtacortical or surface osteosarcoma can be parosteal (low grade), periosteal (intermediate grade), or high grade. A parosteal osteosarcoma may resemble an osteochondroma or chondroma and may be difficult to differentiate from myositis ossificans.[10] Telangiectatic osteosarcoma, ABC, and giant cell tumor can be very similar in their presentation (Fig. 19-19). Therefore, if telangiectatic osteosarcoma is in the differential, a biopsy is recommended before any definitive surgical treatment. **NEWSFLASH! The differential diagnosis between surface osteosarcoma and myositis ossificans can be facilitated by the history (trauma) and by radiographic characteristics, as osteosarcoma shows the most dense part of the lesion in the center and myositis has peripheral ossification** (Fig. 19-20). Chemotherapy has improved the overall survival of localized primary extremity osteosarcoma to approximately 70%. The goal of the chemo is to kill "micrometastasis." The prognosis depends on staging and response to chemotherapy.

> **THE GURU SAYS...**
>
> The overall survival of patients with osteosarcoma has not changed substantially in 30 years. The classic treatment paradigm for high-grade osteosarcoma is preoperative chemotherapy, surgical resection, followed by additional chemotherapy. The prognosis for patients with pelvic osteosarcoma or with metastatic disease is decreased.
>
> KRISTY L. WEBER

> **THE GURU SAYS...**
>
> Like other small round cell lesions, the plain radiographic changes can at times be subtle even when there is a large accompanying soft tissue mass.
>
> KRISTY L. WEBER

EWING SARCOMA

Ewing sarcoma (EWS) is slightly less common than osteosarcoma; it tends to involve the same areas of the growing skeleton, but it has a predisposition for the axial skeleton and diaphyseal region of long bones. EWS may present very similar to an infectious process, including constitutional symptoms such as weight loss, fever, and pain. While most cases are accompanied by a large soft tissue mass, some cases will only have intramedullary changes (see Fig. 19-4). **ORTHOPAEDICS**

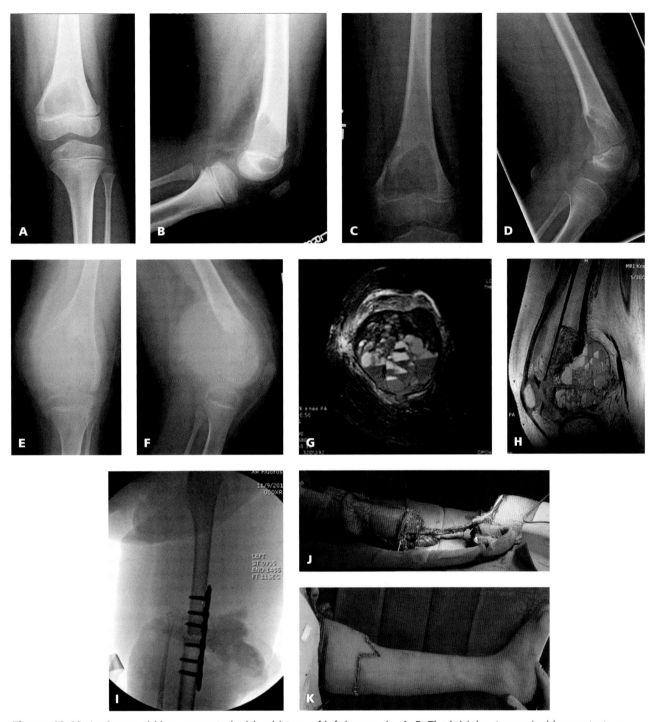

Figure 19-19 An 8-year-old boy presented with a history of left knee pain. **A, B:** The initial radiographs (demonstrate a well-defined lytic lesion in the distal femur metaphysis, without periosteal reaction, cortical disruption, or soft tissue mass, suggesting a diagnosis of a benign cystic lesion such as unicameral bone cyst (UBC) or aneurysmal bone cyst (ABC). **C, D:** Approximately 1 mo later, there is continued pain and slight enlargement of the lesion. **E, F:** Another month later, this lesion has grown significantly, and there is cortical destruction and a soft tissue mass posteriorly with physeal disruption. At that time, sagittal (**G**) and axial (**H**) MRIs showed several fluid levels and significant bone expansion as well as epiphyseal involvement and physeal destruction. **I:** Intraoperative fluoroscopy demonstrating the fixation between femur and tibia. **J:** Intraoperative clinical image demonstrating the sparing of the neurovascular bundle to allow the rotationplasty. **K:** Final clinical appearance at the end of the procedure. (Used with permission of CHOP Orthopedics, Philadelphia, PA.)

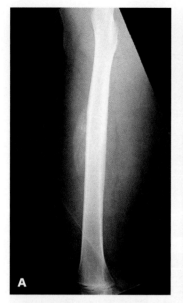
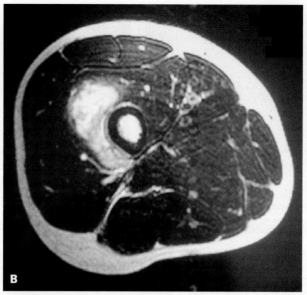
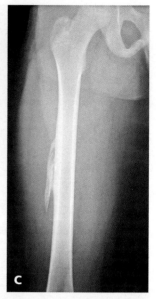

Figure 19-20 Myositis ossificans can have a confusing or even scary appearance. **A:** Lateral radiograph of the femur of a boy presenting after trauma to the anterior thigh shows a calcified mass anterior to the midshaft of the femur. **B:** MRI shows that the calcified mass is in the vastus intermedius muscle and does not emanate from the femoral bone itself. This reassuring image clarified that this was a muscle process and not bone malignancy. Based on this evaluation, the surgeon avoided biopsy and just recommended radiographic follow-up over the next several months. **C:** AP femur radiograph taken 3 mo after initial presentation shows myositis ossificans that has matured and no longer has a concerning appearance.

> **THE GURU SAYS...**
>
> The overall survival of patients with Ewing sarcoma is similar to those with osteosarcoma. For those with isolated extremity lesions, the 5-year survival is about 70%.
>
> KRISTY L. WEBER

101: Biopsy every culture and culture every biopsy. This is especially true in cases where EWS is in the differential. EWS staging includes bone marrow biopsy, as positive marrow metastasis is present in approximately 20% of the children at time of diagnosis. CT of the chest and positron-emission tomography (PET) scan complete the staging. Local control can be achieved with surgery or radiation therapy with similar rates of success.

> **THE GURU SAYS...**
>
> It is important to perform a thorough extremity examination, including for lymph node enlargement, as childhood sarcomas—including synovial sarcoma, rhabdomyosarcoma, and epithelioid sarcoma—can metastasize to the lymph node chain.
>
> KRISTY L. WEBER

> **THE GURU SAYS...**
>
> Although chemotherapy has not been proved effective in most soft tissue sarcomas, it is a standard of care for rhabdomyosarcoma in children. Patients with large synovial sarcomas also often are treated with chemotherapy.
>
> Many soft tissue sarcomas larger than 5 cm, especially when located adjacent to important structures, will be indicated for preoperative radiation therapy.
>
> KRISTY L. WEBER

A Few Facts on Soft Tissue Lesions

- Size matters: Lesions over 5 cm are malignant until proved otherwise.
- Depth matters: Malignant lesions are usually located deep to the deep fascia (Fig. 19-21).
- Examination matters: Most malignant lesions are firm and noncompressible. For superficial and soft lesions, transillumination can be very helpful.
- Pain may matter: Not all malignant tumors are painful (most are not) and not all benign tumors are painless.
- Behavior matters: Lesions that are rapidly growing are more concerning, than lesions that have been stable and not changing in size.
- Rhabdomyosarcoma represents 50% of all malignant soft tissue tumors in children.
- Synovial sarcomas are tumors that can be stable in size for quite a while before demonstrating their aggressive nature, with rapid growth pattern. They are the most common soft tissue tumor of the foot and between ages 20 and 40 years.

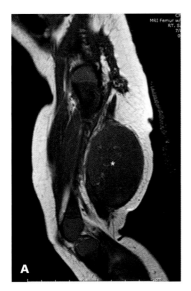
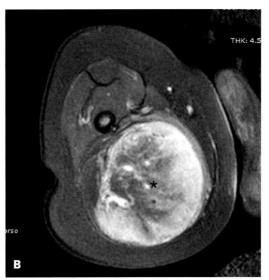

Figure 19-21 MRIs demonstrate a large heterogenous soft tissue mass in the thigh of a 3-year-old boy. Note the size of the mass (*), its depth, and displacement of surrounding structures. Pathology was consistent with a high-grade sarcoma. (Used with permission of CHOP Orthopedics, Philadelphia, PA.)

Staying Out of Trouble With Tumors

* While bone and soft tissue tumors are rare conditions, particularly in children, they will find you regardless of what your subspecialty interest may be.

* Classic red flag symptoms that should raise awareness of treating physician are pain that wakes children from sound sleep, pain resistant to regular analgesics, and pain that has no relationship with the type of physical activity exerted throughout the day.

* Radiographs are the single most useful imaging modality for diagnosis of bone lesions; it should be seen as the stethoscope of the orthopaedist. MRI is the gold standard for soft-tissue lesions and is also very helpful for bone lesions.

* In the metaphysis, "anything can be anything," as this is the most common area for development of bone lesions.

* "Biopsy every culture and culture every biopsy" is a principle that should be followed, as several neoplastic processes may present in a very similar fashion as an infection.

* For active UBCs, close to the adjacent physis, preoperative MRI may be useful to ensure that there is no pretreatment physeal disruption.

* As parents are often extremely anxious when an NOF is noted incidentally after trauma, it is important to discuss the natural history and benign nature of the lesion. These "birthmarks" on the bone should not require any imaging other than plain X-rays.

* The indications for excision of osteochondroma should include chronic pain, impingement on musculotendinous structures, neurovascular symptoms, block to motion, or angular deformities.

* Knee pain is the most common presentation for osteosarcoma, and as this is a very common complaint in teenagers, it is important to keep a healthy level of suspicion and have a low threshold level to obtain radiographs of the involved area if there are atypical pain symptoms.

SOURCES OF WISDOM

1. Cancer Stat Facts: Bone and Joint Cancer. National Cancer Institute Surveillance, Epidemiology, and End Results Program Website. Available at https://seer.cancer.gov/statfacts/html/bones.html. Accessed July 18, 2019.

2. Mankin HJ, Mankin CJ, Simon MA. The hazards of the biopsy, revisited. Members of the Musculoskeletal Tumor Society. *J Bone Joint Surg Am.* 1996;78(5):656-663.

3. Traina F, Errani C, Toscano A, et al. Current concepts in the biopsy of musculoskeletal tumors. *J Bone Joint Surg Am.* 2015;97(1):e7.

4. Kadhim M, Sethi S, Thacker MM. Unicameral bone cysts in the humerus: treatment outcomes. *J Pediatr Orthop.* 2016;36(4):392-399.

5. Stanton RP, Abdel-Mota'al MM. Growth arrest resulting from unicameral bone cyst. *J Pediatr Orthop.* 1998;18(2):198-201.

6. Oliveira AM, Hsi BL, Weremowicz S, et al. USP6 (Tre2) fusion oncogenes in aneurysmal bone cyst. *Cancer Res.* 2004;64(6):1920-1923.

7. Wirganowicz PZ, Watts HG. Surgical risk for elective excision of benign exostoses. *J Pediatr Orthop.* 1997;17(4):455-459.

8. Hosalkar HS, Garg S, Moroz L, et al. The diagnostic accuracy of MRI versus CT imaging for osteoid osteoma in children. *Clin Orthop Relat Res.* 2005;(433):171-177. Erratum in *Clin Orthop Relat Res.* 2005;(436):286.

9. Yasko AW, Fanning CV, Ayala AG, et al. Percutaneous techniques for the diagnosis and treatment of localized Langerhans-cell histiocytosis (eosinophilic granuloma of bone). *J Bone Joint Surg Am.* 1998;80(2):219-228.

10. Yarmish G, Klein MJ, Landa J, et al. Imaging characteristics of primary osteosarcoma: nonconventional subtypes. *Radiographics.* 2010;30(6):1653-1672.

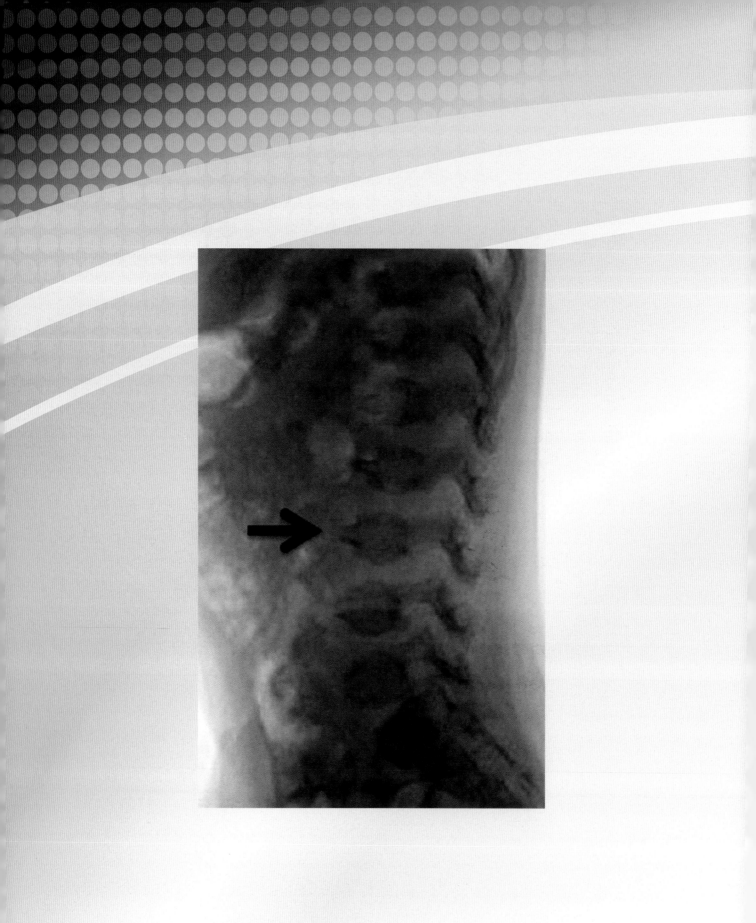

Chapter 20

Skeletal Dysplasias

KLANE K. WHITE, MD, MSc

Guru: Vernon T. Tolo, MD

As a group, these disorders are commonly encountered by the pediatric orthopaedist, but individually, each disorder is quite rare. Orthopaedic training programs often provide little education in the area of skeletal dysplasia, except perhaps a few facts that may appear on in-training or board certification examinations. Many orthopaedists relegate this subject to the arena of orthopaedic trivia. With the growth of support groups and Internet sites for unusual disorders, the skeletal dysplasia patient or parents often know the latest facts about their disorder, a fact that the orthopaedic surgeon can use in their favor. This chapter is designed to suggest a way to approach the evaluation and treatment of your patients with skeletal dysplasia and to help you successfully navigate the world of rare disease.

There are now more than 400 recognized genetic disorders of bone. The skeletal dysplasias, more formally referred to as the "osteochondrodystrophies," represent a subset of this group in which the primary defect is in the function and development of the growth plate. Genetic mutations of the growth plate result in an array of cytokine, enzyme, and structural malfunctions of the tissues in which they are expressed. The genetic aberrations found in the skeletal dysplasias can be broken up into four different groups: (1) proteins that are structural, (2) proteins that regulate developmental signaling pathways, (3) proteins responsible for metabolite processing or transport, and (4) proteins that regulate cell replication and tumorogenesis.

If the skeletal dysplasia diagnosis has not been established or is unclear, the first step is always to do a skeletal survey, which includes radiographic evaluation of the skull, spine, and all extremities. Long-bone radiographs will establish whether there is epiphyseal or metaphyseal involvement, or both—which in turn will help to narrow down the possible diagnoses to consider. If there is platyspondyly, the term *spondylo* appears somewhere in the name of the condition (Fig. 20-1). If there is primarily epiphyseal involvement, early joint degeneration is likely to occur. If there is primarily metaphyseal involvement, angular deformity with growth is often seen, which may mimic rickets. Often, the morphology of the ilium or acetabulum reveals unique finding specific to a particular disorder. Even though the X-rays and the physical findings may seem characteristic for a given skeletal dysplasia, it is mandatory to obtain the opinion of a geneticist for confirmation of diagnosis, which has significant implications with regard to treatment options, health maintenance, and genetic counseling.

There is a paucity of literature on many of these dysplasias as far as effective treatment is concerned. Rather than memorizing obscure names and irrelevant dysmorphology facts (which nowadays can be found on many private and government-funded websites, as well as sites for patient advocacy groups), these patients should be approached in a systematic, anatomical fashion. Using known orthopaedic principles, only then should the orthopaedist pursue the specific findings and concerns for each disorder.

Keeping in mind what is known about the natural history of orthopaedic problems in a particular skeletal dysplasia condition, the best orthopaedic approach often here is to use tested orthopaedic principles for joint problems, spine deformity or instability, and limb realignment in the average-sized person, and then apply them to the dysplastic skeleton. Examples would be decompression for spinal stenosis, custom-made implants for total joint replacement, and guided growth or osteotomies to regain mechanical axis alignment.

There are generalized and specific pitfalls with each of these procedures that can occur more often in patients with skeletal dysplasia, but the underlying orthopaedic principles stay constant. This group as a whole has an increased risk for

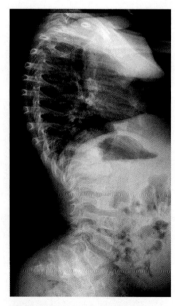

Figure 20-1 Lateral spine radiograph demonstrates the finding of platyspondyly (height of vertebrae less than normal in relation to width) in a child with spondyloepiphyseal dysplasia congenita.

perioperative complications related to the anatomy of their upper airway, abnormalities of tracheal-bronchial morphology and function; deformity of their chest wall; abnormal mobility of their upper cervical spine; and associated issues with general health and body habitus. There is extreme phenotypic variability in this population. When combined with the rarity of each condition, make it becomes important that patients are assessed and managed in facilities that are aware of these potential complications, and have the skill and resources to anticipate and manage them.

Achondroplasia

Achondroplasia is the most common form of skeletal dysplasia and is recognizable at birth. Upregulation of fibroblast growth factor receptor 3 (FGFR3) leads to the growth inhibition here. Rhizomelia is present in all extremities and the facial appearance includes frontal bossing and nasal bridge depression. Head size is large for the body and, while hydrocephalus may be suspected, this is usually not present. Delayed milestones and hypotonia are common and should be compared to published norms available for achondroplasia from the American Academy of Pediatrics. An anteroposterior spinal radiograph will show interpediculate narrowing in the lumbar spine, with short pedicles and thoracolumbar kyphosis, is common on the lateral view in the first few years of life (Fig. 20-2).

The primary orthopaedic concerns in this condition are foramen magnum stenosis and spinal stenosis. As an infant, the main medical concern centers around sleep apnea, which may be due to either upper airway obstruction or hypotonia resulting from foramen magnum narrowing and compression of the upper cervical spinal cord (Fig. 20-3). Sleep studies and regular neurological exams are recommended to detect and follow these issues. Screening MRI should be reserved for infants with upper motor neuron signs, significant hypotonia, or central sleep apnea. Posterior impingement of the cord is common and typically asymptomatic. While published reports have noted improvement in respiratory function after foraminal decompression, there is a substantial morbidity associated with this

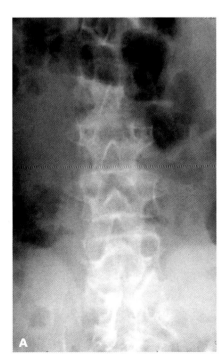
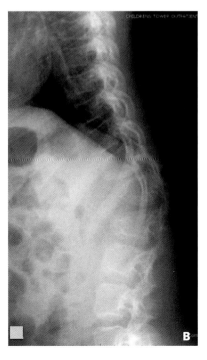

Figure 20-2 Anteroposterior (**A**) and lateral (**B**) spine radiographs of a child with achondroplasia demonstrate the interpediculate narrowing and short pedicles, most obvious in the lumbar spine. The lateral also demonstrates thoracolumbar kyphosis that may persist in children with achondroplasia.

Figure 20-3 A: Sagittal plane MRI of the upper cervical spine demonstrates narrowing of the spinal canal at the foramen magnum and C1 often seen in young children with achondroplasia. **B:** Foramen magnum decompression provides ample space for the spinal cord.

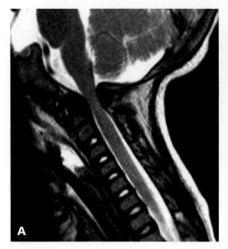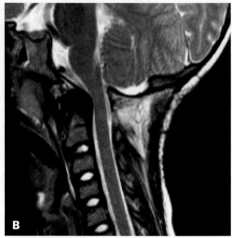

procedure in infancy. If the foramen magnum stenosis is severe enough (anterior *and* posterior impingement or cord signal change), neurosurgical decompression of the foramen magnum is considered. For asymptomatic stenosis, we know that over the first few years of life, there is a predictable enlargement of the foramen magnum relative to the spinal cord so that cord impingement becomes less of a problem by age 3 or so. Unless there is clear-cut and life-threatening respiratory compromise from this foraminal stenosis, it may be wiser to wait to see if mild sleep apnea and hypotonia resolve with time, without surgery.

Other medical issues are often present in early childhood, especially due to the mid-face hypoplasia present in achondroplasia. Respiratory function can be compromised not only by the foramen magnum stenosis, but also by a small thoracic cage and a redundant tissue in the retropharynx. Because of mid-face hypoplasia, drainage of the Eustachian tubes is impaired and otitis media is common. If unrecognized or not treated aggressively enough, these ear infections can result in significant, permanent hearing loss and delay in speech development.

KYPHOSIS

Spinal problems are common in achondroplasia. In infancy, there is nearly always a thoracolumbar kyphosis present, with the kyphosis accentuated clinically when the child is sitting. Independent walking generally does not take place until 18 to 24 months of age in achondroplasia, but the standing position seems to lead to resolution of this thoracolumbar kyphosis in about 90% of the children. As lumbar lordosis increases with standing and walking, sagittal plane balance occurs with improvement in the thoracolumbar kyphosis. Progression of deformity is associated with developmental motor delays or vertebral body wedging beyond that typically seen in achondroplasia. A fraction of these patients will develop symptomatic, fixed deformities requiring surgery. Clinical surveillance (with periodic plain radiographic imaging when concerned) is encouraged to monitor for progression to a symptomatic deformity requiring treatment. Persistence of kyphosis beyond childhood may lead to myelopathy, paraparesis, or back pain. With that said, the majority of thoracolumbar kyphoses occur below the level of the conus medullaris, and consequently the risk of spinal cord compression or other neurologic compromise in young children is extremely low. In older children and adolescents the presence of thoracolumbar kyphosis can exacerbate the symptoms of neurogenic claudication. Intervention for thoracolumbar kyphosis should be reserved for deformities that are progressive or symptomatic (i.e., neurological compromise or secondary muscular back pain). Bracing has not been proven effective. Published indications for surgery are for a thoracolumbar kyphosis exceeding 60° with more than 10° of progression in 1 year.

Successful treatment of symptomatic kyphosis relies on achievement of sagittal alignment at the site of correction and overall spinal balance. For less severe and more flexible deformities, such as those found in young children, isolated posterior fusion and instrumentation can be successful. However, surgical treatment in this group should be an uncommon occurrence.

Typically speaking, older children, adolescents, and adults with symptomatic deformities require a more aggressive surgical correction, using either an anteroposterior approach, or an all-posterior, posterior column shortening. The approach to achieve appropriate sagittal alignment and balance relies less on any prescribed recommendation, and more on the experience of the surgeon and the perceived risk of surgery in that surgeon's hands in attaining appropriate correction. Be aware that the risk of neurologic injury or dural tear is much higher in these patients because of the limited canal size.

The most common problem in achondroplasia is spinal stenosis, which can occur anywhere throughout the spine. It is most commonly symptomatic in the lumbar spine (Fig. 20-4). There is characteristic narrowing of the interpediculate distances in the coronal plane of the spinal canal and pedicle shortening on the sagittal plane. Spinal claudication signs and symptoms can occur at any age but are uncommon before the second decade. In children and adolescents, spinal stenosis is almost always associated with thoracolumbar kyphosis. For adults, spinal stenosis becomes increasingly a problem as degenerative changes occur, further narrowing the spinal canal and compressing either the cauda equina or the spinal cord. Multiple levels of compression may be present, so it is very important to evaluate lower extremity symptoms of spinal stenosis with a magnetic resonance image (MRI) of the *entire* spine.

> **THE GURU SAYS...**
> For young children with achondroplasia and progressive kyphosis, loss of intraoperative neuromonitoring signals is common, and surgical correction should be limited to 50% or less.
> VERNON T. TOLO

> **THE GURU SAYS...**
> Teenagers with achondroplasia who develop spinal stenosis symptoms usually assume a squatting position to increase lumbar spine capacity. Increased squatting time should be a trigger for obtaining a spinal MRI since this is usually associated with worsening spinal stenosis.
> VERNON T. TOLO

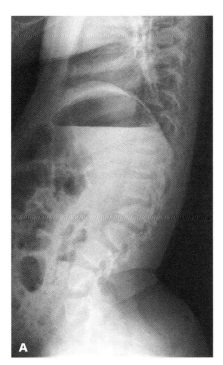
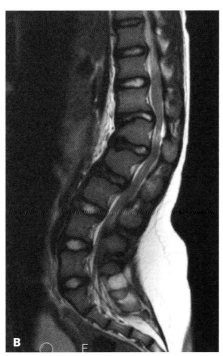
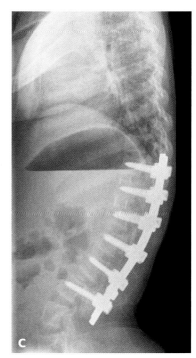

Figure 20-4 Persistent thoracolumbar kyphosis exacerbates spinal stenosis in adolescents with achondroplasia. A 13-year-old girl with neurogenic claudication and modest kyphosis (**A**) has multilevel stenosis (**B**), requiring decompression and instrumented fusion (**C**).

In general, decompression is needed over multiple levels, commonly T11 to S1, to relieve the lower extremity neurologic symptoms. Using a high-speed burr to transect the lamina adjacent to the facet and then lifting the lamina dorsally appears to be a safer technique of laminectomy than placing rongeurs within the tight spinal canal, but neurologic deficit as a complication of laminectomy is not rare, and dural tears occur in up to 40% of surgeries. Fusion is needed after multilevel laminectomy when there is persistent thoracolumbar kyphosis or skeletal immaturity. If thoracolumbar kyphosis is present in the area of laminectomy, this will worsen postlaminectomy. Since the pedicles are of adequate size to accept screw placement, pedicle screw instrumentation and posterior fusion at the time of the laminectomy is required to adequately treat this kyphosis. Placement of hooks into the canal is discouraged.

The most obvious orthopaedic concern to surface in achondroplasia is progressive bowing of the legs. In achondroplasia the fibula is longer than the tibia, and some degree of bowing is present in most with this condition. It is unclear why some get worse and some do not, but it is expected that about 20% of the tibiae in achondroplasia will at some point have corrective surgery. It is a curious finding that for older adults with achondroplasia and mild genu varum, medial compartment degenerative arthritis rarely occurs, and as such does not need to be treated prophylactically. The primary reasons for surgical correction, which usually is done between the ages of 4 and 12, are lateral leg pain with walking or running activity and the physical finding of a lateral thrust of the knee in early and mid-stance. Surgery may be needed in either the femur, the tibia, or both. Gait analysis studies have shown excellent improvement and normalization of gait parameters from this relatively simple proximal tibial/fibular valgus osteotomy. The need to repeat the tibial osteotomy at a later age is uncommon. Guided growth can be attempted at younger ages (<8 years). Because of slow growth in these patients, complete correction may take longer than generally expected (up to 3 years), or may not occur at all (Fig. 20-5).

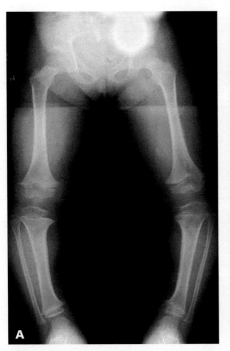
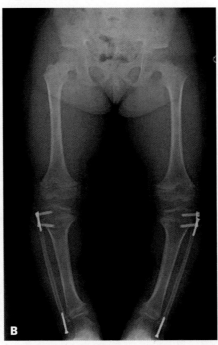
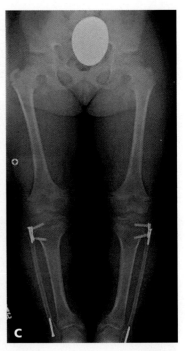

Figure 20-5 Varus deformity is usual in children with achondroplasia. Approximately 20% require surgical intervention for lower extremity symptoms such as pain or instability. In young children (<6 y), guided growth can be attempted, but correction is slow and often incomplete, as in this 5-year-old treated by guided growth of the tibia and fibula. **A:** Preoperative. **B:** One year postoperative. **C:** Three years postoperative.

Addressing the lateral distal femur, proximal tibia, and proximal fibula (by placing a cannulated screw across the growth plate) can be attempted. Older children are less likely to benefit from guided growth as a result of limited growth. In these patients, osteotomy is likely the better option.

The question of limb lengthening for stature in achondroplasia is a complicated discussion of medical and ethical concerns. There are certainly functional benefits that may be achieved with limb lengthening. Humeral lengthening for the achondroplastic dwarf can provide significant functional benefits and should be considered for any child unable to clasp their hands over their head. While adaptive equipment is available for perineal self-care and hygiene, in some individuals with achondroplasia independent self-care can be difficult to achieve with the severe rhizomelia of the arms. As for the lower extremities, one can point to real barriers to independence such as ability to reach counter surfaces, elevator buttons, bathroom sinks, and car accelerator and brake pedals. In Europe and East Asia, there is great enthusiasm for limb lengthening in achondroplasia, in which the femora and tibiae are lengthened up to 35 cm. In these instances, the humera also require lengthening so that the children can reach their feet. Keep in mind that limb lengthening generally takes about 1 month per 1 cm of lengthening, so that the whole process usually takes about 2 to 3 years of lengthening treatment. The Little People of America, the primary support group for patients with skeletal dysplasia in the United States, has not generally supported limb lengthening in achondroplasia, but have rather pushed for societal accommodations to short stature. In the case of children this often requires working with families and the patients' schools. The decision for or against limb lengthening is one the individual family and patient has to make, but the orthopaedist should be able to present the pros and cons objectively to help them form this decision. It should be remembered that the quality of life of achondroplastic individuals is the same as that of average-sized people up to about age 40, at which time the quality of life in achondroplasia deteriorates due to a higher incidence of back pain and symptomatic spinal stenosis, not because of short stature.

Pseudoachondroplasia

As the name would imply, the body proportions of this dysplasia are similar to those seen with achondroplasia; however the genetic defect and clinical manifestations are completely different. The genetic defect for pseudoachondroplasia is in cartilage oligomeric matrix protein (COMP), an important trafficking protein in both growth plate and articular cartilage. In contrast to achondroplasia, the head size is normal, excessive joint laxity is a hallmark, and precocious arthritis is expected. The most common spine problem is atlantoaxial instability, which may require fusion in some. While kyphosis and, more commonly, scoliosis can occur in pseudoachondroplasia, foramen magnum and spinal stenosis are *not* seen.

On a lateral spinal X-ray, there is a characteristic vertebral body shape with a mid-vertebral anterior projection, which is absent in achondroplasia, and is essentially diagnostic for this condition (Fig. 20-6A). Radiographs of the long bones show abnormalities in both the epiphyses and metaphyses (Fig. 20-6B). Varus and valgus alignment of the lower extremities are equally common, and a wind-swept deformity is not unusual.

Realignment surgery is difficult due to the joint laxity and the delayed ossification of the epiphyses, which makes the joint level difficult to see without

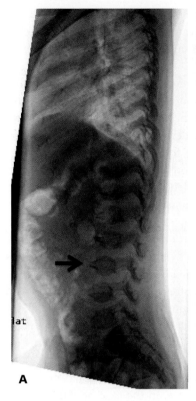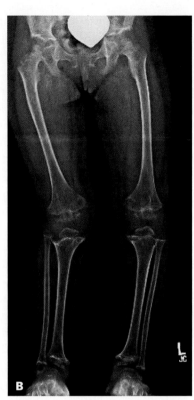

Figure 20-6
Pseudoachondroplasia can be readily recognized by the squared, mid-body anterior projection seen in the lumbar spine (arrow in **A**) and the profound epiphyseal dysplasia and often wind-swept deformity seen in the lower extremities (**B**).

concomitant arthrography. Recurrence of deformity is common. Guided growth may need repeated attempts, with efficacy diminishing with age. The goal is to keep lower extremity alignment as normal as possible with the expectation of realignment osteotomies at skeletal maturity. The hips tend to slowly subluxate and become arthritic, and commonly require total hip arthroplasty in early adult life.

Spondyloepiphyseal Dysplasia Congenita

There are two types of spondyloepiphyseal dysplasia (SED), and they are very distinct from one another. SED congenita is one variation of the type II collagen disorders which also includes forms of Stickler syndrome, Kniest dysplasia, and hypochondrogenesis. SED tarda results from mutations in the SEDL gene, affects only males, and is generally not diagnosed until preadolescence, when degenerative arthritis of the hips begins to develop.

Individuals with SED tarda are typically over 5 feet tall and their diagnosis is usually delayed, while those with SED congenita are very short and usually have the diagnosis made in infancy.

Orthopaedic problems are more widely seen in SED congenita. The trunk is short and X-rays show delayed epiphyseal ossification and platyspondyly. Angular deformity of the knees (primarily genu valgum) may develop with growth. Walking will occur but may be somewhat delayed and characteristically is associated with an external foot progression and accentuated lumbar lordosis, as a result of coxa vara. Abductor fatigue pain is commonly reported as well. Valgus-extension osteotomy of the proximal femur with internal rotation is often very useful in late childhood to improve the gait and trunk position (Fig. 20-7).

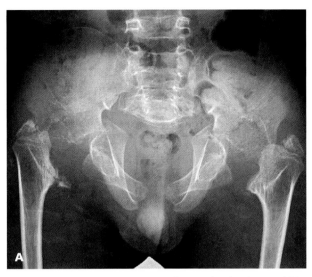
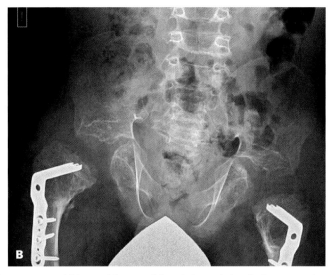

Figure 20-7 Anteroposterior radiograph of pelvis and hips in a 6-year-old boy with spondyloepiphyseal dysplasia congenita demonstrates the marked coxa vara (**A**) and delayed epiphyseal ossification typical of this condition and commonly requiring proximal femoral valgus-extention-internal rotation osteotomy (**B**).

The most common orthopaedic condition needing early treatment is genu valgum, which can be treated by guided growth. Upper cervical spine instability and associated odontoid hypoplasia occur to some degree in many patients with SED congenita and may be seen as young as 1 year of age. Since vertebral ossification is delayed in this condition, the use of flexion/extension MRIs of the cervical spine is useful periodically over the first 10 years of life to assess most accurately the possible need for upper cervical fusion to protect from spinal cord from injury. If instability is demonstrated, posterior occiput to C2 fusion, immobilized in a halo when necessary, is effective treatment (Fig. 20-8).

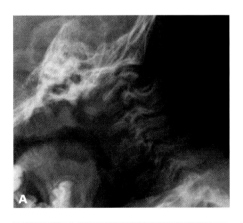
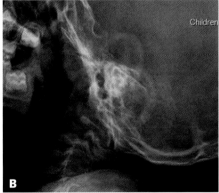
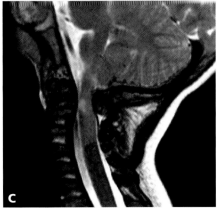
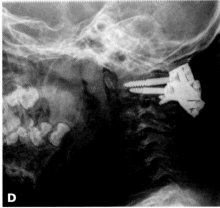

Figure 20-8 A: Lateral flexion radiograph of upper cervical spine in child with spondyloepiphyseal dysplasia congenita demonstrates odontoid hypoplasia and anterior subluxation (arrow) of C1 on C2. **B:** C1 reduces on extension lateral. **C:** Sagittal MRI view of upper cervical spine this 3 year old child demonstrates odontoid hypoplasia and signal changes within the upper cervical spinal cord characteristic of significant C1-C2 instability requiring posterior fusion stabilization. **D:** Lateral cervical spine radiograph obtained 2 y postoperatively illustrates one technique to provide stabilization and fusion for this condition. In younger children, a halo is routinely applied to facilitate fusion.

Mucopolysaccharidoses

The mucopolysaccharidoses (MPS) are a family of lysosomal storage disorders in which specific enzyme deficiencies result in failure of glycosaminoglycan (GAG, formerly mucopolysaccharides) metabolism. Progressive accumulation of these normal cell byproducts results in significant cellular dysfunction, and in all forms of MPS, some degree of skeletal dysplasia. There are seven main types of MPS syndromes. Individually each of these syndromes is rare, but combined the MPS syndromes are as common as other conditions familiar to the orthopaedist, such as muscular dystrophy and spinal muscular atrophy.

Hurler syndrome is the most severe form of MPS type I (MPS I-H). Scheie (formerly type V, now I-S) is the more attenuated form of type I, while Hurler-Scheie is the eponym applied to those with an intermediate phenotype. The other MPS syndromes include Hunter (type II), Sanfilippo (type III), Morquio (type IV), Maroteaux-Lamy (type VI), and Sly (type VII). While all of these have individual differences that are beyond the scope of this chapter, all can have some degrees of occipital-cervical stenosis or instability, thoracolumbar kyphosis, early degenerative hip disease, genu valgum, or carpal tunnel syndrome. Morquio syndrome is probably the most common of these conditions to be seen by the orthopaedist.

The biggest pitfall for orthopaedists in these patients is the failure to recognize and diagnose the condition. Some of the early signs of MPS are developmental delay, generalized joint stiffness even in the fingers, corneal clouding, inguinal and umbilical hernias, and upper respiratory infections. Musculoskeletal abnormalities, such as a gibbus deformity (>90% of children with Hurler syndrome) or bilateral Perthes disease, are often the presenting symptoms for MPS patients and should be considered red flags for diagnosis (Fig. 20-9). A child with more mild forms of MPS may not be as obvious as those with more extensive involvement, and diagnosis may be further delayed.

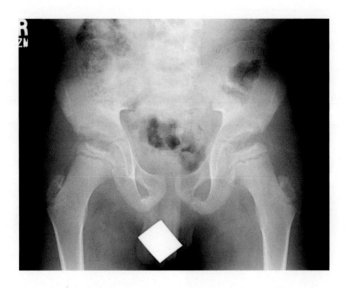

Figure 20-9 Anteroposterior radiograph of the pelvis demonstrates bilateral Perthes-like changes to the proximal femoral epiphyses that often lead to the diagnosis of MPS (mucopolysaccharidoses), as in this 9-year-old boy with MPS IV (Morquio syndrome).

The importance of early diagnosis cannot be overemphasized, as long-term outcomes are largely dictated by the age at which medical therapies are initiated. In the case of Hurler syndrome, the results of hematopoietic stem cell transplant (HCST) are much better if treatment is initiated prior to 2 years of age. Although the benefits to many organ systems are greatly realized by early treatment with HCST or enzyme replacement therapy, orthopaedic abnormalities of this condition still often need ongoing follow-up and surgical treatment.

In infancy or toddler age, children with MPS may present to the orthopaedist because of a "bump" in the back. A lateral spinal radiograph that you take will show a thoracolumbar kyphosis with anterior deficiency of the vertebral body or bodies, often mistaken for congenital kyphosis.

For Hurler, Hunter, and Maroteaux-Lamy syndromes, this deficiency is typically limited to the L1 or L2 vertebrae. In Morquio syndrome, the apical vertebrae of the kyphosis (usually T12-L1)—as well as several adjacent vertebrae—will have a vertebral body projection that extends anteriorly from the inferior aspect of the vertebra; this is not seen in nonsyndromic congenital kyphosis.

If MPS is suspected, the simplest test is a quantitative urine assay for GAGs. Importantly, urine GAG sensitivity decreases with age, so children who are older, typically with milder disease, will have normal levels of urine GAGs. If MPS is truly suspected, a blood test for leukocyte enzyme activity should always be pursued. Radiographic findings are also helpful in establishing a diagnosis. Common findings include odontoid hypoplasia, a shallow sella turcica, platyspondyly, wide ribs, tapering of the ilium, acetabular dysplasia, and "bullet-shaped" metacarpals. In older children, abnormal femoral head ossification, often mistaken for bilateral Perthes disease, may be present.

Surgical management is commonly required for patients with MPS. For Morquio syndrome, particularly in its classic manifestation, spinal cord compression from cervical instability is common, but not universal. Children with myelopathy, significant instability or cord signal change on MRI should be considered surgical candidates. Hip dysplasia is common and progresses in Hurler and Morquio syndrome and may benefit from surgical reconstruction in childhood or custom total hip arthroplasty in adulthood. Genu valgum is very responsive to guided growth techniques in younger children (<8 years), but due to diminished growth potential in older children becomes less effective with age.

Regular nerve conduction studies for carpal tunnel syndrome are recommended, and carpal tunnel releases should be performed when any evidence of reduced nerve conduction is present.

Even though the abnormal thoracolumbar kyphosis present in infancy may be the first reason for orthopaedic consultation, surgical treatment is not always needed for this, as this kyphosis may never progress from that seen at birth. Bracing has not been proven to be effective and, if there is no kyphosis progression, treatment is not necessarily needed. Neurologic deficit is rare with this deformity. If there is kyphosis progression, particularly with MRI evidence of spinal cord or cauda equina compression, spinal instrumentation and fusion is effective. Effective treatment requires adequate deformity correction that can be accomplished through both combined anterior/posterior approaches or all-posterior approaches with osteotomies (Fig. 20-11).

THE GURU SAYS...

In my experience, the most common reason an infant with MPS is seen by an orthopaedist is because of the thoracolumbar kyphosis. It is essential for early MPS diagnosis and treatment to correctly differentiate the MPS vertebral body with an inferior anterior projection at more than one level from congenital kyphosis usually seen at one level (Fig. 20-10).

VERNON T. TOLO

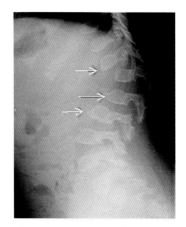

Figure 20-10 Lateral spine X-ray of a 19-month-old with MPS (mucopolysaccharidoses). Note the inferior anterior vertebral projection on multiple vertebrae (arrows). This is different from congenital kyphosis, which typically involves one vertebra.

THE GURU SAYS...

When osteotomy is needed to correct genu valgum, for me distal femoral varus osteotomy, rather than proximal tibial varus osteotomy, is associated with less chance of recurrence of valgus deformity.

VERNON T. TOLO

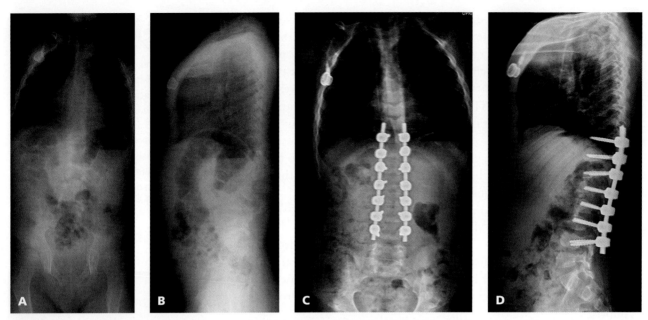

Figure 20-11 Thoracolumbar kyphosis is found in over 90% of children with MPS 1H (Hurler syndrome). Progressive deformity beyond 70° (**A, B**), as seen in this 5-year-old boy, can be treated by combined anterior discectomy and fusion and posterior instrumented fusion (**C, D**). All-posterior approach is advocated by some authors.

Diastrophic Dysplasia

A rarer dysplasia, but one with many orthopaedic manifestations, diastrophic dysplasia (DTD) is recognizable at birth and results from a defect in diastrophic dysplasia sulfate transporter (*SLC26A* gene). Characteristic features include very short extremities, hand differences including the classic hitchhiker's thumb and stiff IP joints (Fig. 20-12), severe club feet, and, within a few weeks of birth, external ear cysts which develop into "cauliflower ears." About 25% have an associated cleft palate. Intelligence is normal.

Several body segments have orthopaedic-related abnormalities. Starting at the top, the cervical spine often has cervical kyphosis at a young age, though most will be resolved with growth and age. If this kyphosis is progressive, associated myelopathy can be fatal if untreated and requires aggressive treatment and fusion if progression is proven. Flexion/extension MRI can be useful to assess the cervical kyphosis on a serial basis and to evaluate possible need for surgical treatment. In the thoracic spine, the primary problem is the development of progressive mid-thoracic kyphoscoliosis, simulating a severe congenital scoliosis, which occurs in about 30% of these children and always is noted before the age of 4. These severe deformities can be controlled with growth-friendly techniques in younger children, facilitating chest growth until 9 or 10 years of age, after which definitive fusion is appropriate. Another 30% to 40% develop lesser degrees of scoliosis, many of which do not require treatment. Definitive fusion may be proceeded by thoracoscopic anterior release, halo-gravity traction, and staged posterior fusion with osteotomies when needed (Fig. 20-13).

There usually is no treatment for the hand deformities present. The IP joints of all fingers are stiff and usually immobile, but the MP joints move normally. Hand function is adequate but without good power grip, due both to the IP stiffness and the thumb deformity.

Casting for clubfoot may result in limited correction. Equinus deformity tends to be recalcitrant and persists. Even with attempted correction of clubfoot

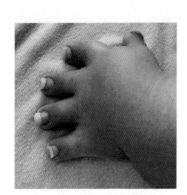

Figure 20-12 The hand of a child with diastrophic dysplasia demonstrates the "hitchhiker's thumb" and stiff interphalangeal joints characteristic of this condition.

THE GURU SAYS...

Despite the severe thoracic kyphoscoliosis that may develop, neurologic deficits are very uncommon unless over-aggressive surgical correction of these stiff curves results in iatrogenic neurologic problems.

VERNON T. TOLO

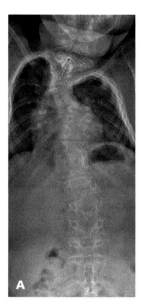 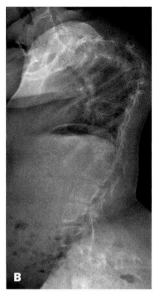 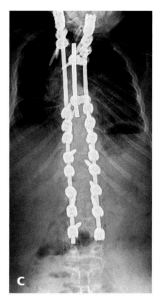 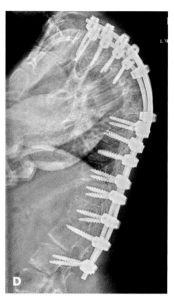

Figure 20-13 A, B: Progressive kyphoscoliosis is common in children with diastrophic dysplasia. Rigid kyphosis in children with skeletal dysplasia responds well to staged anterior thoracoscopic release, halo-gravity traction, and posterior instrumented fusion. **C, D:** Pedicle subtraction osteotomy was abandoned in this case due to intraoperative neurological changes (common in diastrophic dysplasia), but a reasonable outcome was obtained nonetheless.

deformities, many adults with DTD are unable to place their heels on the ground. Thus, they stand solely on their metatarsals and toes and function well with accommodating shoe wear. Typically, the adult with classic DTD stands on his toes with knee and hip flexion deformities and marked lumbar lordosis with limited ambulatory ability. In the rare absence of flexion deformities of the knees and hips, flexion osteotomy of the distal tibia may be indicated to create a plantigrade foot.

Flexion contractures at the knee and hip are also present from birth. Treatment of lateral patellar subluxation has been recommended by some. Early treatment of patellar subluxation may slow flexion deformity progression of the knee and consequently improve and extend ambulatory status in children with DTD. In my experience treatment of patellar subluxation is of little long-term functional benefit. Hip flexion contractures can usually be accommodated and tendon release shouldn't be needed. By early adult life, lateral hip subluxation and degenerative arthritis of the hip may be improved markedly with custom-sized total hip arthroplasty.

Individuals with DTD are able to walk, but are functionally household ambulators. Use of a walker is often required, but prescription of a motorized scooter for longer distances is of greatest benefit. The maintenance of household ambulation improves independence for these individuals, and this should be a goal in the orthopaedic treatment of these patients.

Staying Out of Trouble With Skeletal Dysplasias

✳ Skeletal dysplasias generally will present with disproportion and height below the third percentile.

✳ Physical exam can determine whether limbs or spine or both are involved most.

✳ X-ray skeletal survey can determine whether epiphysis, metaphysis, and spine are involved, which often allows a differential diagnosis.

THE GURU SAYS...

With surgical treatment for the clubfoot and equinus, it is mandatory to have the foot fully plantigrade at the end of the surgery. This may include splitting the syndesmotic ligament to better seat the talus, but hoping to complete correction by postoperative casting will not work.

VERNON T. TOLO

THE GURU SAYS...

Complete lateral dislocation of the patella can be a major factor in knee flexion contracture here. Surgical relocation and muscle balancing can improve knee flexion and leg stability. Diagnosis of patellar dislocation is by ultrasound as the patella is thin and flat and is often difficult to palpate.

VERNON T. TOLO

(continued)

Staying Out of Trouble With Skeletal Dysplasias *(continued)*

✳ Diagnosis can be established by the orthopaedist, but must be confirmed by a geneticist.

✳ Knowledge of the natural history of specific conditions, and what to expect from the orthopaedic abnormalities over time, is critical to surgical decision making.

✳ Early recognition of genetic skeletal disorder helps both the family to obtain genetic information and counseling and the child to receive care.

✳ Because of the rarity of these conditions, it is usually best to refer these children to a pediatric orthopaedic center for ongoing care.

FOR FURTHER ENLIGHTENMENT

Bayhan IA, Abousamra O, Rogers KJ, et al. Valgus hip osteotomy in children with spondyloepiphyseal dysplasia congenita: midterm results. *J Pediatr Orthop*. 2019;39(6):282-288.

Ngo AV, Thapa M, Otjen J, Kamps SE. Skeletal dysplasias: radiologic approach with common and notable entities. *Semin Musculoskelet Radiol*. 2018;22(1):66-80.

Solanki GA, Martin KW, Theroux MC, et al. Spinal involvement in mucopolysaccharidosis IVA (Morquio-Brailsford or Morquio A syndrome): presentation, diagnosis and management. *J Inherit Metab Dis*. 2013;36(2):339-355.

White KK, Bompadre V, Goldberg MJ, et al. Skeletal Dysplasia Management Consortium. Best practices in peri-operative management of patients with skeletal dysplasia. *Am J Med Genet A*. 2017;173(10):2584-2595.

White KK, Bompadre V, Shah SA, et al. Early-onset spinal deformity in skeletal dysplasias: a multicenter study of growth-friendly systems. *Spine Deform*. 2018;6(4):478-482.

Yilmaz G, Oto M, Thabet AM, et al. Correction of lower extremity angular deformities in skeletal dysplasia with hemiepiphysiodesis: a preliminary report. *J Pediatr Orthop*. 2014;34(3):336-345.

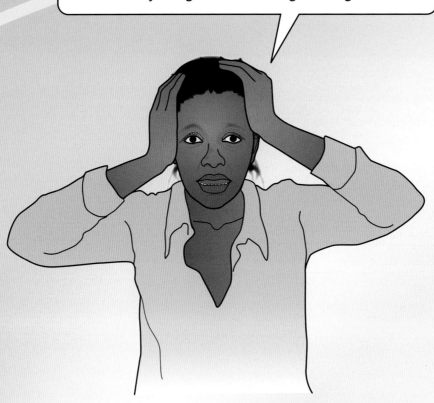

Chapter 21

Spine I: Early-Onset Scoliosis

MICHAEL G. VITALE, MD, MPH, DAVID L. SKAGGS, MD, MMM, and JOHN M. (JACK) FLYNN, MD

Gurus: Suken A. Shah, MD and Lindsay Andras, MD

Early-onset scoliosis (EOS) presents many opportunities for trouble in diagnosis and treatment, even in the most experienced hands. Defined as the development of scoliosis before the age of 10 years,[1] EOS is associated with four general etiologies: congenital or structural, syndromic, neuromuscular, and idiopathic. Remember the most important factors for making decisions about how best to treat children with EOS are the age of the child and the rate of progression. One may observe a 60° curve or even larger curves in young children if progression is very slow. On the other hand, if a curve progresses rapidly and repeatedly, it may be time to intervene even in smaller curves.

EOS is different from adolescent scoliosis because of the relationship between lung development and spinal deformity. Spine deformity in young children can negatively affect lung development and function. Young children with large curves can develop severe respiratory issues that may affect quality and even quantity of life. We all have seen the graph showing how children with severe EOS have decreased life expectancy as they age. Knowing that natural history is often not great, a number of strategies have been developed to try to improve outcomes in these kids, although complications of treatment remain a challenge.[2-6]

As observation of a severe and progressive curve is likely to lead to a bad outcome, we face pressure to "do something." In the past, spine fusion for young children with EOS led to a straight spine, and X-rays surgeons could be proud of. Unfortunately, early fusion also led to a thoracic spine, thorax, and lungs that were stunted in growth. As one could imagine, early fusion of the thoracic spine drastically hurts pulmonary function and is not recommended. "Growth-friendly" techniques such as distraction-based growing rods that are periodically lengthened offer the hope of promoting growth while controlling scoliosis. Unfortunately, we have discovered that anytime metal is put over a long segment of a child's spine, spontaneous fusion is highly likely at somewhere around 5 years after implantation. In addition, growth-friendly techniques do not prevent crankshaft phenomenon, which makes sense if they slow the posterior growth but not the anterior growth. After seeing the problems that occur in these kids over time, many experienced (humbled) EOS surgeons temper expectations of families and surgeons.

Idiopathic Early-Onset Scoliosis

Infantile idiopathic scoliosis (IIS) describes that group of children generally diagnosed within the first 18 months of life, where no other cause is known. Our job in presumed idiopathic EOS is to make certain that there is no underlying cause of the EOS. Truly idiopathic EOS is a diagnosis of exclusion. This means a careful history and physical examination, close inspection of X-rays to look for subtle congenital differences, and in most cases, a screening MRI to rule out underlying intraspinal anomalies. Any change in the skin over the spine (hairy patch, significant dimple above the gluteal cleft, birthmark) should be a warning sign about a potential change underneath as well, prompting an MRI[7] (Fig. 21-1).

When ordering an MRI of the cervical, thoracic, and lumbar spine for EOS, consider ordering limited sequences of only sagittal T1 and T2. This saves lots of time in the MRI, which may reduce anesthesia time in this at-risk population, with no loss in sensitivity.[8]

While progression may be the most important variable affecting the need for treatment, be aware that there can be some "false progression" in X-rays when children transition from lying down or sitting to standing radiographs. X-rays are really comparable only when performed in the same position, and the "clock

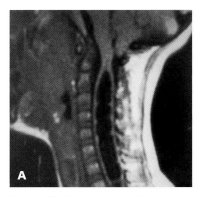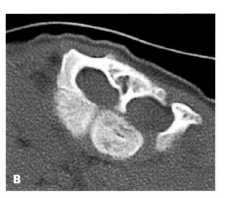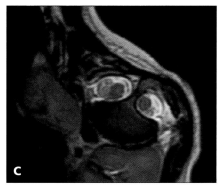

Figure 21-1 Examples of common spinal dysraphism seen in some children with early-onset scoliosis. **A:** MRI demonstrating a large cervical syrinx with Arnold Chiari malformation. **B, C:** CT and MRI, respectively, demonstrating diastematomyelia (split cord malformation).

resets" when the first erect (sitting or standing) X-ray is taken. Warn parents about this to allay anxiety before the first erect X-ray.

Children with idiopathic EOS under age 2 have a roughly 85% chance of spontaneous resolution within the first 18 months of life, and close observation is generally the most appropriate initial treatment. Mehta showed that children with a rib-vertebral angle difference (RVAD) greater than 20° and curves greater than 20° demonstrated higher rates of progression[9] (Fig. 21-2). For patients who show continued progression past 12 to 15 months of age, MRI is obtained to rule out spinal dysraphism.

Congenital Scoliosis

Congenital scoliosis is classified as either a failure of formation (hemivertebra and wedge vertebra) or a failure of segmentation (block vertebra and unilateral bar) or both. If the hemivertebra has growth plates, it is called "segmented" and this

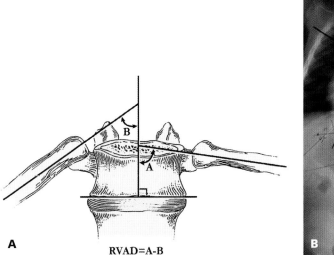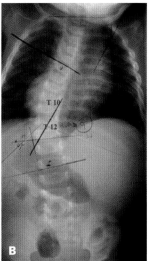

RVAD=A-B

Figure 21-2 A: Measurement of Mehta's rib-vertebral angle difference (RVAD) can be calculated by subtracting the convex value (**B**) from the concave value (**A**) at the apical vertebra of a thoracic curve. **B:** X-ray showing small RVAD in a patient with idiopathic infantile scoliosis. RVAD less than 20° predicts a higher likelihood of spontaneous resolution of the scoliosis. (A: Adapted with permission from Lenke LG, Dobbs MB. Idiopathic scoliosis. In: Frymoyer JW, Wiesel SW, eds. *The Adult and Pediatric Spine.* 3rd ed. Philadelphia, PA: Lippincott Williams & Wilkins; 2004:337-361. Figure 15-3.)

generally has a higher chance of progression. Highest rates of progression are seen with fully segmented hemivertebra (both growth plates intact), especially opposite a contralateral bar. Hemivertebra in the lumbosacral junction causes significant deformity, affecting the overall balance of the spine. This often requires surgical treatment.

The mesodermal layer that is responsible for vertebral body formation is also responsible for the urogenital, cardiac, and pulmonary systems. Perhaps because of this, there is approximately a 15% chance of a cardiac abnormality or renal abnormality in children with congenital scoliosis. Consider a cardiac echo and renal ultrasound in every child with congenital scoliosis. Spinal dysraphism (most commonly a tethered cord or Chiari malformation and less commonly a diastematomyelia) can be present in up to a third of patients with congenital spinal anomalies. An MRI requires general anesthesia in young children, so the downside of anesthesia to the developing brain must be considered. As long as there is no significant progression, or neurologic signs or symptoms, one may delay the MRI as long as there is regular assessment, but it should always be done before surgery, if there are signs or symptoms of neurologic problems, or a curve is rapidly progressive.[10]

TREATMENT

In general, we prefer to stall surgical treatment unless progression is constant and obvious and curves are greater than 50°, or an overall deformity is significantly progressing, such as a hemivertebra above the sacrum. In children less than 2 years of age, bone quality is so soft that anchors can plow through the bone, which can make intraoperative correction challenging, as well as lead to postoperative loss of fixation. Unsegmented vertebra generally demonstrates lower rates of progression, and surgery can often be delayed.

One of the few times surgical intervention is indicated immediately in the young child is in cases of a fully segmented hemivertebra opposite a unilateral bar. (This is a frequent test question.) We know this will progress, and we should prevent it from getting too much worse. If the child is too young and vertebrae too weak for a resection, consider a fusion in situ with cervical implants. You can always come back later and do a resection.

The precise anatomy of congenital scoliosis can be unclear. A CT scan can be very helpful in planning the surgical approach (sometimes with 3D model fabrication). When ordering CT scans in small children, make sure to limit the levels to the area of interest to decrease radiation. In an isolated hemivertebra, we generally perform a complete excision with limited two-level fusion (Fig. 21-3). Results are generally good although the chance of future surgery (generally related to progression above or below the limited fusion) has been reported to be up to 40%, especially in younger children. If a hemivertebra resection is performed, it is important to do a complete resection in all planes and to obtain as much segmental correction as possible. Hooks are sometimes used as an adjunct to obtain correction given the poor quality of pedicle bone.

A technical trick for closing a wedge after removing a thoracic hemivertebra is to place rib hooks above and below the removed segment, and compress the rib anchors, not the spine anchors (Fig. 21-4). Another option is to share the load with both pedicle screws and laminar hooks above and below the removed hemivertebrae. In young kids, laminar hooks often seem to plow less than pedicle screws. Instrumented hemiepiphysiodesis has been used in more extensive anomalies with reasonable, but with mixed results.

THE GURU SAYS...

If the congenital scoliosis is diagnosed before 3 months of age, a spinal ultrasound can be used to evaluate for a tethered cord and does not require anesthesia.

SUKEN SHAH

THE GURU SAYS...

Pay attention to the compensatory (noncongenital curves) also. Progression in these areas with coronal imbalance can be an indication to act on the congenital segment surgically.

SUKEN SHAH

THE GURU SAYS...

Various approaches to congenital hemivertebra are available, with the posterior approach the most popular, but what is most important is complete excision of the abnormal bone and disk on either side to get full correction and complete fusion. This can be your best chance to get a cure for a big problem with a short-segment procedure.

SUKEN SHAH

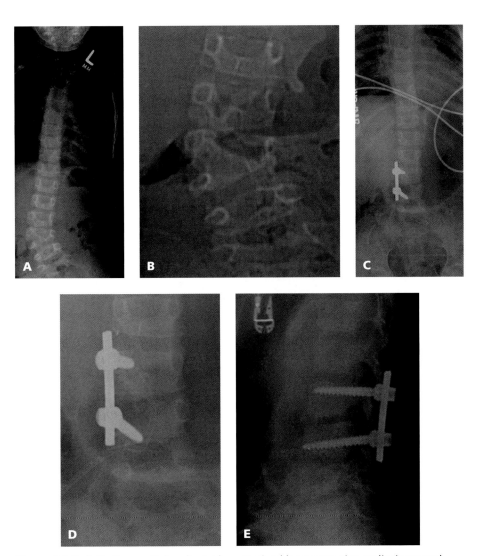

Figure 21-3 A, B: Congenital scoliosis characterized by progressive scoliosis around semisegmented hemivertebra. **C, D:** Treated with isolated hemivertebra resection with instrumentation. Bilateral instrumentation is more often used in most constructs. Complete resection of the hemivertebra is important to get correction, balance, and fusion.

Traditional growing rods and, more recently, the MAGEC (MAGnetic Externally Controlled growing rod) growing rod are a more common treatment option to control a large segment of spine with multiple congenital anomalies (Fig. 21-5). With growing rods, fusion is historically performed when skeletal maturity nears, though there is some thought that formal fusion might be avoided in "graduates" of growing systems. Anytime we put metal in the child's spine, we start a process of slow fusion over a course of about 5 years, so it's really best to prolong intervention when possible.

Congenital kyphosis can progress quite rapidly, especially when related to failure of anterior formation. This is most often a diagnosis that requires surgical intervention. Have a healthy respect for congenital kyphosis. These are the kids at highest risk of paralysis, with or without surgery. In these cases, a posterior fusion done earlier can help forestall rapid progression, complications, and larger, higher risk surgeries at a later date. Again, reoperations rates are high and this needs to be discussed with parents to keep us out of trouble if and when reoperation is necessary.

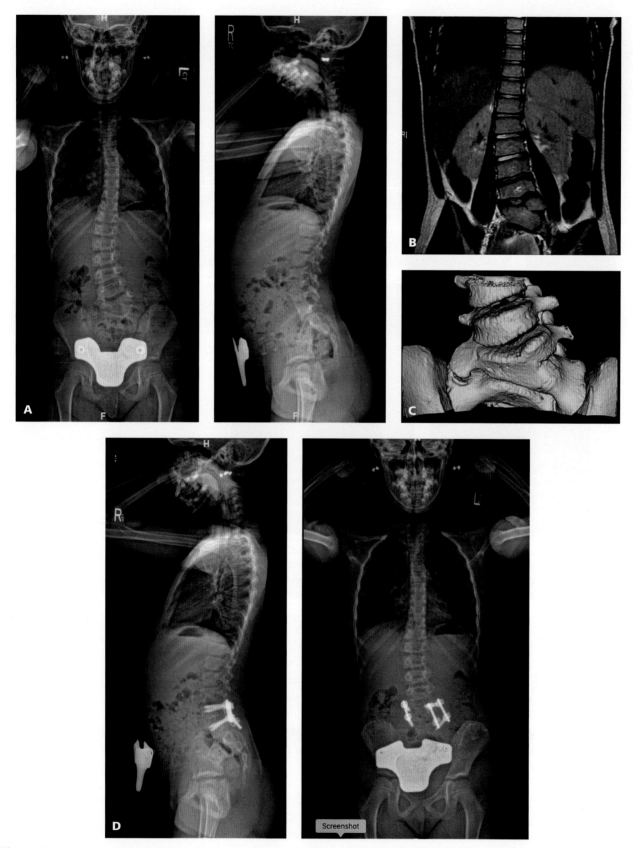

Figure 21-4 A 7-year-old girl with early-onset scoliosis with radiographs (**A**), MRI (**B**), and CT scan (**C**) demonstrating L5A left hemivertebra. This segmented hemivertebra was progressive and caused significant trunk shift. **D:** Postoperative imaging 2 y after hemivertebral resection and L5-S1 fusion. Midline supplemental hook construct was used to assist in closing the osteotomy gap without risking screw plow.

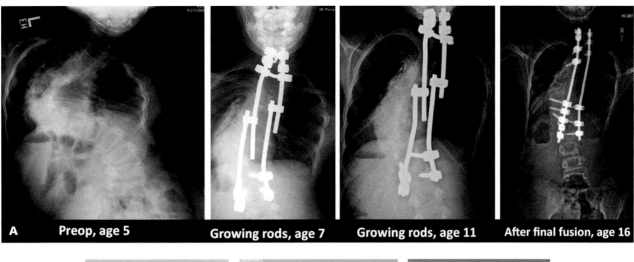

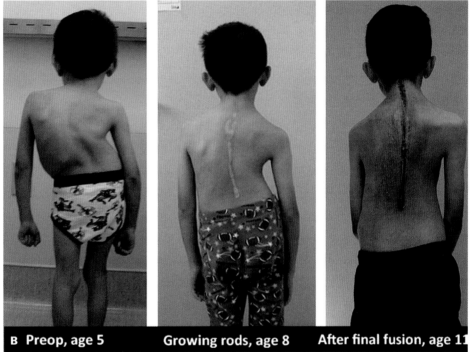

Figure 21-5 Use of a growing rod to treat large complex congenital scoliosis resulting from multiple hemivertebrae opposite bar. Preoperative curve was 137° at 5 y of age. Radiographs (**A**) and photos (**B**) show follow-up until 16 y of age, 5 y after fusion.

NEUROMUSCULAR EARLY-ONSET SCOLIOSIS

There are numerous neuromuscular disorders that result in neuromuscular EOS. Neuromuscular scoliosis is often a long, sweeping, C-shaped curve at times with pelvic obliquity. Children with spinal cord dysraphism may experience improvement in the scoliosis once the spinal cord issue is treated (detethering or decompression of the Arnold Chiari formation), especially when the curve is less than 35°.

Cerebral palsy is the most common cause of neuromuscular scoliosis; comorbidities and high tone in these children present challenges to scoliosis treatment. Optimization of preoperative comorbidities and nutrition is paramount in these kids, and we often employ a plastic surgeon to optimize closure in these fragile children who may undergo multiple spinal surgeries. In children younger than about 8 years with progressive scoliosis greater than 50° to 70°, "growth-friendly" surgery can be considered. Be aware that you are entering into a "contract" with the family where both parties need to be realistic about the relatively high rate of complications and have realistic expectations. S or U hooks are sometimes used for pelvic fixation in the very young or medically fragile patient as they are relatively minimally invasive to insert. However, if significant pelvic obliquity is present, a formal fusion at the caudal base of the construct consisting of screws at L4, L5, S1, and S2AI is effective and perhaps a better option.

Children with low tone include those with spinal muscular atrophy (SMA), and there are some special considerations in treating this group of children. With the advent of Spinraza and other medications in development that may need to be given intrathecally, it is important to consider options to allow continued intrathecal drug delivery after fusion. While catheters and pumps are in development for this purpose, our practice has been to "skip" one or two levels or doing a laminectomy and "marking" the area with a "C-ring" or other implant visible on X-ray when doing a fusion in patients with SMA (Fig. 21-6). Rib fixation in these children has the theoretical advantage of propping up the ribs and potentially slowing the parasol deformity (Fig. 21-7).

Syndromic Early-Onset Scoliosis

Syndromic EOS is related to a genetic anomaly and comorbidities are common. The following list of syndromes responsible for EOS has some tips to stay out of trouble.

Arthrogryposis: Scoliosis develops in only a subset of patients with this heterogenous disorder, but it can involve very stiff curves and can progress rapidly. Growing strategies can be a challenge, and these kids may benefit from fusion somewhat earlier than other children.

Neurofibromatosis: Some of the most challenging patients with EOS. Can progress very quickly with sharp, short-segment deformity with dramatic rotation. Pedicle fixation can present great challenges and vertebral body screws can be a salvage. MRI/CT to assess rib intrusion into spinal canal and presence of neurofibroma in spinal canal important. In neurofibromatosis, because of the potential for such rapid worsening, and disappearance of pedicles over time, consider early fusion. A "one and done" for a 70° kyphoscoliosis at age 8 is likely better than dealing with a 100° deformity with no pedicles 3 years later. Because the bone is weak, consider preoperative traction, and even postoperative halo vest for upper thoracic curves.

Marfan syndrome: Flexible curves that can progress rapidly. Good candidates for growing strategies though can add on above/below constructs. Need workup to include aortic ultrasound.

Osteogenesis imperfecta: Terrible bone quality requires higher density growing constructs. Consider staging surgery to allow anchor sites to fuse prior to insertion of growing rods.

Achondroplasia: Thoracolumbar kyphosis most often resolves without active treatment. Spinal stenosis is a major issue in quality of life and decompression sometimes necessary.

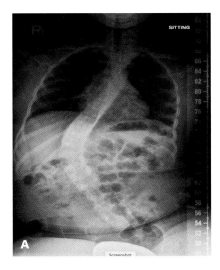
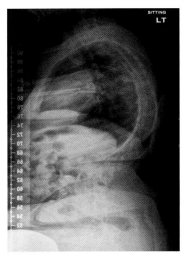
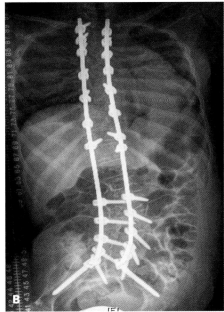
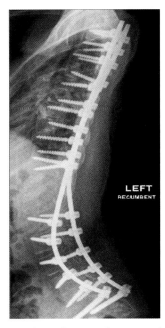
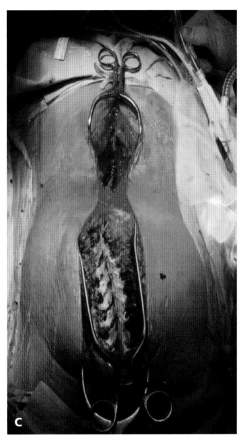

Figure 21-6 A: A 12-year-old with progressive kyphoscoliosis and type 2 spinal muscular atrophy (SMA), undergoing intrathecal injection of nusinersen (Spinraza). **B:** Postoperative X-rays showing fusion from T2 to pelvic "skipping" L1 and L2 levels to allow continued intrathecal injections. Other pharmacological treatments will likely require intrathecal injection and this must be considered when planning definitive fusion in patients with SMA. **C:** Intraoperative photo showing how two levels are not exposed nor decorticated to allow future delivery of drug. Rods are tunneled submuscularly at this level. (Courtesy Michael Vitale, MD; Columbia University Medical Center.)

Nonoperative Treatment

While most parents hope that stretching or therapy will help EOS, there is no good evidence that it does. Mehta style casting (also known as elongation, derotation, flexion casting) can be helpful to decrease and even potentially fully resolve the curve in some patients. Mehta casting is technique dependent, and usually requires multiple cast changes under anesthesia at roughly 2-month intervals.[9] Just as with clubfoot casting, success of Mehta casting requires fastidious attention to details of casting.

Even if casting does not "cure" the scoliosis, slowing progression and delaying surgery has significant benefits. After about 5 years of growing rods, spontaneous

> **THE GURU SAYS...**
>
> The length of time for each cast is determined by how fast the child is growing and how successful the parents are with keeping the cast clean. A good rule of thumb is 2 months for 2 year olds, 3 months for 3 year olds, and 4 months for 4 or over.
>
> LINDSAY ANDRAS

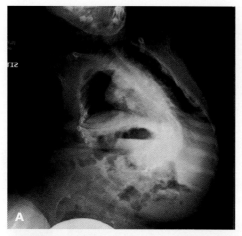
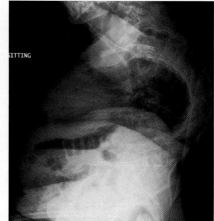
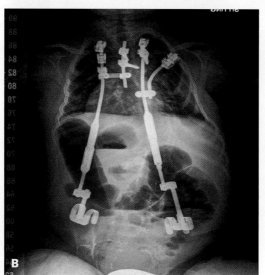
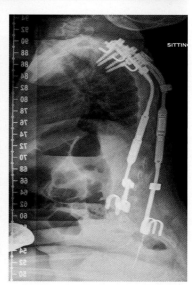

Figure 21-7 Use of hybrid fixation (rib hooks and pedicle screws) in a 7-year-old with large and progressive scoliosis in setting of spinal muscular atrophy in an attempt to control rib parasol. Even in large curves, deformity can be generally controlled with adequate proximal fixation. (Courtesy Michael Vitale, MD; Columbia University Medical Center.)

Dr Flynn Adds

Children deserve a sagittal plane too. It's often hard to find the right place on a young child's back (especially if kyphosis is part of the deformity) for the ramrod-straight 7-cm acuator.
If you take away all the child's kyphosis with MCGR, they will make it somewhere else—often with PJK.

fusion should be expected, so delaying surgery is a worthy goal. Children are often transitioned to a brace when the curve is less than 15° to 20°, though there is variability regarding how and when to exit serial casting.

The role of bracing in children with EOS is still controversial. Compliance is hard and it's not absolutely clear that bracing young children is so effective. There is a major opportunity to improve care here through well-done research. For now, decisions regarding bracing young children with scoliosis need to be made on a case-by-case basis with families.

Surgical Treatment

If curves progress past about 60° and patients have many years of growth remaining, "growth-friendly" surgical treatment should be considered. If curves are very stiff, or very rotated, consider surgery sooner.

Growth-friendly options hold the promise of minimizing spinal deformity and maximizing growth, but in reality they generally do not lead to normal growth, and complication rates have been reported at over 200%. Growth-friendly options include posterior-based distraction rods (e.g., traditional growing rods,

VEPTR, and MAGEC), and strategies that attempt to guide growth (e.g., SHILLA system, Luqué trolley). Strategies that modulate growth (e.g., anterior vertebral body tethering) are generally not used in EOS. In most surgeons' hands, SHILLA results in a small fraction of normal growth, and this technique is not commonly used in EOS. SHILLA may be indicated if patient follow-up is questionable as there are fewer operations needed than other techniques, and it could even be a "one and done" operation. VEPTR taught us a lot about the philosophy of respecting lung growth and rib fixation, but its use is largely limited to thoracic insufficiency patients (e.g., Jeune's syndrome) these days.

In normal adults, two-thirds of air movement during breathing is generated by the diaphragm, and one-third by the bucket handle motion of the ribs. Although popular for a while, thoracotomy (or cutting between ribs), and placing metal devices across ribs should be very rarely performed, perhaps only if there are five or more fused ribs. Preventing rib motion, and stiffening of the chest with metal and scar tissue must take a toll on respiration (Fig. 21-8).

The MAGEC has largely replaced traditional growing rods and has led to less surgeries compared to standard growing rods. While magnetically lengthening rods have the obvious advantage of avoiding an incision for every lengthening, they do not allow for any bending through the portion with the magnet. Try to center this straight portion on the thoracolumbar junction as much as possible to allow for rod bending above and below this to create a harmonious sagittal profile.

There is probably less force generated by MAGEC rods than traditional growing rods, and non-lengthenings are surprisingly frequent, so carefully evaluate if a lengthening actually took place or not. If lengthening did not occur, or was disappointing, try again a couple of months later, after forces have dissipated and lengthening may be successful. MAGEC rods should not be used if an MRI of

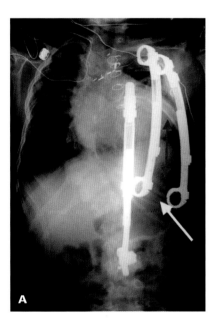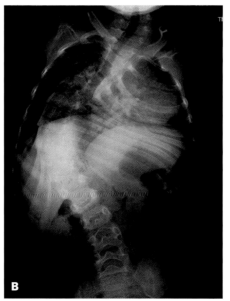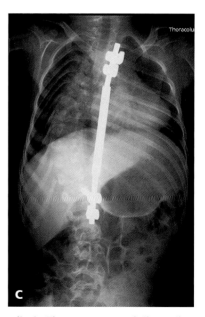

Figure 21-8 Use of VEPTR devices after thoracostomy in effort to control early-onset scoliosis. Thoracotomy and rib-to-rib devices are rarely indicated except perhaps in the rare patients with primary thoracic insufficiency. **A:** Creating large areas of separation between some ribs (red arrow) and crunching up other ribs (yellow arrow) cannot be good for breathing. **B, C:** A growing rod across concave side separates ribs evenly.

the thoracic or lumbar spine will be needed prior to fusion as they create 10 to 15 cm of darkness on MRI. Do not oversell families on the benefit of continued lengthening of the spine implants or you may find them begging for more lengthenings in young teenagers who should probably have been fused years earlier. Set the expectation of a fusion around age 10 from the onset of treatment though the "right" time to fuse is dependent on many variables.

Set parental expectations that the rate of unplanned return to operating (UPROR) may be up to 40% at 2 years even with MAGEC rods. Most common complications involve failure of lengthening, proximal junctional kyphosis, hardware migration, and rod fracture (Figs. 21-9 and 21-10). Small patients with

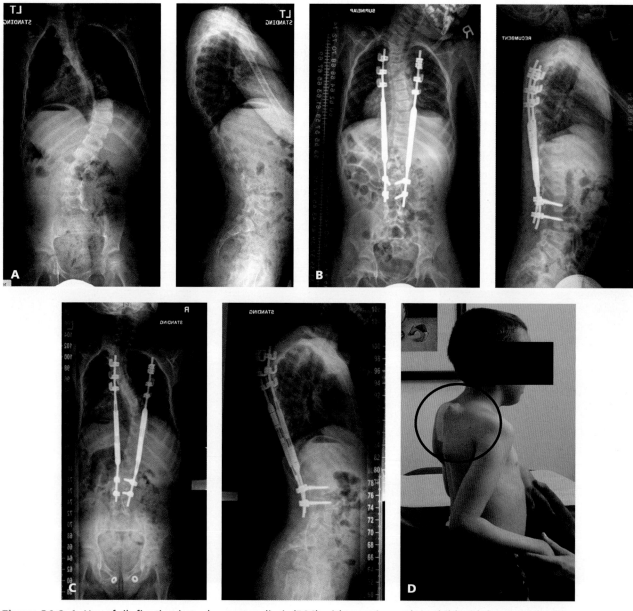

Figure 21-9 A: Use of rib fixation in early-onset scoliosis (EOS) with growing rods in child with large syndromic progressive scoliosis with kyphosis in normal range (s3NP2). **B:** Use of rib fixation in EOS with growing rods. Excellent 3D control of spinal deformity. **C:** Note development of proximal junctional kyphosis less than 2 y after initial surgery, threatening skin. **D:** Clinical appearance of proximal junctional kyphosis. (Courtesy Michael Vitale, MD; Columbia University Medical Center.)

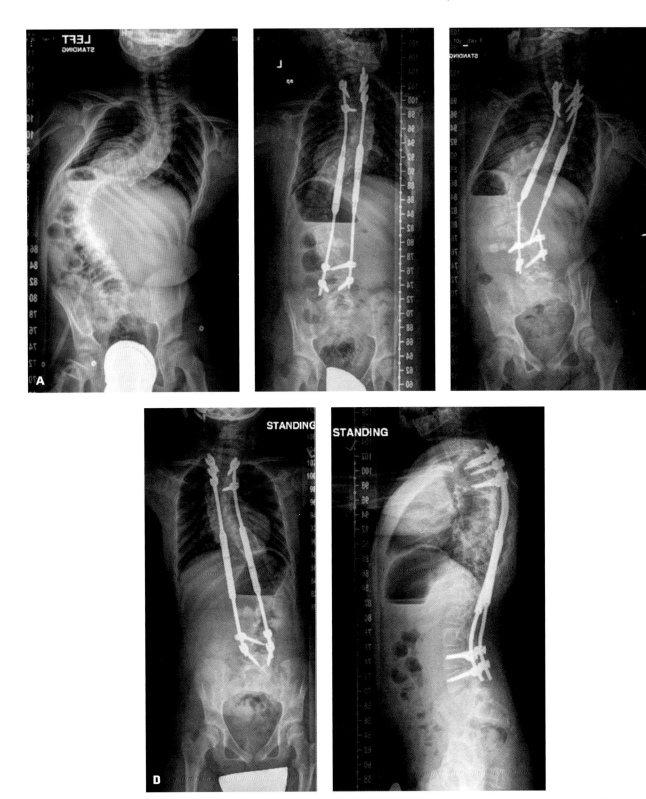

Figure 21-10 A: Large curve in a 6-year-old high-tone syndromic patient (S3NP2) treated with a 4.5-mm MAGEC (MAGnetic Externally Controlled growing rod) with good curve correction and successful lengthening until rod fracture. **B:** The patient was successfully converted to 5.5 MAGEC. (Courtesy Michael Vitale, MD; Columbia University Medical Center.)

hyperkyphosis, and patients with high tone, may be better candidates for traditional growing rods.

Every time you swallow, you have to hold your breath for a moment so the food goes down the right tube. In children with pulmonary dysfunction, the work of eating may come close to the energy gained by eating, so many of these children are extremely thin. Placing anchors on hooks, rather than ribs, has some proven and some theoretical advantages over spine anchors such as better soft-tissue coverage, less rod breakage, a safe mechanism of failure far from the spinal cord, and at least not an intentional fusion (Fig. 21-11).

Placing anchors at or above the sagittal end vertebrae minimizes the risk of proximal junctional kyphosis. Many surgeons prefer the use of multiple (ideally five or six) proximal rib anchors as use of more anchors is associated with less loss of fixation. Rib hooks can easily be converted to pedicle screws at the time of final fusion (see Fig. 21-9).[11]

Especially in young kids, consider a brace for 2 to 3 months after instrumentation to protect against early implant failure. This is especially important in short-segment implants, such as a hemivertebrectomy. There have been reports of proximal screw migration in young children. If one is going to use pedicle screws as the proximal anchors, use at least four good ones (Fig. 21-12).[12]

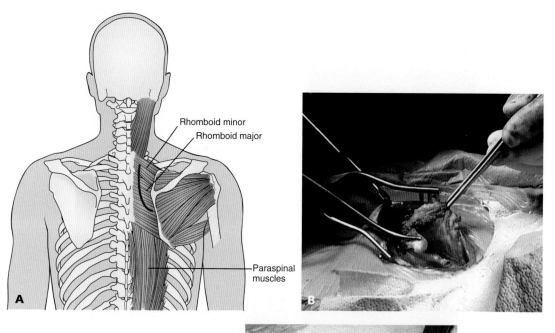

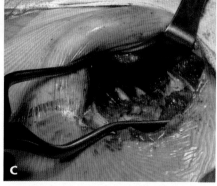

Figure 21-11 Placement of rib fixation in growing constructs. Through a single midline skin incision (**A**), a paraspinal J-shaped flap in the rhomboids reveals the paraspinal muscles, which run longitudinally (**B**). **C:** Once split, ribs are immediately below and easily accessible. This approach allows excellent exposure and excellent coverage. (Courtesy Michael Vitale, MD; Columbia University Medical Center.)

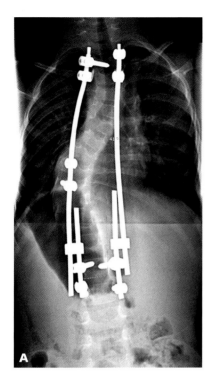

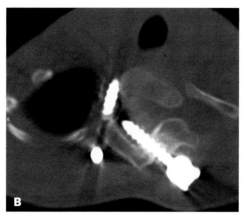

Figure 21-12 Example of migration of pedicle screw with lengthening in hands of an experienced senior surgeon. Adequate proximal anchors are essential for a firm base of lengthening in growing rods. Consider rib-based constructs in the very young, kyphotic patients or when bone quality is poor. The patient developed transient weakness and urinary incontinence that eventually resolved after revision. (Reprinted with permission from Skaggs KF, Brasher AE, Johnston CE, et al. Upper thoracic pedicle screw loss of fixation causing spinal cord injury: a review of the literature and multicenter case series. *J Pediatr Orthop.* 2013;33(1):75-79.)

When placing rib hooks, make certain you are immediately adjacent to the transverse process to minimize lateral drift along the rib and most effectively exert force on the spine. Use a wide hook to maximize metal/bone contact area and minimize the chance of the hook migrating through the rib. If the hooks do migrate through the rib, it is easy to deal with surgically. The rib generally hypertrophies, with lots of new bone at the site of migration, and an even bigger hook can be placed there, providing an even stronger anchor.

It is rather embarrassing that after all these years we still do not have great evidence proving growing rods in EOS help pulmonary function. However, our pulmonary colleagues use %tile weight gain as a proxy for overall health and pulmonary function in young kids, and studies show we help improve weight gain, particularly in the thinnest kids.

Congenital Muscular Torticollis

Congenital muscular torticollis (CMT) is a relatively common disorder, presenting soon after birth. Roughly 80% of cases of CMT resolve spontaneously. Physical therapy is commonly used as it may be useful in speeding up resolution, in managing cases that present in a delayed fashion, and in assisting in recalcitrant cases. If significant plagiocephaly is present, consider a molding helmet. This requires a good orthotist! Botox has been used as an adjunct to physical therapy, but this is illogical and could be harmful. The pathology is likely scarring from compartment syndrome, not from an overactive muscle.

The need for surgical release of the sternocleidomastoid is rare and consideration of surgical treatment should be limited to older children with significant persistent deformity despite conservative treatment. In a lot of cumulative years of experience treating CMT, the authors have done very few surgical releases. It's important to differentiate between CMT and torticollis which may arise from other causes as the differential diagnosis is broad and includes Klippel-Feil syndrome, Grisel syndrome, neurological causes, neoplasms, infection, and congenital scoliosis. If CMT is not resolving with physical therapy, consider spine radiographs.

Dr. Skaggs Adds

Never do a sternocleidomastoid release unless you feel an obvious tight muscle. If a tight muscle is not obvious, search for other causes. C1-occipital anomalies are frequently recognized only on CT scans. When doing a release, I suggest a bipolar release, and take out 1 cm of muscle at both ends. I have never seen overcorrection be a problem, nor have I seen a defect at the sight of resection, but I have seen undercorrections that needed a second surgery.

Staying Out of Trouble With Early-Onset Scoliosis

* EOS is defined as spinal deformity that is present before 10 years of age.

* Severe and progressive early-onset spinal deformity can result in cardiopulmonary insufficiency and increase mortality.

* MRI is necessary on most children with EOS to rule out associated spinal dysraphism.

* It is generally better to stall surgical intervention unless curves are clearly progression. As soon as spinal implants are placed, the clock is ticking toward auto-fusion, commonly within 5 years of the implants.

* The RVAD can help predict progressive and resolving curves in idiopathic EOS.

* Casting can be helpful in progressive cases of EOS in the young child.

* Low-dose, limited cut CT scan is useful in preoperative planning of congenital scoliosis.

* While magnetically controlled growing rods avoid repetitive operative lengthening, unplanned return to the operating room continues to be common, and families need to understand this reality ahead of time.

* Treatment of children with EOS requires a multidisciplinary approach, attention to comorbidities, and grit on the part of the family and surgeon.

SOURCES OF WISDOM

1. Williams BA, Matsumoto H, McCalla DJ, et al. Development and initial validation of the Classification of Early-Onset Scoliosis (C-EOS). *J Bone Joint Surg Am.* 2014;96(16):1359-1367.
2. Pehrsson K, Larsson S, Oden A, Nachemson A. Long-term follow-up of patients with untreated scoliosis: a study of mortality, causes of death, and symptoms. *Spine.* 1992;17(9):1091-1096.
3. Olson JC, Takahashi A, Glotzbecker MP, Snyder BD. Extent of spine deformity predicts lung growth and function in rabbit model of early onset scoliosis. *PLoS One.* 2015;10(8):e0136941.
4. Davies G, Reid L. Effect of scoliosis on growth of alveoli and pulmonary arteries and on right ventricle. *Arch Dis Child.* 1971;46(249):623-632.
5. Fernandes P, Weinstein SL. Natural history of early onset scoliosis. *J Bone Joint Surg Am.* 2007;89(suppl 1):21-33.
6. Dimeglio A, Canavese F. The growing spine: how spinal deformities influence normal spine and thoracic cage growth. *Eur Spine J.* 2012;21(1):64-70.
7. Riseborough EJ, Wynne-Davies R. A genetic survey of idiopathic scoliosis in Boston, Massachusetts. *J Bone Joint Surg Am.* 1973;55(5):974-982.
8. Murgai RR, Tamrazi B, Illingworth KD, et al. Limited sequence MRIs for early onset scoliosis patients detected 100% of neural axis abnormalities while reducing MRI time by 68%. *Spine.* 2019;44:866-871.
9. Mehta MH. The rib-vertebra angle in the early diagnosis between resolving and progressive infantile scoliosis. *J Bone Joint Surg Br.* 1972;54(2):230-243.
10. Hedequist D, Emans J. Congenital scoliosis: a review and update. *J Pediatr Orthop.* 2007;27(1):106-116.
11. Vitale MG, Matsumoto H, Feinberg N, et al. Proximal rib vs proximal spine anchors in growing rods: a multicenter prospective cohort study. *Spine Deform.* 2015;3(6):626-627.
12. Skaggs KF, Brasher AE, Johnston CE, et al. Upper thoracic pedicle screw loss of fixation causing spinal cord injury: a review of the literature and multicenter case series. *J Pediatr Orthop.* 2013;33:75-79.

FOR FURTHER ENLIGHTENMENT

McMaster MJ, Ohtsuka K. The natural history of congenital scoliosis: a study of two hundred and fifty-one patients. *J Bone Joint Surg Am.* 1982;64(8):1128-1147.

Yang S, Andras LM, Redding GJ, Skaggs DL. Early-onset scoliosis: a review of history, current treatment, and future directions. *Pediatrics.* 2016;137(1). doi:10.1542/peds.2015-0709.

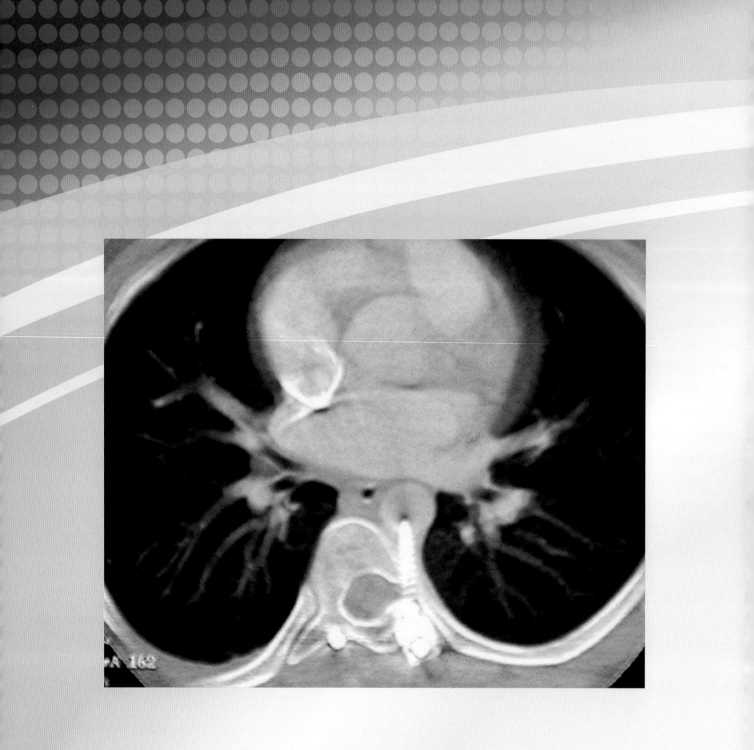

Chapter 22

Spine II: Adolescent Scoliosis and Kyphosis

JOHN M. (JACK) FLYNN, MD, DAVID L. SKAGGS, MD, MMM, and MICHAEL G. VITALE, MD, MPH

Guru: John B. Emans, MD

Adolescent Idiopathic Scoliosis

Adolescent idiopathic scoliosis (AIS) is a very common condition presenting to the pediatric orthopaedist. About 3 million new cases are diagnosed in the United States each year. Most of these children just need a thorough evaluation, complete (but low radiation) imaging, monitoring through the rapid adolescent growth spurt, and reassurance. A smaller subset will need bracing and counseling to prevent surgery. A very small subset will need their serious spine deformity corrected surgically.

The pediatric orthopaedist needs to be mindful of a few key principles when dealing with AIS:

- Be sure you are actually treating idiopathic scoliosis, not an imposter (Fig. 22-1).
- Remind yourself repeatedly that puberty is a high stress, high drama time for humans, when body image and peer pressure are at a lifetime maximum. This dominates all treatment discussions.
- AIS is highly genetic. In clinic, you may be walking into a room with parental guilt hiding in the background. Be particularly alert if one of the parents or grandparents had a "Harrington rod" or a "Milwaukee brace."
- There are many unscrupulous characters out there spreading misinformation and trying to bilk the families out of large sums of money for useless treatments. They run $5000 per week "scoliosis cure" camps. They make braces out of cloth straps. They offer growth-driven surgical treatments for teens who are done growing (as long as the family pays in cash). Some of them are orthopaedists.
- What we offer for treatments (plastic body braces or screws in the vertebra) work really well, have strong scientific evidence behind them and a well-established track record of success, but are enough to make a teenager collapse with anxiety when they think about the consequences.
- The results of modern spine deformity correction are so spectacular and durable that few changes have been made in the past two decades. However, there are persistent risks of infection, neurologic injury, and need for reoperation

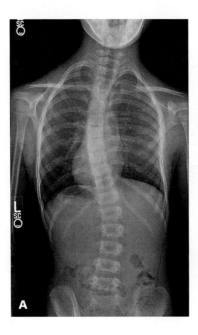 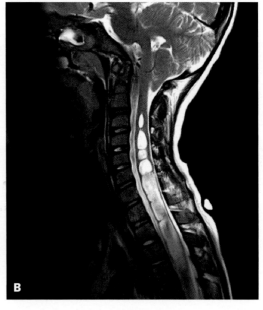

Figure 22-1 A: This boy presented with a 33° left thoracic curve and an asymmetric umbilical reflex. **B:** MRI revealed Chiari I malformation and holocord syrinx, requiring neurosurgical intervention.

that are unacceptably high. Some of these complications are more preventable than others. Pediatric spine surgeons need to be mindful of the factors driving a great long-term result, rather than just the factors that drive a great-looking postoperative X-ray.

In the pages ahead, we've collected many decades of wisdom to allow the pediatric orthopedist to navigate these very common clinic visits and spine deformity correction operations. In all these areas—evaluation, imaging, bracing, and surgery—we've seen lots of trouble resulting in patient harm and lawsuits and are determined to continue the downward trend in "trouble" for the many adolescents whose lives are affected by scoliosis.

HISTORY

There are several key pieces of information that should be collected on every single AIS new patient visit:
- Who discovered the scoliosis—primary care doctor, school nurse, parent, patient, peer, boyfriend/girlfriend?
- Is there a family history of scoliosis? Parse out kyphosis caused by osteoporosis that many will say their grandmother has. Also learn if anyone needed treatment for scoliosis, which suggests a much more significant family history.
- Are there any concerning symptoms (neurologic, pain, etc.)? **NEWSFLASH! Although you must ask about back pain, be careful not to open a Pandora's Box into the teenage psyche.** Scoliosis (when mild) does not cause back pain (if it did, they wouldn't have to screen for it). But, most teenagers have some back aches, especially the ones whose primary form of exercise is video gaming or who are depressed or anxious. Most back pain in teenagers is caused by weak core muscles, not small curvatures of the spine. Of course, pain that awakens the teen at night, or that is localized to a specific part of the spine (especially the lumbosacral junction in the midline), is worth noting and evaluating.

PHYSICAL EXAMINATION

Although a "complete physical exam" is the motherhood and apple pie of medicine, and is always the right answer, realize that you're not expected to be documenting the volume of cerumen in each ear canal for every one of your idiopathic scoliosis patients. So be thorough, but focus on a few key elements: a careful neurologic exam, a complete documentation of the deformity (Adams forward bend test, flank creases, shoulders and pelvis, spinal balance), abnormal skin findings (especially café au lait spots), gait, and leg lengths. Also, look at the bare feet and be sure there is no significant cavus deformity or claw toes. To stay out of trouble with a teenager of the opposite sex from you, keep them as well covered as possible.

Announce your need to do certain aspects of the exam (such as the abdominal reflex) and be considerate of privacy and exposure concerns in front of parents, trainees who are shadowing you, and others. **NEWSFLASH! Do the abdominal reflex with their finger not yours (nobody can tickle themselves).**

One very helpful trick is to do the Adams forward bend test so that the teen is bending their head directly toward their seated parents. This allows the parent to "sight down" their teenagers back, and get a real appreciation for the magnitude and location of the rotational deformity. Especially for less sophisticated families who were told by the pediatrician to be seen quickly for deformity that on first visit may be in surgical range, it is helpful for the mother to see the deformity before treatment is discussed.

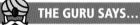
THE GURU SAYS...

Help achieve a sense of security for adolescent girls during the exam by tying the gown at the neck and holding the sides of the gown during the forward bend test. The test may be more accurate too, as the patient isn't twisting her spine trying to keep herself covered.

JOHN EMANS

IMAGING

Full-length PA and lateral radiographs of the entire spine are the standard of care for initial images. The recent availability of slot scanning technology has revolutionized pediatric spine imaging. With microdose slot-scanning on follow-up, the radiographs are often less than 5% of the radiation that a child would get from a standard radiograph. In addition, with proper positioning of the hands beside the face (Fig. 22-2), a free bone age can be obtained on every visit, dramatically improving the ability to make high-quality, data-driven decisions for the rapidly growing patient.

Look at those initial PA and lateral radiographs carefully (Fig. 22-3). Look for congenital anomalies of the spine. Look for spondylolysis or spondylolisthesis. Look at the shoulders and pelvis on the radiographs and consider issues such as leg length inequality.

One big red flag is the spine that looks like it is "windblown." Instead of the typical idiopathic right thoracic or left lumbar spine deformity with significant associated rotation, the "windblown" spine is often a curve to the left with very little rotation and involving both the thoracic and lumbar spine. If it seems to have a neurologic look, you are likely right: this is the appearance of a spine deformity caused by a huge syringomyelia, Chiari malformation, spinal cord tumor, or some other rare but dangerous interest spinal condition (Fig. 22-4).

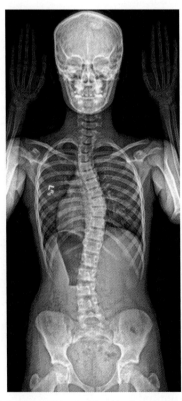

Figure 22-2 Using this positioning innovation, every scoliosis patient gets a free Sanders bone age score. This saves time and money for the family and greatly enhances the skeletal maturity information needed to make sound clinical decisions.

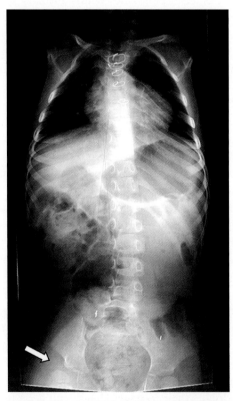

Figure 22-3 Remember to look beyond the spine on each radiograph. The need for this is aptly demonstrated here: the child's right hip was noted to be at risk (arrow). This is easy to overlook during a scoliosis evaluation, but may be made to appear obvious to a jury years later.

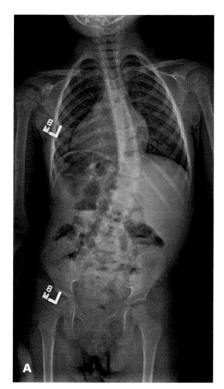
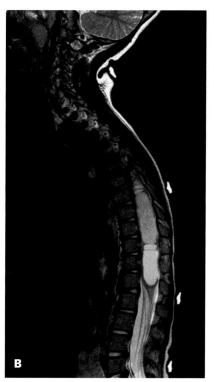

Figure 22-4 **A:** Although this is not the infamous "left-sided curve," it has several concerning features—long sweeping pattern and little or no rotation. It looks like the wind is blowing the spine. As soon as we saw this girl's X-ray, we sent her for an MRI. **B:** The MRI revealed a pilocytic astrocytoma of the spinal cord, requiring urgent neurosurgical management.

SKELETAL MATURITY AND GROWTH REMAINING

Skeletal maturity and growth remaining are absolutely essential to proper scoliosis care. Historically, Risser sign and menarche were all we had, and while they offered basic milestones for growth, wild variability led to some bad medical decisions. In general, females have their peak growth acceleration the year before menarche and continue to grow at a slower pace for about 2 years after menarche; however, menarche can be altered (endocrine abnormality, female athlete Triad). The Risser sign was useful mostly because we could see the pelvis on scoliosis radiographs. However, the most dangerous time for scoliosis progression occurs before Risser 1, and lots of growth can occur after Risser 4.

Fortunately, the work of Jim Sanders and others has greatly improved our skeletal maturity information precision in the last decade. Now, tracking Sanders scores and growth since last visit help us decide when a brace should be started, when it should be tapered down, when it should be finished, and when it should be avoided altogether. **NEWSFLASH! Beware: height measurements done by busy MAs can be inaccurate, or recorded inaccurately.**

One way to know that a family has stopped worrying about the scoliosis: they turn their full attention and passionate emotion into arguing that the Sanders score and the growth chart are wrong, because their son or daughter could not possibly be finished growing: "I kept growing well into college." A simple scoliosis visit can be turned into a tense and emotional realization about final adult height.

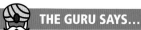
THE GURU SAYS...

Electronic medical records have made the growth chart readily available to even orthopaedists! Growth displayed on the chart is the best measure of all (unless the curve is so large that height is being lost). Growth velocity is readily visible independent of menarche or Risser sign.

JOHN EMANS

THE GURU SAYS...

Have an open mind toward alternative therapies. You may not believe they work and there may be no evidence, but parents are likely going to do it anyway. If you denigrate their chosen alternative treatment, you may deprive the child of a chance of the effective conventional treatment you prescribe.

There is evidence that some AIS patients are vitamin D deficient. There's no harm in suggesting prophylactic vitamin D and calcium supplements.

JOHN EMANS

THE GURU SAYS...

During scoliosis follow-up it looks to most families as if we are doing nothing except ordering radiographs. Explain the need for continued follow-up and that curves may worsen later in growth even though they haven't yet.

JOHN EMANS

THE GURU SAYS...

Take the time to be complete and honest in your discussion of bracing outcomes. Keep some radiographic examples handy—someone who started with a big curve and ended with a small curve, someone who ended up about the same with an acceptable curve, and someone who did everything right and still ended up with surgery. Explain why big curves are offered prophylactic surgery. Explain briefly the downside of a spine fused T3-L3.

JOHN EMANS

THE GURU SAYS...

Twice a year works for the perfect patient and family, but every 3 months for a check of compliance, brace fit, and dose of encouragement may be better for those at risk of losing enthusiasm for wearing the brace. An X-ray is not needed every time. Someone else (orthotist, PA, nurse) can do this.

JOHN EMANS

At that moment, when the boy realizes he's only going to be 5 feet 6 inches tall, the wise clinician reminds him he will never have to pay extra for legroom on an airplane, perhaps saving many thousands of dollars throughout his life. It seems to resonate every time, and the visit ends with everyone happy and laughing, rather than depressed and crying.

TREATMENT

Compared to many other pediatric orthopaedic conditions, treatment decisions are quite simple in idiopathic scoliosis (although families might find that fact depressing):

- Observation for curves less than 25° (or 25°-50° in skeletally mature teens)
- Bracing for growing (Sanders <8) children between 25° and 45° to 50°
- Spine deformity correction surgery for scoliosis greater than 50° (in some rare cases of documented rapid progression, 45°-50°)

From the very first visit, it's important to communicate the limited options clearly to patient and family. Explain that there are no foods, medicines, mattresses, exercises, or musical playlists that can stop scoliosis from progressing, or make it go away. Explain that it is a genetic and growth condition, and neither the child nor the parents can control either of those factors. Once everyone in the room is on the same page about the options: observation/bracing/surgery, then it is simply a matter of using the maturity and radiographic data to help the family make a good decision.

Bracing

We've experienced a nonoperative scoliosis care revolution in the last decade. There is now overwhelming evidence that a well-made corrective scoliosis brace, that is worn snugly and for at least 16 hours a day, can prevent the progression of AIS to surgical range for most children. It is essential that in the treatment decision discussion, the teenager with scoliosis voices a commitment to wearing the brace. It cannot be the doctor's decision or the parent's decision—that will fail in most cases. The teenager has to wrap their head around an amazing fact: scoliosis bracing is one of the rare chances that a human gets to use a treatment which will prevent surgery. A Sanders 3 girl who presents with 35° of scoliosis can choose to have her spine fused in a year or two, or she can "wear the stupid brace" and graduate high school with scoliosis in the 30s and no rods and screws in her back (in most cases). Taking the teenager and the family on this journey can be time-consuming. **NEWSFLASH! It's not unusual for a successful brace conversation to take even longer than a surgical conversation.** The pediatric orthopedist and the parents need to demonstrate empathy to the patient about the sensitivity of wearing a brace to school, the body image issues, and how cruel teen peers can be. Encourage the patient to engage other local teens who are going through the same bracing care, and to consider joining scoliosis support groups which can be extremely helpful. A nurse who is an expert in scoliosis can provide education, and ongoing support is worth their weight in gold and frees the surgeon from countless hours of counseling.

The most successful brace initiation protocol: measurement for the brace on the day it is prescribed, then a follow-up visit in 6 to 8 weeks (after the patient has reached fulltime wear) with an X-ray in the brace to measure correction, and an initial analysis of the compliance button data to see exactly how many hours a day the patient is actually wearing a brace. More counseling is often necessary at that visit. Thereafter, bracing patients are usually seen twice a year, with an X-ray taken with the brace removed for a day or two before the visit ("brace holiday").

To stay out of trouble, make sure your X-rays during bracing use this brace holiday concept. If every X-ray is taken in the brace, the actual deformity progression and size will be masked.

Scoliosis-specific exercises are becoming increasingly popular; the exercises improve posture, core strength, and breathing. The impact on deformity progression is under investigation, but it is much harder to study than the effect of bracing, because the "dose effect" of the exercises is hard to quantify. We've found that the exercises help many kids tolerate the brace better. These exercise programs can be very expensive and time-consuming, so they do not work for every family.

Surgery

Preoperative Family Discussion

A careful and thorough preoperative discussion with the family is absolutely essential to ensure proper informed consent, set expectations, and engage the patient and family in the perioperative care. Be sure the family understands that the primary goal of the surgery is to prevent future health problems, especially pulmonary demise as thoracic scoliosis progresses beyond 70°. The cosmetic benefits are powerful, but secondary. Spine deformity correction is not designed as a pain relieving operation, although some teens with large deformities do report a reduction in their pain after deformity correction.

Of course, a comprehensive discussion of all the risks is mandatory. This can be combined with a discussion of all the precautions that are taken to prevent

> **THE GURU SAYS…**
>
> The Schroth technique is by far the most popular scoliosis-specific program currently. Most Schroth-trained therapists endorse and encourage bracing for curves in the same range we do, or even for lesser curves. Try to establish a line of communication with your local Schroth therapists—they have the same overall goals you do.
>
> JOHN EMANS

> **THE GURU SAYS…**
>
> Most families have trouble understanding why we need to do something now about larger curves over 50° that are currently asymptomatic. Explain the concept of continued curve progression beyond maturity.
>
> JOHN EMANS

> **Dr. Skaggs Adds**
>
> Beware that when children are taught to stand in certain positions, they can change the Cobb angle at the moment the X-ray is taken, which may hide curve progression. One may question if this position can be maintained for the rest of the patient's life (Fig. 22-5).

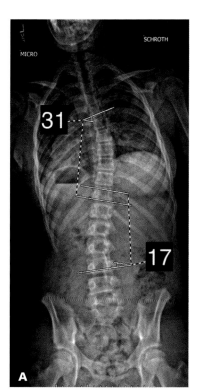 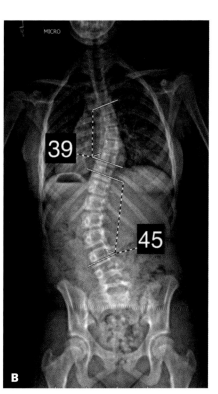

Figure 22-5 Be aware that patients may be coached to stand in ways that can change the Cobb angle enough that it could alter your treatment plan. You may not know this unless you ask the patient. **A:** A 12-year-old girl standing in a position her Schroth therapist told her to stand for the X-ray. **B:** The same girl, moments later, after the physician asked her to stand in her normal position. (Used with permission of the Children's Orthopaedic Center, Los Angeles.)

such complications as infection, implant failure, neurologic injury, and need for reoperation. A well-illustrated booklet that describes indications and procedure and answers all common questions is extremely valuable. **NEWSFLASH! You can't expect the family to remember everything they're told during a stressful visit. Have it in a booklet that you can hand out.**

Surgical Planning

Thoughtful surgical planning is essential for staying out of trouble with AIS correction surgery. This is best done several days before the procedure in a quiet room away from clinic and other distractions. Review the history and imaging. Mark-up an X-ray or a printout of the X-ray, numbering the vertebrae, drawing the CSVL (center sacral vertical line), marking the Cobb angles and how much they each correct on the bending film, noting the neutral/stable/end vertebrae, and studying the lateral X-ray carefully for sagittal plane characteristics and anomalies. Getting a routine full spine MRI for idiopathic scoliosis is controversial; however, every year we find several anomalies which are worth evaluating, and occasionally one that needs neurosurgery. There is great value in synthesizing the surgical planning, a picture of the patient and family, and the key elements of the informed consent discussion onto one document to be saved in the medical record. This can be reviewed on the day of surgery and has powerful medical-legal value.

Selection of fusion levels is famously an art of scoliosis surgery, whose details and published evidence are far beyond this book. However, there are a few key principles to follow to avoid trouble:

- The goal: Fuse the fewest number of vertebra to correct the deformity, balance the spine, and avoid reoperation.
- Choose levels that will optimize spinal balance. Using the first touched vertebra rule is valuable.
- Never *ever* end a fusion at any apex in any plane.
- The lowest instrumented vertebra should never be L4, unless L3 will yield a bad result.
- Always do a selective thoracic fusion when criteria are met (the thoracic curve is bigger, stiffer, and more rotated and translated from the CSVL).
- Protect the shoulder balance when T1 tilts to the right preoperatively (Fig. 22-6).
- For large curves, consider correction over time with either traction or temporary distraction rods.

Avoiding Intraoperative Trouble

Although routine for pediatric spine surgeons, posterior instrumented spinal fusion for significant deformity is a procedure with many dangers. Obvious risks are neurologic injury from technical errors or instrumentation, wrong site surgery (errors in level identification), wound contamination causing later SSI, forgotten surgical steps (such as final tightening), and failure to control blood loss. To stay out of trouble, standardize steps of the procedure as much as possible and engage a Dedicated Team to provide consistency and expertise for this common but complex procedure. Develop checklists, such as a preincision checklist and timeout, and end-of-procedure checklist to be certain all steps have been completed, and checklists for complications such as response to loss of neurologic monitoring data (Fig. 22-8). Communication is key. The surgeon of record should be able to make direct eye contact with the neuromonitoring technician, the anesthesiologist, and patient's vital signs (now on a wall-mounted flat screen in most spine ORs).

Dr. Skaggs Adds

It's easy to forget the sagittal plane when planning for scoliosis surgery. If the center of lower instrumented vertebral body is not in front of the posterior sacral vertical line, distal junctional kyphosis is much more likely (Fig. 22-7).

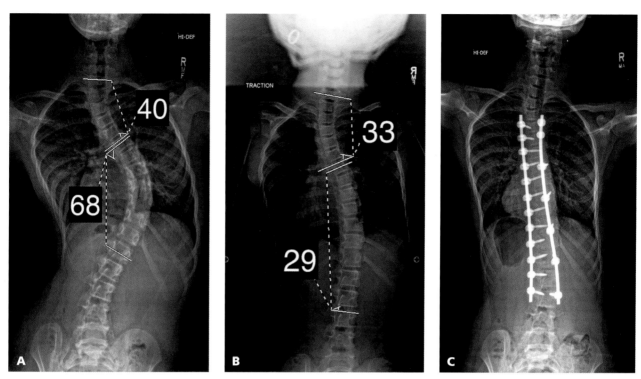

Figure 22-6 A: Respect the structural upper left thoracic curve. **B:** It can be even more rigid than the "main" right thoracic curve as demonstrated in this traction X-ray. The authors planned an upper instrumented vertebra (UIV) of T2. The mother chose to have surgery in a less expensive setting; the UIV was T4. **C:** This postoperative X-ray demonstrates if a structural upper left thoracic curve is not included in the fusion, a high left shoulder will result. The mother was very unhappy with the patient's appearance. (Used with permission of the Children's Orthopaedic Center, Los Angeles.)

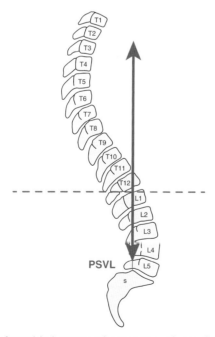

Figure 22-7 Stay out of trouble by remembering to evaluate the lateral X-ray when choosing the lower instrumented vertebrae (LIV). To minimize the chances of distal junctional kyphosis, the center of the vertebral body of the LIV should be anterior to the posterior sacral vertical line. In this case the LIV could safely be L1 or below. PSVL, posterior sacral vertical line. (Used with permission of the Children's Orthopaedic Center, Los Angeles.)

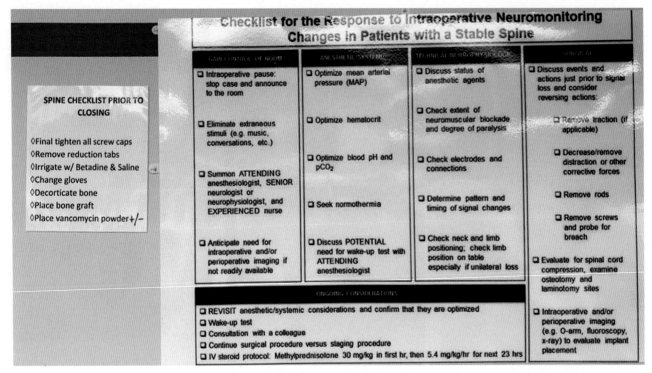

ONGOING CONSIDERATIONS
❑ REVISIT anesthetic/systemic considerations and confirm that they are optimized
❑ Wake-up test
❑ Consultation with a colleague
❑ Continue surgical procedure versus staging procedure
❑ IV steroid protocol: Methylprednisolone 30 mg/kg in first hr, then 5.4 mg/kg/hr for next 23 hrs

❑ Intraoperative and/or perioperative imaging (e.g. O-arm, fluoroscopy, x-ray) to evaluate implant placement

Figure 22-8 Two checklists on the wall in the spine room. The "Prior to Closing" checklist is used for every case by the team to ensure no steps are missed. The "Response to NM Changes" checklist is used on the rare occasions that neuromuscular signal changes occur. (Used with permission of the Children's Orthopaedic Center, Los Angeles.)

To stay out of trouble with blood loss, use TXA and develop anesthesia protocols to keep the mean arterial pressure in the 60s during exposure and low 70s instrumentation. Careful subperiosteal tissue dissection and an overall time-efficient procedure are among the best ways to keep blood loss low.

To stay out of trouble with neurologic injury, the pedicle screws must be in the pedicle and nowhere else (Figs. 22-9 to 22-12). Navigation is becoming increasingly popular (Fig. 22-13), as it gives real-time confirmation of pedicle screw location. Freehand technique can be used, but the screw should be

Figure 22-9 Although penetration of pedicle screws is usually benign, in this case the child had nerve-root pain and paresthesias. Removal of screw was accompanied by immediate improvement of nerve-root somatosensory evoked potentials and complete relief of symptoms. In the lumbar spine, palpating the pedicle from inside the canal with a Penfield #4 may help identify such a protrusion if you are uncertain when palpating from within the pedicle.

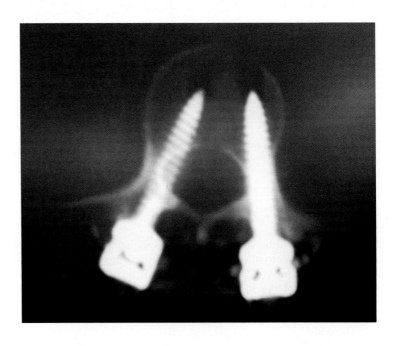

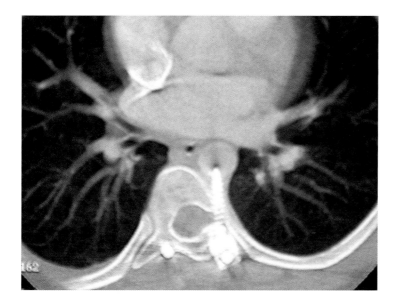

Figure 22-10 Following surgery for idiopathic scoliosis, this child had discomfort deep in the chest. The screw was removed and a bypass graft of the aorta was placed across the damaged part of the aorta.

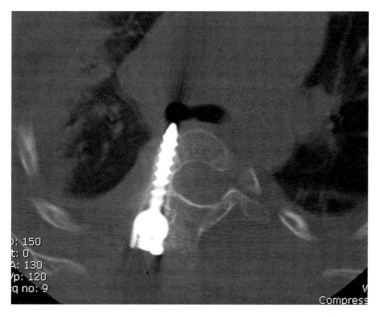

Figure 22-11 The smallest pedicle screw in the set was 25 mm, which was too long for this 3-year-old, which resulted in impingement on the right mainstem bronchus. Either the screw could have been cut shorter with a bolt cutter or an alternative fixation could have been used.

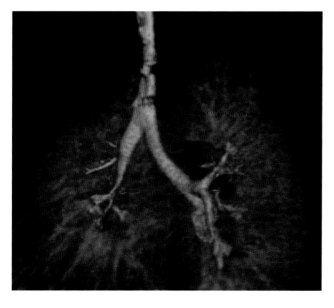

Figure 22-12 Yes, those are screw threads in a child's trachea. This is type of surgical error that can be prevented with navigation but go undetected with EMG or fluoroscopic monitoring.

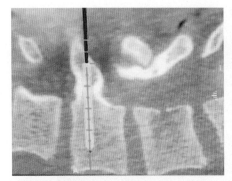
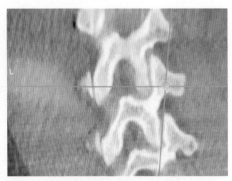
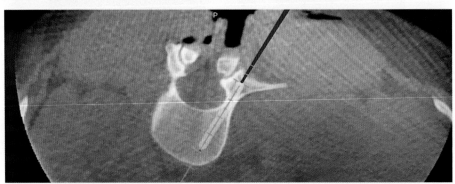

Figure 22-13 Image-guided navigation not only improves screw placement accuracy, but also allows the surgeon to select the screw diameter and length that precisely matches the actual pedicle size. Here, the blue line is the navigation probe a few millimeters into the pedicle, and the yellow is the projection of estimated screw diameter and length (5 mm × 40 mm).

checked radiographically after insertion and tested with EMG. If the right and left screw tips cross on radiographs, one or both may be within the spinal canal. If Ponte osteotomies are performed, it is wise to leave the ligamentum flavum intact until the very last step, to limit the risk of anything (screw driver, Cobb, suction tip, etc.) inadvertently entering the canal. If there is a change in neuromonitoring, pause the surgery, assure that it is not a neuromonitoring technical issue, and raise the mean arterial pressure to 80 to 90. Reverse the last surgical step performed before the neuromonitoring change if the timing suggests a temporal relationship. If there is not an immediate return to baseline, it is usually better to end the surgery and come back another day, but only after feeling certain that nothing is impinging on the cord. In rare instances in very large, sharp curves, the cord may be impinged by the concave pedicles; pedicle resection may restore neuromonitoring data.

To stay out of trouble with surgical site infection, delay operating on very high BMI teens if possible until they have lost a satisfactory amount of weight. Keep instrumentation covered until it needs to be used. Change gloves frequently. Limit OR traffic. Aggressively scrub the entire wound and instrumentation at the end of the procedure (we prefer using both saline and betadine for this step). About 25% of posterior spinal fusion wounds are culture positive at the time of closure; the surgical team should be focused and determined to scrub it clean before closure. Using Dedicated Spine Teams keeps the procedure as short and efficient as possible.

To stay out of trouble with wrong site surgery, do comprehensive preoperative planning and mark up the preop X-ray, and note the lowest rib (it can be T11). Use an intraoperative marking image to confirm levels before placing pedicle screws. Ask the whole surgical team to assess the levels, and welcome anyone who can dispute the initial level determined, and recheck until all in the room are confident.

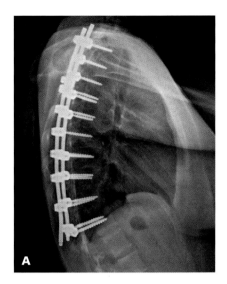
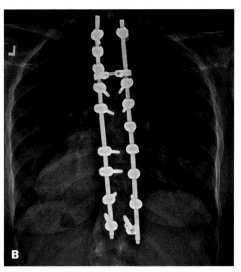

Figure 22-14 This 19-year-old soccer player presented for a second opinion 1 y after PSF (done by an excellent scoliosis surgeon at another center). The caps were dislodged from the distal screws. At the revision surgery, we found that every cap in the construct was loose, suggesting a missed step before closure. Use an end-of-case checklist, as shown in Figure 22-8. Preferably, post it on the wall in the OR and review before closing. Read the steps out loud to the OR team to be sure nothing was missed.

The best time to adjust the position of a concerning screw, improve correction, improve shoulder balance with instrumentation changes, and change fusion levels is while the patient is asleep and the wound is open for the initial operation. If there is any question as to the purchase of pedicle screws on the lowest instrumented vertebrae (LIV). Do not hesitate to add an upgoing laminar hook as a third anchor point, particularly if the patient is eager to return to sports. Everything is harder if a problem is discovered on a postoperative X-ray. Navigation and intraoperative imaging is currently sophisticated and available enough to allow a comprehensive evaluation of the implant and correction prior to closure. And, finally, remember to go through that end-of-case checklist before closing to avoid missing a simple step, like final tightening (Fig. 22-14).

Avoiding Postoperative Trouble

Dramatic advances have been achieved in standardizing postoperative recovery after surgical correction of idiopathic scoliosis. Most centers now have a rapid recovery pathway that standardizes pain management, diet, physical therapy, wound management, antibiotics, and discharge planning. The weeklong stays of the 20th century have been replaced by 48- to 72-hour stays for the vast majority of posterior spine fusions for idiopathic scoliosis. To stay out of trouble in the early postoperative period, standardize the pathway and surround the patient with experienced nurses and nurse practitioners.

NEWSFLASH! The postop recovery goes much better if the family is engaged and well educated at the preoperative consent visit. If the family knows what to expect (yes, your teenager will have some pain, they won't eat as much as they usually do, and they'll need frequent naps), on the first and second postoperative days, they can say, "You told us this would happen." Postoperative nausea and vomiting are worse in kids who arrive dehydrated on the day of surgery; encourage the teens to hydrate for a day or two before surgery as though they are running a marathon through the desert. NEWSFLASH! The only thing worse than having a really sore back after surgery is having a really sore back and throwing up for 2 or 3 days. Another area of critical family education and expectation is immediate postoperative spinal balance. When a giant spine deformity is instantly corrected in the operating room over a few minutes, it takes weeks or months for the teen to completely rebalance. Warn the family that their teenager will likely have shoulder imbalance and maybe some trunk asymmetry (depending on the

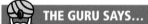
THE GURU SAYS...

Another way to protect against pullout of the questionable LIV screw (usually the convex LIV screw on a lumbar curve) is a doubled sublaminar braided cable passed beneath the LIV lamina and around the rod proximal to the screw.

JOHN EMANS

THE GURU SAYS...

Consider reinforcing expectations post op with a "road map" of the pathway and checklist at the bedside.

JOHN EMANS

specific preoperative deformity) that will be very visible when they first sit in a chair on postoperative day 1, when they are first walking down the hall in the hospital, and when they are at home for the first few weeks or months. We've completed a long-term, comprehensive study of nearly 1000 AIS fusions showing that the vast majority of teenagers achieve rebalancing within 6 months after surgery. Sometimes scoliosis-specific exercises can speed the rebalancing process if the families are particularly concerned and the patient very invested.

To stay out of trouble, keep the postoperative wound management really simple. Don't take off the surgical dressing until the family is heading for the car at discharge. Keep the surgical site dry for at least 7 days. The family could send photographs of the wound about once a week for 3 weeks or more frequently if there are any concerning signs.

It's critical to limit the narcotic prescription at discharge. Most teenagers can be completely off narcotics about 5 days after discharge, managing their pain with only ibuprofen and acetaminophen. We are not far from a complete "no-opioid" pathway for the entire idiopathic scoliosis correction recovery. **NEWSFLASH! Teens die from opioid addiction, not scoliosis surgery pain.** Families have become woke to this message now, making a no-opioid recovery within reach.

The return to impact loading and collision sports after posterior fusion for AIS is controversial, data are limited, and recommendations are all opinion. Biologically, the bone graft should develop into a solid fusion by 6 months after surgery. However, with modern instrumentation (pedicle screw fixation of every vertebra in the construct), scoliosis surgeons have increasingly pushed the limits on return to sports. Recoveries are different, depending on the patient's preoperative conditioning, the length of their fusion, and the nature of their athletic activity. However, most fit athletic teenagers can begin sports rehab after the 6-week postoperative visit, and progress from low-impact cardio conditioning and sport-specific activities (shooting baskets or throwing a baseball) through full running, scrimmaging, and then competitive play in 3 to 4 months after surgery. Some subset will break the LIV screw, but it is rarely symptomatic and rarely requires reoperation. Actual pseudoarthroses causing pain or rod fracture are extremely rare in healthy teens without kyphosis and have not been correlated with premature return to high-level athletic activity. **NEWSFLASH! The most likely injury to an athletic teen after spine fusion is not to their spine. The young athlete who is deconditioned as they recover from spinal fusion surgery is much more likely in the first 6 to 9 postoperative months to sustain a stress fracture of their tibia or foot or overuse injury around the knee or hip, than they are to break their rods or screws.**

Scheuermann Kyphosis

Many of the principles used to stay out of trouble with idiopathic scoliosis apply to Scheuermann kyphosis as well. One fundamental aspect that is different is nonoperative care. The only thing more miserable than a teenager wearing a scoliosis corrective brace is a teenager wearing a corrective brace for thoracic kyphosis. In the mid-20th century, the Milwaukee brace was popular; you won't see that in high schools today—compliance approaches 0%. Exercise can help with symptoms. Core strengthening and hamstring stretching can relieve the back discomfort.

Many parents can become frustrated as they follow Scheuermann kyphosis and "nothing is being done." Deep in their consciousness is an elderly relative with osteoporosis and kyphosis who is truly debilitated, and they are nauseated picturing that future for their child. It is reasonable for these families to see a kyphosis brace—at least a picture of one. Some will actually give it a try for a few years. Evidence is also quite lacking on the efficacy of kyphosis bracing, because it is so poorly tolerated in teenagers. In very motivated teenagers with very flexible kyphosis, we have seen a few successes, but they are very rare.

Another difference of Scheuermann kyphosis is the surgical indications, which are much less well-defined than for idiopathic scoliosis. On one hand, kyphosis of 60° or 70° that is flexible and stable is completely harmless. It does not impact pulmonary function as the three-dimensional deformity of severe thoracic scoliosis can. However, "life is kyphosing": humans tend to progress toward spinal kyphosis, not lordosis, as they age. If a teenager goes off into life with 70° of kyphosis, and their bone density deteriorates in midlife, they are likely to have a debilitating kyphotic deformity when they are elderly. True Scheuermann kyphosis (three consecutive vertebra wedged at least 5°) over 70°, that is progressing even late or after skeletal maturity, is a reasonable place to begin surgical discussion. One other piece of data that can be helpful is the patient's height. We've seen teenagers who finished growing literally get shorter by an inch or more as their kyphosis progresses from 65° to 85°. It is important to assure that the change is just not "bad posture during measurement" which we do see, but a real loss of height due to kyphosis progression. **NEWSFLASH! A shrinking teenager with a worsening deformity makes the surgical indications and conversation much easier for the patient and family.** Surgical expectations should be clear in the minds of the teenager and parents. The goal of the surgery is to prevent a worsening collapse in the kyphosis during midlife and beyond. "The rods will act as a brace inside" is a very helpful picture for the family. Frankly, the teenager just wants to get taller, but can also appreciate the concept of a progressive deformity when they think about their grandparents.

Surgical correction of Scheuermann kyphosis is famously a bit more risky than correction of similar scoliotic deformities. The incidence of intraoperative neurologic monitoring changes is higher, as is the incidence of wound problems and postoperative junctional issues (junctional kyphosis or loss of fixation/implant failure). These need to be considered and discussed with the patient and family. Careful preoperative planning that takes into account pelvic incidence, deformity flexibility, the exact location of the kyphosis, and achievement of sagittal balance are essential. In general, the LIV should be the first lordotic vertebra. Apical osteotomies are helpful to shorten the posterior column during correction. Screw fixation is not of value at the apical vertebra, and in fact can be an issue with implant prominence in low BMI patients. A very successful construct is a cluster of anchors in the proximal thoracic spine, three apical vertebrae with no anchors, and reduction screws or serial reducers in the lumbar spine. A slow, progressive cantilever correction is safe and very effective. Often the correction can be improved by removing one of the rods after both are in, contouring to a bit more correction, then reinserting one by one. It is wise to pause for a few moments after final correction to assure maintenance of neurologic monitoring data. If there are neuromonitoring changes, back off on the kyphosis correction and assure that the MAPs are maintained in the 80s and 90s to get good spinal cord perfusion. Come back another day if any concerns persist.

To lower the risk of junctional kyphosis, three strategies have been helpful: do not overcorrect the deformity (if the teenager has been walking around with a 90° kyphosis for few years, correcting it to 30° is guaranteed to cause junctional kyphosis—especially in this era of chin-to-chest texting all day); contour the top of the rod with a bit extra kyphosis; and use hooks on the UIV (upper instrumented vertebra) to create a more gentle mechanical transition zone between the rigid thoracic screw fixation and the more flexible unfused thoracic vertebra.

> **THE GURU SAYS...**
>
> I've been impressed with modern kyphosis bracing (not Milwaukee) such as a thoracic lumbar sacral orthosis with anterior uprights or the "kypho-logic" variation for curves less than 60° to 75°. Night and evening use is requested. Braces are easier for some teens than compliance with exercises.
>
> JOHN EMANS

Staying Out of Trouble With Adolescent Scoliosis and Kyphosis

* Be sure you are actually treating idiopathic scoliosis, not an imposter.

* Remind yourself repeatedly that puberty is a high stress, high drama time for humans, when body image and peer pressure are at a lifetime maximum. This dominates all treatment discussions.

* Look at those initial PA and lateral radiographs carefully. Look for congenital anomalies of the spine. Look for spondylolysis or spondylolisthesis. Look at the shoulders and pelvis on the radiographs and consider issues such as leg length inequality.

* Use the hand film for a Sanders bone age to make treatment decisions (bracing, etc). The Risser sign is poor measure of peak height velocity (before Risser I) and the end of growth (much scoliosis progression can occur at Risser IV).

* X-rays during brace treatment should use the brace holiday concept (have the brace off for a day or so before the clinic visit). If every X-ray is taken in the brace, the actual deformity progression and size will be masked.

* Be sure the family understands that the primary goal of the surgery is to prevent future health problems, especially pulmonary demise as thoracic scoliosis progresses beyond 70°. The cosmetic benefits are powerful, but secondary.

* To stay out of trouble with scoliosis surgical planning:
    * Fuse the fewest number of vertebra to correct the deformity, balance the spine and avoid reoperation.
    * Never, ever end a fusion at any apex in any plane; the lowest instrumented vertebra should never be L4, unless L3 will yield a bad result.
    * Always do a selective thoracic fusion when criteria are met (the thoracic curve is bigger, stiffer, and more rotated and translated from the CSVL)
    * Protect the shoulder balance when L1 tilts to the right preoperatively.

* Develop checklists, such as a preincision checklist and timeout, and end-of-procedure checklist to be certain all steps have been completed, and checklists for complications such as response to loss of neurologic monitoring data.

* About 25% of PSF wounds are culture-positive at the time of closure. The surgical team should be focused and determined to scrub wounds clean before closure.

* When a giant spine deformity is instantly corrected in the operating room over a few minutes, it takes weeks or months for the teen to completely rebalance. Warn the family that their teenager will likely have shoulder imbalance and maybe some trunk asymmetry (depending on the specific preoperative deformity) that will be very visible in the initial phase of recovery.

* Life is kyphosing: humans tend to progress toward spinal kyphosis, not lordosis, as they age. If a teenager goes off into life with 70° of kyphosis, and their bone density deteriorates in midlife, they are likely to have a debilitating kyphotic deformity when they are elderly. True Scheuermann kyphosis (three consecutive vertebra wedged at least 5°) over 70° that is progressing relentlessly is a reasonable place to begin surgical discussion.

Staying Out of Trouble With Adolescent Scoliosis and Kyphosis (continued)

* After final kyphosis correction, it is wise to pause for a few moments to assure maintenance of neurologic monitoring data. If there are neuromonitoring changes, reduce the kyphosis correction and assure that the MAPs are maintained in the 80s and 90s to get good spinal cord perfusion. Remove the rods and come back another day if any concerns persist.

* To lower the risk of junctional kyphosis, two strategies have been helpful: do not overcorrect the deformity and contour the top of the rod with a bit extra kyphosis.

FOR FURTHER ENLIGHTENMENT

Gornitzky AL, Flynn JM, Muhly WT, Sankar WN. A rapid recovery pathway for adolescent idiopathic scoliosis that improves pain control and reduces time to inpatient recovery after posterior spinal fusion. *Spine Deform*. 2016;4(4):288-295.

Ughwanogho E, Patel NM, Baldwin KD, et al. Computed tomography-guided navigation of thoracic pedicle screws for adolescent idiopathic scoliosis results in more accurate placement and less screw removal. *Spine*. 2012;37(8):E473-E478.

Vitale MG, Riedel MD, Glotzbecker MP, et al. Building consensus: development of a Best Practice Guideline (BPG) for surgical site infection (SSI) prevention in high-risk pediatric spine surgery. *J Pediatr Orthop*. 2013;33(5):471-478.

Vitale MG, Skaggs DL, Pace GI, et al. Best practices in intraoperative neuromonitoring in spine deformity surgery: development of an intraoperative checklist to optimize response. *Spine Deform*. 2014;2(5):333-339.

Weinstein SL, Dolan LA. The evidence base for the prognosis and treatment of adolescent idiopathic scoliosis: the 2015 Orthopaedic Research and Education Foundation Clinical Research Award. *J Bone Joint Surg Am*. 2015;97(22):1899-1903.

Weinstein SL, Dolan LA, Wright JG, Dobbs MB. Effects of bracing in adolescents with idiopathic scoliosis. *N Engl J Med*. 2013;369(16):1512-1521.

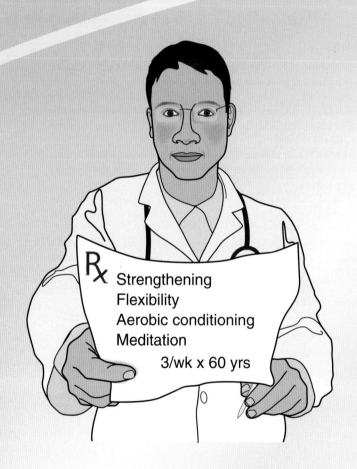

Chapter 23

Spine III: Back Pain, Spondys, and Other Issues

DAVID L. SKAGGS, MD, MMM, JOHN M. (JACK) FLYNN, MD, and MICHAEL G. VITALE, MD, MPH

Gurus: Daniel J. Sucato, MD, MS and Laurel Claire Blakemore, MD

We should approach back pain with humility; it is very poorly understood and treated by modern medicine. Back pain is estimated to occur in 60% to 80% of adults, and the rate in older adolescents seems to be approaching this.

Traditional teaching has been that normal children do not have back pain, so if a child presents with pain, it is our responsibility to find the underlying pathology. More contemporary studies report that over 80% of adolescents presenting with back pain have no definitive diagnosis. The truth probably lies somewhere in between for those patients who make it to your office.[1]

Back pain is difficult for orthopaedic surgeons to treat. We like to fix something that is broken, and back pain is usually not that simple. A comprehensive negative workup or technically perfect surgery can result in continued or worse physical and psychological pain, with a family who is disappointed in you. Make it your mission to not be discouraged by the possibility of failure and to do your best to find any treatable cause of back pain. Taking a child out of pain and returning them to normal activities is one of the most rewarding things we can do.

Back Pain

HISTORY

Perhaps start by asking if the pain is getting better or worse. If it is getting better, is that because of rest? Does it hurt if they return to their sport? If so there is still a problem unless they want to stop the sport. Just because pain has been constant for years, does not mean there is not an underlying cause. Spondys (meaning spondylolysis and spondylolisthesis) can cause someone years of constant pain and remain undiagnosed after years of various health care evaluations. Progressively worse pain despite no activities must be taken seriously.

Be very suspicious of an underlying problem in young children who have stopped playing normally or patients who have any constitutional symptoms. Having the patient draw a pain diagram before seeing them can be helpful (Fig. 23-1). One complaint that is almost always benign is a young child who complains of pain primarily when sitting in a car seat. One treatment is to let them pick out their own new seat.

> ▶ **Red Flags: Ask These Questions of Every New Back Pain Patient and Document the Answers**
>
> ▶ Night pain, defined as pain that wakes the patient up from sleep
> ▶ Loss of bladder control
> ▶ Numbness, tingling, weakness, or pain radiating down arms, legs, or buttocks

Many studies report a strong association between psychosocial factors (stress, anxiety, depression, loneliness) and back pain,[2,3] and that psychosocial factors may be even more important than mechanical factors such as carrying a backpack.[4] One can ask about a mental history gently, such as, "Do you see any other doctors, or therapists, or take any other medications?" Families are often welcome to this discussion, as they often suspect a link. Also inquire about other somatic complaints, such as headaches, stomachaches, and sore throats, which are associated with low-back pain.[5] In a child with multiple complaints, a physical, treatable cause of back pain is less likely to be found. These children and adolescents

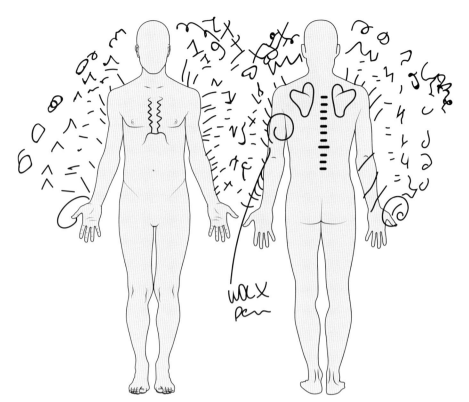

Figure 23-1 Actual drawing by patient showing most of her "back pain" is outside of the body. It is unlikely that an orthopaedic cause of pain will be found.

may benefit from a comprehensive pain service with psychological support. If there are family members eager to talk about their on-going medical problems, a certain amount of pain and somatic complaints may be the family norm.

EXAMINATION

Observe the patient's movements and emotional state. Are they appropriate? histrionic? smiling or flat? Do they look like they are in pain when getting on and off the table?

Ask them to point to where their pain is with one finger. If they point to one specific location of pain (a positive finger test; Fig. 23-2), take that seriously; it is your job to prove there is nothing wrong there. Consider ordering imaging studies, including an MRI and CT, to prove that area is free of pathology. If they have pain over a widely distributed area, you may be much less rigorous in pursuit of discreet pathology.

Beware that in some patients chronic, undiagnosed pain may lead to seemingly exaggerated symptoms over time. When someone seems depressed, histrionic, or has pain all over the back, this can be a cry for help. This is particularly true if the patient feels "blamed" for their pain, feels no one believes them, or has lost touch with their friends as they stop participating in sports. We have seen this many times in the former star athlete with physician visits and MRIs that have missed a posterior element fracture.

Have the patient bend forward as if to touch their toes. This compresses the vertebrae and discs, and if it causes localized pain, this is notable. If bending forward causes modest discomfort over a wide distribution, welcome them to adulthood—this is common and usually not worrisome. Then ask them to bend

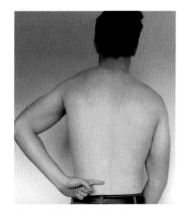

Figure 23-2 Positive finger test. The patient points to one well-localized area of pain. If they point around L5, think spondy.

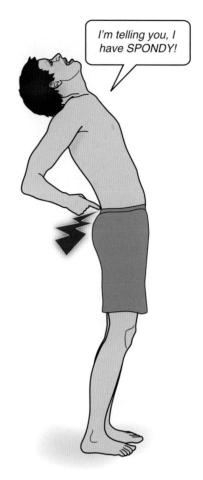

Figure 23-3 Patient bends backward, causing pain at the lowest part of spine.

backward. If this causes localized pain, assume there is a posterior element fracture, usually a spondy and less commonly a facet fracture (Fig. 23-3).

Sacroiliac (SI) joint tenderness is fairly specific and sensitive for SI joint problems such as infection. Localized tenderness over a spinous process is consistent with a fracture or ligament injury, such as a clay shoveler's fracture (avulsion of C7 usually or a Chance fracture).

The 60-Second Neuro Spine Examination (Fig. 23-4)

- Hop on each foot three times
- Walk on the heels
- Umbilicus, patella, and Achilles reflex
- Verify no claw toes or cavus feet
- Ankles dorsiflex with normal tone, no excessive clonus
- Sensation intact over medial knee, medial malleolus, great toe, lateral foot
- Popliteal angle <60°
- Dr. Blakemore also asks her patients to squat and stand from a squat

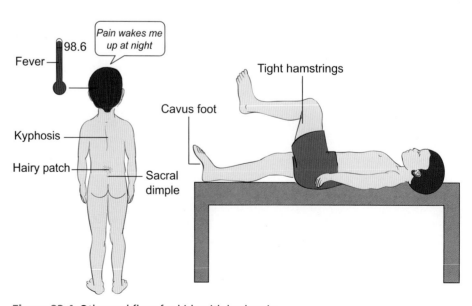

Figure 23-4 Other red flags for kids with back pain.

IMAGING

If there are no red flags on history or physical, imagining may not be needed. If imaging with low-radiation doses is available, that may influence the decision. Discuss the pros and cons with the family. If any red flags are present, imaging is necessary. Radiographs are usually first, perhaps due to availability. If there are neurologic signs or symptoms, or a tumor is suspected, it may be reasonable to get an MRI. The default MRI is of the cervical, thoracic, and lumbar spine unless the pain is well localized.

> **THE GURU SAYS...**
>
> Sometimes plain X-rays reassure both parents and the surgeon that nothing very terrible is going on. This may be a false sense of security. Because advanced imaging studies may require general anesthesia in children younger than 8 years of age, as well as expose them to larger radiation doses in the case of CT or bone scan, some caution is appropriate when ordering. Everyone's fear—yours and the families—is missing a neoplastic process. Red flags like night pain, limited activity, and limited motion can help you decide. Discuss pros and cons with family. I find they usually agree with a reasonable approach with a plan for escalating evaluation if symptoms persist or worsen.
>
> LAUREL BLAKEMORE

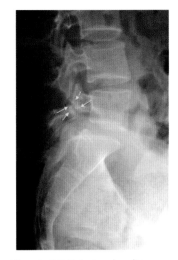

Figure 23-5 Lateral radiograph demonstrates a spondylolysis, the dark band between the yellow arrows. It is usually not this easy to see.

> **THE GURU SAYS...**
>
> MRI can show edema in the pedicle adjacent to a spondy when an actual break in the pars isn't seen. It's worthwhile to learn the MRI findings as your review may show more positive findings than a radiologist report from someone who is not trained in musculoskeletal radiology.
>
> LAUREL BLAKEMORE

When a patient has well-localized pain with back extension, you are looking for a posterior element fracture (Fig. 23-5). MRIs and X-rays (Fig. 23-6) will frequently miss posterior element fractures,[6] so have a low threshold to order a limited CT scan of the few vertebrae in question. If you are at a center where technique is tightly controlled, a localized CT scan of one or two vertebrae can require as little radiation as AP and lateral radiographs of the lumbar spine.[7] Sagittal and 3D reconstructions are particularly helpful in looking for spondys and facet fractures. Oblique radiographs are not recommended; they add radiation with no additional information.[8] Similarly, while flexion-extension radiographs may be common in the world of adult low-back pain, there is no benefit of this additional radiation in children and adolescents.

Bone scans should be ordered only rarely, as they expose the entire body to significant radiation and usually do not add information that cannot be obtained from other studies.

> **THE GURU SAYS...**
>
> I still use bone scan when the pain is concerning but not well localized enough to guide other imaging. If you're confident where to look, then MRI or CT can be first choice. If identified, an osteoid osteoma can often be managed with minimally invasive techniques, such as radiofrequency ablation.
>
> LAUREL BLAKEMORE

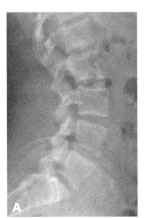
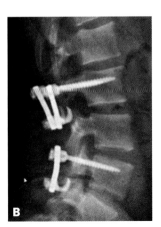
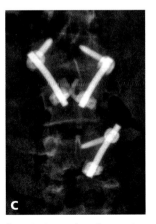

Figure 23-6 A 16-year-old athlete with back pain on extension. **A:** Lateral radiograph was negative. CT showed spondylolysis bilateral at L2 and unilateral at L4. **B, C:** Direct repair led to 100% pain relief and return to sports. While this case turned out wonderfully, direct repairs are not as reliable for pain relief as fusion.

TREATMENT OF BACK PAIN WITHOUT A CLEAR DIAGNOSIS

First, set expectations that most of us have back pain at some point. Elimination of all back pain is not a reasonable goal. In terms of medications, ibuprofen seems to work best,[9] with very little risk or side effects in the short term. The patient will likely have to get through the present episode of pain and then work on prevention. There is some evidence to suggest exercise helps.[10] Back extension exercises anecdotally seem to work well in the motivated (Fig. 23-7).

Physical therapy comes with a significant time and financial commitment, and may help in the short term but is not a long-term solution. The most effective treatment is the one that is most likely to actually happen, so see what the child might find *fun*. We encourage an activity that the child wants to do, perhaps with friends or family, and perhaps under the supervision of a "cool" athletic trainer, rather than something that feels related to disease. You can partner with local gyms and trainers to ensure quality and alignment of mission and print "prescriptions" for training.

Dr. Flynn Adds

Families and kids are busy. Co-pays are high. Too often, "PT" ends up being some time laying on the therapist's table with a warm pack on the back followed by some hamstring stretching next time the therapists happens by the table. There is a free and effective alternative: isometric core strengthening at home. Test the patient in your office up on the examination table. Put them in plank position, start the timer on their smartphone, then resume talking with parents. If the patient can hold a plank for 3+ minutes like most fit teen athletes, they don't have a core strength problem. Much more commonly, they collapse after 30 seconds and say, "My muscles are burning!" You suddenly have a diagnosis and a cure. At home, on the living room floor, in between games of Fortnight, they should do three sets of planks per day and post their record on the fridge. The goal is to increase their plank time by 5 seconds per week. With engaged parents, this solves the problem about 90% of the time.

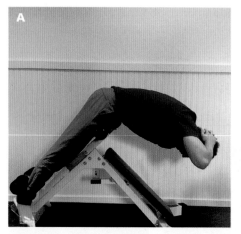 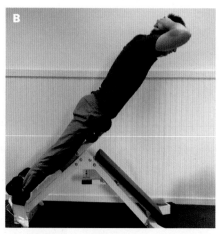

Figure 23-7 Roman chair. While many patients are eager to work on their six-pack, back extension exercises are at least as important in the prevention of back pain. This is good for surgeons too!

Spondylolysis and Spondylolisthesis

These words have too many syllables, so let's just call them spondys. Spondys are present in about 1 in 20 people, and most people probably do not even know they have one. The golden rule of treating a spondy is that if it is not bothering the patient, it is not a problem (Fig. 23-8). When treating a spondy, the most important thing for the family to understand is that the goal is to improve pain, not necessarily heal the fracture. Rarely if ever do they progress to the point of harm without symptoms.

A symptomatic spondy is one that hurts with extension right over the spondy. Conversely, just because someone has a spondy does not mean that it is the source of pain. Avoid this pitfall! Stress reactions around the pars of L5 are quite common in even asymptomatic high-level athletes, such as pitchers and tennis players.[12] So again, it is only a problem if there is pain.

NONOPERATIVE MANAGEMENT

Let's consider how to approach a few scenarios. If a spondylolysis is hot on MRI and the gap is not bigger than a few millimeters on CT, this may be an opportunity to heal a fracture. Keeping the patient out of sports that cause discomfort likely maximizes chances of healing, but it may take many months. Use of a brace is controversial and may actually increase movement and stress at L5. Healing over time may be assessed with some combination of MRI (look for decreased signal) and CT of that vertebra only (look for bony healing). Families should be warned that bony healing is not even close to predictable, and sometimes the fracture gap actually widens despite rest (Fig. 23-9). If a spondylolysis is not hot on MRI or if the fracture gap is greater than a few millimeters, it is very unlikely to heal. Simply keeping the patient out of sports until they feel better is an option, though playing through pain is unlikely to cause injury.

> **THE GURU SAYS...**
>
> An acute history of sudden pain with an extension-type activity together with an acute appearing spondy on CT indicates an acute fracture. Especially when these are at L4, healing is possible with a correct program of activity modification, antilordotic bracing, and maintenance of core strengthening with exercises (Fig. 23-10).
>
> DAN SUCATO

> **THE GURU SAYS...**
>
> Radiographic evidence of healing isn't a requisite for return to activity. I use symptoms as a guide and try to avoid obtaining repeat studies for this reason. The evidence on bracing is minimal, and I recommend it less, but would for persistent pain after 6 weeks of PT, in an effort to decrease activity if nothing else.
>
> LAUREL BLAKEMORE

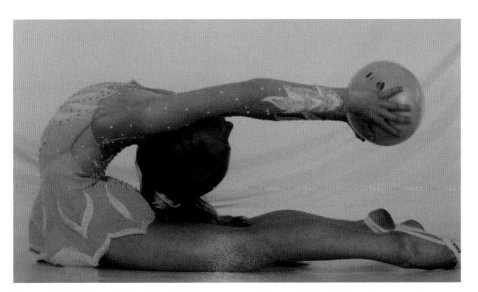

Figure 23-8 Olympic-level rhythmic gymnast with spondyloptosis and no symptoms. No treatment is needed.

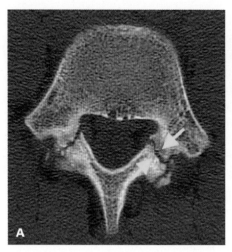
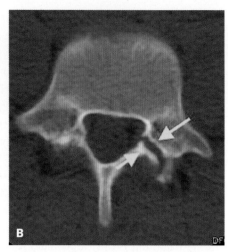

Figure 23-9 **A:** A 16-year-old lacrosse player presented with bilateral spondylolysis at L5, as seen on CT. The family wanted to try everything that could help heal the spondylolysis with conservative care. **B:** After 14 wk of rest, bracing (lumbosacral orthosis [LSO] with thigh cuff), and electrical stimulation, the fracture gap is larger (arrows). The other side is worse as well but seen best on other cuts.

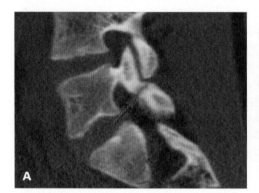
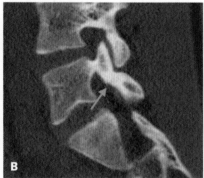

Figure 23-10 This 16-year-old male soccer player with acute symptoms and left-sided low-back pain with a unilateral pars defect (red arrow) (**A**) treated with combination physical therapy, bracing, and ibuprofen had excellent healing at 3 mo (green arrow) (**B**). (Courtesy of Dan Sucato, MD.)

Core strengthening is believed to help all spondys, but there are little data on this. Tight hamstrings should be thought of as a symptom of the spondy from nerve root irritation. It is not necessarily mechanical irritation; it can be chemical irritation from inflammation. There is no evidence that treating tight hamstrings improves a patient with back pain due to a spondy. I have had many patients complain that physical therapy hurt them and even seemed to make the problem worse. Bracing can be used if it relieves symptoms. Most kids with symptomatic spondys treated conservatively will be able to return to sports for many years to come, but warn families there may be with periods of pain that can interfere with activities at times.[13]

After conservative measures have been exhausted, an athlete with a painful spondy will have to face the following options: (1) Play through pain, which may be minor and intermittent, or significant (Steve Nash in the National Basketball Association took this approach over a long and successful career); (2) stop activities that cause pain; or (3) surgery. There is resistance to hearing this, so I put it in writing.

In some patients with spondys, the pain is truly affecting them so much that they cannot sit in school and concentrate on studies. There may be buttock or leg pain. If there is no significant improvement after 6 to 12 months of conservative therapy, surgery is likely to greatly improve their quality of life.

SURGICAL TREATMENT

Please pause for a moment to reflect on the fact that the great, great majority of people with spondys will never need surgery and may in fact never even know they have a spondy. However uncommon the need for surgery, there are so many opportunities for trouble in the operative treatment of spondys that some technical points are worth discussion. Direct repair of a spondylolysis has the advantage of not fusing across a joint, but it probably has a lower rate of success than a fusion. In cases of multiple levels of spondylolysis, an attempt at direct repairs is preferable to fusing multiple levels (see Fig. 23-6). For an L5 spondylolysis, if the L5-S1 disc is degenerated, fusing across the joint is indicated. Otherwise, following repair of the bone defect, the patient may still have pain from the disc. While degenerated discs are generally rare in adolescents, they seem much more common in association with spondys, possibly because of the abnormal stresses due to the fracture.

When thinking about doing a posterior-only fusion for a spondy, there is not a lot of bone proximal to the spondy to fuse to. Robust fusions along the transverse process are more common in theory than reality. A posterior-only approach (with or without a transforaminal lumbar interbody fusion) seems to fail more often in adolescents than adults, perhaps because adolescents returning to sports probably place more demands on their spine than adults. Especially in athletes who want to return to sports, strongly consider an anterior interbody fusion through an anterior approach. This almost guarantees an early, robust fusion in a young, healthy population (Fig. 23-11). While translaminar interbody fusions (TLIFs) in adults may have good results, a high rate of failure has been reported in the adolescent population.[14]

Stay out of trouble with posterior instrumentation by ensuring that the pedicle screw at the top of the construct (most commonly L5) does not touch the L4-L5 joint. To help ensure the screw avoids the joint, use an inferior and lateral starting point and make sure the screw head is left well proud of the joint (Fig. 23-12).

> ⊕ **THE GURU SAYS...**
> Repair is less likely to succeed at L5-S1, and so I would offer a frank discussion with the parents regarding repair versus L5-S1 fusion, neither of which guarantees success.
>
> LAUREL BLAKEMORE

> ⊕ **THE GURU SAYS...**
> Erectile dysfunction is a low but real risk with an anterior fusion at L5-S1, so that has to be included in your discussion with the family and may affect their decision.
>
> LAUREL BLAKEMORE

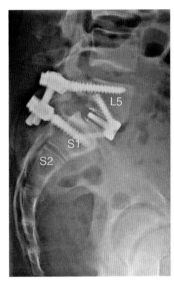

Figure 23-11 Example of an anterior lumbar interbody fusion with posterior instrumentation. Anterior fusion is reliable, and athletes can return to sports 3 to 6 mo postoperatively. I have personally never seen this construct fail (D.L.S.). (Courtesy of David Skaggs, MD, Children's Orthopaedic Center, Los Angeles.)

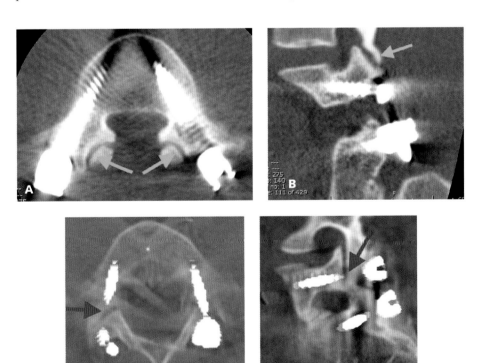

Figure 23-12 A, B: Good examples of a pedicle screw with a lateral and inferior entry point to avoid the adjacent facet joint (arrows) with the screw tulip left proud of the joint. **C, D:** Violation of the facet joint (arrows) by pedicle screws.

THE GURU SAYS...

High-grade spondylolis-
thesis is a very rare condition
that carries very high risk, so the
treatment should be tailored to
the experience of the team managing the patient. A 360° fusion/
partial reduction is technically
demanding and requires some
experience and lots of patience
to trace out the L5 nerve root
over time to avoid complications.

No matter which technique
is used to manage a patient with
a high-grade spondylolisthesis, it
is critical to turn the patient to
the supine position from the OR
table with the hips slightly flexed
(20°-30°) and the knees flexed
(60°) to take tension off the L5
nerve root. This position should
be maintained in the first 18 to
24 hours and then lessened if the
L5 nerve root is functioning well.

DAN SUCATO

THE GURU SAYS...

Assessment of pelvic
parameters is changing how
some think of treating spine
deformity, but we still don't
know how this should affect
treatment recommendations.

LAUREL BLAKEMORE

Beware that minimally invasive surgery (MIS) is not always so minimally invasive. A haunting study of experienced MIS surgeons found 58% of lumbar pedicle screws violated facet joints.[15] Consider a midline skin incision, then split the fascia and muscles just lateral to the pedicles on each side, so you have one skin incision and two fascial incisions. This offers a direct visualization of L5 and S1 pedicle screw starting points with minimal dissection, and compared with a midline muscle dissection, there is less lateral soft tissue you have to retract as you try to aim the pedicle screws a bit medially.

Unless there is imaging evidence of stenosis about the nerve root, elimination of motion with a solid fusion in spondylolysis or low-grade spondylolisthesis is highly likely to relieve the nerve root symptoms. When decompressing nerve roots, decompress aggressively all the way out past the pedicle. You never want to go back there or worry if postoperative nerve pain is from an inadequate decompression. Beware that there is an increased rate of spina bifida occulta with spondylolisthesis, so be particularly careful during dissection. It is surprisingly easy to cut or cautery sacral nerve roots during exposure of a high-grade spondylolisthesis. This devastating complication has resulted in at least one lawsuit. One may consider a preoperative neurosurgical consult in patients presenting with nerve root symptoms, depending on institutional norms.

Quite often in low-grade slips, reduction occurs with positioning, and this poses little risk to the nerves. Kyphosis at the spondylolisthesis is often improved with hip extension. In contrast, in slips greater than 50%, nerve injury rates are over 10% in many series of surgical correction.[16] There was a period when the rate of nerve injuries increased in the Scoliosis Research Society Morbidity and Mortality Reports, during which time many thought leaders were promoting aggressive reduction of high-grade slips from the podium. Most of the strain on L5 and risk of nerve root injury occurs during the second half of reduction,[17] so keeping surgeon ego in check and going for partial reduction is a good way to stay out of trouble.[13] Concentrate on correction of kyphosis, which is relatively safe and is likely to improve patient outcome more than correction of the slip. Fusing high-grade slips in situ has the greatest chance of minimizing complications, and Helenius found better clinical outcomes in patients fused in situ than in those undergoing reductions[18] (Figs. 23-13 and 23-14).

Figure 23-13 This 8-year-old boy presented with severe constant back pain. **A:** Lateral radiograph shows a high-grade slip with chronic changes of L5 and S1. The family asked for the surgery with the small-est chance of nerve injury as the child's dream was to play college basketball. **B:** Following correction of kyphosis with patient positioning, in situ fusion was performed, with the S1 pedicle screws extend-ing into the body of L1. The patient went on to play 4 y of Division I basketball on scholarship without significant back pain. If we were to do this again, we would consider more distal fixation, such as S2 or sacral alar iliac screws.

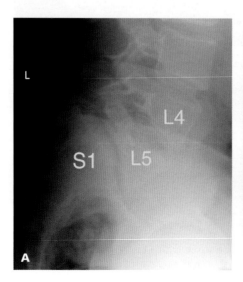
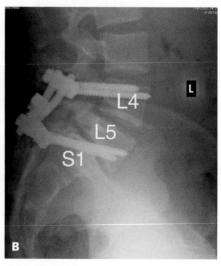

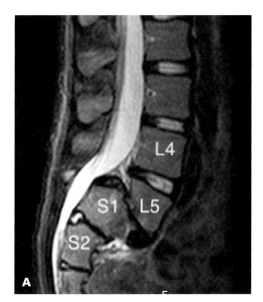
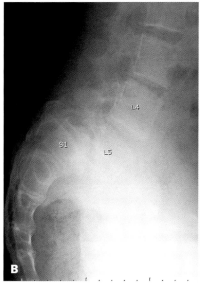
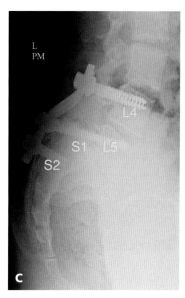

Figure 23-14 MRI (**A**) and lateral radiograph (**B**) of a 14-year-old with high-grade slip, back pain, and no nerve symptoms. C: Lateral radiograph after in situ fusion. Note S1 pedicle screw extended into the body of L5.

Facet Fractures

Facet fractures of the lumbar and sacrum are a rare injury but an important diagnosis not to miss, because treatment can lead to remarkable pain relief. The diagnosis is suspected if the patient has localized pain with extension. These fragments are usually missed on plain radiographs, bone scans, and MRI, though sometimes MRI shows inflammation (usually in hindsight). CT confirms the diagnosis (Fig. 23-15). Treatment is removal of the intra-articular fracture fragments through a small (<2 cm) incision and muscle-splitting approach. Rely heavily on intraoperative imaging before making the incision. Minimize dissection; there is no reason to open the facet joint beyond what is needed to see the fragment. The fragment is often surrounded by inflammatory tissue and can be identified by its mobility. Pain relief is usually almost 100% after recovery form surgery; it is like taking a piece of sand out of your eye. In theory, intra-articular fragments could cause joint destruction, so if they cause focal pain with extension, we recommend resection sooner rather than later.

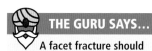

THE GURU SAYS...

A facet fracture should be considered in patients who present with persistent localized pain with extension but other radiographic studies are negative.

LAUREL BLAKEMORE

Transitional Lumbar-Sacral Vertebrae

Consider transitional lumbar-sacral vertebrae (aka Bertolotti syndrome) as a normal variant that is present in 10% to 20% of the population. They are rarely a cause of back pain in the pediatric population. However, if there is focal pain off midline directly over unilateral transitional vertebrae when a patient is in extension, consider an MRI to look for inflammation at the pseudoarthrosis (Fig. 23-16). This is best seen in a coronal STIR sequence but may be seen on T2 as well. Bone scans are hot as well but generally not indicated to avoid radiation. Symptomatic transitional vertebrae are analogous to the more well-known tarsal coalition, which may become painful as a teenager, presumably as the cartilage ossifies and the pseudoarthrosis becomes more rigid. A mechanical engineer father of the patient in Figure 23-15 pointed out that such unilateral transitional vertebrae would cause large forces across the pseudoarthrosis. In these rare cases,

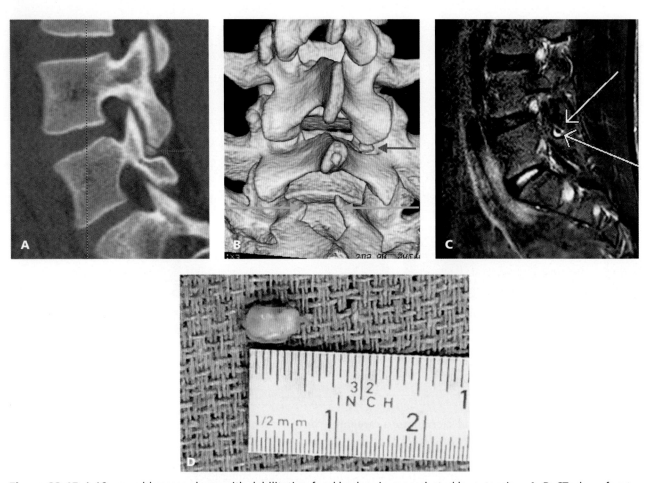

Figure 23-15 A 16-year-old soccer player with debilitating focal back pain exacerbated by extension. **A, B:** CTs show facet fracture (red arrows). Note spina bifida occulta (blue arrows). **C:** MRI showed edema about fragment (arrow). **D:** Removal of fragment cured pain, with full return to sports at 4-year follow-up.

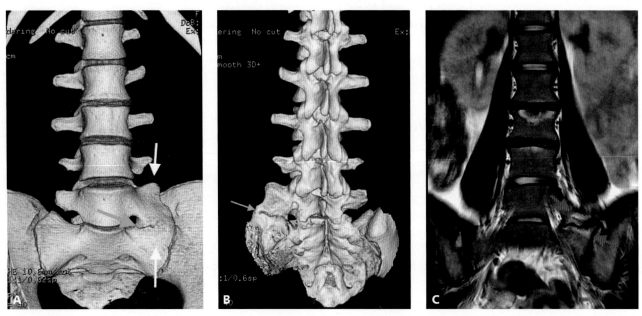

Figure 23-16 A 10-year-old swimmer with focal pain over transitional vertebrae. **A, B:** 3D CT shows pseudarthrosis (blue arrows, partial fusion between L5 and sacrum). **C:** MRI T2 coronal sequence shows inflammation on both sides of the pseudarthrosis (red arrows).

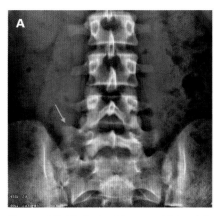
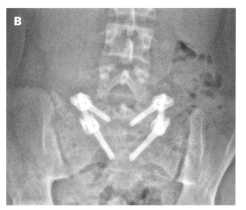

Figure 23-17 A: An 11-year-old level-9 gymnast with 18 mo of focal back pain, worse in extension, at transitional vertebrae (arrow). **B:** Three weeks after minimally invasive surgery involving in situ instrumentation and fusion, she returned to back handsprings free of her previous pain.

instrumented fusion can be curative and does not decrease motion (Fig. 23-17). Bony resection may stress facet joints that have never experienced much motion or load.

Spina Bifida Occulta

Spina bifida occulta is a very common condition, seen in about 10% of the population, in which the posterior elements are open (see Fig. 23-16B). It is usually in S1, but can be in L5 and even in the cervical spine. It never causes pain for the child but has caused panic among families who look up "spina bifida" on the internet after a reading their child's radiology report.

It is vitally important for a spine surgeon to be aware if there is any chance of encountering spina bifida occulta during exposure of the spine.

Disc Disease

Fortunately, true disc disease in the pediatric population is quite rare. Most of the time an MRI reading of bulging disc, particularly when readings come from "adult" centers, is not clinically relevant. The rare case of a true disc herniation is usually something like an adolescent who is trying to set a personal best in dead lifts when he feels a pop and has sudden pain running down his leg. Referral to specialists who deal with disc herniations on a regular basis is probably best for the patient and pediatric orthopaedic surgeon.

A classic pitfall is an endplate fracture read on an MRI as a bulging disc (Fig. 23-18). Patients with endplate fractures usually have a sudden onset of pain and pain out of proportion to a relatively modest "budging disc" seen on MRI. On physical examination, they are very stiff, and in so much pain, they can seem histrionic. A CT scan makes the diagnosis. CT scans see bone better than MRIs, no matter what MRI sequences are used. The old doctor books say these can be treated conservatively, but I have never seen a child choose conservative treatment, as they are in so much pain.

In the adult world, epidural steroid and other injections of the spine are quite common. We have not seen such injections lead to significant meaningful improvement in children or adolescents.

> **THE GURU SAYS...**
>
> The vast majority (>90%) of pediatric patients who have a herniated disc will have success with conservative management! The parents and patient need to recognize this fact and need to be patient to optimize the overall success of conservative treatment to avoid the long-term health problems with removal of the disc.
>
> DAN SUCATO

> **THE GURU SAYS...**
>
> Apophyseal ring fractures will not improve as often as in a disc herniation. Especially in the presence of neurologic symptoms, I move to surgical resection, usually with a surgeon who routinely treats disc herniations.
>
> LAUREL BLAKEMORE

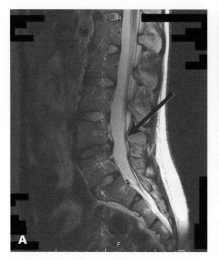
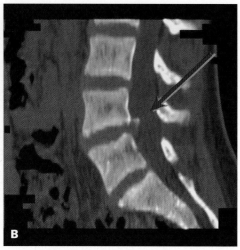

Figure 23-18 This 14-year-old girl presented with back pain and sciatica. **A:** The MRI showed a mild "bulging disc" at L4, with some canal effacement (arrow). **B:** The CT showed the bony endplate fragment that had displaced from the inferior endplate of L4 (arrow). She had complete relief after fragment excision.

Staying Out of Trouble With Back Pain, Spondys, and Other Issues

* Be concerned when back pain is progressive, well localized, or the patient stops doing fun activities.

* One will not cure all back pain, particularly when it is associated with other chronic pain conditions or psychologic overlay.

* For back pain without red flags, a sustained exercise program can do wonders for a patient's physical and mental states.

* If there is localized pain in the lumbar spine with back extension, it is a posterior element fracture until proved otherwise.

* Spondylolysis is frequently missed on X-rays and MRI. CT limited to the suspected vertebrae can make the diagnosis while minimizing unnecessary radiation.

* Spondylolysis generally has a benign natural history; surgery is not often indicated.

* Bulging discs are commonly read on MRIs but uncommonly the cause of back pain in children.

SOURCES OF WISDOM

1. Yang S, Werner BC, Singla A, Abel MF. Low back pain in adolescents: a 1-year analysis of eventual diagnoses. *J Pediatr Orthop*. 2017;37:344-347.
2. Batley S, Aartun E, Boyle E, et al. The association between psychological and social factors and spinal pain in adolescents. *Eur J Pediatr*. 2019;178(3):275-286.
3. Hestbaek L, Leboeuf-Yde C, Kyvik KO, Manniche C. The course of low back pain from adolescence to adulthood: eight-year follow-up of 9600 twins. *Spine*. 2006;31:468-472.
4. Watson KD, Papageorgiou AC, Jones GT, et al. Low back pain in schoolchildren: the role of mechanical and psychosocial factors. *Arch Dis Child*. 2003;88:12-17.
5. Jones GT, Watson KD, Silman AJ, et al. Predictors of low back pain in British schoolchildren: a population-based prospective cohort study. *Pediatrics*. 2003;111:822-828.
6. Yamaguchi KT Jr, Skaggs DL, Acevedo DC, et al. Spondylolysis is frequently missed by MRI in adolescents with back pain. *J Child Orthop*. 2012;6:237-240.
7. Fadell MF, Gralla J, Bercha I, et al. CT outperforms radiographs at a comparable radiation dose in the assessment for spondylolysis. *Pediatr Radiol*. 2015;45:1026-1030.

8. Beck NA, Miller R, Baldwin K, et al. Do oblique views add value in the diagnosis of spondylolysis in adolescents? *J Bone Joint Surg Am*. 2013;95:e65.

9. Clark E, Plint AC, Correll R, et al. A randomized, controlled trial of acetaminophen, ibuprofen, and codeine for acute pain relief in children with musculoskeletal trauma. *Pediatrics*. 2007;119:460-467.

10. Michaleff ZA, Kamper SJ, Maher CG, et al. Low back pain in children and adolescents: a systematic review and meta-analysis evaluating the effectiveness of conservative interventions. *Eur Spine J*. 2014;23:2046-2058.

11. Zapata KA, Wang-Price SS, Sucato DJ. Six-month follow-up of supervised spinal stabilization exercises for low back pain in adolescent idiopathic scoliosis. *Pediatr Phys Ther*. 2017;29(1):62-66.

12. Alyas F, Turner M, Connell D. MRI findings in the lumbar spines of asymptomatic, adolescent, elite tennis players. *Br J Sports Med*. 2007;41:836-841.

13. Sousa T, Skaggs DL, Chan P, et al. Benign natural history of spondylolysis in adolescence with midterm follow-up. *Spine Deform*. 2017;5:134-138.

14. Nielsen E, Andras LM, Siddiqui AA, et al. 40% reoperation rate in adolescents with spondylolisthesis. *Spine Deform* 2020. In press.

15. Patel RD, Graziano GP, Vanderhave KL, et al. Facet violation with the placement of percutaneous pedicle screws. *Spine*. 2011;36:e1749-e1752.

16. Kasliwal MK, Smith JS, Shaffrey CI, et al. Short-term complications associated with surgery for high-grade spondylolisthesis in adults and pediatric patients: a report from the scoliosis research society morbidity and mortality database. *Neurosurgery*. 2012;71:109-116.

17. Petraco DM, Spivak JM, Cappadona JG, et al. An anatomic evaluation of L5 nerve stretch in spondylolisthesis reduction. *Spine*. 1996;21:1133-1138.

18. Skaggs DL, Avramis I, Myung K, Weiss J. Sacral facet fractures in elite athletes. *Spine*. 2012;37:e514-e517.

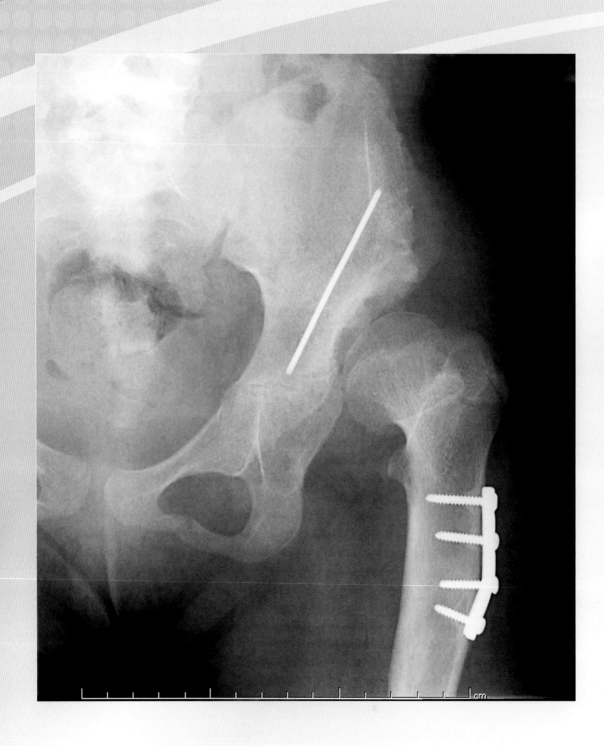

Chapter 24

Hip I: Developmental Dysplasia of the Hip

JOHN M. (JACK) FLYNN, MD

Guru: Wudbhav N. Sankar, MD

Diagnosis

Perhaps most important aspect of staying out of trouble with developmental dysplasia of the hip (DDH) is making the diagnosis early. Delay in diagnosis may lead to a worse outcome, more invasive treatment, and legal action. For instance, it's well recognized that treating a dislocated hip beginning after 7 weeks of age has a worse outcome than treatment earlier. For the pediatric orthopaedist, the vast majority of cases are referred when an abnormality has been detected by the pediatrician or neonatologist either on the physical examination or in the patient's family history. It is incumbent upon the pediatric orthopaedist to either prove that the newborn or child has a completely normal hip, or carefully characterize the extent of pathology and the treatment or surveillance that is appropriate.

DDH is the most common hip disorder in children with the typical rate of 1% to 3% for all newborn babies. Included in this large number is a wide spectrum of pathology, from hip laxity and acetabular dysplasia to frank fixed hip dislocation.

Taking a few moments to obtain an infant's history, including the associated risk factors for DDH such as breech delivery, family history of DDH and torticollis, is essential. While the presence of risk factors should heighten a clinician's suspicion of DDH, remember that the majority of cases of DDH have no risk factors present, and the majority of infants with risk factors do not have DDH.

> **► Pearls and Pitfalls of Physical Examination**
>
> ► In the newborn with bilateral dislocated hips, the Galeazzi test is normal and abduction equal and possibly normal. With bilateral dislocated hips in a newborn, absence of normal hip flexion contractures may be the only finding that suggests DDH on physical examination. In an older child, lordosis and a waddling gait suggest bilateral DDH.
> ► Examine the baby on a table when performing the Galeazzi and abduction test for maximum accuracy. A screaming baby is easier to examine on the mother's lap, but the examination will not be as accurate.
> ► Gently perform the Ortolani and Barlow tests multiple times—it can take a few iterations to sense the sliding of the cartilaginous femoral head in and around the acetabulum.
> ► The Ortolani and Barlow tests will not pick up fixed dislocations, as may occur in older children, nor will they unveil teratologic dislocations. For this reason, be sure to look for asymmetric abduction and a positive Galeazzi test in all cases.

RADIOLOGY

The role of ultrasound screening is quite complex and controversial from a public health standpoint. In some European countries, ultrasound screening of all newborns is routine. In the United States and many other countries, ultrasound evaluation is reserved primarily for babies at risk (history of breech position or DDH in the baby's family).

The femoral head begins to ossify in most children between 4 to 7 months of age. Prior to 6 months of age, ultrasound is ideal for DDH evaluation because it provides both morphometric information as well as a test of hip stability. The femoral head position, acetabular depth, and capsular laxity can be objectively assessed in one simple study with no radiation to the baby. An AP pelvis radiograph is used after 6 months of age, when ossification of the femoral head makes ultrasound more difficult, and stability information is less of a factor. Plain radiographs of infants can be misleading if one confuses an absence of a frank dislocation to be a sign of a normal hip.

THE GURU SAYS...

Getting baseline ultrasounds in my practice for patients with known DDH has shown me that I have often missed subluxations and dislocations on the contralateral side. Keep in mind that an irreducible hip dislocation will have a negative Barlow and Ortolani test! While it may not be consistent with AAP recommendations or cost-effective, I think the only way to stay out of trouble with the diagnosis of DDH is to get an ultrasound in any baby in whom DDH is at all a concern. Pediatric orthopaedists simply cannot miss this diagnosis.

WUDBHAV N. SANKAR

THE GURU SAYS...

The Barlow and Ortolani maneuvers should be performed very gently in order to prevent the infant from guarding and allow you to pick up what can be a subtle finding. I tell residents that if the blood leaves your capillary beds of your fingers, then you are squeezing the child's thighs too hard!

WUDBHAV N. SANKAR

THE GURU SAYS...

The appearance of an ossific nucleus is often delayed in hips with DDH. In these cases, judge the position of the medial and midportion of the proximal femoral metaphysis to determine if the hip is located.

WUDBHAV N. SANKAR

It is important to understand the significance of femoral rotation on a hip radiograph. Shenton line breaks with external rotation and may suggest DDH. Another pitfall of external rotation of the hip on a hip radiograph is that it creates the illusion of hip valgus.

Treatment

For all involved—parents, grandparents, the referring pediatrician, and the pediatric orthopaedist—it is helpful to talk about DDH as a spectrum, and a 1 to 10 scale adds value to the conversation. A "1" would be a hip click felt or skin fold asymmetry seen, but imaging looks normal—this is a normal hip. A "10" would be the older school-age child with completely missed DDH/dislocation. In general, we successfully treat lots of "2 and 3" with observation, lots of "3 to 6" with Pavlik harness and Ilfeld braces, and "7 to 9" with surgery. But everyone involved should know that the journey is much longer the higher the number, and risks increase based on what presents to the pediatric orthopaedist's office on day 1. Early detection is obviously optimal, but even children who are privileged to be born in a nation with an outstanding health care system can walk in at age 3 with both hips dislocated and a presenting complaint of "toe walking" (Fig. 24-1). **NEWSFLASH! Babies who were in the breech position have about four times greater chance of rapid resolution of newborn hip dysplasia than babies who have a family history, or no apparent predisposition to DDH.**

PAVLIK HARNESS

The Pavlik harness is the first-line treatment for babies up to 6 months of age. The sooner the Pavlik is started, the better the results. Although many parents will have Googled "Pavlik" before arrival, expect tears from many as they

> **A Scale for Communicating DDH Severity to Parents**
>
> 1. Hip click felt or skin fold asymmetry seen, but imaging looks normal—This is a normal hip
> 2. Hip click felt or skin fold asymmetry seen, but imaging shows slight immaturity
> 3. Usually a breech baby, normal examination—Ultrasound shows mild laxity and dysplasia
> 4. Usually a breech baby, normal examination—Ultrasound shows moderate laxity and dysplasia
> 5. Positive Barlow
> 6. Positive Ortolani and Barlow
> 7. Infant with incompletely/irreducible hip
> 8. Walking DDH, hip partially reducible, associated dysplasia
> 9. Walking DDH, irreducible, severe dysplasia
> 10. Older school-age child with completely missed DDH/dislocation

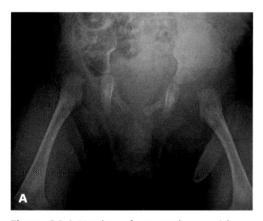 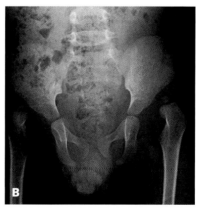

Figure 24-1 Newborn from rural area with no pediatric orthopaedist in area. **A:** "Hip click" was evaluated and the examination seemed normal, but as a precaution they sent the infant for an AP pelvis radiograph, which was read by the local radiologist as "normal." **B:** Seen at a children's hospital at age 2 for another neglected problem. The pediatrician did a comprehensive evaluation, thought a follow-up hip image was wise, and sent the child for urgent orthopaedic evaluation when the new X-ray showed both hips were dislocated. LESSONS: (1) The examination may seem normal in an infant with bilateral fixed hip dislocations. (2) Use ultrasound not radiographs on infants. (3) If you see a toddler who has potentially unresolved concerns of hip dysplasia, get new X-rays. Cost is low and the findings may be very important.

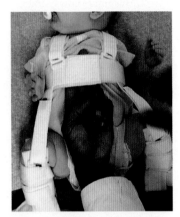

Figure 24-2 There should always be two-finger space under the chest strap. (Courtesy of Meg Morro, MD and Wudbhav N. Sankar, MD. Used with permission of CHOP Orthopedics, Philadelphia, PA.)

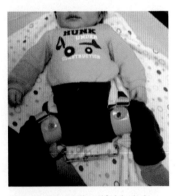

Figure 24-3 The Ilfeld abduction brace is an excellent solution for many babies when the Pavlik fails. Many parents find it easier to use. The abduction and anterior push, without the flexion, is just the solution that many DDH hips need. (Used with permission of CHOP Orthopedics, Philadelphia, PA.)

anticipate their newborn strapped into the device. A few lines of discussion really help ease the emotional strain that the new parents are feeling. First, be sure the families understand that a dislocated hip (and the process of relocating the hip) is completely painless for the babies. It's logical to think their infant is in pain; disabuse them of this notion. Secondly, put things in perspective for them. The Pavlik harness can be 95% successful if started early and used properly. It has saved countless hips over the past three generations. The alternative is weeks or months in a body cast, or perhaps surgery. Painting this picture of high success and avoidance of surgery before they lay eyes on the velcro and cloth straps of the Pavlik makes the whole initial fitting less stressful, and treatment compliance much more likely.

The anterior straps should flex the hip 90° to 100° and posterior straps should limit adduction to no more than neutral, which should maintain the hips in a reduced position and reduce likelihood of re-dislocation. The anterior and posterior straps should be taped into position to prevent an unwanted change in hip position by caretakers "adjusting" the straps. Be sure caregivers know that there should be "room for two fingers" under the chest strap at all times (Fig. 24-2).

Too much hip flexion can cause a femoral nerve palsy or inferior subluxation of the femoral head. Be sure to observe that the knees actively extend at each office visit (legs kicking) while in the harness to demonstrate a functioning femoral nerve. If femoral nerve palsy is noted, it is best to stop use of the harness for a short period of time, then switch to an alternative method such as an Ilfeld brace (Fig. 24-3). Brachial plexus injury has been reported with Pavlik harness use that promptly resolved when the harness was removed.

Avascular necrosis (AVN) has been reported with Pavlik harness treatment and may be related to the initial magnitude and position of hip displacement rather than the method of treatment. Extreme abduction in the harness may lead to AVN, though it is rare.

To stay out of trouble, abandon the Pavlik harness if it's not working. A very successful protocol is to obtain a no stress ultrasound in the Pavlik harness about 2 weeks after initial harness placement to confirm reduction of the hips. If the ultrasound shows that the position of the hip is improving but it is not perfectly reduced after 2 weeks in the harness, adjust the straps (perhaps a bit more abduction), then repeat the ultrasound about 2 weeks later. If the hips are now well reduced, then initiate 6 weeks of treatment. **NEWSFLASH! If the hips cannot be reduced with the use of a Pavlik harness, an Ilfeld brace can be successful for**

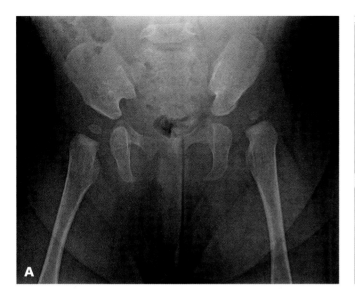
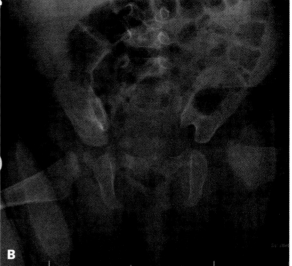
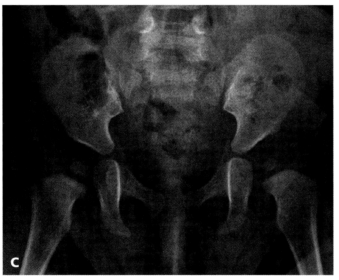

Figure 24-4 A: This 6-month-old girl on initial presentation for developmental dysplasia of the hip has high left hip dislocation, a clearly defined false acetabulum, and a moderate abduction contracture. The hip did not feel completely reducible on examination. Sounds like three trips to the OR and 18 wk of spica casting, right? **B:** Instead, we try an Ilfeld brace. Here is an in-brace X-ray after 3 wk. It looked encouraging, so we persisted. **C:** Taken at 12 mo of age, this image shows hip reduction and early improvement in the severe acetabular dysplasia that was seen at presentation. While it is too soon to know whether this baby will ever need left hip surgery, the early results show how remarkable the Ilfeld can be for some hips that in the past were automatically "CR, arthrogram, spica × 18 wk."

many, avoiding closed reduction and casting for all Pavlik failures (Fig. 24-4). The best DDH treatment ladder: Pavlik harness, then Ilfeld brace for Pavlik failures, then Spica cast for Ilfeld brace failures.

CLOSED REDUCTION AND CASTING

Closed reduction and casting is used after Pavlik/Ilfeld failure in infants, or as initial treatment in children from 6 months old to about 18 months of age (successful closed reduction alone becomes increasingly difficult after 9-12 months). Reduction, assessment of reduction, and creation of an optimal spica cast, requires as much skill and judgment as many big open operations we do. Under general anesthesia, an arthrogram is performed and gentle reduction attempted. If the

> **THE GURU SAYS...**
>
> I think the notion of "Pavlik harness disease"—the dogma that a Pavlik should be abandoned after 3 to 4 weeks if the hip has not reduced because it can lead to erosion of the posterior acetabular rim—is a bit overstated. As long as serial ultrasounds are showing some improvement, I am not afraid to use a Pavlik for longer than a month in order to get a hip to reduce.
>
> WUDBHAV N. SANKAR

medial dye pool is less than 5 to 7 mm and the reduction appears concentric, application of a well-made cast leads to success in most. Modern waterproof liners, when used correctly, greatly improve care and skin protection. It's wise to use plaster as the deepest layer to assure a great mold on the dislocation side, and then cover with fiberglass for waterproof durability.

> ### THE GURU SAYS...
>
> In practical reality, it is hard to measure the exact size of the medial dye pool intraoperatively. Ideally the dye pool is thin and concentric, but equally important is judging the "sharpness" of the chondrolabral complex. If dye reveals an infolded labrum, with poor coverage of the head, then that closed reduction should not be accepted.
>
> WUDBHAV N. SANKAR

> ### THE GURU SAYS...
>
> Placing a well-molded spica cast for DDH is truly an art. I prefer using plaster with several strips placed front to back to provide ischial support and create an upward trochanteric mold. I hold the hips myself and have several assistants cast around my hands as I constantly check and recheck the position of the hips and the adequacy of the mold.
>
> WUDBHAV N. SANKAR

Hip flexion is often as important as abduction in keeping the hip reduced. It is often a technical challenge to maintain Salter's recommended 100° of hip flexion during casting. The application of padding and cast material into the anterior hip crease tends to extend the hip.

AVN is associated with excessive hip abduction (>55°) in the spica (Fig. 24-5), yet the hip may need 50° to 60° of abduction to stay reduced. The surgeon must weigh the risks and benefits of more hip abduction in a closed reduction versus an open reduction, by assessing the safe-zone (at what amount of adduction does the femoral head dislocate). Certainly, abduction of 80° to 90° should be avoided. A pitfall in spica cast application is assuming hip abduction is OK because the combined hip abduction is less than 110°. As the surgeon pushes up on the greater trochanter, the infant's pelvis has a tendency to tilt upward on that side, and one hip may end up abducted 90° and the other at 20°. Keeping the patient's pelvis level on the spica cast table is important to judging abduction. **NEWSFLASH! IF you are losing hip flexion during spica cast application, or there is asymmetric hip abduction, or too much hip abduction, take off the casting material and start again. It is a lot better to redo the spica cast during the first anesthesia than the second.**

Following closed reduction of the hip and application of a spica cast, CT or MRI should be used to confirm reduction. Many centers use MRI to check both reduction and perfusion. **NEWSFLASH! Hip perfusion on MRI can be underestimated in**

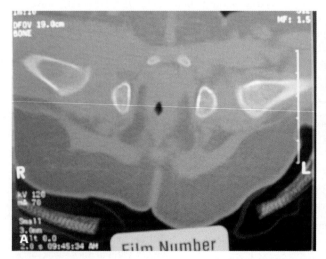
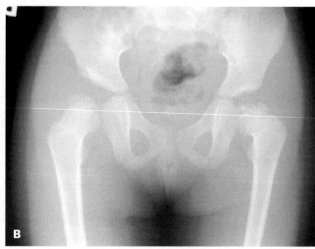

Figure 24-5 A: Note the position of excessive abduction of both hips in this CT scan following closed reduction of the right hip and spica casting. **B:** Three years later there is iatrogenic avascular necrosis in the *left* hip, which was not the dislocated hip. Immaturity of the patient's right acetabulum may be noted.

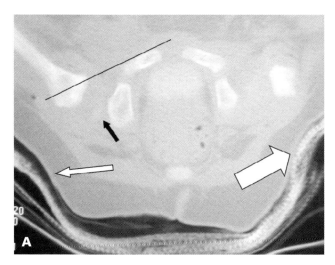

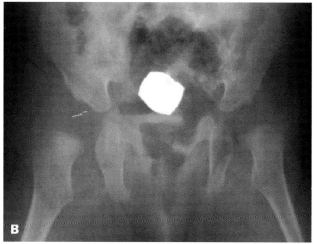

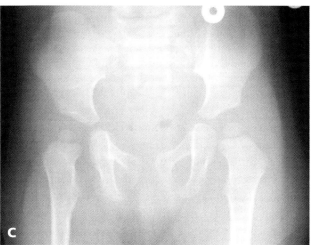

Figure 24-6 A: CT scan following closed reduction and arthrogram of the right hip. The hip is located as judged by a line along the anterior cortex of the pubis intersecting the proximal femoral metaphysis (black line). The black arrow demonstrates the characteristic apparent posterior subluxation of the femoral head within the acetabulum, which is present even when the hip is located. The small white arrow demonstrates mediocre molding of the cast under the greater trochanter to help keep the hip reduced. The trochanteric molding on the other hip (large white arrow) is actually better in this patient. A substantial trochanteric mold can help maintain the hip in a reduced position. **B:** AP radiograph 3 mo after closed reduction and casting. **C:** AP radiograph 12 mo after closed reduction. The right femoral head is smaller than the contralateral unaffected side, which may persist for a long time despite correct treatment.

an infant or toddler who is emerging from general anesthesia with blood pressure different from their normal baseline; beware of the false-positive. Use of the anterior Shenton line aids judgment of hip reduction (Fig. 24-6). When it remains dislocated, it is usually clear (Fig. 24-7).

It the child seems to be experiencing increasing irritability in a spica cast, the skin must be fully examined. This may be accomplished with a flashlight, but if necessary the spica cast may need to be removed. Preverbal children cannot always communicate where they are feeling pain, and severe ulceration and infection can develop under the cast, particularly in casts soiled by feces and urine.

OPEN REDUCTION

A hip that requires open reduction is, by definition, on the far end of the DDH severity spectrum, and everyone involved—parents, grandparents, and the surgeon—should girt their loins for a potentially long course of multiple procedures over a course of

> **THE GURU SAYS...**
>
> If you're just looking for positional information, MRI protocols can be pared down to include quick axial and coronal sequences through the hip joints. These "rapid" protocols can often be completed in 5 to 10 minutes and can avoid the need for sedation or a second anesthetic after the initial surgical procedure. Compared to CT, MRI can provide useful anatomic information about residual blocks to reduction and also avoid radiation exposure.
>
> WUDBHAV N. SANKAR

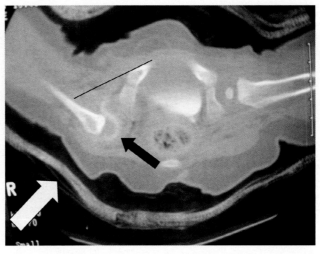

Figure 24-7 CT scan following arthrogram and closed reduction of the right hip. Note that obtaining the CT scan shortly after the intraoperative arthrogram helps outline the femoral head (thick black arrow). The right hip is dislocated as judged by a line along the anterior cortex of the pubis *not* intersecting the proximal femoral metaphysis (black line). The casting technique is quite poor, so it's no surprise this hip is dislocated. There is no molding under the greater trochanter (white arrow). The extreme abduction of the contralateral hip is undesirable and could result in avascular necrosis.

years. However, experienced DDH surgeons will tell you that some of their very best, "one and done" results were with the toddler who presents with a complete dislocation at age 2, a well-formed ossific nucleus and a false acetabulum that with a well-executed reconstruction created a 5 year old with a reduced hip indistinguishable from the opposite unaffected side, and equal leg lengths, and forever grateful parents (and pediatrician malpractice defense teams). What approach is chosen is probably of secondary importance to what surgery is done under the skin.

THE GURU SAYS...

The best chance for a well-reduced hip is the first chance, so do everything in your power to release all the normal impediments to reduction (tight psoas, inverted labrum, tight transverse acetabular ligament, etc.), and be sure you have a well-reduced hip before you leave the operating room. If the hip still doesn't medialize, check the inferior capsule as this is an underappreciated block to reduction. I always confirm the adequacy of my open reduction with intraoperative fluoroscopy to be sure I'm happy with the hip before starting to close.

WUDBHAV N. SANKAR

Staying Out of Trouble With Open Reduction

Medial Approaches

✳ Do not use a medial approach for high dislocation, as a capsulorrhaphy or other procedures cannot be done.

✳ Avoid ligating the medial circumflex artery, as it may increase the risk of AVN.

Anterior Approaches

✳ Release the psoas and adductor tendons early during the procedure—it makes the next steps easier.

✳ Reduce the hip into the real acetabulum, not the false acetabulum.

Staying Out of Trouble With Open Reduction *(continued)*

* A true inverted limbus is uncommon, and it is rare for this to impede reduction. If you think this is impeding reduction, look for other causes, like an incomplete release of the transverse acetabular ligament or psoas tendon.

* Be sure to divide the transverse acetabular ligament completely. Many failed open reductions result from insufficiently released. It is deep in the wound, but may be safely excised (Fig. 24-8).

Femoral Procedures

* Femoral shortening in combination with an open hip reduction decreases the risk of AVN.

* Consider a femoral shortening if the hip rests superior to the acetabulum in an unreduced position, or if reduction of the hip requires force. Shorten the hip by the number of millimeters that the femoral head is above its ideal resting location in the acetabulum. 1.0 to 1.5 cm shortening is common. Leg lengths, long term, are not usually impacted significantly.

> **THE GURU SAYS...**
>
> The decision to perform a femoral osteotomy is usually made intraoperatively. If traction is necessary to reduce the hip, you should probably shorten the femur. In most cases, derotation of the femur is not necessary, and can even increase the risk of a posterior dislocation. However, I assess each patient's femoral version preoperatively and do consider derotating the femur if I estimate the femoral anteversion to be greater than 50°.
>
> WUDBHAV N. SANKAR

* Be cautious not to overderotate the femur, which it can lead to posterior dislocation.

If in Doubt

* Do a femoral shortening.
* Do pelvic osteotomy in kids older than 18 months.

> **THE GURU SAYS...**
>
> Plates used for femoral shortening osteotomies should always be removed as DDH patients are at high risk of needing a total hip replacement later in life. Leaving the implants in for several years will lead to some intramedullary plates.
>
> WUDBHAV N. SANKAR

> **THE GURU SAYS...**
>
> For most walking-aged patients in need of a femoral osteotomy, I use a one-third tubular plate cut down to four holes. The proximal two holes can be predrilled with the most proximal screw inserted loosely. The plate can then be rotated out of the way to allow the osteotomy to be performed before being rotated back into position and fixed proximally. The distal fragment then just needs to be reduced to the plate.
>
> WUDBHAV N. SANKAR

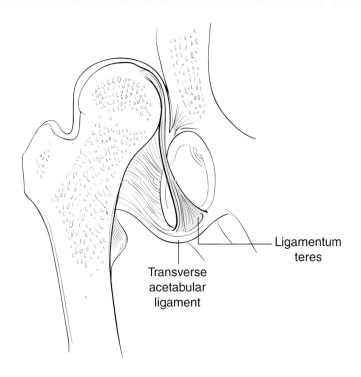

Transverse acetabular ligament

Ligamentum teres

Figure 24-8 The transverse acetabular ligament may be found by following the ligamentum teres to its origin in the inferior medial edge of the acetabulum, on the transverse acetabular ligament. The transverse acetabular ligament is often hypertrophied in dislocated hips, and must be incised to allow full reduction of the hip.

PELVIC OSTEOTOMIES

When dissecting periosteum off the outer table in very little kids, the sciatic notch may be surprisingly close. A Cobb should never be directed anywhere but anteriorly toward the hip. In the Dega osteotomy, be sure that you are high enough above acetabular rim when starting your cut. The osteotome tends to drift downward and leaves too little bone to push against when wedging open the osteotomy. Rotation of the superior acetabulum occurs in part through the triradiate cartilage, so consider other procedures if the triradiate cartilage is closed.

FOLLOW-UP

One of the more difficult judgments in pediatric orthopaedics is determining whether acetabular development is sufficient following reduction of a hip. An acetabular index of 35° or more 2 years after reduction of the hip was associated with an 80% probability of becoming a Severin grade III/IV hip in one series, so this may serve as some objective measure. Unfortunately, the acetabular index is subject to significant variability. A subjective criterion we have found useful to confirm maturation of the acetabulum is increased concavity of the acetabulum over time.

Avascular Necrosis (aka Proximal Femoral Growth Disturbance)

Most AVN in reality is a minimal growth disturbance, often of no clinical consequence. Have patience and observe without panicking, as there is little that can be done at early stages anyway. A particular type of AVN to be aware of is a lateral arrest, which occurs at a mean age of 9 years. This further emphasizes the importance of long-term follow-up for children with DDH.

For proximal femoral undergrowth, and relative overgrowth of the greater trochanter, avoid a useless operation by remembering that a greater trochanter physeal arrest will only be of benefit under age 8, as in older children there is not sufficient growth remaining for an epiphysiodesis to have a meaningful effect. In children 8 years old and older, a trochanteric transfer is preferable to an epiphysiodesis. A technical point for a trochanteric transfer is to plan on extensive release of soft tissues to allow for sufficient movement of the greater trochanter.

THE GURU SAYS...

Most DDH experts agree that continued follow-up until skeletal maturity is warranted after closed or open reduction because of the risk of residual dysplasia. When to intervene surgically for a patient with asymptomatic dysplasia, however, is more controversial. That being said, subluxation or the development of subchondral cysts are poor prognostic signs and almost always indicate the need for surgery.

WUDBHAV N. SANKAR

Staying Out of Trouble With Developmental Dysplasia of the Hip

* Do an ultrasound of the hips in infants with the following risk factors for DDH: breech position in utero, family history, and congenital muscular torticollis.

* The Ortolani and Barlow tests may take a few tries to feel the movement. Do not hesitate to repeat these tests multiple times. If a baby is crying or irritable, try a pacifier, or Mom's little finger, or a bottle.

* With Pavlik harness treatment, confirm reduction of hips within 1 to 3 weeks of placement of harness. If hips cannot be reduced, abandon Pavlik harness treatment and try and Ilfeld brace.

Staying Out of Trouble With Developmental Dysplasia of the Hip *(continued)*

* Avoid abduction of more than 55° of either hip in a spica cast, as this increases the risk of AVN of the femoral head.

* Confirm reduction with an MRI (for closed reduction) or CT (for open reduction). Beware of the false-positive MRI ischemia test when the infant is emerging from anesthesia

* In an open reduction for "walking DDH," if in doubt, shorten the femur.

SOURCES OF WISDOM

1. Gornitzky AL, Georgiadis AG, Seeley MA, et al. Does perfusion MRI after closed reduction of developmental dysplasia of the hip reduce the incidence of avascular necrosis? *Clin Orthop Relat Res.* 2016;474:1153-1156.
2. Sankar WN, Nduaguba A, Flynn JM. Ilfeld abduction orthosis is an effective second-line treatment after failure of Pavlik harness for infants with developmental dysplasia of the hip. *J Bone Joint Surg Am.* 2015;97(4):292-297.
3. Sankar WN, Tang EY, Moseley CF. Predictors of the need for femoral shortening osteotomy during open treatment of developmental dislocation of the hip. *J Pediatr Orthop.* 2009;29(8):868-871.
4. Sarkissian EJ, Sankar WN, Baldwin K, Flynn JM. Is there a predilection for breech infants to demonstrate spontaneous stabilization of DDH instability? *J Pediatr Orthop.* 2014;34(5):509-513.
5. Sarkissian EJ, Sankar WN, Zhu X, et al. Radiographic follow-up of DDH in infants: are x-rays necessary after a normalized ultrasound. *J Pediatr Orthop.* 2015;35(6):551-555.
6. Suzuki S, Kashiwagi N, Kasahara Y, et al. Avascular necrosis and the Pavlik harness: the incidence of avascular necrosis in three types of congenital dislocation of the hip as classified by ultrasound. *J Bone Joint Surg Br.* 1996;78(4):631-635.
7. Upasani VV, Bomar JD, Matheney TH, et al. Evaluation of brace treatment for instant hip dislocation in a prospective cohort. *J Bone Joint Surg.* 2016;98:1215-1221.
8. Wang TM, Wu KW, Shih SF, et al. Outcomes of open reduction for developmental dysplasia of the hip: does bilateral dysplasia have a poorer outcome? *J Bone Joint Surg Am.* 2013;95(12):1081-1086.

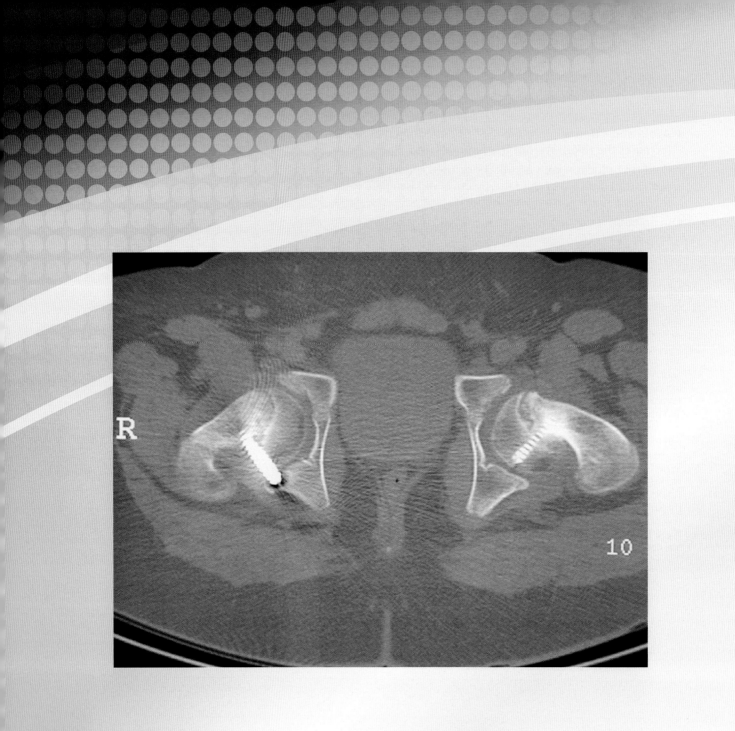

Chapter 25

Hip II: Legg-Calvé-Perthes Disease, Slipped Capital Femoral Epiphysis, and Transient Synovitis Versus Septic Arthritis

JOHN M. (JACK) FLYNN, MD

Guru: Wudbhav N. Sankar, MD

Legg-Calvé-Perthes Disease

Legg-Calvé-Perthes is an idiopathic avascular necrosis (AVN) of the capital femoral epiphysis in a young child. The condition tends to run a fairly predictable time course. It affects both hips in about 10% of cases and is much more common in boys (about 4:1). Children with Legg-Calvé-Perthes disease most commonly present between the ages of 4 and 8 years, but the condition may be seen in children less than 2 years old and as old as skeletal maturity. Most of the trouble with Legg-Calvé-Perthes disease revolves around making the diagnosis, dealing with the parents, and being selective about surgical treatment. Without careful selection, the orthopaedist can get into trouble by overtreating the young or the mildly affected, or the untreatable severe cases, or conversely, get into trouble by missing the more involved older child who would really benefit from surgical management (Fig. 25-1).

The key to staying out of trouble and making the diagnosis of Legg-Calvé-Perthes is to recognize that the presentation can be very subtle and may be mistaken for transient synovitis in the early stages. The most common experience of

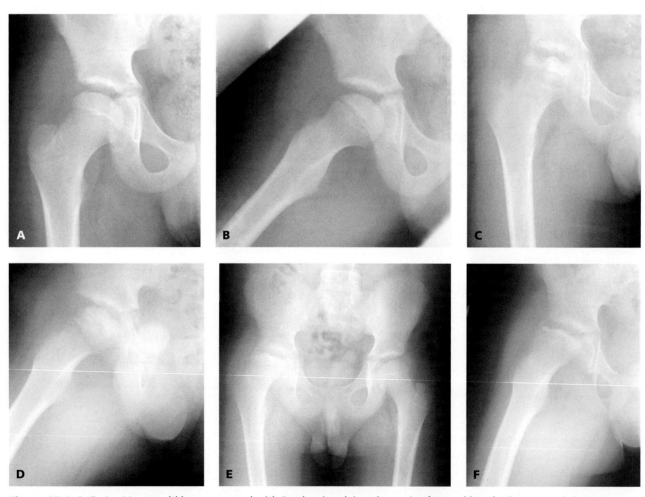

Figure 25-1 **A, B:** An 11-year-old boy presented with Perthes involving the entire femoral head. His prognosis is poor. Although it may be premature to assign a Herring type, it is not too early to intervene. No treatment was offered. **C, D:** Six months later, the hip is still contained. Most would call it a Herring B/C. No treatment was offered. **E, F:** Ten months after presentation, there is subluxation. He has very little motion. Now the family was offered surgical management. Could the surgeon have stayed out of trouble with surgical management at presentation?

the orthopaedist at diagnosis is a mom who says "I notice a slight limp at the end of the day, but he wasn't complaining of pain."

Another source of trouble with Perthes is being fooled by conditions that imitate it.

On physical examination, the only sign of a problem may be a subtle asymmetry in hip motion, typically a loss of hip abduction and/or internal rotation. In a young child in the early stages of the disease, the examiner should carefully control the pelvis during examination to avoid missing subtle asymmetry between the hips.

In later stages of the disease, the child may have a flexion contracture and a positive Thomas test. Contracture or spasm of the adductor tendon can also be seen. Just as it is easy to miss a subtle loss of hip motion, it is easy to miss gait abnormalities early in the condition. If there is a subchondral fracture or a hip effusion, the child may walk with either an antalgic gait or with the foot somewhat externally rotated. Later in the condition, the child may develop a Trendelenburg gait and have a Trendelenburg sign.

To stay out of trouble, order an anteroposterior and frog lateral plain radiograph at the first visit for any child who presents complaining of hip or thigh pain.

If there is a synovitis, the pelvis is shifted to the affected side because the X-ray technician is trying to abduct that side but since the hip won't abduct, the child elevates that pelvis and it appears "catawampus," or out of line. Be aware that even high-quality plain radiographs may be normal at the first visit.

On initial radiographs, look for the extent of involvement of the femoral epiphysis, paying particular attention to the lateral pillar, the key to prognosis. Increasingly, MRI is becoming essential in the management of Perthes. Although radiographs are always the starting point, MRI can "predict" what future radiographs will look like, as gadolinium-enhanced and diffusion-weighted MRI can identify the ischemic areas of the femoral head early in the disease process.

The treatment of Legg-Calvé-Perthes disease remains controversial and has been dominated in the past more by personal preference and local customs than good data. There are several keys to staying out of trouble when treating Perthes. **NEWSFLASH! It is important to understand how much the concept of a "dead hip" terrifies parents. Parents who present to you, especially for a second opinion, can be bewildered by information on the web and the multiple varying opinions that they get from experienced "experts."** To stay out of trouble you will need more time with these families to explain the pathophysiology of the condition, the expected time course, and the limited amount of long-term natural history and treatment data. It is disconcerting to families to learn how uncertain the experts are about definitive treatment.

It is clear that the orthopaedic surgeon should focus attention on children 8 years and older, and on those with moderate hip involvement (Herring B, or B/C). Surgeons and children get in trouble when a complication occurs in the process of overtreating one of the 60+% of children who would do perfectly well without ever seeing a doctor.

Trying to rest the hip of an active (often hyperactive) boy or girl with Legg-Calvé-Perthes can create trouble for the family and the doctor. Children younger than 7 years cannot use crutches effectively. Even older children capable with crutches will be highly noncompliant, especially considering that the request is to use crutches for many months. Therefore, when resting the hip seems important, many prefer to use abduction (Petrie casts) for a period of 6 weeks, followed by physical therapy to work on hip and knee range of motion. To stay out of trouble with Petrie casts, be careful to pad carefully around the Achilles tendon, as this is

Perthes Imitators

- Transient synovitis
- Septic arthritis
- Sickle cell disease
- Osteomyelitis of the femoral neck
- Chondrolysis
- Gaucher disease/mucopolysaccharidosis
- Juvenile rheumatoid arthritis
- Multiple epiphyseal dysplasia
- Spondyloepiphyseal dysplasia
- Meyers dysplasia

THE GURU SAYS...

More research is needed, but the amount of hypoperfusion of the femoral head on perfusion MRI seems to correlate with the amount of radiographic deformity down the road. Early perfusion MRI, therefore, may offer the best chance to identify those patients most at risk for femoral head deformity and allow early intervention in certain patients.

WUDBHAV N. SANKAR

THE GURU SAYS...

In your initial discussion with a family dealing with a new diagnosis, take time to explain the condition, what is known and what is unknown about the disease. Be sure to inform families that dealing with Perthes is a "marathon not a sprint" and that continued attention over months to years of active disease is necessary to optimize results. And focus on overarching principles (containment, range of motion, etc.) rather than treatment specifics at least at the start.

WUDBHAV N. SANKAR

a common site of cast pressure sores. Also, prepare the family for a child who is difficult to transport and move around the house.

Should the orthopaedist choose a surgical option, there are certainly several areas that can be sources of trouble for any of the operations: shelf arthroplasty or varus derotational osteotomy (VDRO). Each of these surgical options has one or more champions who promote it as the best option for most kids. Each method has pros and cons and sources of trouble. A common theme for any procedure is to avoid surgery on a very stiff hip.

Staying Out of Trouble in the Surgical Management of Legg-Calvé-Perthes Disease

Shelf Arthroplasty

* Be certain the child has full hip motion preoperatively, and use an arthrogram to check that the hip is congruent.
* A shelf is better early in the diagnosis, not during the late remodeling stages.
* Be certain not to block hip flexion with the shelf.

Varus Derotational Osteotomy

* Warn the family preoperatively that either real or apparent limb shortening may be seen postoperatively.
* Be certain the child has full hip motion, and use an arthrogram to check that the hip is congruent.
* Do the osteotomy fairly early after the diagnosis, not during the remodeling stage.
* Warn the family that a valgus osteotomy may be needed later to improve hip abduction.
* Do not create too much varus. Keep the neck shaft angle at 115° (or more) or the child will limp for a long time (warn the parents!).

Slipped Capital Femoral Epiphysis

Slipped capital femoral epiphysis (SCFE) is the most common adolescent hip disorder, estimated at 1 per 10 000 in the United States, and is probably increasing with the epidemic of pediatric obesity. About 80% of the cases occur during the adolescent growth spurt (at ~12 years of age for girls and 13.5 years of age for boys). The condition is said to be more common in obese African American boys, and more common on the left side. In northern climates, presentation is most common in late summer/early fall, perhaps due to months of low sunlight followed by more active summer months.

One key to staying out of trouble with SCFE is to recognize the child who is an outlier in terms of these demographic criteria. If the child is 11 years old or younger, consider a possible underlying cause such as renal osteodystrophy, hypothyroidism, panhypopituitarism, and hypogonadal conditions. These require an endocrine evaluation and also increase the risk of subsequent contralateral slip. About 25% of the cases of SCFE are bilateral, although some experts believe that up to 60% to 80% are bilateral, many being silent cases that are not discovered until much later. Perhaps the greatest source of trouble with SCFE is a delay in diagnosis (Fig. 25-2). Remember that in SCFE associated with renal failure, the SCFEs are bilateral in 95% of cases.

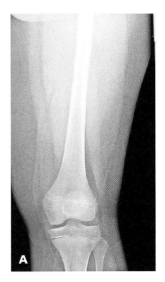
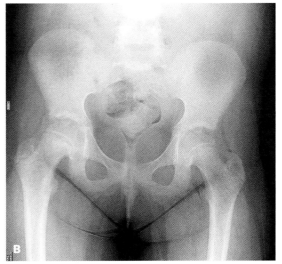
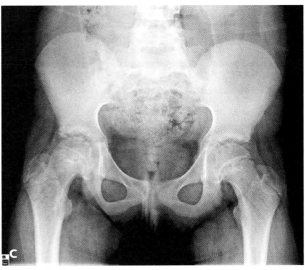
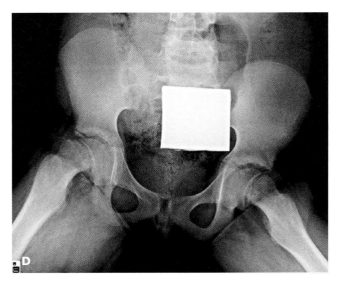

Figure 25-2 This 9-year-old girl presented to her primary care doctor with a 4-month history of left hip and knee pain. The physician obtained knee (**A**) and hip (**B**) films, but relied on the radiologist to detect a problem. Unfortunately for the child and doctor, the radiologist read the films as "normal examination." **C, D:** The child was finally referred to the pediatric orthopaedist 2 mo later, with what had become moderately displaced SCFE bilaterally.

At presentation, the child will usually have hip, groin, or thigh pain, often for a long time. Although many reports have described the challenges that primary care doctors face in diagnosing SCFE, the diagnosis is missed by orthopaedic surgeons missing the diagnosis. These include stories in which the surgeon first thinks of SCFE while trying to get the externally rotated hip into the leg holder for a knee arthroscopy, or worse, discovering a SCFE at one of the knee arthroscopy postop visits (Fig. 25-3). On physical examination, these children will often have an abductor lurch or an antalgic gait. The foot is usually externally rotated. On the table-top examination, the patient will demonstrate obligate external rotation and abduction with attempts to flex the hip. To stay out of trouble, recognize the signs of an unstable SCFE. Children will not be able to walk and may have pain just with gentle log-rolling of the hip.

Poor imaging, or the misreading of good imaging, can be a source of trouble with SCFE. An AP and frog lateral of both hips should be obtained. Although some believe that the true lateral radiograph is more sensitive, it is much harder to

> **THE GURU SAYS...**
>
> Making the diagnosis early in SCFE is key. Most patients will have groin or thigh pain or pain referred to the knee, but some will just have a painless limp. Have a very low threshold for getting hip X-rays in an adolescent to rule out the diagnosis.
>
> WUDBHAV N. SANKAR

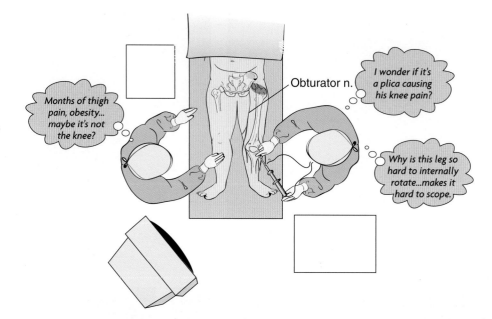

Figure 25-3 "It's an SCFE, stupid!!" SCFE can present as knee pain instead of hip pain. The reason this is thought to occur is that the obturator nerve picks up the inflammation around the hip and refers the pain to the medial thigh. If the physician examines the knee instead of the hip, the child may be subjected to unnecessary knee arthroscopy when in fact the proper diagnosis is SCFE in the hip.

obtain in a morbidly obese adolescent with hip pain. Often, the AP view will show important signs of a mild SCFE for the careful observer, such as subtle physeal widening, a break in Klein line (Fig. 25-4), or a decrease in femoral epiphyseal height of the involved side compared to the opposite side.

More advanced imaging, such as an MRI, is rarely necessary in SCFE. In some select cases, when there is a very high clinical suspicion, but no confirming evidence on good quality plain radiographs, an MRI can be helpful to make the diagnosis (Fig. 25-5). The surgeon should look for edema on either side of the physes. Other signs on MRI may be slight widening of the physes and a hip effusion. Beware, however, that an obese adolescent with a hip effusion could certainly have other conditions.

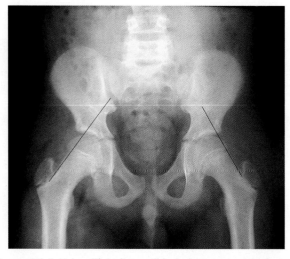

Figure 25-4 Using Klein line will help keep you out of trouble. The line drawn along the superior neck on the AP radiograph intersects less epiphysis on the left (SCFE) side.

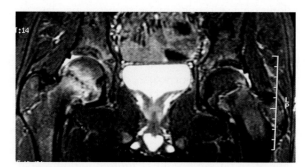

Figure 25-5 An MRI is rarely needed, but can keep you out of trouble on the most questionable cases. This image of a child with a right early SCFE shows slight physeal widening and edema on both sides of the physis. (Courtesy of L. Wells, MD.)

The goals of treatment of SCFE are to stabilize the physis before more epiphyseal displacement occurs and avoid AVN or some procedure or hardware-related complication. Timing of treatment of unstable SCFE has gained increased attention. In the past, unstable SCFE was felt to require urgent reduction and treatment. Unfortunately, many cases don't arrive at the treatment center within 24 hours of the onset of symptoms, so even if the surgery is within hours after arrival in the ED, it is more than 24 hours after the unstable SCFE occurred. Increasingly an AVN "danger zone" has been identified at 1 to 7 days after occurrence. Until definitive data are available, timing of treatment cannot be standardized in a way to guarantee avoidance of AVN. There is not enough evidence to make the kid who arrives 2 days after first symptoms lie in bed for 5 more days to get out of the "AVN danger zone." The reality is that we prioritize unstable SCFEs as urgent add-ons, but it is not clear that such prioritization improves outcomes. Stable SCFEs should not be discharged and returned for elective fixation. Every institution has stories about mild stable SCFE patients who went home for the weekend and had significant progression.

In stabilizing a slipped capital femoral epiphysis, the surgeon should aim to have a screw (≥7 mm) into the center of the femoral head on every radiographic view, perpendicular to the physis, stopping about 5 mm from the subchondral bone of the epiphyseal articular cartilage. To stay out of trouble, avoid the posterior, superior portion of the femoral head where the blood supply enters the epiphysis. If you are going to miss in one direction or another, miss with your screw inferior to the center of the head.

> **THE GURU SAYS...**
>
> To facilitate potential screw removal in the future in cases that need further surgery, always use full threaded screws. Most partially threaded screws have a narrower unthreaded portion and are not reverse cutting—both of which make them extremely difficult to remove when the bone is hard.
>
> WUDBHAV N. SANKAR

Good intraoperative imaging is essential to staying out of trouble. You must be able to clearly visualize the femoral head on both the AP and lateral views. Many surgeons have discovered that it is easier to obtain good visualization of the femoral head on the lateral view in an obese adolescent using a radiolucent table. Using the radiolucent table is a somewhat more demanding technique, because it is easy to bend the guide pin as the hip is taken into the frog lateral position.

Classic descriptions of the surgical technique recommend entering the anterior femoral neck as proximal as is necessary in order to place the guide in perpendicular to the physes. If you use the same technique as for pinning an adult hip fracture, you may not be perpendicular to the physis and you risk subtrochanteric fracture (Fig. 25-6). Such recommendations, however, can lead to several sources of trouble in severe SCFEs. As the entry site for the screw gets closer and closer to the physis, there is less metaphyseal bone of the femoral neck to hold the screw. This can lead to cutout of the screw, progression of the slip after pinning, or femoral neck fracture. Likewise, the anterior screw can also abut against the edge of the acetabulum (Fig. 25-7) during flexion and extension, leading to damage.

Hard bone can be a problem as well (Fig. 25-8). In chronic SCFE, the bone just distal to the physes can become very dense, as the region is subjected to high shear forces during the progression of the slip. When drilling your guide pin, don't

> **THE GURU SAYS...**
>
> A cannulated depth gauge can be used to protect the guidewire from bending when the hip is frogged for a lateral. The assistant must push down against the skin with the depth gauge as the hip is being moved.
>
> WUDBHAV N. SANKAR

> **THE GURU SAYS...**
>
> To prevent impingement from the head of the screw try to avoid inserting the screw medial to the intertrochanteric region. While you should still aim for the center of the femoral head, a more distal and lateral starting point may mean that your screw won't cross the physis perfectly perpendicular—but that's better than tearing up the joint or the labrum with an intra-articular screw head.
>
> WUDBHAV N. SANKAR

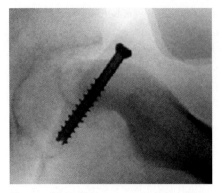

Figure 25-7 This screw was left a little proud, and it abuts the acetabulum when the hip is flexed.

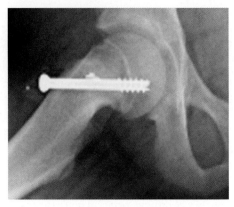

Figure 25-8 Obese teenagers can have extremely hard bone. This image demonstrates a metal fragment adjacent to the screw. The fragment was the thread of the first attempted screw that unraveled in the hard bone of the calcar portion of the femoral neck. (Courtesy of R. Davidson, MD.)

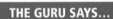

Figure 25-6 This SCFE was stabilized using an adult hip fracture technique, with a very low subtrochanteric starting point for two screws. The screws were not perpendicular to the physis, and they created a stress-riser leading to a subtrochanteric fracture.

THE GURU SAYS...

In extremely hard bone, don't be afraid to tap across the physis. This takes the pressure off the screw and minimizes the chance of stripping the head during insertion.

WUDBHAV N. SANKAR

THE GURU SAYS...

The approach-withdrawal technique uses live fluoroscopy to assess the distance between the screw tip and the edge of the femoral head. Move the hip in all positions, and find the point at which the screw is closest to the edge of the joint, but then moves away. This is the true position of the screw in relation to the joint.

WUDBHAV N. SANKAR

---

allow it to stop in this dense bone: it can be very difficult to restart the guide pin. Judicious use of live fluoroscopic imaging and continuous drilling can avoid this problem. In most cases, it is unnecessary to overdrill the guide pin. **NEWSFLASH! If you like to overdrill, be very alert that any bend in the pin can drive pin migration, or could lead to shearing of the pin or during overdrilling.** Although there is controversy about how far the screw should be across the physis, most experts and studies recommend 4 to 5 threads into the epiphysis. Finally, after the screw is in place, it is essential to be certain that the most proximal tip of the screw is not in the joint itself. Use of the approach and withdrawal technique can assure proper screw positioning at the end of the case (Fig. 25-9).

Special considerations may be necessary to stay out of trouble in atypical SCFE in young children. If the SCFE is related to renal osteodystrophy, stay out of trouble with combined medical management and surgery with custom-machined pins preventing slip progression while allowing continued physeal growth. Warn parents of children with Down syndrome that there is a much higher incidence of AVN in Down syndrome kids, and look for hypothyroidism.

After surgery, partial weight bearing is recommended, although most adolescents will stop using crutches within about 2 weeks. **NEWSFLASH! Persistent hip pain more than 2 weeks after surgery should be a red flag! Because most patients experience a rapid relief of their preoperative symptoms, the surgeon should carefully look for problems if the patient returns for a follow-up visit and there is persistent hip pain.**

Potential Causes for Persistent Hip Pain After Fixation of SCFE

- Persistent instability of the physis with inadequate fixation
- Pin penetrating into the joint (Fig. 25-10)
- Superficial or deep infection
- AVN of the capital femoral epiphysis

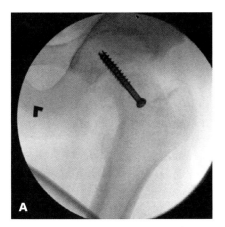
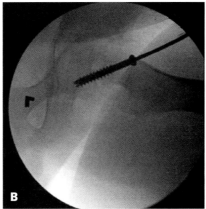
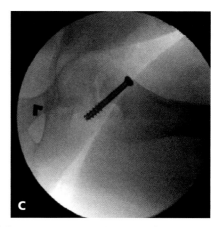

Figure 25-9 An essential part of staying out of trouble after SCFE fixation is careful intraoperative evaluation of the screw placement. Importance of a true lateral approach-withdrawal technique. This screw looks perfect on the AP (**A**) and semi-lateral (**B**). **C:** This image shows threads out, however. The time to discover this is in the operating room, not months later in the clinic (see Fig. 25-10).

To stay out of trouble and avoid a sometimes difficult, unsatisfying (broken screw), and unnecessary operation, advise the family during that very first post-operative discussion that the screw never needs to be removed in the vast majority of patients.

Another important counseling discussion regards whether the asymptomatic side should be stabilized with a screw. Families may recoil when told that it would be a good idea to put a screw in a hip that is currently "normal" to prevent a future problem—it sounds like fixing something that is not broken. Depending on age and underlying conditions (especially endocrine disorders), the probability of contralateral SCFE can be more than 30%. Maturity is a critical predictor, and though many studies have been done over the years, the long-standing wisdom still holds: if the triradiate cartilage is open, fix the contralateral "normal" hip. To stay out of trouble, if the child is from a typical demographic group and follow-up will be reliable, observation is generally preferred to the risk of creating a complication on the asymptomatic side (which is uniformly unappreciated by families and exploited by plaintiff attorneys). On the other hand, if the child has an open triradiate cartilage, renal osteodystrophy, hypothyroidism, or some other endocrine problem, it is probably best to offer bilateral internal fixation at the time of the initial presentation.

THE GURU SAYS...

When weighing the pros and cons of prophylactic pinning of the contralateral side, it's best to involve the family in the discussion to allow "shared decision making." For those patients who fall in a gray area, discuss the pros and cons of both approaches and allow the family to make their own choice.

WUDBHAV N. SANKAR

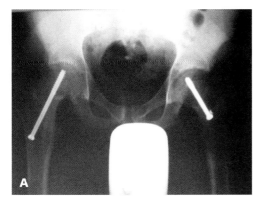
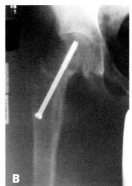
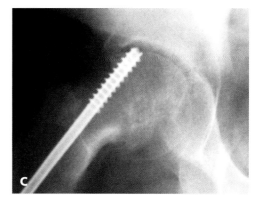

Figure 25-10 Persistent hip pain after internal fixation of an SCFE requires careful evaluation. This AP pelvis image (**A**) and this AP of the right hip (**B**) do not show a clear source of the pain. **C:** This oblique image shows the screw in the joint, with damage to the acetabulum. That certainly explains this patient's persistent pain.

Although only about 5% to 10% of SCFEs are unstable, they certainly cause at least 5% to 10% of the problems. To stay out of trouble, an unstable SCFE should be treated urgently (with the 1- to 7-day danger window caveat previously discussed), and the family should be counseled at the time of presentation about the high risk of AVN. A second screw for additional internal fixation is wise, and the child should be followed up very closely in the postoperative period.

Reduction of the unstable SCFE is a favorite source of discussion and debate. In the hands of an expert, the Modified Dunn procedure can give a perfect anatomic result with relatively low rates of AVN. Others show similar results with "inadvertent reduction" and capsulotomy, or the Parsch technique of mini-open manual reduction, evacuation of hematoma, and pinning. Considering that Level 1 evidence from a randomized controlled trial of many thousands of unstable SCFEs is unlikely, follow the principles to stay out of trouble—get the best possible, unforced reduction, evacuate the intra-capsular hematoma, and assure stable fixation. Increasingly, surgeons are checking the femoral epiphyseal perfusion after fixation (Fig. 25-11), although how to handle the unperfused head after reduction and fixation is a conundrum. Internal fixation of a valgus slipped capital femoral epiphysis presents certain challenges. The perfect trajectory for a pin may put the neurovascular bundle at risk (Fig. 25-12).

GETTING OUT OF TROUBLE IN SCFE

If symptoms and plain radiographs suggest possible improper fixation of a slipped capital femoral epiphysis, or possible loss of reduction, a CT scan can be a very valuable study to understand the problem in three dimensions (Fig. 25-13). It may be necessary to exchange screws or add a second screw for further fixation. Any time a screw is removed, protective weight bearing should be considered to avoid a pathologic fracture. This is particularly true if the screw entered the subtrochanteric area of the femur, where it can create a stress-riser, leading to fracture. Infection around the screw fixing a SCFE is rare, but has been reported. These children will often present with persistent pain and possibly an elevated C-reactive protein (CRP) and radiolucency around the screw on plain radiographs. Early after surgery, every effort should be made to avoid removing the screw. The area should be cultured and the child should be placed on appropriate antibiotics. If that fails, the screw should be removed, the area debrided, and a new screw should be placed in a different position.

AVASCULAR NECROSIS

The surgeon should have a high index of suspicion for AVN in acute SCFE, and consider a bone scan or MRI early after surgery. Non–weight bearing is recommended until the presence or absence of AVN is confirmed. If AVN occurs, the decision to change screws depends on the status of the physis. If the physis is closed, any penetrating screws should be removed promptly. If the physis is still open, any penetrating screws should be backed off or a new screw should be placed in a different position. Treatment of AVN in SCFE with a vascularized fibula graft has been recommended by some. Success depends on many factors, particularly the experience of the person performing the vascularized fibular grafting. In most cases, AVN after SCFE is treated with protective weight bearing, activity restrictions, and use of nonsteroidal anti-inflammatory drugs. In most cases, the final result is disappointing. A redirecting osteotomy is an option if there is just a small segment of the head affected.

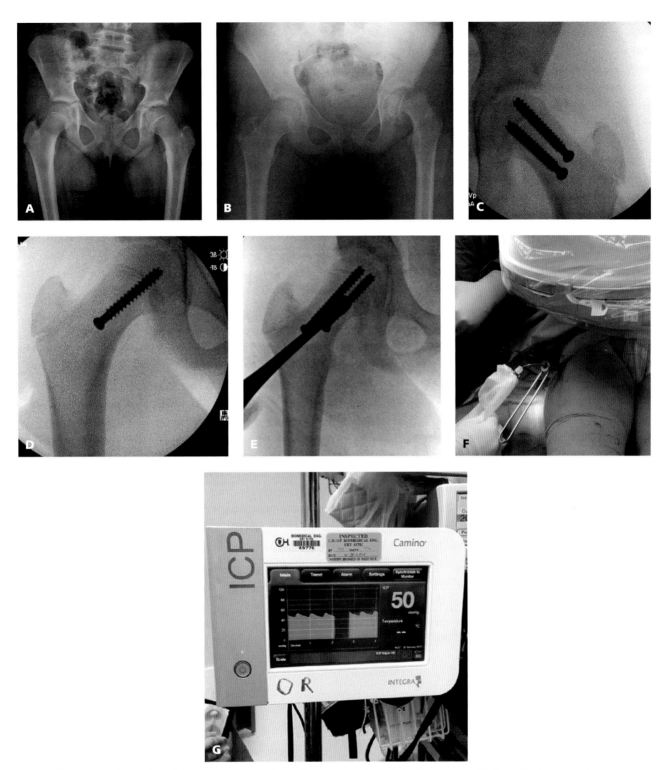

Figure 25-11 **A:** After a fall, this patient was evaluated at another hospital, diagnosed with "nondisplaced avulsion fracture," and sent home. **B:** Three weeks later, the patient experienced sudden onset of left hip pain while hopping. **C:** Gentle closed reduction (Leadbetter maneuver) and fixation was undertaken with two screws on the left. **D:** Single-screw prophylactic fixation was done on the right. **E:** Capsulotomy was performed with a Cobb elevator to decompress. **F:** An intracranial pressure probe was placed down the screw shaft of the left unstable SCFE side and into the femoral head. **G:** Waveforms should have a pulse pressure and should be synchronous with the patient's heart rate. Absolute value of pressure is not important.

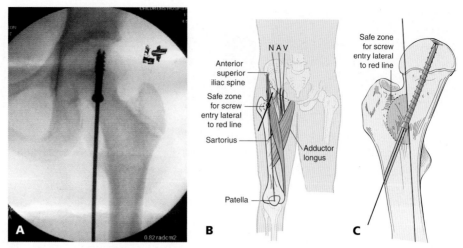

Figure 25-12 The "valgus SCFE" can be trouble. **A:** The fluoroscopic image shows the screw oriented perpendicular to the physis. **B:** The relationship between the guidewire trajectory and the neurovascular bundle. **C:** Staying out of trouble pinning a valgus SCFE. The safe zone for the screw is just lateral to the red line drawn here between the anterior-superior iliac spine and the center of the patella. The femoral head sits very superiorly and almost laterally on the neck of the femur. A very vertical track should be taken from distal to proximal in order to get a screw across the physis.

Chondrolysis is much less frequent than in the past. It is clear now that many previous cases were related to intra-articular hardware. The surgeon should be certain when making the diagnosis of chondrolysis that there is no persistent pin penetration. A CT scan may be best for this assessment. Otherwise, the treatment of chondrolysis is physical therapy, anti-inflammatory drugs, and possibly an epidural anesthetic with physical therapy.

Persistent limited motion is common after stable or unstable SCFEs, especially if SCFE is severely displaced. Observation only is recommended for the first 18 to 24 months, because remodeling of the femoral neck can occur. However, there is also a growing body of evidence that the displaced metaphysis of a severe slip damages the acetabular cartilage, leading to degenerative changes. A variety of proximal femoral osteotomies have been proposed for the proximal femoral deformity that occurs after an SCFE. Many of these osteotomies restore internal

> **THE GURU SAYS...**
>
> Femoroacetabular impingement from residual SCFE deformity is being increasingly recognized after in situ pinning. It remains unclear why certain patients become symptomatic from FAI while others do not, but it's best to explain the potential for this condition at the time of in situ pinning. Reconstructive surgery can then be offered to those that become symptomatic over time.
>
> WUDBHAV N. SANKAR

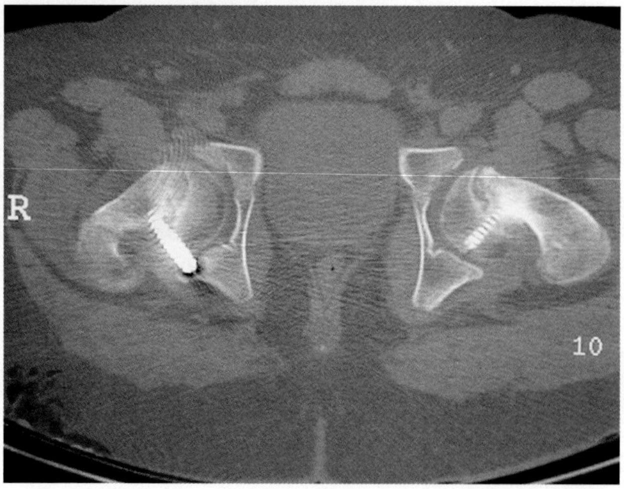

Figure 25-13 This CT cut demonstrates why this boy had so much pain and stiffness after SCFE fixation. Persistent postoperative pain must be investigated.

rotation and flexion. Some of them may be able to alter the likelihood of osteoarthritis. The closer the osteotomy is to the physis, the better the correction of the deformity, but also the higher risk of complications. Intertrochanteric osteotomy with internal/external fixation has been the most widely used. However, this creates a very complex shape to the proximal femur and may challenge our total hip colleagues in the future.

Transient Synovitis Versus Septic Arthritis

Transient synovitis is the most common cause of hip pain in school-age children. Conversely, septic arthritis of the hip is rare but is a potentially crippling disaster if the diagnosis is delayed or not made at all. Distinguishing transient synovitis from septic arthritis is an essential skill for staying out of trouble in pediatric orthopaedics. Although clinical prediction rules using physical examination findings and lab results abound, they are no substitute for experience, good judgment, and a careful history and physical examination.

In septic arthritis, the child is usually sick, getting worse by the hour, and will not bear weight on the involved side. There is usually pain with simple log-rolling of the hip. Usually the CRP is up even early in the condition. **NEWSFLASH! To stay out of trouble, use CRP not ESR when encountering an early presentation of potential septic arthritis.** The key to diagnosis is history and physical examination followed by an aspiration of every hip that is suspicious for septic arthritis. Beware that in the early hours of septic arthritis, there may be very little hip effusion, the CRP may be low but on the rise, and the ultrasound unimpressive. If there is a concern in this scenario, admit, continue serial examinations, repeat labs and ultrasound, and perhaps even err on the side of a hip I&D if there is clinical worsening (examination, fever). Like appendicitis, there will be an occasional false-positive and unnecessary operation to avoid failure to drain the most subtle cases.

The surgical technique for draining septic arthritis is familiar to most pediatric orthopaedists. To stay out of trouble, it is important to avoid the blood supply to the capital femoral epiphysis, which enters posteriorly. For this reason, the approach is anteriorly through the tensor fascia lata/sartorius interval. It is important to have a very definite capsulotomy. It is important to irrigate the joint aggressively and decompress the femoral neck if there is associated femoral neck osteomyelitis. A drain is usually placed around the femoral neck and pulled a few days later. Without a drain, the hip arthrotomy can close quickly and there can be a reaccumulation of the fluid, necessitating repeat surgery.

The child should rest in bed for a couple of days to keep the drain in and allow the hip to quiet down. **NEWSFLASH! Bedrest is needed until the drain is removed. You don't want a kid walking with a drain in their hip—it can dislodge, become trapped in the joint, or sheared off. We recommend "free cage activity" (i.e., rolling around in bed only) until the hip drain is out.** CRP is the most valuable test to follow in the postoperative period. As soon as CRP begins to drop in a child who is afebrile, the drain can be removed, IV antibiotics can be switched to oral, and the child can be discharged. Infectious disease experts tend to recommend 3 to 6 weeks of antibiotic management, depending on length and severity of symptoms before diagnosis, and the organism cultured.

> **THE GURU SAYS...**
> In general, the higher the CRP, the higher the acuity and the concern for systemic sepsis. In patients with markedly elevated CRP, be on the lookout for thrombosis and clinical decompensation.
> WUDBHAV N. SANKAR

> **THE GURU SAYS...**
> Another mimicker of septic hip arthritis is Lyme disease (in certain regions of the country). While a child with Lyme may have a large effusion with a WBC well in excess of 50 000, they usually appear nontoxic, are able to bear weight, and usually have only slightly elevated CRPs.
> WUDBHAV N. SANKAR

> **THE GURU SAYS...**
> Depending on your local pathogens and patterns of antibiotic resistance, consider getting an MRI on all patients suspected of having a septic arthritis before going to surgery (as long as it doesn't lead to treatment delays!). Several studies have shown high rates of concomitant osteomyelitis and periarticular abscesses that may also need to be addressed at the time of surgery.
> WUDBHAV N. SANKAR

> **THE GURU SAYS...**
> It can be helpful to excise a small part of the capsule to allow continued drainage and prevent the capsulotomy from closing too quickly.
> WUDBHAV N. SANKAR

THE GURU SAYS...

In deciding whether or not to take a child back to the operating room for a repeat I&D, it's best to rely on clinical information: persistent fevers, increased pain, rising CRP, etc. Getting an MRI after surgery can be very misleading as postsurgical changes are nearly indistinguishable from persistent infection.

WUDBHAV N. SANKAR

To stay out of trouble, beware when C-reactive protein does not rapidly normalize in the first week after surgery. In the face of either persistent symptoms or an elevated CRP, the surgeon reflects on these questions: Could there be another collection in another area? Could the fluid have reaccumulated? Is the diagnosis right? Are the antibiotics right?

After septic arthritis, follow-up for at least a few years is valuable, to study growth and the risk of AVN. **NEWSFLASH! For neonates who experience sepsis, it is the orthopaedist's job to prove that there are not two septic hips or septic arthritis elsewhere.** Multifocal septic arthritis is very common in the neonate and can be a major source of trouble. It is best to aspirate both hips and perhaps other joints in order to make the diagnosis as soon as possible.

Staying Out of Trouble With Hip Conditions

Legg-Calvé-Perthes Disease

* The key to staying out of trouble making the diagnosis of Legg-Calvé-Perthes is to recognize that the presentation can be very subtle and may be mistaken for transient synovitis in the early stages.

* Order an anteroposterior and frog lateral plain radiograph at the first visit for any child who presents complaining of hip or thigh pain.

* It's disconcerting to families to learn how uncertain the experts are about definitive treatment. Get ready to spend lots of time during the visit when the diagnosis is made and the options explained.

* Focus attention on children 8 years and older and on those with moderate hip involvement (Herring B, or B/C). Surgeons and children get in trouble when a complication occurs in the process of overtreating one of the 60% or more of children who would do perfectly well without ever seeing a doctor.

Slipped Capital Femoral Epiphysis

* For SCFE, recognize the child who is an outlier in terms of typical demographic criteria. If the child is 11 years old or younger, consider a possible underlying cause such as renal osteodystrophy, hypothyroidism, panhypopituitarism, and hypogonadal conditions.

* Stable SCFEs should not be discharged and returned for elective fixation. Admit and fix, to avoid risk of preventable progression.

* Aim to have your SCFE screw (7 mm or bigger) into the center of the femoral head on every radiographic view, perpendicular to the physis, stopping about 5 mm from the subchondral bone of the epiphyseal articular cartilage.

* To stay out of trouble, avoid the posterosuperior portion of the femoral head, where the blood supply enters the epiphysis. If you are going to miss in one direction or another, miss with your screw inferior to the center of the head.

* When drilling your guide pin, don't allow it to stop in this dense bone: it can be very difficult to restart the guide pin. Judicious use of live fluoroscopic imaging and continuous drilling can avoid this problem.

Staying Out of Trouble With Hip Conditions *(continued)*

* Persistent hip pain more than 2 weeks after SCFE fixation should be a red flag. Because most patients experience a rapid relief of their preoperative symptoms, the surgeon should carefully look for problems if the patient returns for a follow-up visit and there is persistent hip pain.

* Advise the family during that very first postoperative discussion that the SCFE screw never needs to be removed in most patients.

Septic Arthritis

* Use CRP not ESR when encountering an early presentation of potential septic arthritis.

* After septic hip washout, bedrest is needed until the drain is removed. You don't want a kid walking with a drain in their hip—it can dislodge, become trapped in the joint or sheared off.

* Beware when C-reactive protein does not rapidly normalize in the first week after a septic hip is drained. It could be a sign that there is another source of infection, like a psoas abscess, osteomyelitis, etc.

* For neonates who experience sepsis, it is the orthopaedist's job to prove that there are not two septic hips or septic arthritis elsewhere.

FOR FURTHER ENLIGHTENMENT

Caird MS, Flynn JM, Leung YL, et al. Factors distinguishing septic arthritis from transient synovitis of the hip in children: a prospective study. *J Bone Joint Surg Am*. 2006;88(6):1251-1257.

Kim HK, Burgess J, Thoveson A, et al. Assessment of femoral head revascularization in Legg-Calvé-Perthes disease using serial perfusion MRI. *J Bone Joint Surg Am*. 2016;98(22):1897-1904.

Kohno Y, Nakashima Y, Kitano T, et al. Is the timing of surgery associated with avascular necrosis after unstable slipped capital femoral epiphysis? A multicenter study. *J Orthop Sci*. 2017;22(1):112-115.

Laine JC, Martin BD, Novotny SA, Kelly DM. Role of advanced imaging in the diagnosis and management of active Legg-Calvé-Perthes disease. *J Am Acad Orthop Surg*. 2018;26(15):526-536.

Loder RT, Schneble CA. Seasonal variation in slipped capital femoral epiphysis: new findings using a National Children's Hospital database. *J Pediatr Orthop*. 2019;9(1):e44-e49.

Novais EN, Maranho DA, Heare T, et al. The modified Dunn procedure provides superior short-term outcomes in the treatment of the unstable slipped capital femoral epiphysis as compared to the inadvertent closed reduction and percutaneous pinning: a comparative clinical study. *Int Orthop*. 2019;43(3):669-675.

Parsch K, Weller S, Parsch D. Open reduction and smooth Kirschner wire fixation for unstable slipped capital femoral epiphysis. *J Pediatr Orthop*. 2009;29(1):1-8.

Perry DC, Metcalfe D, Lane S, Turner S. Childhood obesity and slipped capital femoral epiphysis. *Pediatrics*. 2018;142(5):e20181067.

Schmitz MR, Blumberg TJ, Nelson SE, et al. What's new in pediatric hip? *J Pediatr Orthop*. 2018;38(6):e300-e304.

Shah H. Perthes disease: evaluation and management. *Orthop Clin North Am*. 2014;45(1):87-97.

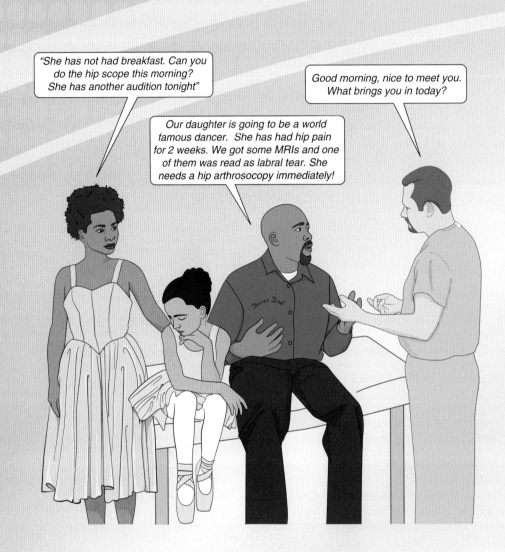

448

Chapter 26

Hip III: Adolescent Hip

ERNEST L. SINK, MD

Guru: Ira Zaltz, MD

Since the description of femoroacetabular impingement (FAI) by Professor Ganz in 2000 as a cause of hip pain and eventual arthritis, the field, now known as hip preservation, has grown exponentially. With the introduction of surgical dislocation as an approach to manage intra-articular hip pathology, there has been tremendous growth of surgery for the prearthritic hip. The surgical dislocation approach enabled elucidation of the pathology of certain hip disorders. With the expanding knowledge of FAI and improved techniques of hip arthroscopy, arthroscopic procedures have increased exponentially. Also, with increased adolescent sports participation, many more adolescents are being evaluated for hip pain. A labral tear diagnosed by hip MRI is now an epidemic in adolescent athletes. Because there is a "tear" of the labrum, patients have been referred for arthroscopic labral repair often without a complete understanding of the underlying pathology or an effort to promote nonoperative care. A labral tear is not always a true tear like a knee ligament, but the word creates significant angst in patients and parents. The labral tear can be seen in many asymptomatic hips and in most cases does not need an isolated repair. A better description would be labral irritation present in deformities such as FAI or hip dysplasia. Surgeons should be aware that hip pain and labral findings may be instability or dysplasia that is not recognized or inappropriately diagnosed as FAI. **NEWSFLASH! It's not always about the labrum but the *true cause* of hip pain, which may be abductor weakness, hip flexor overuse in adolescents associated with growth, version abnormalities of the femur or acetabulum, FAI, or instability and dysplasia.** Focusing of the labrum and arthroscopic repair has resulted in many patients improperly diagnosed and treated. Therefore, a careful history, examination, and three-dimensional imaging are often necessary.

THE GURU SAYS...

It is accepted that labral damage confirmed as a source of pain, especially in younger patients, is associated with abnormal anatomy that predisposes the hip to mechanical aberrations. Prior to considering any form of treatment, a systematic and comprehensive evaluation of the radiographic and clinical properties of each hip is required to arrive at an appropriate differential diagnosis.

IRA ZALTZ

THE GURU SAYS...

Subtle deformities of the hip are highly prevalent and may, in certain settings, predispose a patient to hip dysfunction and pain. Since many recognized deformities may be associated with both instability and impingement, it is imperative to make the correct mechanical diagnosis. Failure to perform the appropriate procedure mechanically worsens the hip joint.

IRA ZALTZ

THE GURU SAYS...

As mentioned in the previous section, the biggest issue with arthroscopic hip surgery in incorrect diagnosis of FAI, underappreciation of femoral torsional disorders, and females with limited hip motion but dysplastic acetabuli.

IRA ZALTZ

Three Important Components of Evaluation and Treatment of the Prearthritic Hip

Finding the Correct Diagnosis

- This is sometimes a challenge as many patients can have significant discomfort with subtle deformities.
- The correct diagnosis is still evolving as FAI is not always the diagnosis, and the true pathomechanics of hip discomfort can be debated among experts.
- The pain may be associated with spinal pathology or muscular injury to the pelvis such as athletic pubalgia.

Determining the Best Treatment

- When it comes to operative treatment there are only a few treatments and approaches that surgeons utilize: hip arthroscopy, surgical dislocation, periacetabular osteotomy (PAO), femoral osteotomy, or a combination of any of the above.
- While the surgical treatment option may be straightforward in a patient with significant dysplasia (PAO) or a male with a large cam lesion (hip arthroscopy), the best option is not always clear (for example, a female with a mild dysplasia and radiographic criteria of impingement or patients with version abnormalities of the acetabulum and/or femur).

Technical Implementation

- Hip arthroscopy is a technically challenging procedure. Not only are the indications for its use still evolving, but how to manage the labrum, rim, and capsule is still debated. Hip arthroscopy has a very steep learning curve where training and volume is necessary. Unfortunately hip arthroscopy is not a large portion of residency training. A majority of those performing hip arthroscopy receive some training during a 1-year sports medicine fellowship, and a majority of those performing hip arthroscopy are doing only a handful a year.

- The same applies for the PAO, for which volume, training, and mentorship are essential.
- The surgical dislocation has the fastest technical learning curve. Management of the acetabulum and femur present many options and making the appropriate decision, e.g., repair the labrum, rim resection, trochanteric resection, proximal femoral osteotomy, is challenging and often a point of controversy. Furthermore, we are now recognizing that extra-articular deformities are a cause of hip pain that may need to be addressed by trochanteric osteoplasty and even femoral osteotomy.

> **THE GURU SAYS...**
>
> The original descriptions of FAI, CAM, and pincer are often oversimplifications of what is now considered a complex problem often related to versional abnormalities of the femur and acetabulum.
>
> IRA ZALTZ

Causes of Adolescent Hip Pain

MUSCULAR

After a period of rapid growth, the pelvis and hip muscles have to accommodate the forces to move and support a longer leg. This creates problems, particularly in teens who are high-intensity, year-round athletes or dancers. The gluteal and core muscles (abdominal rectus, obliques, proximal hamstrings) are underdeveloped and not coordinated. This can also be a cause of anterior knee pain. It can be accentuated with anteversion of the femur giving the abductor mechanics a disadvantage.

OVERUSE SYNDROMES AND APOPHYSITIS

Apophysitis of the anterior inferior iliac spine is common from rectus femoris overuse in sprinters and soccer players. Iliac apophysitis is common in runners and will often take months to become asymptomatic. Iliac apophysitis is common in abductor overuse and occasionally is an early symptom of hip dysplasia.

Impingement disorders: The most common is FAI from a decreased offset between the femoral head and neck (cam lesion) that appears to develop during the final growth of the proximal femur in response to overload. With hip motion this "bump" can damage the anterior labral cartilage junction. **NEWSFLASH! FAI is much more common in males than females. It is more subtle in females, and surgeons should be aware of dysplasia or instability as the main reason for pain in females.** Impingement can result from an overly deep hip socket, but this diagnosis of pincer impingement was overdiagnosed previously in adolescents. Extra-articular impingement can also occur where aspects of the greater and lesser trochanter impinge on the pelvis. This is not an easy diagnosis but needs to be considered prior to jumping in to treat intra-articular FAI.

DYSPLASIA

This is more common in females. A wise mentor has a saying that "all female hips are unstable until proven otherwise." Our center has a complex case conference each week that composed mostly of female patients who had prior hip arthroscopy that failed due to missed acetabular dysplasia. Historically, the lateral center edge was the primary measurement used to diagnose hip dysplasia. We now know that acetabular deficiency is highly variable and anatomically complex and a normal lateral center edge angle is not sufficient to exclude dysplasia. Undercoverage can also be posterior-superior, anterior only, global, or nearly normal associated with ligamentous laxity or iatrogenic instability from prior hip arthroscopy.

> **THE GURU SAYS...**
>
> "Growing pains" of the adolescent hip are underappreciated. As the skeleton elongates, forces that are generated at muscular origins, insertions, and myotendinous junctions increase exponentially. The high variability of labral morphology can lead to misdiagnosis. Adjusting activity to enable adaptation is frequently required.
>
> IRA ZALTZ

> **THE GURU SAYS...**
>
> Understanding the relationship between structure, range of movement, and stability is essential. In addition to traditional forms of impingement, the practitioner needs to evaluate acetabular and femoral version before deciding upon treatment. Extra-articular impingement associated with versional problems can cause labral damage.
>
> IRA ZALTZ

Physical Examination and Imaging

Adolescents with hip pain should not be diagnosed by just looking at the MRI or X-ray. Adolescent hip pain is a symptom complex that requires the classic doctor-patient interaction taught in medical school in which surgeons listen completely to the patient's symptoms. It is important to understand what activities exacerbate pain and how the pain affects patient activities. Try to understand whether the pain is associated with other concerns common in adolescent life, including anxiety and depression. Unlike much of pediatric orthopaedics, which evaluates deformity, we are evaluating pain, which has many factors.

Evaluating Adolescent Hip Pain

Keep in Mind

- Acute symptoms and a pop associated with running or soccer are avulsion injury of the anterior iliac spine or ischial apophysis, not acute labral tear.
- A patient's activities can be crucial to understanding their symptoms. It is common to evaluate dancers who place their hips in the extremes of motion. Dancers may have coexistent impingement and instability. It is also very challenging for those involved in dance to modify or decrease their activities.
- Rule out dysplasia or instability in a female patient who has complaints of pain "when I sit or stand too long."
- A sharp stabbing pain while standing from a sitting position in male athlete is more likely FAI. They often move in positions in sitting to extend the hip.
- For mild deformities find out what nonoperative treatment patients have done and for how long. Impatience with nonoperative treatment is common. Patients and families want their problem "fixed" where commonly more extensive nonoperative treatment would be the least invasive and most appropriate approach.
- Unfortunately, it is common to see patients with prior failed surgery. Understand what was done (rim trimming, labral repair, capsular closure, psoas tendon release) as well as how their symptoms have changed after the surgery.

Perform a Full Physical Examination

- Have patients walk. Observe gait looking for a limp and version abnormalities. Check for abductor weakness with single leg squat.
- Examine the hip range of motion supine: hip flexion, internal rotation, and external rotation in 90° of flexion. Femoral version is the greatest contributor to hip range of motion and a decreased internal rotation does not necessarily mean there is FAI.
- The FADIR (flexion, adduction, and internal rotation test) or "impingement test" is a sign of hip irritation and does not mean patient has FAI—it means the anterior aspect of their hip (labrum, capsule, psoas sheath) is irritated.
- In a patient with increased hip flexion and internal rotation, FAI is less common.
- Provocative tests: FADIR, apprehension, PART can assess what hip positions recreate symptoms.

Imaging

- Screening images are the AP, false profile, and Dunn lateral.
  - The AP pelvis can give general information such as lateral center edge angle, the position of the anterior and posterior walls of the acetabulum, sourcil shape and coverage, Shenton line, and proximal femoral shape.
  - An AP in standing will often affect the perceived acetabular version. My prefer-ence is to get the standing AP.
  - The false profile view does not give a full picture of anterior coverage when it was studied with a CT and cadaver.
  - A Dunn lateral has less abduction than a Lowenstein lateral so will show the longer view of the head and neck junction.

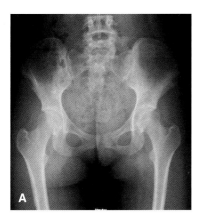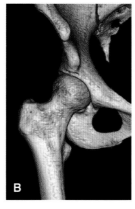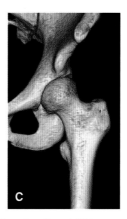

Figure 26-1 A: A 16-year-old girl with 2 y of bilateral hip pain. The standing AP hip radiograph does not indicate significant deformity. **B, C:** CT scans of the right and left hip with a femoral anteversion of 25° and inadequate acetabular anterior coverage of the femoral head. The chronic anterior hip pain is due to anterior overload. Correction may be better by reorienting the acetabulum rather than hip arthroscopy, which was unsuccessful on the right.

- Secondary imaging includes MRI, 3D CT, and ultrasound.
  - If routine imaging is not obvious with regard to the diagnosis and surgical treatment is being considered, obtain a 3D CT. The gives a better analysis of the acetabular and proximal femoral anatomy. Acetabular coverage may be deficient anterior only, posterior lateral only, or globally (Fig. 26-1). CT also allow the calculation of femoral and acetabular version which may impact the diagnosis and treatment. For example, the outcomes of hip arthroscopy may be affected by excessive femoral anteversion or retroversion. Finally, the presence of a real cam lesion or decreased offset can be better visualized on CT.
  - MRI is helpful to evaluate soft tissue and look for other diagnosis such as synovitis or osteoid osteoma. **NEWSFLASH! A large number of MRI readings are dictated as a "labral tear." Do not just treat this MRI diagnosis. First, the term "tear" is not what is really what has occurred. More likely the labrum may be inflamed, separated from the bone, or a normal finding. Figure out whether the labral pathology is the result of a bony morphologic issue. The reading on labral tear on MRI has resulted in patient and family anxiety and incorrect surgical treatment.**

> **THE GURU SAYS...**
>
> MRI interpretations are frequently a source of misinformation and misdiagnosis. Variations in labral morphology and elevations of alpha angle are not disorder-specific.
>
> IRA ZALTZ

Treatment

Determining the cause of adolescent hip pain can be the first challenge, with the second being: what is the best treatment? In clear DDH or FAI cases, the decision of PAO and hip arthroscopy/dislocation can be straightforward. Extensive nonoperative treatment including physical therapy is recommended in the majority of hips with the exception of a dysplastic hip with a lateral center edge angle less than 16° and a break in Shenton line. The natural history of this hip is poor and should be treated with a PAO once the patient starts to have symptoms.

> **THE GURU SAYS...**
>
> Become familiar with other measurable characteristics of the acetabulum and warning signs associated with progressive deterioration causing a poor natural history. Intervening at the appropriate time, especially for dysplasia, truly preserves the native hip.
>
> IRA ZALTZ

Because the adolescent is still developing after a period rapid growth, the hip symptoms may improve with physical therapy and training. Unfortunately, there is no uniform nonoperative protocol. A period of activity modification and physical therapy focusing on gluteal and abdomen strength (core strengthening) is what is prescribed. Getting the sport specialized adolescent to rest can be a real challenge and not what families want to hear.

A treatment focused on "labral repair" may sound effective to families, but the focus should be on understanding the cause of pain and treating the pathomechanics rather than the quick hip arthroscopy and labral repair.

> **THE GURU SAYS...**
>
> Beware of trying to "just repair the labrum" that can leave the hip more difficult to treat since subsequent procedures are rarely as efficacious as a comprehensive approach.
>
> IRA ZALTZ

Hip arthroscopy would be a good option for patients with clear FAI pathomechanics with anterior hip pain, a cam lesion on 3D imaging, and no evidence of hip dysplasia. Key to the indication: symptoms despite 3 to 6 months of nonoperative care. This is more common in male athletes although it can occur in females who do not show any ligamentous laxity or dysplasia. In many cases, avoid a lot of bony resection of the acetabular rim as this may lead to iatrogenic instability, especially in female hips. A complete cam resection improves outcomes as residual cam lesion is the most common cause of revision hip arthroscopy. In most cases, *do not* perform an iliopsoas lengthening. This will result in hip flexor weakness and may exacerbate instability as the iliopsoas tendon can be a secondary stabilizer of the hip especially in anteverted or dysplastic hips.

PAO can be considered in hips with dysplasia as diagnosed with both plain radiographs and 3D imaging (Fig. 26-2) who fail extensive conservative treatment (6 months). Adjuvant hip arthroscopy to evaluate the labrum at the time of PAO can be safely performed, although how this affects the long-term outcomes of a PAO is unknown.

Proximal femoral derotation may be considered in hips with excessive anteversion or retroversion. These patients should exhibit gait or range of motion alterations that results in symptomatic functional limitations. The proximal femoral derotation may be included with a PAO for dysplastic hips or a surgical dislocation in complex impingement hips. Surgeries such as hip arthroscopy and PAO are technically demanding, are associated with a known steep learning curve, and have evolving indications. It is critical to receive specialized training and mentorship to understand hip morphology, clinical analysis, and execution of

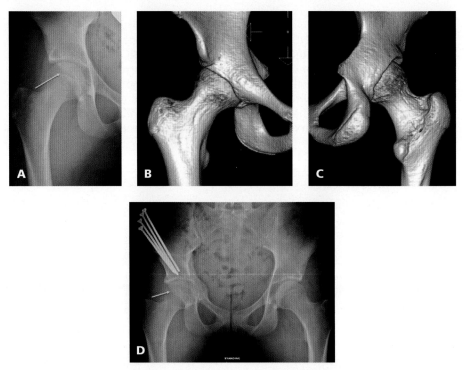

Figure 26-2 A: A 17-year-old girl with right hip pain and no relief after hip arthroscopy. The image indicates there may be acetabular deficiency in the posterior-superior portion of the acetabulum (arrow). **B, C:** CT scans highlighting good acetabular anterior coverage, but poor posterior-superior coverage of the femoral head. There is also a decreased offset of the anterolateral femoral head/neck junction. **D:** The hip symptoms resolved after acetabular reorientation with an anteversion PAO. The posterior wall is now just lateral to the femoral head (arrow).

these procedures. Cadaveric work and postgraduate training are recommended. Continued collaboration and communication with a mentor or other hip surgeons will improve the learning curve and patient care.

Staying Out of Trouble With the Adolescent Hip

* While the labrum is often blamed for hip pain, the true cause may be abductor weakness, hip flexor overuse in adolescents associated with growth, version abnormalities of the femur or acetabulum, FAI, or instability and dysplasia.

* The biggest issue with arthroscopic hip surgery is incorrect diagnosis of FAI, underappreciation of femoral torsional disorders, and females with limited hip motion but dysplastic acetabuli.

* Adolescents with hip pain should not be diagnosed by just looking at the MRI or X-ray. Adolescent hip pain is a complex symptom that requires the classic doctor-patient interaction taught in medical school where surgeons should listen completely to the patient's symptoms.

* FAI is much more common in males than females. It is more subtle in females, and surgeons should be aware of dysplasia or instability as the main reason for pain in females.

* If routine imaging is not obvious with regard to the diagnosis and surgical treatment is being considered, obtain a 3D CT. This gives a better analysis of the acetabular and proximal femoral anatomy.

* A large number or MRI readings are dictated as a "labral tear." *Don't* just treat this MRI diagnosis. Figure out if the labral pathology is the result of a bony morphologic issue. The reading of labral tear on MRI has resulted in patient and family anxiety and incorrect surgical treatment.

* Hip arthroscopy could be a good option for patients with clear FAI pathomechanics with anterior hip pain, a cam lesion on 3D imaging, and no evidence of hip dysplasia. Key to the indication: symptoms despite 3 to 6 months of nonoperative care. This is more common in male athletes, although it can occur in females who do not show any ligamentous laxity or dysplasia.

SOURCES OF WISDOM

1. Bedi A, Ross JR, Kelly BT, Larson CM. Avoiding complications and treating failures of arthroscopic femoroacetabular impingement correction. *Instr Course Lect.* 2015;64:297-306.
2. Ganz R, Gill TJ, Gautier E, et al. Surgical dislocation of the adult hip a technique with full access to the femoral head and acetabulum without the risk of avascular necrosis. *J Bone Joint Surg Br.* 2001;83(8):1119-1124.
3. Ganz R, Klaue K, Vinh TS, Mast JW. A new periacetabular osteotomy for the treatment of hip dysplasias: technique and preliminary results, 1988. *Clin Orthop Relat Res.* 2004;(418):3-8.
4. Ganz R, Leunig M, Leunig-Ganz K, Harris WH. The etiology of osteoarthritis of the hip: an integrated mechanical concept. *Clin Orthop Relat Res.* 2008;466(2):264-272.
5. Ganz R, Parvizi J, Beck M, et al. Femoroacetabular impingement: a cause for osteoarthritis of the hip. *Clin Orthop Relat Res.* 2003;(417):112-120.
6. Howie DW, Beck M, Costi K, et al. Mentoring in complex surgery: minimising the learning curve complications from peri-acetabular osteotomy. *Int Orthop.* 2012;36(5):921-925.
7. Kalhor M, Gharehdaghi J, Schoeniger R, Ganz R. Reducing the risk of nerve injury during bernese periacetabular osteotomy: a cadaveric study. *Bone Joint J.* 2015;97-B(5):636-641.
8. Larson CM, Clohisy JC, Beaule PE, et al. Intraoperative and early postoperative complications after hip arthroscopic surgery: a prospective multicenter trial utilizing a validated grading scheme. *Am J Sports Med.* 2016;44(9):2292-2298.

9. Larson CM, Ross JR, Stone RM, et al. Arthroscopic management of dysplastic hip deformities: predictors of success and failures with comparison to an arthroscopic FAI cohort. *Am J Sports Med.* 2016;44(2):447-453.

10. Leunig M, Ganz R. The evolution and concepts of joint-preserving surgery of the hip. *Bone Joint J.* 2014;96-B(1):5-18.

11. Lynch TS, Minkara A, Aoki S, et al. Best practice guidelines for hip arthroscopy in femoroacetabular impingement: results of a delphi process. *J Am Acad Orthop Surg.* 2020;28(2):81-89.

12. Mannion AF, Impellizzeri FM, Naal FD, Leunig M. Fulfilment of patient-rated expectations predicts the outcome of surgery for femoroacetabular impingement. *Osteoarthritis Cartilage.* 2013;21(1):44-50.

SECTION 6

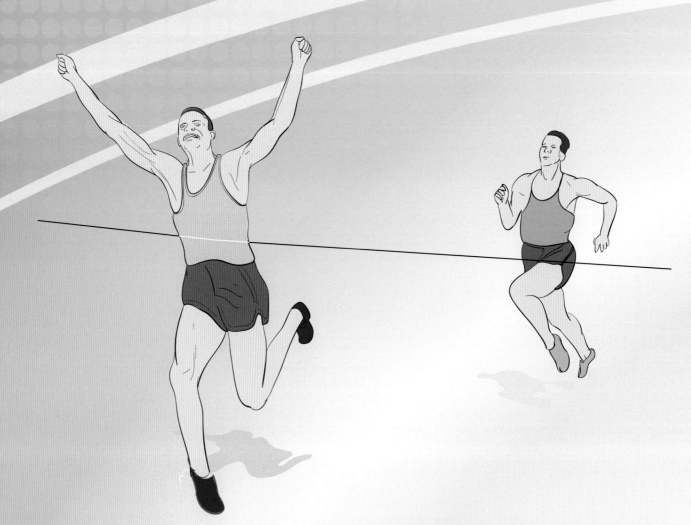

Our champion again reflects how lucky he is the Dennis Brown Bar didn't work.

LOWER EXTREMITY

Chapter 27

Knees Bow Out, Feet Turn In, Who Cares?

KENNETH J. NOONAN, MD, MHCDS

Guru: Michelle S. Caird, MD

At some point in their career, every pediatric orthopaedist has a portion of their practice where they are asked to help parents who are concerned about their child's limb development. Often they aren't sure that what they are seeing is normal development or the beginning of some horrific condition that will affect their child's life. Our jobs are to detect the few pathologic conditions and provide appropriate treatment. Just as important, in the majority of cases, we educate and assuage the fears of young parents and tell them that their child is developing normally. The young orthopaedist will stay out of trouble if they remember a few important things about the "worried well":

- Confirm with the family what they are seeing and their concerns. Empathize with their worry. Never tell a mom not to worry; unless you want to get punched.
- Educate them on the range of normal development.
- Explain why braces and homeopathic treatments usually can't change what they are seeing even if they don't like it.
- Make the families feel welcome to come back to clinic if anything changes.

ORTHOPAEDICS 101: Remember to maintain a high level of vigilance as you evaluate these apparently normal children. "You may not have seen a host of rare disorders, but they may have seen you."

Angular Deformities of the Legs

Most children seeing an orthopaedic surgeon for angular deformities of the legs are within normal limits. To stay out of trouble, the physician must be able to pick out the "abnormal" alignment by understanding normal physiologic progression of limb alignment.[1,2]

Several general rules of thumb exist:
- Maximum genu varum (bowlegs) occurs at birth (Fig. 27-1A)
- Legs straighten at 18 months (Fig. 27-1B)
- Maximum genu valgum (knock knees) occurs around age 4 years (Fig. 27-1C)
- Alignment is straight to slight valgus at maturity (Fig. 27-1D)

A few important historical questions can help guide whether you should worry that a child has pathologic limb deformity and requires further consideration. Try to assess whether the child was a product of normal pregnancy and delivery. Does the child have nutritional rickets as result of being African-American and who lives in the northern climates (little sun exposure and decrease endogenous production of vitamin D) with a mom who breastfeeds him (lower calcium)? At what age did the child begin walking (Blount disease tends to occur in early walkers)? Is there a past history of infection or trauma that could lead to growth arrest or growth stimulation? Is deformity unilateral (possibly worrisome) or bilateral (less worrisome)? How is the child growing? Is he overweight, as this is a known factor leading to Blount disease in early walkers? A good screening tool is to know the child's height on a growth curve (Fig. 27-2). A child with abnormal angulation of the legs, whose height is more than two standard deviations below normal, should be evaluated for an underlying condition such as rickets or a skeletal dysplasia. Are there any significant past history of surgical procedures (Fig. 27-3)? Is there a family history of bent or rotated bones, such as sex-linked hypophosphatemic rickets? These questions will not only demonstrate that you are concerned but will also help to discern possible pathology from the families that are convinced that Junior won't make the Olympics unless the legs are fixed.

Dr. Skaggs Adds

Perhaps the most important question in angular deformity of the legs is "Is it getting better, worse, or staying the same?" From Figure 27-1, we know normal development should never lead to things getting worse, so worsening deformity is always concerning. If things are getting better, it is unlikely there is physical pathology requiring treatment, though follow-up may make everyone feel better.

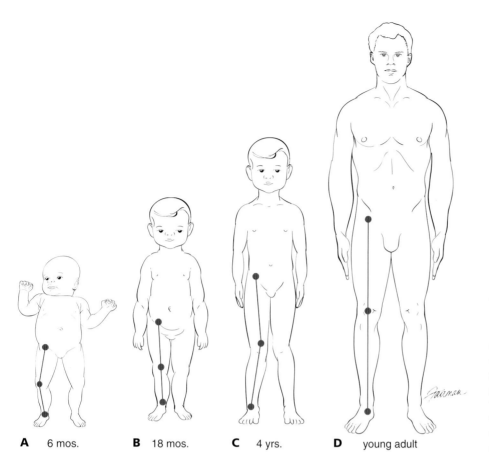

A 6 mos.   **B** 18 mos.   **C** 4 yrs.   **D** young adult

Figure 27-1 A: A 6-month-old with genu varum. **B:** An 18-month-old with straight legs. At some point in most children, usually around 18 mo of age, the legs are perfectly straight as their developmental stage passes from genu varum to genu valgum. **C:** A 4-year-old with genu valgum. **D:** An adult with nearly straight legs, erring on the side of slight valgus.

A couple of measures can be made on physical examination when trying to detect abnormal alignment and also can be used to record progression of alignment. If you are uncertain as to whether the angulation is physiologic, measure the intermalleolar distance (for knock knees) or intercondylar distance (for bowlegs). The graph in Figure 27-4 can help you decide if this is within 2 standard

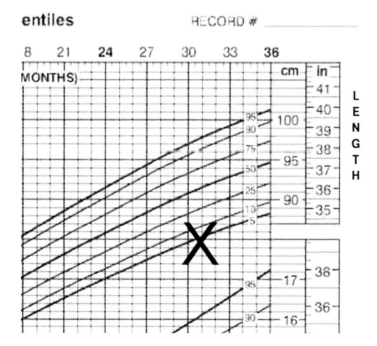

Figure 27-2 Any child with abnormal angulation of the legs, whose height is more than 2 standard deviations below normal, probably has an underlying condition such as rickets or a skeletal dysplasia.

Figure 27-3 A 13-year-old boy presented to clinic with concerns about how his knees look and with activity-related knee pain. He was shorter than his peers but otherwise healthy except for a remote history of "bladder surgery" at age 2. **A:** His alignment film demonstrated valgus with mechanical axis falling outside his knees. **B, C:** The careful clinician looked closely at the growth plates and noticed widening and cupping of the epiphysis (red arrows). A quick general chemistry test revealed a creatinine of 10.3. Unfortunately, he came to clinic with knee problems but left with a diagnosis of renal failure as a result of failed reconstruction for past ureter-pelvic junction obstruction.

 D: Nine months after renal transplantation, his knees are finally corrected with guided growth.

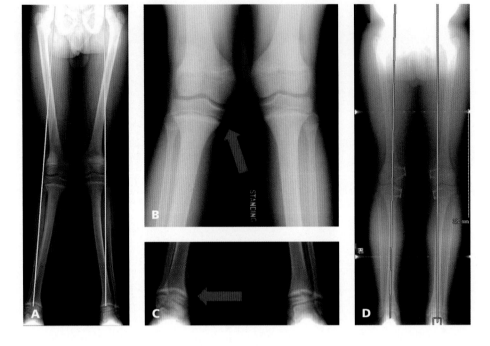

Figure 27-4 For each of the 12 age groups, mean values (solid circles) and 2 standard deviations (pen circles) were plotted for knee angle (**A**) and intercondylar or intermalleolar distance (**B**). Lines and shaded areas show general trends. (From Heath CH, Staheli LT. Normal limits of knee angle in white children—genu varum and genu valgum. *J Pediatr Orthop*. 1993;13(2):259–262.)

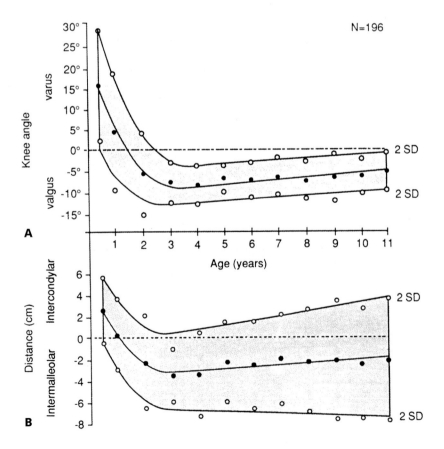

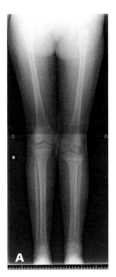
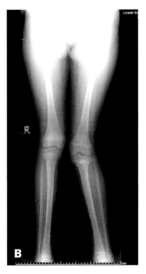
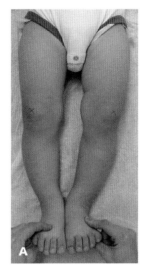
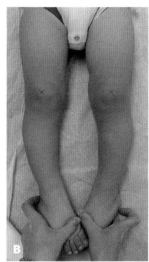

Figure 27-5 A: This radiograph was taken of a child with clinical unilateral genu valgum of the left leg, but the leg was externally rotated and the genu valgum is not evident. **B:** After the doctor drew an X on the patella and instructed the radiology technician to take the radiograph with the X pointing forward, the true genu valgum was evident radiographically.

Figure 27-6 A: Child demonstrating the apparent genu varum of tibial torsion. The chief complaint of this child's parents was bowed legs. With the feet pointing forward the legs have the appearance of genu varum when the child is supine or walking. The apparent "bowing" is a product of the knees pointing laterally, so knee flexion gives the appearance of bowing.
B: When the child's patellas point anteriorly, it is clear that there is no significant genu varum present. This demonstration often helps alleviate parental anxiety.

deviations. This measurement can be assessed 6 months later to provide some objective evidence regarding progression or improvement. The technique of measurement can be readily taught to the family members; they will then feel that the situation is being monitored and taken seriously. In younger children, the distances may have to be measured supine, and future measurements must occur in the same position for consistency.

Radiographs may be obtained for documentation and could be used for longitudinal comparison, provided they are of similar technique. Comparing a supine radiograph at 9 months with a weight-bearing film at 15 months is like comparing apples to oranges. The weight-bearing status of the radiographs has to be the same, or differences in deformity may be falsely attributed to progression or improvement. While taking radiographs, it is important that the patellas (not feet) are pointing forward (Fig. 27-5). In the case of a child with tibial torsion, if the feet point forward, the patellas point laterally and may give a false impression of genu varum radiographically and clinically (Fig. 27-6A). Clinically, the parents (and even clinician) may mistakenly think a child with tibial torsion is bowlegged. As Figure 27-6B demonstrates, turning the legs inward so the patella points straight anterior allows assessment and demonstration of varus/valgus alignment.

Two useful facts to remember from Heath and Staheli's study are (1) normal children aged 2 to 11 years may have knock knees up to 12° and an intermalleolar distance up to 8 cm and (2) the existence of bowlegs after age 2 years is abnormal.[2]

GENU VARUM

Here is the classic scenario: 18-month-old boy named Babe Ruth with bilateral bowlegs is accompanied to clinic with mom, dad (wearing his tattered Major League baseball jersey), and both grandmothers who have menacing looks for the "young-looking" doctor. The first step is to determine whether Babe is growing well; if he is of normal stature and height, you can rule out skeletal dysplasia and metabolic bone disease. Now you have to differentiate between physiologic genu varum (>95% likely) and Blount disease, which at this age is often quite difficult. On physical examination, you cover up the foot and rotate the knee until the patella is pointing to the ceiling. If he has valgus knees, he has internal tibial torsion that looks like varus when he walks and not Blount disease. If the knee "might be" in a bit of varus, the child could still have either diagnosis. Radiographs are unlikely to show "definitive" signs of Blount disease (metaphyseal beaking and epiphyseal fragmentation) until after 2 years of age. This may be problematic with respect to confirming the diagnosis and selecting the optimal timing and method of treatment (Fig. 27-7). Radiographs at 18 months of age may be "predictive" for developing Blount disease. A metaphyseal-diaphyseal angle greater than 16° increases the likelihood of a diagnosis of Blount disease but is by no means definitive. Stay out of trouble by not relying too heavily on a radiographic diagnosis of Blount disease in children less than 2 years of age. Radiographs do still have value at this time point; a standing alignment film could be taken as the child leaves clinic and could be compared to future films should Babe fail to straighten out. **NEWSFLASH! Today's smartphones are a useful tool for parents to follow their children. Have them take a frontal picture of the child standing in a diaper and set the alarm for 6 months. When the alarm goes off, they can pull up the picture and compare to the child. If the kid is worse, they should come back for comparative X-rays.**

Genu Varum: Suspect Blount Disease When...

- Child is older than 2 years
- There is lateral thrust (as weight is placed on a leg during the stance phase of gait, the knee abruptly translates laterally) (Fig. 27-8A)
- Focal angulation on examination and radiograph at proximal tibia is observed (Fig. 27-8B)
- There is medial beaking and downward slope of the proximal tibial metaphysis on radiographs. These radiographic changes cannot be detected before 2 years of age (Fig. 27-8C)
- Parents report it is not improving

These Associations Raise Level of Suspicion
- Obesity
- African-American ethnicity
- Early walker
- Unilateral occurrence

Genu Varum Is Likely Physiologic Bowing When...

- Parents report it is improving
- It's symmetrical
- Generalized bowing on examination and radiographs over femur and tibia is observed (see Fig. 27-7B)

TREATMENT OF INFANTILE BLOUNT DISEASE

The use of orthotics to unload medial compressive forces may, according to some investigators, alter the natural history of infantile Blount disease. Others recognize that these straight leg braces (no knee joint) are very challenging for parents and children as they are hard to fit on obese children and that have to be worn during the day. While many aspects of orthotic treatment are controversial, bracing proponents feel that this should be started before the age of 3 years.[3]

Two surgical options exist for the child older than 3 years with progressive varus and radiographic changes consistent with infantile Blount disease—growth

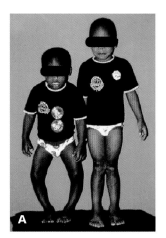 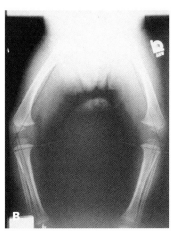 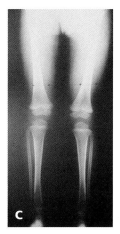

Figure 27-7 A: A 3-year-old with bowed legs next to his older brother. The mother reported the older brother had bowed legs just as bad as his younger brother but grew out of it without any treatment. **B:** Radiograph of the 3-year-old shows generalized bowing of the femurs and tibia. There is not a focal deformity of the proximal tibia that would be expected with Blount disease, and the physes appear normal. Given the child's severity of bowing and age, treatment would generally be indicated for genu varum. In the context of the family history and radiographs suggestive of physiologic bowing, however, the child was followed up with close observation only. **C:** Radiograph of the same child at age 5 y demonstrates resolution of the genu varum without treatment. (Courtesy of John T. Killian, MD.)

plate modulation and osteotomy. The choice requires shared decision-making with the family. Guided growth with temporary hemiepiphysiodesis of the lateral (Fig. 27-9) may correct the deformity.

To stay out of trouble, the patient should be less than 4 years of age, and no bony bar should be present in the medial physis. Modular screw and side plate constructs are preferred as standard Blount staples don't get as good as purchase in the immature tibia and its preponderance of unossified cartilage (Fig. 27-10).

> **THE GURU SAYS...**
>
> To really set expectations, it is helpful to be clear with families that with guided growth surgery, the leg will not immediately be straight after surgery, but that this method "elegantly" works with the child's own growth to straighten the bones over time.
>
> MICHELLE CAIRD

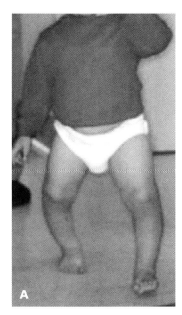 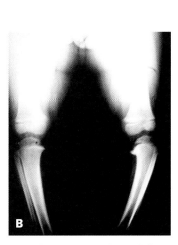 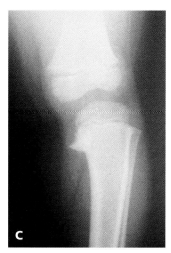

Figure 27-8 Signs of Blount disease. **A:** During weight bearing, a lateral thrust of the knee is suggestive. **B:** Focal angulation at the proximal tibia and medial beaking of the tibia are suggestive. **C:** Medial tibial beaking and downward sloping of the metaphysis are characteristic.

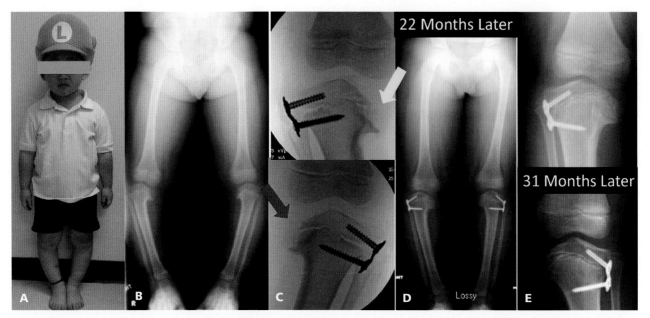

Figure 27-9 A, B: A 3½-year-old boy with bilateral infantile Blount disease. **C:** He underwent guided growth after MRI demonstrated no bony bar, even though the right growth plate (yellow arrow) looks more affected than the left growth plate (red arrow). Modular plate and screw implants were placed. **D, E:** Follow-up at 22 and 31 months reveals asymmetric improvement. To stay out of trouble, the surgeon must continue to follow the patient until full correction and consider implant removal versus complete epiphysiodesis to avoid the high chance of recurrence, especially on the right.

THE GURU SAYS...

With tibial osteotomy, prophylactic release of the anterior compartment and avoidance of epidural or intrathecal anesthetics can help prevent unrecognized compartment syndrome.

MICHELLE CAIRD

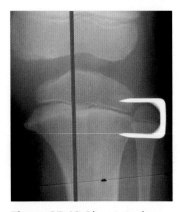

Figure 27-10 Blount staple extrusion in a young tibia. To stay out of trouble, the surgeon could have used a modular screw plate device. Conversely the rigid device may be preferred in older patients with limited growth available for correction. In these cases, the Blount device seems to retard growth quicker.

The child with infantile proximal tibia vara and excessive internal tibial torsion may not be a good candidate for guided growth as it is debated that guided growth actually changes rotation.

When contemplating osteotomy, there are some common areas of potential trouble that the surgeon should be aware of. The best outcomes from osteotomy are found in children who are younger than 4 years to minimize the risk of recurrence of deformity.[4,5] To stay out of trouble in children who are older than 4 years; obtain an MRI to rule out a bony bar (Fig. 27-11). A child with deformity and a bony bar could be treated with bar excision in addition to osteotomy. Proximal tibia and fibula osteotomies have significant risk of compartment syndrome. The anterior tibial artery passes through the interosseous membrane near the level of the osteotomy. Acute correction through the osteotomy site is believed to cause occlusion of the artery and lead to compartment syndrome at times. Acutely lessening the degree of correction has relieved signs of ischemia in some cases.[6] Anterior compartment release at time of correction should be performed, and careful postoperative monitoring is essential. It may be wise to avoid an epidural catheter because it might mask symptoms of compartment syndrome.

When considering correction of deformity, the surgeon has to consider three important things; how they are going to cut the bone, how are they going to reduce the deformity, and how are they going to stabilize the osteotomy. The location of the osteotomy is not at the site of the deformity (the growth plate) and thus pure angular correction will introduce a secondary translation deformity. This is not as critical to account for in infantile Blount disease as it is in adolescent Blount disease where remodeling is not as likely.

Make a lateral approach to the fibular shaft halfway down the leg and cut the fibula in an oblique fashion that allows the two ends to bayonet when the varus is corrected. There are two benefits to this approach: (1) cutting the fibula at a different level than the tibia provides some stability to the leg and (2) by cutting the fibula first, it's easier to detect when the tibia cut is completed later. There are many successful osteotomy techniques described in the treatment of Blount disease. To stay out of trouble, perform a straight osteotomy below the tubercle (to avoid apophysis injury and later recurvatum) by predrilling the bone and completing the osteotomy with an osteotome. Externally rotate the distal tibia and translate the distal segment laterally *before* correcting the angular deformity. If you correct angulation first, it's difficult to rotate and translate the bone. After overcorrecting the leg into slight valgus, the osteotomy is stabilized with simple K-wire fixation and long-leg casting. Assess the mechanical axis in the operating room with a Bovie cord and C-arm. When the cord is over the center of the hip and ankle, it should pass just through the center of the knee or just lateral to this to achieve slight overcorrection.

Late-onset Blount disease may share the same name as infantile Blount disease and the tibia in both disorders can be treated with guided growth (provided there is at least 2 years of growth remaining) and osteotomy, but there are more differences than similarities:

- Late-onset Blount disease occurs in children 9 years and older.
- It is usually associated with obesity.
- Classic radiographic metaphyseal beaking and epiphyseal fragmentation slope that are encountered in the infantile form are rarely seen (Fig. 27-12).
- Varus deformity is always in the tibia, and half patients also have distal femoral varus. With substantial growth remaining, any varus of the femur greater than 8° is best treated with guided growth. If little growth remains, a distal femoral osteotomy with plate fixation is preferred.
- The Afghan percutaneous osteotomy described by Paktiss and Gross[7] is safe and effective, with less postoperative pain allowing for earlier mobilization. This technique using a Gigli saw and two 1- to 1.5-cm incisions is well described in the cited reference (Fig. 27-13).
- When tibial osteotomy is performed in late-onset Blount disease, the best form of fixation is usually an external fixator with acute or gradual correction capabilities.

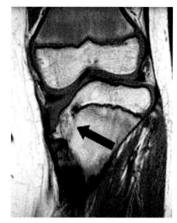

Figure 27-11 MRI of a child with Blount disease demonstrating that a bony bridge has formed. An osteotomy alone is not sufficient treatment, as the deformity will recur relatively rapidly when there is growth remaining.

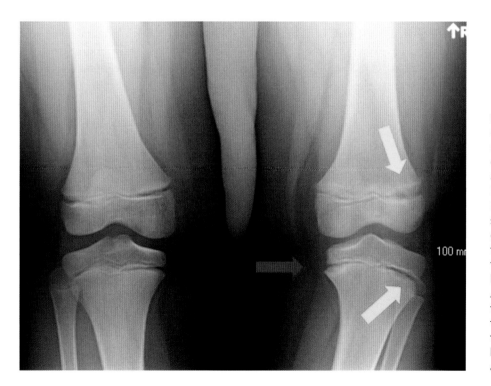

Figure 27-12 AP radiograph of a 12-year-old boy with unilateral late-onset Blount disease. The fragmentation and sloping seen in infantile Blount disease is not seen here. Radiographs demonstrate widening of the lateral growth plate of the femur and tibia (yellow arrows) and that the medial tibia epiphysis is blunted in height (red arrow). Although not present here, the surgeon who stays out of trouble knows that half the time late-onset Blount disease has distal femoral varus as well as proximal tibial varus.

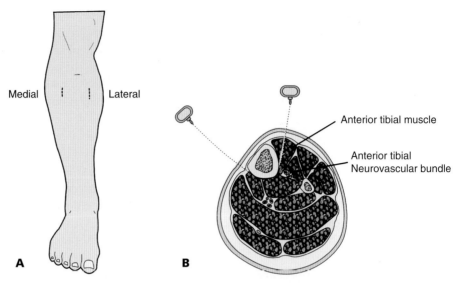

Figure 27-13 A: Location of incisions for proximal tibial osteotomy. **B:** Position of the Gigli saw just before performance of the osteotomy. (From Paktiss AS, Gross RH. Afghan percutaneous osteotomy. *J Pediatr Orthop.* 1993;13(4):531–533.)

OTHER CAUSES OF VARUS ANGULATION

Rickets may be due to many conditions and can be associated with genu varum or genu valgum. Nutritional rickets or genetic causes of metabolic bone disease usually result in progressive varus as the normal postnatal varus alignment continues to progress. In contrast, a child who develops renal rickets after age 4 years (when the legs are in valgus) will usually progress into more valgus (see Fig. 27-3). In patients with metabolic bone disease, radiographs may demonstrate widened and cupped physes, though this is difficult to discern at times.

In cases of rickets, it is unwise to consider surgery until the child's underlying condition is medically controlled or the deformity is likely to recur. In some cases of severe rickets in very young children, merely correcting the metabolic deformity can allow the bones to fix themselves (Fig. 27-14). In patients with longstanding metabolic deformity, the growth plates can accommodate to maintain a neutral mechanical axis despite obvious anatomic deformity. For example, a child with hypophosphatemic rickets may have obvious femoral shaft bowing that is balanced by progressive distal femoral valgus (Fig. 27-15). Simply correcting the femoral shaft with an osteotomy and intramedullary fixation will fix the varus bow but will leave the limb is excessive

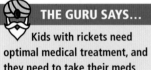

THE GURU SAYS...

Kids with rickets need optimal medical treatment, and they need to take their meds throughout growth or the deformity can come back again!

MICHELLE CAIRD

Figure 27-14 A, B: This 2-year-old child was born without kidneys and was on peritoneal dialysis when referred for treatment. The author considered osteotomy and intramedullary fixation techniques that are occasionally used in osteogenesis imperfecta after the planned kidney transplant. **C:** Five years later, the child returned to clinic never having orthopaedic treatment. The author harkens back to his residency when his mentor Richard Brand once said, "Don't just do something—sit there."

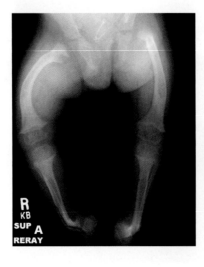
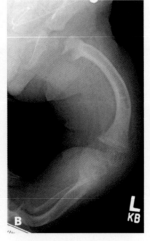
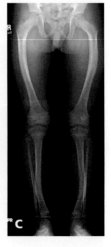

valgus. **ORTHOPAEDICS 101: When considering deformity correction anywhere in the body, the cautious surgeon will understand that when faced with an obvious anatomic deformity and an intact mechanical alignment, a compensatory deformity exists. For example, severe kyphosis of the spine is usually balanced with excessive lordosis (watch for a spondylolysis with excessive lordosis), excessive hindfoot valgus leads to forefoot supination, and distal femoral valgus can be compensatory to longstanding hip varus. Should compensatory deformities become rigid, correcting the primary deformity alone will lead to imbalance.**

THE GURU SAYS...

Kids may not heal their osteotomies or may have delayed union if their rickets is not controlled or if their doses of medications are not adequate for their weight. Work closely with their endocrinologists!

MICHELLE CAIRD

Other causes for varus include focal injury to the growth plate from trauma, infection (especially neonatal infection or meningococcemia) should be suspected, particularly in deformities outside of the usual age and type. One cause of angulation deserving of special mention is focal fibrocartilaginous dysplasia. In this condition, there is focal indentation of bone, most often the medial proximal tibia, which may be confused with Blount disease, though involvement of the distal femur and upper extremities has been reported as well (Fig. 27-16). The physis and epiphysis appear radiographically normal. The deformity associated with focal fibrocartilaginous dysplasia has been shown to resolve spontaneously in at least 45% of tibial cases, so initial observation may be warranted.[8]

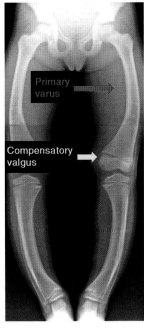

Figure 27-15 This boy with hypophosphatemic rickets demonstrates primary femoral shaft varus with secondary distal femoral compensatory valgus. Growth plates are smart—they try to balance things out if they're given enough time.

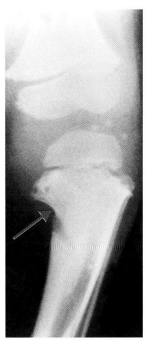

Figure 27-16 Radiograph in a 39-month-old boy shows a characteristic focal defect in the medial aspect of the proximal tibia (arrow). Note that there is no sloping of the medial metaphysis, which helps differentiate this from Blount disease. (From Choi IH, Kim CJ, Cho TJ, et al. Focal fibrocartilaginous dysplasia of long bones: report of eight additional cases and literature review. *J Pediatr Orthop*. 2000;20(4):421–427.)

GENU VALGUM

Symmetric genu valgum reaches its maximal degree of deformity at 3 to 4 years of age in normal children and demonstrates spontaneous resolution to 5° to 9° of anatomic valgus. If genu valgum is severe, or seen in children of other age groups, suspect underlying disorders such as renal osteodystrophy, skeletal dysplasias, or a posttraumatic origin following an incomplete tibial metaphysis (Cozen) fracture (Fig. 27-17). The natural history for uncorrected genu valgum is not known but is likely better than that for patients with equal amounts of genu varum. While there is no good science to suggest when genu valgum should be corrected operatively, we consider it when children are symptomatic (gait or running problems, pain) or for a mechanical axis passing lateral to middle of the lateral femoral condyle. Gait analysis has demonstrated objective improvement in gait following hemiepiphysiodesis for correction of genu valgum.[9] Adolescents with severe genu valgum report difficulty running and may have associated patella pain and subluxation; these symptoms may resolve with normalization of the mechanical axis via hemiepiphysiodesis of the distal femur.[10]

Guided growth via hemiepiphysiodesis is a powerful way of correcting deformity in growing children and can be done with a single screw (Metaizeau method; Fig. 27-18), modular plates and screws (Figs. 27-19 and 27-20), or with Blount staples. Consider permanent hemiepiphysiodesis with great caution, as overcorrection has been reported in 12% of children treated with a permanent hemiepiphysiodesis.[11]

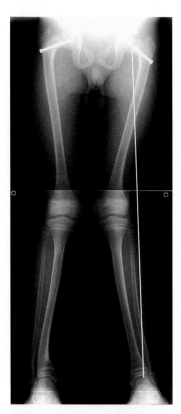

Figure 27-17 Radiograph of a 14-year-old boy with renal osteodystrophy. Widened growth physis is characteristic of rickets. The mechanical axis drawn from the center of the hip to the center of the ankle is lateral to the knee. This child also had bilateral slipped capital femoral epiphysis, which is also associated with renal osteodystrophy.

> **THE GURU SAYS...**
>
> Remind families that guided growth methods are very powerful and it is important to follow-up regularly while the plates or screws are in place to avoid overcorrection or opposite deformity.
>
> MICHELLE CAIRD

Dr. Skaggs Adds

When using the modular screw plate technique, placing screws eccentrically away from the growth plate will cause compression of the growth plate as they are tightened, similar to compressing a fracture site with dynamic compression plates. Theoretically this may help stop growth sooner.

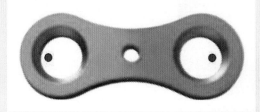

Dr. Skaggs Adds

Guided growth with modular screw plate techniques in which screws are inserted parallel to the growth plate results in optimal correction when compared with screws inserted divergently.[12]

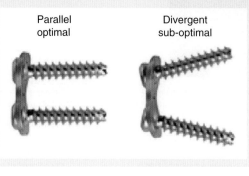

Parallel optimal   Divergent sub-optimal

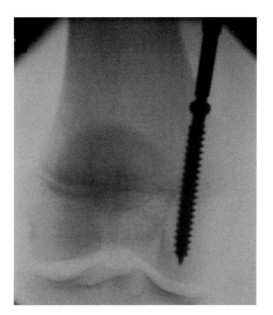

Figure 27-18 A single threaded screw can be used as a method of hemiepiphysiodesis when placed across the periphery of a growth plate. This method is very effective for distal tibia valgus deformity and works well in the distal femur. Some report fewer effective results in the proximal tibia, as the epiphysis is too small to gain much screw purchase. To stay out of trouble, don't use this method in the proximal tibia.

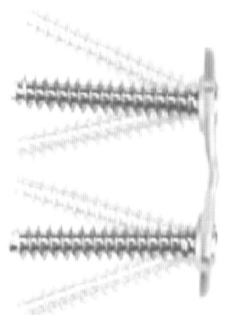

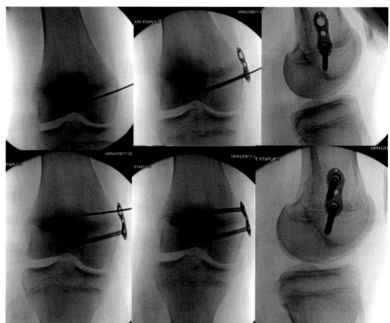

Figure 27-19 An "8" plate is specifically designed for hemiepiphysiodesis. Growth is prevented at the plate, but angulation of the screws within the plate permits asymmetric growth of the physis and angular correction.

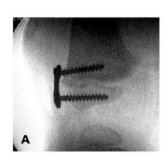

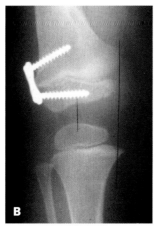

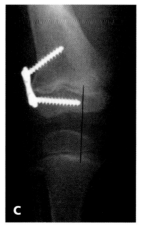

Figure 27-20 With asymmetric growth of the physis, progressive angulation of the screws (or staples) is expected with angular correction. **A:** Intraoperative image at time of implantation of "8" plate. **B:** Same patient 2 months after surgery. **C:** Same patient 9 months after surgery.

Staying Out of Trouble With Guided Growth

✳ Plan on a temporary hemiepiphysiodesis only in children likely to return to follow-up appointments (Fig. 27-21).

✳ Just because a growth plate is open doesn't mean the growth plate is growing. This is important in considering patients with metabolic disorders (Fig. 27-22) and especially patients with skeletal dysplasia and extreme short stature.

✳ If you divide the knee into quadrants in the frontal plane, the goal is to restore the mechanical axis to neutral, or within the middle two quadrants (physiologic range). Consider slight overcorrection in children under the age of 10 years as rebound growth can be expected after the implant is removed.[10,13,14]

✳ Implants can break under strain and thus consider solid screws in the metaphysis where fractures of screws tend to occur (Fig. 27-23).

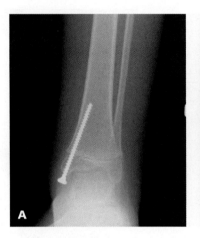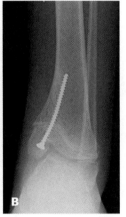

Figure 27-21 This 12-year-old boy with spina bifida had a medial malleus screw placed to perform a temporary hemiepiphysiodesis for a valgus ankle. **A:** The ankle is almost in a neutral position after some correction has already occurred. **B:** The child was lost to follow-up and returned 4 y later with this radiograph. Temporary hemiepiphysiodesis is perhaps best reserved for patients likely to comply with follow-up instructions.

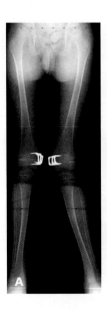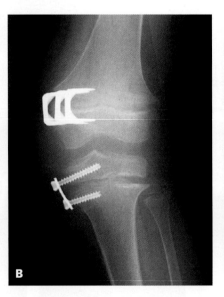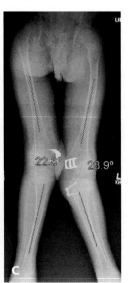

Figure 27-22 This 13-year-old boy with Lowe syndrome had guided growth at another institution. **A, B:** The author recommended adding proximal tibia–guided growth on the left side. **C:** Twenty months later, his valgus is worse. Just because a child has growth plates doesn't mean he's growing. Results may be unpredictable in patients with skeletal dysplasias or in children with generalized retarded growth.

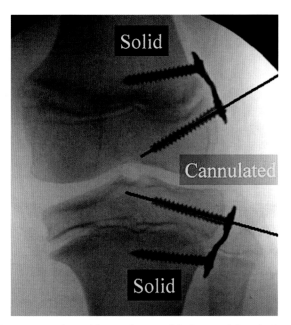

Figure 27-23 To stay out of trouble, perform guided growth by placing cannulated screws in the epiphysis first over a wire (precise placement is needed here) and use a solid screw in the metaphysis (strength is needed here).

BOWING OF TIBIA

Posteromedial bowing is relatively benign condition in comparison to anterolateral bowing of the tibia described below. There is almost always an associated calcaneovalgus foot in which the dorsum of the foot often touches the skin over the tibia, and this makes the deformity initially very scary for the parents (Fig. 27-24). Thankfully the foot deformity rapidly resolves with stretching, and the bowing spontaneously improves greatly within the first year or two of life. The most frequently encountered problem needing treatment (both in real life and standardized tests) is a leg length discrepancy of 3 to 5 cm at maturity, of which the parents should be forewarned.

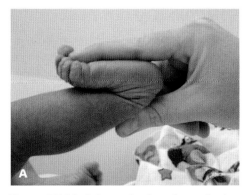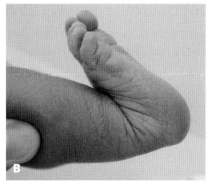

Figure 27-24 Calcaneal valgus foot—looks very scary, but resolves very quickly. (Used with permission of the Children's Orthopaedic Center, Children's Hospital Los Angeles.)

In contrast to posteromedial bowing, the natural history of anterolateral bowing of the tibia can be much more severe. Stay out of trouble by recognizing that these patients have equal trouble healing established psuedarthrosis as well as an osteotomy performed by the ill-advised orthopaedist who tries to straighten and bone graft the bent bone. Fractures are common in children with anterolateral bowing, so help prevent them with an ankle-foot orthosis (AFO) or knee-ankle-foot orthosis (KAFO) to be used whenever the child is weight bearing. If pseudarthrosis is not congenital (present at birth), it may ensue following fracture.

About 50% of patients have neurofibromatosis; early recognition of neurofibromatosis can help a child receive early treatment for problems associated with it. Beware that many of the cutaneous manifestations of neurofibromatosis, such as axillary and inguinal freckling and café-au-lait spots, may not be present in infancy, so it may be reasonable to consider a genetics referral for all infants with anterolateral bowing of the tibia.

While there is not a clearly established "best" surgical treatment for established psuedarthrosis, try to hold off surgery as long as possible with braces. When surgery becomes inevitable, make certain the parents understand that multiple surgeries are possible. **ORTHOPAEDICS 101: It's always a good idea to paint realistic and sometimes pessimistic outcomes from treatment of difficult problems. In the best-case scenario, the family is thrilled treatment worked; in the worst-case scenario, the consulting physician is respected for providing prophetic guidance.**

Most agree that the best initial procedure is resection of the psuedarthrosis and intramedullary fixation with a rod that spans the subtalar and ankle joints. The resected area is bone grafted with recombinant bone morphogenetic protein (BMP), and in older patients, iliac crest bone can also be harvested. If technically feasible, it's also a good idea to rod the fibula. The patient is casted until healed and then a solid-ankle AFO is needed until the patient grows enough such that the rod is no longer in the ankle joint. Although there is no level 1 data to support electrical stimulation, it can't hurt. Despite doing everything possible, this initial treatment may fail and salvage options include external frame correction, bone transport, and even vascularized fibular grafting. Prior to these extensive treatments, this is the time to point out that amputation may provide better function and less psychological trauma than multiple heroic procedures.

Torsional Deformities

BUT DOCTOR, YOU HAVE TO *DO* SOMETHING ABOUT THIS!

Rotational differences between children are a common source of parental consternation, and this concern can challenge even the most patient and empathetic provider. It's always a good idea to explain to families that all physical characteristics run a spectrum. A few statements can help frame the discussion, such as, "Blonde, brown, red and black hair are distinctly different...but they are all normal." And, "The average man is 5 foot 9, yet the jockey and the basketball star are also normal."

A common perception of the parents, grandparents, and panicked soccer coaches is that you are not taking the torsional problem seriously enough (see Chapter 1, *Partnering with Families*). To avoid this, simply verbalize the logical risk/benefit analysis we consider obvious and the parents almost always come to the same conclusion you do, and choose observation. But letting them make the choice may make all the difference between a satisfied and disgruntled family.

Some families seeking second opinions demand treatment because the first doctor would not do anything. To the best of our knowledge, there is no evidence that bracing influences the natural history of torsional deformities.

> **THE GURU SAYS...**
>
> With physiologic bowing, it is helpful to acknowledge that we used to brace for this (they may remember a family member who was braced), but luckily for this child, now we know that it improves with growth alone and we don't have to put the child and family through this unneeded and unhelpful method.
>
> MICHELLE CAIRD

While it may be tempting to placate demanding family members, it has shown that even corrective shoes have detrimental psychological effects on children, with lasting lowered self-esteem as adults[15] (Fig. 27-25). Maintaining a good relationship with the family is important but cannot be at the expense of the child. On occasion, a family will demand surgical treatment for physiologic intoeing. One approach is, "Yes, Sally's feet certainly *do* turn in. I can surgically *snap* her thighbones and reset them. On the *other* hand, this problem usually resolves over time by itself without surgery."

One may consider assigning the parents "homework" of watching a professional basketball game on television. There is usually a lot of intoeing going on, but the players nevertheless seem to function adequately. Symmetric torsional deformities are different from angular deformities in that torsional deformities are not associated with long-term problems in otherwise-normal children. Thus measuring the extent or progression of deformity is usually a moot point.

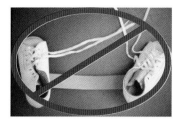

Figure 27-25 There is no evidence to suggest that bracing affects the natural history of torsional deformities.

FEMORAL TORSION

While femoral anteversion is maximal at birth, there are also soft-tissue external rotation contractures present at birth that may mask bony torsion. Thus, intoeing may appear to worsen during the normal resolution of external rotation contractures of the hip. Femoral anteversion and hip rotation decreases spontaneously over the first decade[16,17] (Fig. 27-26). When running, knees point in and feet fly outward, and it looks very clumsy. The truth is, there is very little trouble one can get into over symmetric excessive femoral anteversion and there is little evidence that persistent excessive femoral anteversion causes problems. A cadaveric study of adult 110 cadavers from Africa reports an association of arthritis of the distal femur with *decreased* anteversion.[18] Other studies (conducted on live adults) have found no association between increased femoral anteversion and abnormal patellofemoral characteristics.

On the other hand, asymmetric femoral anteversion is not normal, and a pelvis radiograph should be obtained to rule out hip dysplasia. Finally, excessive external rotation of the hips with a decrease in internal rotation can be manifested as severe outtoeing and has been associated with acetabular protrusio and certain genetic disorders such a Sticker syndrome. Stay out of trouble and get a pelvis X-ray when femoral torsion is asymmetric or if there is severe external rotation with no internal rotation in the prone position.

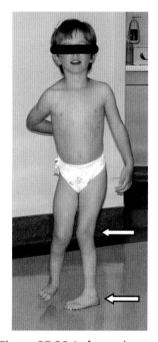

Figure 27-26 In femoral anteversion, the knee and foot both point inward.

TIBIAL TORSION

Tibias can be internally rotated (intoeing) and can also have external rotation (outtoeing). Up to 30° of internal tibial rotation is present at birth normally, and spontaneous improvement can be expected in most children.[17] Acknowledge to

> **THE GURU SAYS...**
>
> In older kids with lots of external rotation and limited internal rotation and groin, knee, or thigh pain, these can be signs of slipped capital femoral epiphysis (SCFE), and pelvis X-rays are needed to evaluate.
>
> MICHELLE CAIRD

parents that this may lead to more tripping in young children. It has been demonstrated that high-performance sprinters have more internal tibial torsion than controls. Once the parents understand the true nature of their child's superior genetic gift, they may leave your office with pride.[19]

Pitfalls for Torsion

▶ If feet turn outward, consider a SCFE or coxa vara, or tibial torsion.

▶ If one foot turns in, consider hemiplegia or other neuromuscular disorder.

▶ Limping: Torsion usually does not cause a limp, which by definition is an asymmetry of gait. Search for other causes of the limp.

▶ Pain: Torsional disorders generally are not painful, so search for other causes with one exception: miserable malalignment syndrome. This is defined by excessive femoral anteversion, excessive tibial outward rotation, and patellofemoral pain. There are two reports of a total of 40 extremities treated by ipsilateral femoral and tibial osteotomies with good results.[20,21]

Staying Out of Trouble With Knees That Bow Out and Feet That Turn In

✳ Suspect rickets or skeletal dysplasia if a child with bowed legs is of small stature.

✳ For Blount disease, surgery should be done by age 4 years to minimize the risk of recurrence of deformity.

✳ The most common pitfall of torsional deformities is the parental perception of you not taking the problem seriously enough.

✳ Residual inward tibial torsion may be associated with faster running.

SOURCES OF WISDOM

1. Salenius P, Vankka E. The development of the tibiofemoral angle in children. *J Bone Joint Surg Am.* 1975;57(2):259-261.
2. Heath CH, Staheli LT. Normal limits of knee angle in white children—genu varum and genu valgum. *J Pediatr Orthop.* 1993;13(2):259-262.
3. Zionts LE, Shean CJ. Brace treatment of early infantile tibia vara. *J Pediatr Orthop.* 1998;(1):102-109.
4. Loder RT, Johnston CE II. Infantile tibia vara. *J Pediatr Orthop.* 1987;7(6):639-646.
5. Doyle BS, Volk AG, Smith CF. Infantile Blount disease: long-term follow-up of surgically treated patients at skeletal maturity. *J Pediatr Orthop.* 1996;16(4):469-476.
6. Steel HH, Sandrow RE, Sullivan PD. Complications of tibial osteotomy in children for genu varum or valgum: evidence that neurological changes are due to ischemia. *J Bone Joint Surg Am.* 1971;53(8):1629-1635.
7. Paktiss AS, Gross RH. Afghan percutaneous osteotomy. *J Pediatr Orthop.* 1993;13(4):531-533.
8. Choi IH, Kim CJ, Cho TJ, et al. Focal fibrocartilaginous dysplasia of long bones: report of eight additional cases and literature review. *J Pediatr Orthop.* 2000;20(4):421-427.
9. Stevens PM, MacWilliams B, Mohr RA. Gait analysis of stapling for genu valgum. *J Pediatr Orthop.* 2004;24(1):70-74.
10. Stevens PM, Maguire M, Dales MD, et al. Physeal stapling for idiopathic genu valgum. *J Pediatr Orthop.* 1999;19(5):645-649.
11. Ferrick MR, Birch JG, Albright M. Correction of non-Blount's angular knee deformity by permanent hemiepiphyseodesis. *J Pediatr Orthop.* 2004;24(4):397-402.
12. Schoenleber SJ, Iobst CA, Baitner A, Standard SC. The biomechanics of guided growth: does screw size, plate size, or screw configuration matter? *J Pediatr Orthop B.* 2014;23:122-125.
13. Fraser RK, Dickens DR, Cole WG. Medial physeal stapling for primary and secondary genu valgum in late childhood and adolescence. *J Bone Joint Surg Br.* 1995;77(5):733-735.
14. Mielke CH, Stevens PM. Hemiepiphyseal stapling for knee deformities in children younger than 10 years: a preliminary report. *J Pediatr Orthop.* 1996;16(4):423-429.

15. Driano AN, Staheli LT. Psychosocial development and corrective shoewear use in childhood. *J Pediatr Orthop*. 1998;18(3):346-349.
16. Svenningsen S, Apalset K, Terjesen T, et al. Regression of femoral anteversion: a prospective study of intoeing children. *Acta Orthop Scand*. 1989;60(2):170-173.
17. Staheli LT, Corbett M, Wyss C, et al. Lower-extremity rotational problems in children. Normal values to guide management. *J Bone Joint Surg Am*. 1985;67(1):39-47.
18. Eckhoff DG, Kramer RC, Alongi CA, et al. Femoral anteversion and arthritis of the knee. *J Pediatr Orthop*. 1994;14(5):608-610.
19. Fuchs R, Staheli LT. Sprinting and intoeing. *J Pediatr Orthop*. 1996;16(4):489-491.
20. Delgado ED, Schoenecker PL, Rich MM, et al. Treatment of severe torsional malalignment syndrome. *J Pediatr Orthop*. 1996;16(4):484-488.
21. Bruce WD, Stevens PM. Surgical correction of miserable malalignment syndrome. *J Pediatr Orthop*. 2004;24(4):392-396.

FOR FURTHER ENLIGHTENMENT

Kline SC, Bostrum M, Griffin PP. Femoral varus: an important component in late-onset Blount's disease. *J Pediatr Orthop*. 1992;12(2):197-206.

Lincoln TL, Suen PW. Common rotational variations in children. *J Am Acad Orthop Surg*. 2003;11(5):312-320.

Salenius P, Vankka E. The development of the tibiofemoral angle in children. *J Bone Joint Surg Am*. 1975;57(2):259-261.

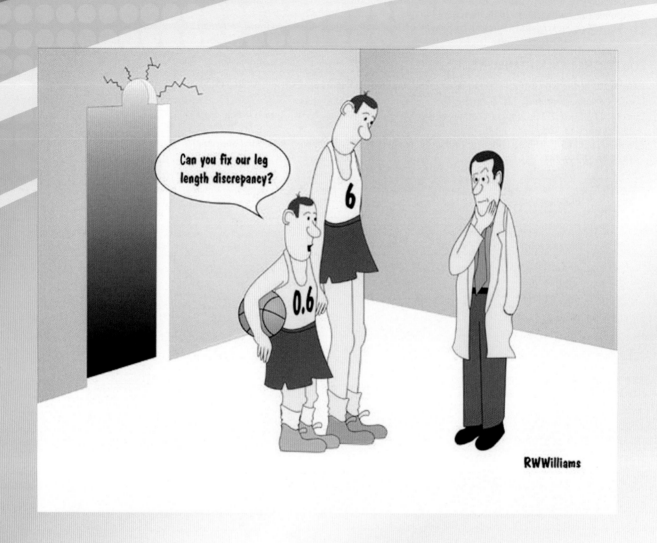

Chapter 28

Leg Length Discrepancy

KENNETH J. NOONAN, MD, MHCDS

Guru: Christopher Iobst, MD

General Considerations

A modest leg length discrepancy (LLD) is common and may be considered a normal variant. A study of 600 military recruits found an LLD of 0.5 to 1.5 cm in 32% of recruits, and 4% had a difference of over 1.5 cm.[1] While a few small studies report an increased incidence of back or hip problems with modest LLD, most large series do not report an increased incidence of long-term problems with LLD of less than 1 inch. However, the long-term effect of LLD is not certain. Nor is there convincing evidence to support the position that an LLD less than 1 inch is acceptable while LLD larger than 1 inch warrants treatment. Clearly a 2-cm discrepancy in a 6-foot 10-inch NBA player may not be as much of an issue as it would be in a 5-foot 2-inch jockey. Gait analysis has shown that children with LLD less than 3% do not use compensatory strategies.[2] A 3% LLD in an average adult is about 1 inch. Conversely and in some cases, a small LLD may actually be beneficial; in patients with a stiff ankle or a drop foot from hemiplegia, a leg that is 1 to 2 cm shorter will accommodate an ankle foot orthosis and be able to clear the toe better in swing phase.

Even though small to moderate LLD may not lead to functional issues; sometimes patients and parents are more concerned about the cosmetic appearance of a short limb gait and seek treatment for this issue. To stay out of trouble, it is important to recognize that equaling out the leg length in a child with cerebral palsy will not relieve the spastic components of their gait. Similarly, limb lengthening will not improve the Trendelenburg sway from a child with coxa vara from severe Perthes disease.

Assessment

It is important to make an accurate diagnosis of LLD so you can to predict the eventual discrepancy at maturity and also rule out serious underlying causes, such as neurofibromatosis, bone or soft tissue tumors, and neurologic disorders that may require additional medical treatment. The first pitfall to recognize is determining which leg is abnormal. Is one leg too short, or the other one too long? While making this distinction sounds simple, this point is not just academic. For example, recognizing that the long limb is abnormal in an infant with idiopathic hemihypertrophy can be critical. If the patient has a variant of Beckwith-Wiedemann syndrome, regular ultrasounds of the abdomen at 3- to 6-month intervals for the first 6 to 8 years of life to rule out associated Wilm or other abdominal tumors are necessary. In some instances, the orthopaedic surgeon may be the first person to make this diagnosis.

Looking at the proportions of the legs to the body can be helpful in determining which limb is abnormal. Hint: pathologically short limbs often have associated musculoskeletal abnormalities such as coxa vara, bowing, absence of an anterior cruciate ligament (ACL), lateral femoral hypoplasia, fibular hemimelia, tumorous conditions such as fibrous dysplasia, etc. In contrast, pathologically long limbs are often associated with cutaneous or vascular anomalies as seen in Proteus syndrome (Fig. 28-1), Klippel-Trenaunay syndrome, neurofibromatosis, or Beckwith-Wiedemann syndrome.

PHYSICAL EXAMINATION

On physical examination, there are numerous pitfalls in the assessment of LLD. **ORTHOPAEDICS 101: Any joint contracture will affect the functional discrepancy of the limb in gait even if there is no anatomic difference in the**

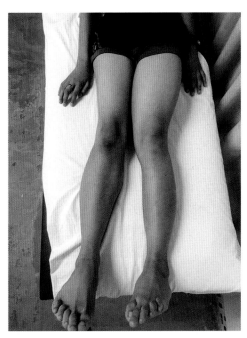

Figure 28-1 A 13-year-old Honduran boy with likely Proteus syndrome showing asymmetric enlargement of his right thigh and left leg and variable macrodactyly. (Used with the permission of the University of Wisconsin Division of Pediatric Orthopaedics.)

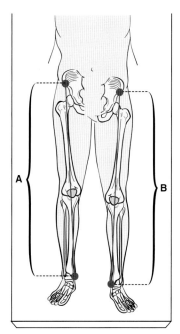

A=B

Figure 28-2 Pelvic obliquity can cause an apparent leg length discrepancy; patient supine on examining table.

length of the bones. An adducted hip makes the leg appear shorter, while an abducted hip makes the leg appear longer. In fact, an apparent discrepancy of 3 cm is created for each 10° of hip adduction/abduction.[3] Similarly, a knee flexion contracture will functionally shorten the leg while an equinus contracture will make it functionally longer. Because of this, simply looking at the position of the feet of a supine patient is not accurate (Fig. 28-2). Measuring leg lengths from the anterior superior iliac spine to the medial malleolus is subject to extreme variability and will not account for any difference in foot height that can be seen in children with congenital limb deficiency or overcorrected clubfoot (Fig. 28-3). A good way to measure LLD on physical examination is to have the patient stand up, with knees straight, and place the examiner's fingers on the iliac crest. Placing blocks of various sizes under the short leg until the pelvis is level provides a reasonable estimation of the LLD. This test is less accurate in the circumferentially challenged (obese) child, as the pelvis is more difficult to palpate. Beware that previous pelvic surgery, such as a Salter osteotomy in which part of the iliac crest has been removed, may make this test inaccurate. Another pitfall in evaluating for LLD by the standing method is that a chronically short leg often develops an equinus contracture. Make certain both feet are flat on the floor. Similarly children with significant LLDs will automatically bend the knee of the longer leg to level the pelvis—this is another pitfall.

> **THE GURU SAYS...**
>
> Placing a patient prone on the examining table with the knees flexed 90° allows both the hip to knee and knee to plantar foot segment lengths to be evaluated. Family members are usually appreciative that you can demonstrate the size and location of the discrepancy with this simple technique.
>
> CHRISTOPHER IOBST

> **THE GURU SAYS...**
>
> Have the patient stand on blocks placed under the short limb until they feel the leg lengths are equalized. If blocks are not available, a stack of magazines or books work equally well. The patient will usually feel most comfortable with the short limb length slightly undercorrected.
>
> CHRISTOPHER IOBST

> **THE GURU SAYS...**
>
> In thin patients, the posterior sacral dimples are easily visible and can be used to demonstrate any pelvic obliquity to the parents.
>
> CHRISTOPHER IOBST

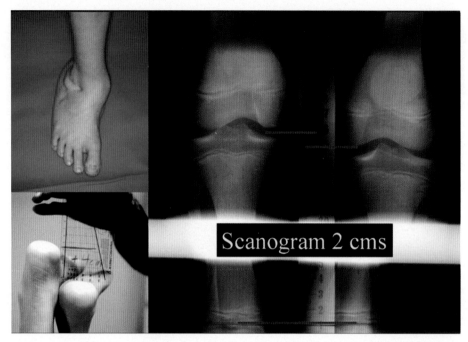

Figure 28-3 This 14-year-old boy presented with a 4-cm clinical leg length discrepancy (LLD). The scanogram revealed 2 cm at the tibial level. The remaining 2 cm is due to the loss in foot height as a result of pantalar release for clubfoot. Key point: Scanograms don't identify all levels of LLD. (Used with the permission of the University of Wisconsin Division of Pediatric Orthopaedics.)

A good general musculoskeletal examination of the child is also critical. In children for whom lengthening may be considered, pay particular attention during the physical examination to evaluate joint stability of the hips, knees (is the ACL missing?), patella and ankles (valgus/varus). An unstable joint is best discovered and corrected before it dislocates during lengthening. Does the femur have rotational asymmetry that could be derotated after osteotomy? Are there scars or soft tissue contractures that would limit bone lengthening? Does the limb have normal vascular flow or is there altered vascular status? What is the neurologic function? Does the child have a drop foot that would be best accommodated with the limb being slightly shorter?

RADIOGRAPHIC STUDIES

Plain radiography is the most common method used to quantitate LLD; yet it is still subject to a variety of errors, such as patient positioning and unrecognized joint contractures. A standing teleoroentgenogram (AP radiograph of the lower extremities including the hips, knees, and ankles on one film with the patella facing forward) has value as the initial screening examination for all patients with LLD. This study provides information about the entire lower extremity length from the pelvis to the bottom of the foot and allows each limb to undergo deformity analysis. This study can also detect any lesions within the bones of the lower extremities. Unfortunately, the X-ray beam of the teleoroentgenogram is at an angle to the hip and ankle and any subtle hip dysplasia or ankle abnormalities may be missed; the parallax can also introduce some magnification error. However, because the effect is symmetric to both limbs, a 10% magnification error does not likely effect clinical decision-making. It is a great tool for following small children that won't stay still for the multiple exposures required during a scanogram (which is preferable to follow the LLD in children who can lie still).

THE GURU SAYS...

If deformity is suspected in the hip or ankle after a standing lower extremity radiograph, obtain dedicated radiographs centered on the joint in question. A more accurate deformity analysis can then be performed.

CHRISTOPHER IOBST

THE GURU SAYS...

Although the standing lower extremity radiograph is the preferred study to analyze limb lengths, some radiography suites may not have the capability to acquire long leg films. A scanogram should be achievable in any radiology setting and is the next best option.

CHRISTOPHER IOBST

Scanograms can give the clinician very accurate data on the length of the femur and tibia provided there are no hip or knee contractures. If contractures are present, computed tomography (CT) scanograms more accurately assess limb lengths in these children and can also quantitate differences in rotational profile. Because scanograms center on the joints, it also allows one to detect hip dysplasia or other joint abnormalities. One pitfall of the scanogram is that the foot is not included, so a foot deformity that contributes to the overall LLD will not be recognized by the scanogram (Fig. 28-4). In these patients, standing lateral foot radiographs

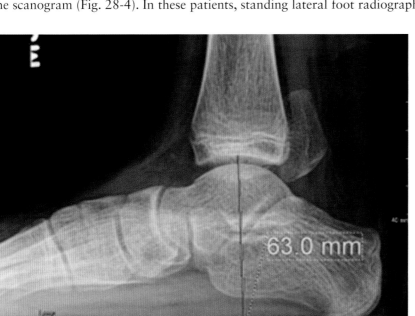

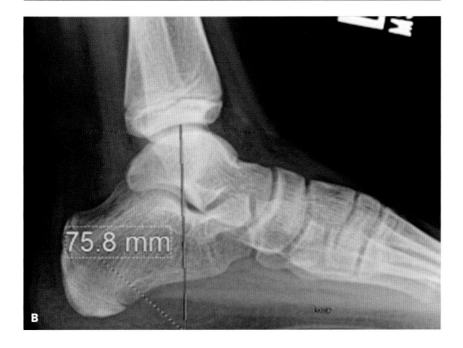

Figure 28-4 This patient with fibular hemimelia has a loss of foot height (**A**) in comparison to the contralateral foot (**B**). In my experience, one can see up to 2 cm of leg length discrepancy in foot deformities, which has to be accounted for in treatment strategies. (Used with the permission of the University of Wisconsin Division of Pediatric Orthopaedics.)

TABLE 28-1 Useful Chart for Reading a Scanogram

	Length of Femur	Length of Tibia	Length of Tibia + *Femur*
Right	32.7 cm	26.8	59.5
Left	35.0	22.3	57.3
Difference	(−2.3)	4.5	2.2 = LLD

When reading a scanogram, making a chart such as this helps to avoid errors, as the total leg length discrepancy (LLD) difference is calculated two ways. One is by subtracting the total leg lengths in the last column, and the other is by verifying the calculation by adding the differences of the femoral and tibial limb length in the last row.

are helpful to quantitate the deformity. A second pitfall of the scanogram that is used as an initial screening tool is that the diaphysis of the femur and tibia are not imaged, so a midshaft lesion, deformity, or other cause of the LLD may be missed.

When interpreting a scanogram, chart the lengths and differences of the femur and tibia individually (Table 28-1), then confirm that the lengths and differences give the same total LLD for the entire limb independently. This can be written directly on the scanogram (Fig. 28-5) or dictated in the chart, so the accuracy may be later verified. While this sounds elementary, most errors in LLD surgery are from miscalculations. Two studies looking at epiphysiodesis found high rates of failure due to errors in timing surgery. One review of 57 patients[4] found 71%

THE GURU SAYS...

Scanograms are not weight-bearing films. Therefore, any contribution to the limb deformity from ligament instability will not be appreciated.

CHRISTOPHER IOBST

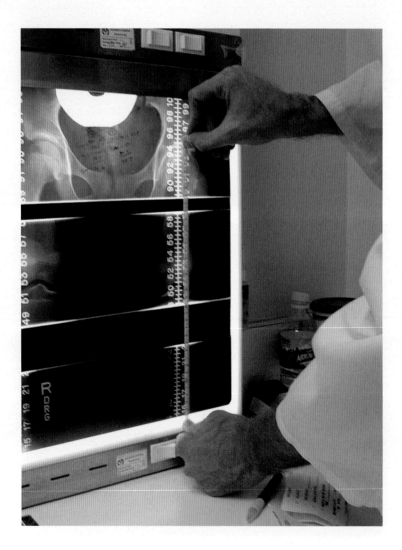

Figure 28-5 A quick way to double-check your calculated leg length discrepancy (LLD) from the scanogram: Measure the length from the top of the femur to the bottom of the tibia of both legs with a tape measure. The difference of these measurements should equal the formally calculated LLD.

of patients had a final LLD of more than 1.5 cm. Another review of 67 patients[5] found that 51% had a final LLD greater than 1.0 cm.

Recently, low-dose standing biplanar radiographic imaging systems have been used for assessment of spinal deformity. Known as EOS, this technology has also been used to assess lower limb alignment and limb length discrepancy. It is expensive and is currently not available in most hospitals, but studies suggest that they have lower radiation exposure with greater accuracy then CT scanograms and standard radiographic measures. Another advantage is the ability to quantify limb alignment and deformity at the same time measurements of length are determined.

NORMAL GROWTH

It is important to recognize that growth is not static, and thus, discrepancies in length in growing children can change over time. The family and the clinician should consider what the LLD will be at skeletal maturity, so having a few rules of growth is helpful in predicting what the ultimate LLD will be. For instance, a rule of thumb for prediction of a child's final height is summation of parental height/2 +6.5 cm for boys and −6.5 cm for girls. A rough estimate of the growth of the physes of the lower extremity is proximal femur 4 mm/y, distal femur 10 mm/y, proximal tibia 6 mm/y, and the distal tibia 5 mm/y (Fig. 28-6).

> **THE GURU SAYS...**
> Smartphone applications (Multiplier, Paley Growth) have been developed to help the clinician make growth assessments quickly and conveniently. They contain multiple platforms that allow a comprehensive evaluation of growth. The formulae and tables available in the applications include calculating limb length discrepancy at maturity (congenital, developmental), growth remaining (femur, tibia, entire leg), and bone length at maturity for both the upper and lower extremity.
> CHRISTOPHER IOBST

> **THE GURU SAYS...**
> As a quick reference, the standing height of a 2-year-old child is 50% of the final adult height. At the age of 5 years, the standing height is 60% and at the age of 9 years it is 80% of the final adult height.
> CHRISTOPHER IOBST

Lower extremity skeletal growth generally ends at age 14 years in girls and age 16 years in boys. Keep in mind that the age of growth cessation is also dependant on medical comorbidities. For example, patients with skeletal dysplasia, metabolic and nutritional disorders, and history of malignancy and chronic chemotherapeutic treatment may not follow the normal growth patterns. Also, beware that underlying disorders may affect maturation, for example, one third of children with spina bifida may have precocious puberty and that children with Blount disease often have an advanced skeletal age.

One of the biggest challenges in pediatric orthopaedics is to assess a child's growth remaining. Qualitatively the experienced pediatric orthopaedist can gain some general insight by the radiologic appearance of physis, comparison of child's height to the parents and their growth patterns (e.g., dad grew 4 inches in college), and comparison to siblings. Quantitatively we can use the patient's chronologic age or the skeletal age using the Greulich-Pyle atlas. Bone age using the Greulich-Pyle method is subject to significant variability. In one study, 60 hand radiographs

> **THE GURU SAYS...**
> Make sure the patient can stand still for at least 30 seconds before ordering an EOS image of the lower extremities. Any movement during the exposure will interfere with the image quality.
> CHRISTOPHER IOBST

> **THE GURU SAYS...**
> The femoral and tibial lengths should remain constantly proportional after the age of 5 years. The tibial length is 80% of the femoral length.
> CHRISTOPHER IOBST

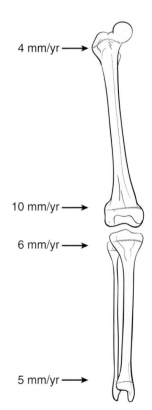

4 mm/yr →

10 mm/yr →

6 mm/yr →

5 mm/yr →

Figure 28-6 Estimate of growth of the physes of the femur and tibia: proximal femur 4 mm/y, distal femur 10 mm/y, proximal tibia 6 mm/y, and distal tibia 5 mm/y.

were read by four radiologists, and 50% of the children were assigned a skeletal age that differed by more than 1 year between radiologists; 10% varied by more than 2 years.[6]

As skeletal age is subject to inaccuracies, one should consider comparing the skeletal with the chronologic age. When the chronologic age is the same as the skeletal age, they may give the most accurate picture and one can be reasonably confident in the skeletal age reading. **NEWSFLASH! When the chronologic age and the bone age differ by more than 2 years, one should take pause in planning different limb equalization procedures like permanent epiphysiodesis that depend on years of growth remaining.**

PREDICTING LEG LENGTH DISCREPANCY

At the risk of being too simple, remember the LLD we are treating is the LLD predicted at maturity, not the current LLD. The three traditional methods of predicting LLD are the arithmetic method, the growth-remaining method, and the straight-line method. These three all use data from one database by Anderson and Green. A potential pitfall in using only the growth-remaining method is that tall children obtain more correction than short children after an epiphysiodesis, because they will have more growth. Of these three methods, the Moseley straight-line method has several advantages to help minimize errors, such as using multiple measurements at different times and considering growth percentiles.[7] While the Moseley straight-line method has been the gold standard, multiple measurements should be obtained to use it, and there are many potential sources of error. Remember to use the appropriate gender-specific Moseley growth chart. The multiplier method is an alternative method of assessing growth remaining. The multiplier method characterizes the pattern of normal human growth by using an age- and gender-specific coefficient. The multiplier for each age and gender is a measure of the percentage of growth remaining. It is, therefore, viewed as a universal method for predicting lower limb length because it is independent of percentile, regional, racial, ethnic, and generational differences in growth data. An advantage of the multiplier method is that it allows prediction of LLD with one measurement of limb lengths, without the need for bone age or graphing and is quite simple for predicting LLD in congenital discrepancies.[8]

Beware that one-time events can cause a bone to shorten by slowing or shutting down the growth of a bone, and thus, the above growth predication methods are unreliable. This is particularly important to remember in patients with a history of neonatal sepsis and multiple levels of old osteoarticular infections (Fig. 28-7). In these patients, the growth plates may grow slower than the contralateral side and even shut down years before the other growth plate closes. Growth plates can also grow faster from juxtaphyseal inflammation (chronic juvenile inflammatory arthritis) infection, tumor, or traumatic events, and the degree and duration of growth stimulation is very unpredictable. Also remember that growth plates can increase growth in the face of acute malunion such as a femur fracture healing 3 cm short (Fig. 28-8). To stay out of trouble, it's important to remember that ultimate LLD in acquired cases is really only predictable in cases of complete physeal arrest. Because growth is constant in congenital limb deficiencies, one can use the Moseley growth chart and the multiplier method to predict LLD with good reliability. **NEWSFLASH! The rate of growth in congenital conditions can be affected by treatment. Femoral lengthenings may increase growth rate of the distal femur while tibial lengthenings may slow the growth rate of the proximal tibia.**[9]

THE GURU SAYS...

For first-time consultations, the ability to predict the ultimate limb length discrepancy at skeletal maturity is highly valuable. Based on this prediction, a life plan can be devised for the patient and the family that outlines the number of procedures necessary to obtain normalized limb lengths.

CHRISTOPHER IOBST

THE GURU SAYS...

When attempting to understand the growth dynamics of a patient, the ideal approach should use multiple methods that complement each other. For example, checking the Anderson-Green-Messner growth-remaining chart in addition to the Menelaus rule of thumb or the multiplier method is better than using any one method alone. If the different methods are in agreement, then one can feel comfortable that the calculations are probably reliable.

CHRISTOPHER IOBST

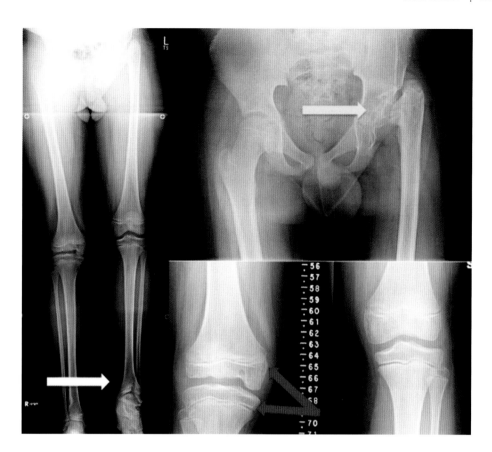

Figure 28-7 This 12-year-old boy had a history of neonatal sepsis and likely multifocal joint infections. He had complete growth arrests in his left ankle (white arrow) and growth retardation at his right knee (red arrows). All of these problems led to a significant challenge in planning for the future as there was no way to predict final anatomic leg length discrepancy. Complicating matters further, his left hip never developed properly (yellow arrow) and his hip instability and Trendelenburg gait resulted in functional discrepancy during gait as well. (Used with the permission of the University of Wisconsin Division of Pediatric Orthopaedics.)

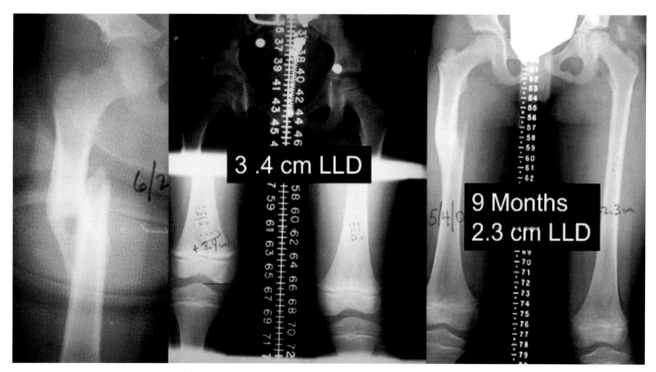

Figure 28-8 An 8-year-old girl with a femoral fracture malunion of 3.4 cm. After 9 mo, the leg had accelerated growth to recoup more than 1 cm of leg length discrepancy. Her mother refused to come in for a follow-up X-ray at maturity because "her legs are fine." (Used with the permission of the University of Wisconsin Division of Pediatric Orthopaedics.)

Treatment

GENERAL PRINCIPLES

Traditional guidelines for the treatment of LLD are outlined in Table 28-2. Most children can tolerate an LLD of 4 to 5 cm by flexing the knee of the long leg or walking on the toe of the short leg. On occasion, a shoe lift is requested by the family over concern that the LLD will cause hip or spine arthritis (*not!*). Perhaps a more reasonable indication for a shoe lift is when the child wants it or if the child is getting a fixed equinus contracture on the short leg. In these cases, the child may feel better and may prevent a gastrocsoleus contracture. Be aware that lifts more than 5 cm may be more difficult to control and can lead to ankle sprains. It is wise to use the standing teleoroentgenogram as a judge of what the functional discrepancy is as opposed to the scanogram. Consider a lift that is 1 to 2 cm less than this value, especially if the child has a contracture of the knee or a drop foot, which makes swing-through difficult during ambulation.

When performing surgery for an LLD, stay out of trouble and aim at 0.5 to 1.0 cm of undercorrection as discrepancies less than 2 cm are well tolerated. Families may be quite unhappy if the long leg was shortened too early via an epiphysiodesis and the child's long leg is now the short one. Similar to orthotic use, it is important to plan for a leg to end up shorter if the knee can't bend well and is in extension during swing phase of gait. In cases with fixed lumbar-sacral obliquity, an LLD may be an important compensation; in this case, equalizing the leg lengths could result in a functional leg length discrepancy with further spine imbalance.

TABLE 28-2 Traditional Guidelines for the Treatment of Leg Length Discrepancy[a]	
Projected Discrepancy at Maturity	**Guideline**
<2 cm	No treatment or consider shoe lift if symptomatic
2-6 cm	Epiphysiodesis if enough growth remains
	Acute skeletal shortening if mature
	Lengthening if osteotomy is required for deformity correction
6-20 cm	Limb reconstruction with 1-3 lengthenings with or without growth arrest
>20 cm	Amputation and prosthetic fitting

[a]Must be modified to individual patient's condition and goals.

EPIPHYSIODESIS

One of the challenges of epiphysiodesis is explaining the procedure to families and how it works. Many times, families are not too excited about shortening the "good leg" even if it's the correct option. One way to help them is to have the child stand on just the long leg and then just the short leg and ask if that difference is an issue. In addition, the family thinks that you are shutting down the child's entire growth. Finally, it can be challenging to explain the goals of epiphysiodesis and the importance of timing.

> **THE GURU SAYS...**
>
> It is important to stress that determining the timing of epiphysiodesis is an educated guess about the amount of growth remaining. The goal is to get the leg lengths back to an acceptable limit with the short leg ideally just slightly shorter than the opposite limb.
>
> CHRISTOPHER IOBST

> **THE GURU SAYS...**
>
> Having a long leg radiographic image available where each of the four major lower extremity physes are visible makes it easier to demonstrate to the family that the epiphysiodesis will only stop the growth at one (or two) areas, not the entire limb.
>
> CHRISTOPHER IOBST

The author used to practice in the land of NASCAR racing and uses the following analogy to explain epiphysiodesis (which is enhanced with a number of "gosh dangs" and appropriate references to oil filter companies/sponsorships): "Consider your child's two legs as race cars running a race until they both run out of gas (growth). Dale's [popular NASCAR driver name] left leg is a V8 engine and is now 3 miles ahead of his right leg, which is a V6 engine. Our goal is for both legs to cross the finish line at the same time (photo-finish is highly desirable for both patient and fans alike). In order to do this, we need to remove one or two cylinders (growth plates) from the V8 (left leg) so that the V6 (right leg) catches up at and they coast over the line together. The key is making sure we take the pistons out at the right time; too early and the V6 wins, but too late and the V8 wins." Note: Similar scenarios can be used for international providers by referencing Formula One racing.

The key point to staying out of trouble is to *double check all calculations*, as this operation can be permanent. There are numerous methods to halt the growth of a physis via open and percutaneous techniques with or without implants.[10] Different methods and implants have their advantages.

> **THE GURU SAYS...**
>
> Remember that in cases of limb length discrepancy caused by a physeal arrest, epiphysiodesis of the corresponding contralateral physis only prevents the current limb length discrepancy from getting worse. It does not correct the limb length discrepancy unless an additional physis is closed in the long limb.
>
> CHRISTOPHER IOBST

Blount Staples

Rigid Blount staples can be used for a spell when one wants to temporarily slow the growth of a child (8-12 years of age) with a gigantism type of syndrome such as Klippel-Trenaunay-Weber. This method is beneficial if the current discrepancy is more than 6 to 8 cm, but the child is not a limb lengthening candidate, and they are too young to consider permanent growth arrest. In this case, the implants are placed on the medial and lateral sides of the femur and tibia and kept in place for up to 2 years and then removed. Be aware of rebound growth after the staples are removed. Rebound growth is well described in temporary hemiepiphysiodesis for angular deformity, and we suspect it is underappreciated in the treatment of LLD. Stay out of trouble by using two or three staples on each side of the distal femur and one or two staples on each side of the proximal tibia. Most important, *do not use* modular plate and screw constructs (tension band plates) as they can lead to deformity or screw fracture.

Percutaneous Epiphysiodesis With Transphyseal Screws

This is a good method for closing the growth plate of the distal femur or fibula. It is minimally invasive and is less painful that percutaneous growth plate ablation with a drill. To stay out of trouble, do not use in the proximal tibia (higher failure rates) and use fully threaded screws that are 6.5 mm diameter. Because this technique has a tendency to undercorrect, it may need to be instituted a few months earlier than the calculated start date to achieve full correction.

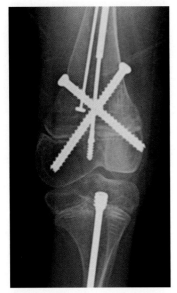

Figure 28-9 This boy with osteogenesis imperfecta and a leg length discrepancy underwent epiphysiodesis with percutaneous epiphysiodesis with transphyseal screws. Percutaneous epiphysiodesis would have been a challenge with the existing implant and with worries for pathologic fracture. (Used with the permission of the University of Wisconsin Division of Pediatric Orthopaedics.)

> **THE GURU SAYS…**
>
> For epiphysiodesis of the distal femur, use a curved curette to reach up through your entry hole to the undulating physis on the medial and lateral edges.
>
> CHRISTOPHER IOBST

Fluoroscopic Percutaneous Drill Epiphysiodesis

This is the gold standard for growth plate ablation. Use of rigid staples or screws for definitive closure, although effective, does not immediately shut down growth as quickly as the fluoroscopic drill method. On the other hand, it may be preferable to use staples or screws in children with brittle bone disease such as osteogenesis imperfecta (Fig. 28-9). Stay out of trouble and use a Kirschner wire (K-wire) introduced into the growth plate as a guide for a cannulated drill bit. One can use a 7-mm cannulated reamer for the femur and tibia and could use cannulated 3.5- or 4.5-mm drill bits for use in the distal tibia and fibula (Fig. 28-10). Technically, when ablating the physis with a drill and curette, there is a tendency for the instrument to fall into the softer adjacent cancellous bone. Stay out of trouble with liberal use of images to make certain you are ablating the physis. The distal femoral physis in particular is not flat; make certain the ablation follows the undulations of the physis.

> **THE GURU SAYS…**
>
> To avoid the possibility of overcorrection with the percutaneous drill method, add a few months' time to the predicted age for epiphysiodesis. It is better to end up slightly short than to overcorrect the short limb.
>
> CHRISTOPHER IOBST

> **THE GURU SAYS…**
>
> Use suction to remove all of the fluid from the epiphysiodesis site just prior to obtaining a fluoroscopic image. The path of your fluid-free epiphysiodesis site will be more visible on the screen.
>
> CHRISTOPHER IOBST

Most surgeons make medial and lateral incisions for this method in the distal femur and proximal tibia. Others have performed epiphysiodesis from only one side with predictable good results. If performing an epiphysiodesis from one side, it is essential not to miss the corners of the growth plate adjacent to the incision (Fig. 28-11). When performing a proximal tibial epiphysiodesis in a child with

Figure 28-10 After an ankle fracture this 9-year-old girl with a partial growth arrest (yellow arrow) underwent bilateral distal tibia growth arrests with a cannulated 4.5-mm drill. The fibular growth plates were closed with 4.5-mm cannulated screws via percutaneous epiphysiodesis with transphyseal screws method. (Used with the permission of the University of Wisconsin Division of Pediatric Orthopaedics.)

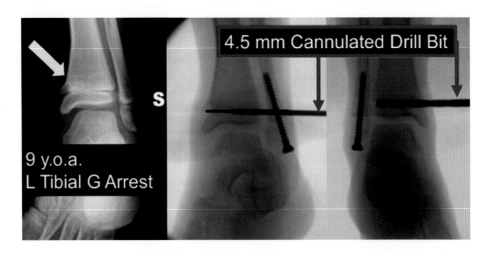

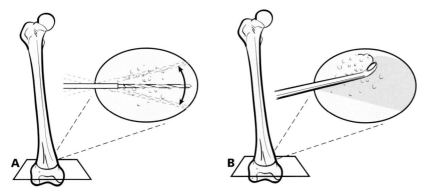

Figure 28-11 Minimalist technique of percutaneous epiphysiodesis. Drill from one side. Drill across the physis almost to the other side, and then repeat with multiple passes at slightly different angles within the plane of the physis. When most of the physis is drilled, begin to windshield the drill back and forth. If too much force is used, the drill may break. A key part of staying out of trouble with this technique is to then use a curette to remove the portion of the physis adjacent to entrance of the drill.

many years of growth remaining, consider concomitant epiphysiodesis of the proximal fibula to avoid a prominent fibular head. With proper respect for the peroneal nerve, this procedure has been shown to be safe.[11]

Complications of Epiphysiodesis

Inadequate epiphysiodesis may lead to angular growth, or continued normal growth. These complications should usually be noted by growth arrest lines within 6 months by serial radiographs. Stay out of trouble by recognizing a partial growth arrest early, before significant angular deformity develops. If recognized early, a repeat epiphysiodesis may be all that is necessary, and the need for an osteotomy avoided.

ACUTE SHORTENING

Acute shortening for LLD is usually done when insufficient growth is available to recoup the LLD from a growth arrest; knee heights will often end up different, but that is not a functional problem and patients who expect it ahead of time do not seem to be bothered. If possible, it is recommended to perform shortening in the femur and not in the tibia. Tibial shortenings are challenging because of the need to address the fibula and the increased risk for compartment syndrome. Femoral shortenings may be performed open or closed with an intramedullary saw. Femoral shortening should be performed proximally. Shortening in the diaphysis, below the origin of much of the quadriceps muscle, weakens the knee extensor mechanism more than a proximal shortening. In general, avoid shortening more than 15% of the original bone length or about 5 to 6 cm, as this may also lead to muscular weakness. When the skeletal shortening is performed open, the final site of the osteotomy is proximal and the bones are stabilized with an intramedullary rod, blade plate or locking plate fixation is most appropriate for children and small-statured adolescents. Remember to pay attention to rotational alignment when applying fixation to the segments.

   Closed femoral shortening with intramedullary stabilization seems seductive at first glance, but there are lots of opportunities for complications. These are difficult operations to perform, and there are multiple pitfalls (Fig. 28-12). First is determining the appropriate patient as an intramedullary saw has to fit down a 12-mm diaphysis, which makes this technique applicable only for older patients. In patients with an appropriately sized canal, there are some pitfalls with the saw.

> **THE GURU SAYS...**
> Intraoperative ultrasound can identify the relation of the peroneal nerve to the fibular physis allowing a safe, percutaneous approach to proximal fibular epiphysiodesis.
>
> CHRISTOPHER IOBST

> **THE GURU SAYS...**
> Acute shortenings of several centimeters will tend to make the limb segment more sausage shaped. Make sure you discuss this cosmetic result with the patient beforehand.
>
> CHRISTOPHER IOBST

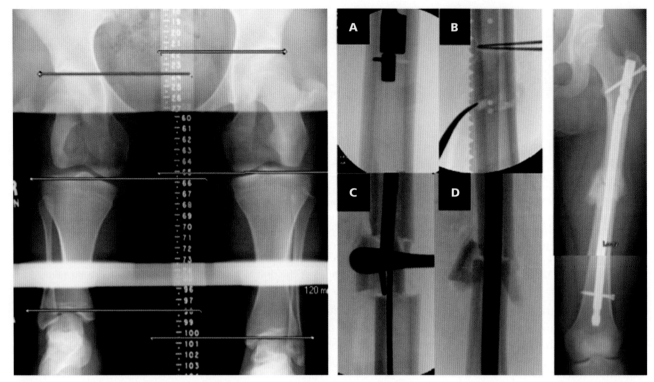

Figure 28-12 A 16-year-old girl with fibular hemimelia and a 3.5-cm leg length discrepancy underwent closed femoral shortening. **A:** The initial intramedullary cut was made. **B:** The distance to be shortened is confirmed with a radiopaque ruler. After the second osteotomy is made the fragment needs to cut and manipulated out of the way. **C:** The intramedullary nail stabilizes the osteotomy site. **D:** Follow-up radiograph at 4 mo shows good healing. In retrospect, the osteotomy could have been more proximal to avoid weakness. Looks easy, but these are "futzy" procedures. (Used with the permission of the University of Wisconsin Division of Pediatric Orthopaedics.)

To stay out of trouble and to avoid fat emboli syndrome with reaming a closed femoral shaft, it's important to vent the femur before reaming with fluted reamers. (One way to do this is to percutaneously drill multiple holes at the site of the planned distal osteotomy site.) The first osteotomy is performed distally through the previous vent sites. This is the easiest cut, as the intact femur can be held while the saw is rotated. A technical trick to help complete the second cut (proximal cut) is to use the distal femur as a (well-controlled) battering ram against the proximal piece. The posterior portion of the cut along the linea aspera may need to be completed with a percutaneously placed osteotome.

LIMB LENGTHENING

Preparation of Expectations for Surgery

Unless you are a very experienced limb reconstruction surgeon, it may be unwise to recommend limb reconstruction with multiple lengthenings in patients with expected LLD greater than 20 cm (or in cases less than this but with severe joint instability or other comorbidities). The morbidity and psychological impact of a childhood full of hospitalizations, operations, and complications may be profound. A relatively simple amputation and prosthetic fitting could be better than years of treatment required to produce a stiff, painful, reconstructed limb. Sometimes the best way to stay out of trouble is to avoid a heroic procedure in favor of an amputation. Birch et al.[12] showed that young adults who underwent a Syme amputation in childhood showed no difference from normal adults in psychological testing, quality of life, or self-esteem, and all 10 adults had no difficulty walking or running. However, before taking the irreversible step of amputation, consider recommending second and third opinions.

THE GURU SAYS...

A typical life plan for a congenital limb length discrepancy projected to be 20 cm at skeletal maturity would be:

1. Preparatory surgery to stabilize the hip/knee/ankle at age 2 years
2. First limb lengthening at age 4 years with goal of 4 to 5 cm
3. Second lengthening at age 8 years with goal of 5 cm
4. Third lengthening combined with epiphysiodesis to correct final 10 cm at age 12 years, or no epiphysiodesis at age 12 years but a fourth lengthening at maturity to complete the correction

CHRISTOPHER IOBST

Each patient with an LLD greater than 5 or 6 cm who desires a limb lengthening will have unique characteristics that will require individualized treatment strategies. Patient and family selection is critical for this treatment, both from a psychological and physiologic perspective.

Unstable parents provide inadequate support for the program. It is absolutely essential that the patient and family understand that when a limb has a predicted LLD that requires lengthening, the treatment for correcting this will be a *process* and one that could consist of a series of operations. For instance, a child with congenital short femur and a predicted LLD of 6 cm may require a pelvic osteotomy (for severe dysplasia) prior to lengthening and a medial distal femoral hemiepiphysiodesis (for femoral valgus) during limb lengthening.

THE GURU SAYS...

The concept of preparatory surgery is essential, especially in congenital causes of limb length discrepancy. Before any lengthening procedure is considered, the joints above and below the bone of interest need to be evaluated for stability and function. Restoring the joints to (near) normal stability should be undertaken prior to any lengthening surgery.

CHRISTOPHER IOBST

Even in cases in which one routine distraction osteogenesis is performed, it's still not a *procedure*; but a *process* that includes surgery, limb lengthening over weeks, and then callus maturation which can take months. In cases of congenital limb deficiencies, one should only expect to lengthen a bone 20% of its length before complications/pain become overwhelming. If the family wants a "heroic" lengthening, and you feel uncomfortable with this, refer the family to a surgeon with a similar philosophy as the family.

Not only should families understand the steps of the treatment and the stages of limb lengthening, but in cases in which external fixation is used, they should expect a 100% complication rate, with a need for additional unplanned surgery. Within the past 5 years, the use of intramedullary magnetic rods for limb lengthening has revolutionized the process of limb lengthening in the United States. This device has reliably lengthened bone with much less soft tissue complications and without pin tract infection and scarring. If such a device can be used the complication rate is much lower. In retrospect, the historical recommendation that limb lengthening only be considered for LLD greater than 5 cm was probably made in light of the high rate of complications of standard distraction osteogenesis with external fixation. If you're going to put a kid through 6 months of torture, might as well do it for only larger discrepancies. With the use of intramedullary lengthenings and the lower complication rate, we wonder if the LLD considered for limb lengthening may become less (Fig. 28-13).

Regardless of the device that lengthens the bone (external fixation or intramedullary nail), complications are usually a result of the tension in the soft tissues that begins to increase after a 10% increase in bone length. Except in lengthenings for stature (achondroplasia bones, which can be lengthened more than 30%), the "wheels start falling off the bus" when you reach 20% or 6 cm in cases with congenital LLD. The pain and problems of limb lengthening are *significantly* greater

THE GURU SAYS...

Family support for lengthening patients is critical and needs to be assessed prior to surgery. Family members will need to help patients at home with daily activities, fixator or lengthening nail adjustments, wound/pin care, monitoring of the weight-bearing activity, and encouraging daily range of motion exercises. In addition, adequate transportation to and from weekly clinic visits will be required for an extended period of time.

CHRISTOPHER IOBST

THE GURU SAYS...

For substantial leg length discrepancies, multiple small, safe lengthenings are preferable to one large lengthening that risks regenerate fracture, joint contracture or joint subluxation.

CHRISTOPHER IOBST

THE GURU SAYS...

Acceptance of complications is easier if the patient and family are prepared for them beforehand. Let them know preoperatively that pin site infections are an expected but manageable aspect of the treatment. Explain there will be three surgeries along the way: one to apply the frame, one to remove the frame, and one in between to address any potential complication that may arise.

CHRISTOPHER IOBST

THE GURU SAYS...

From a pain standpoint, lengthening with an intramedullary nail should result in minimal discomfort for patients. However, they need to be prepared for an extended period of time with limited weight bearing.

CHRISTOPHER IOBST

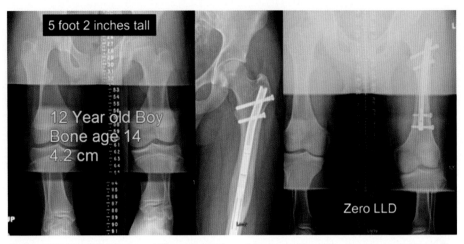

Figure 28-13 This 14-year-old boy was 5 foot 2 inches tall and had a 4.2 cm leg length discrepancy. He refused to consider a growth arrest ("I am short enough!"). At the age of 16 y, he returned and requested limb lengthening with an external fixator. Fortunately, the Precice magnetic lengthening device had gained US approval and his femur was lengthened without complications. (Used with the permission of the University of Wisconsin Division of Pediatric Orthopaedics.)

with external fixation when the soft tissues are tethered by the transfixing pins and wires needed with external fixation.

> **THE GURU SAYS...**
>
> Assessment of joint flexibility before surgery is key. A tight muscle is only going to become tighter with bone lengthening. Anticipating trouble by recessing the hamstrings or gastrocsoleus prophylactically can alleviate some of the soft tissue tension. For femoral lengthening, consider releasing the iliotibial band at the level of the proximal patella.
>
> CHRISTOPHER IOBST

Common Problems With External Fixation

Bone fixation can be performed with half pins and/or transfixing wires. Acute injuries to nerves or blood vessels during wire and half pin insertion are uncommon but potentially serious. Review of cross-sectional anatomy is essential. As Dr. Vernon Tolo teaches, "You can invent an operation, but not anatomy." In older patients, it's a good idea to use three pins proximal and distal to the distraction site. In smaller children, two pins may suffice. Hydroxyapatite coated pins are preferable for limb lengthening, and they should be removed only in the operating room. If removal is attempted in clinic, the patient and surgeon will endure much pain.

As a bone lengthens, the tension in the muscles can become excessive. This soft tissue tightness first manifests itself as a decrease in joint motion but can progress to permanent contractures and/or joint dislocation. Stay out of trouble by avoiding bifocal lengthenings[13] and ipsilateral lengthenings, as these increase muscle tension and increase pressures across the knee joint. If the hip is potentially unstable, which can conceivably be found in congenital short femur cases, a pelvic osteotomy prior to lengthening to increase acetabular coverage should be performed to normalize the center edge angle (CEA <20°). Spanning the knee with an external fixator or reconstructing the ligaments prior to lengthening may be needed as congenital LLD cases are often cruciate deficient. Similarly, the ankle may need to be spanned in fibular hemimelia to prevent equinus or lateral ankle subluxation. It's a good idea to keep the spanning device in place for at least 4 weeks after the lengthening phase.

> **THE GURU SAYS...**
>
> Bring a cross-sectional anatomy atlas with you to the operating room for every case. You can refer to the appropriate image prior to placing a fixation element to identify the safe corridors.
>
> CHRISTOPHER IOBST

> **THE GURU SAYS...**
>
> Because the hydroxyapatite (HA) pins are designed to bind to the bone, they can be difficult to remove. There can also be a fair amount of bone bleeding at the time of removal. For this reason, HA pin removal is best handled in the operating room. A fixator with non-HA pins could potentially be removed in the office if the patient and family was amenable to it.
>
> CHRISTOPHER IOBST

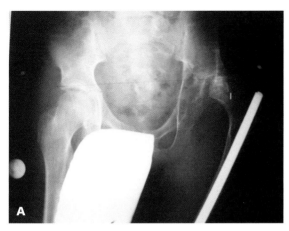
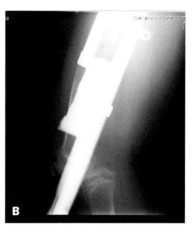
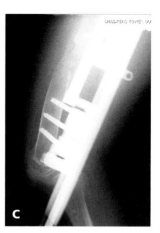

Figure 28-14 A: This child sustained a dislocated hip after a perhaps overenthusiastic femoral lengthening over an intramedullary rod in the setting of an abnormal hip. Note the severe osteopenia of the lengthened femur. **B:** After approximately 3.5 cm of lengthening, posterior subluxation of the knee was noted. Note that the lengthening apparatus may obscure the view of the knee, so extra attention to the adjacent joints is important in evaluation of radiographs.

Whether you have chosen an external fixator or an intramedullary device; to stay out of trouble, always get an X-ray 1 week after the process is begun to ensure the bone is lengthening. As lengthening progresses, stay focused on the soft tissues—this is the point at which most troubles occur. At follow-up visits, look at joint above and below for subluxation; the hip and knee are at risk (Fig. 28-14). Knee subluxation is always preceded by a loss of full extension. Make sure the joint centers line up on the lateral radiograph and haven't changed alignment compared to previous images. At the point of persistent significant lack of knee extension, stay out of trouble by stopping lengthening and even consider shortening. Surgical treatment in the form of soft tissue releases may be needed.

> **THE GURU SAYS...**
>
> Nothing is more embarrassing than to find your patient has an incomplete osteotomy preventing distraction. Spend extra time in the operating room to confirm that the osteotomy is complete. If the bone ends can translate on each other, the osteotomy must be complete.
>
> CHRISTOPHER IOBST

> **THE GURU SAYS...**
>
> Do not ignore gradually worsening range of motion by continuing to lengthen. Hoping it will go away will not work. An immediate intervention is required to prevent potentially devastating injury to the joint.
>
> CHRISTOPHER IOBST

Staying Out of Trouble With Femoral Lengthening With External Fixation

* Label direction of turning on the device, such as drawing an arrow on a piece of tape.
* Start in some valgus and expect to drift into varus with lengthening. Consider prophylactic release of iliotibial band to help minimize varus drift.
* Ensure there is good knee motion after fixator placement. By acutely flexing the knee the tensor fascia lata will release around the tethering pins (Fig. 28-15).
* Expect poor knee ROM during femoral lengthening (Fig. 28-16). Maintain knee extension.

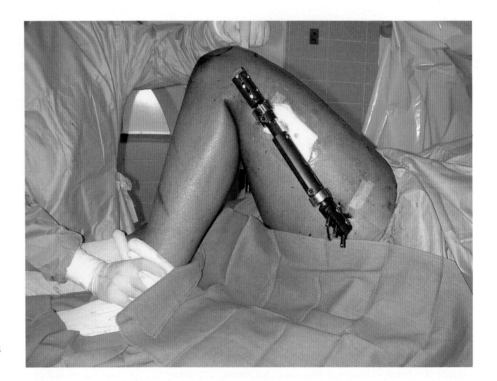

Figure 28-15 Following placement of an external fixator for femoral lengthening, the knee is taken through a full range of motion. This minimizes soft-tissue tethering of the pins, in this case probably by allowing the distal pins to split the fibers of the iliotibial band.

THE GURU SAYS...

If the tibial lengthening is being performed with a hexapod circular external fixator, add valgus and procurvatum deformity parameters to your preoperative deformity program. As the lengthening progresses, the frame will then counteract the natural tendency for the regenerate bone to bend in those directions.

To deal with the expected valgus and procurvatum that occurs during tibial lengthening with threaded rods, use hexapod rings as part of your initial frame construct. At the end of lengthening, you can swap the threaded rods for struts and gradually correct the alignment back to neutral.

CHRISTOPHER IOBST

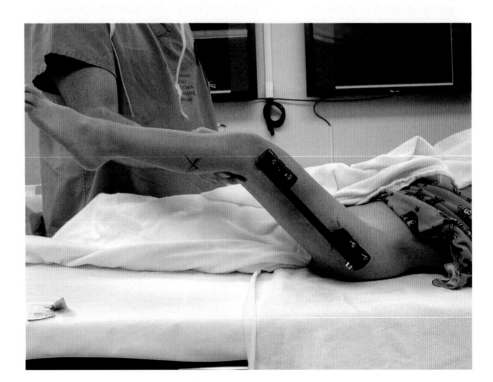

Figure 28-16 Despite physical therapy, and a modest 3-cm lengthening, the patient's maximum knee flexion is 30° even under anesthesia. With physical therapy, this patient's knee flexion returned to near normal within 6 mo.

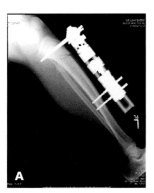 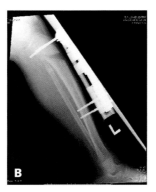 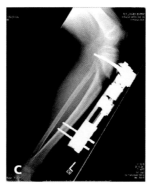

Figure 28-17 The patient is undergoing a lengthening through a normal tibia and fibula. **A:** Immediately postoperative period. Note that a fibular osteotomy was performed, but a section of the fibula was not removed. **B:** Patient 3.5 wk later. There is more opening anteriorly at the tibial osteotomy site, and the pins are beginning to bend. These two findings should make one suspect that something is wrong. The fact that the fibula osteotomy has healed was not recognized at this time. **C:** Lengthening was continued, and 40 days later, radiographs show that a separation of the proximal fibular physis has occurred. The bent pins and fibular healing were noted in this radiograph, but unfortunately the physeal separation was not appreciated. A second (and unneeded) fibula osteotomy was performed, but nothing needed to be done as the lengthening was proceeding nicely through the separated fibular physis.

Staying Out of Trouble With Tibial Lengthening With External Fixation

* Remove 1-cm section out of the fibula to avoid consolidation (Fig. 28-17).
* Use a transfixion wire or screw across ankle syndesmosis to prevent proximal migration of distal fibula.
* The tibia tends to drift into valgus and procurvatum. If this happens, consider overlengthening 1 to 1.5 cm and then manipulate the callus in the OR to a straight alignment.

The best management of pin sites is uncertain, and a strong case has been made for nothing but showering with antimicrobial soap.[14] Avoid doing harm by recommending caustic agents. A reasonable primary treatment of infected or inflamed pin sites is 10 days of an oral antibiotic (cephalexin). Expect pin site infections, and give the family a prescription for oral antibiotics, so they can fill it when needed (Figs. 28-18 and 28-19). Change the antibiotics if they are not working. Remember that periarticular pin site infections can lead to septic arthritis, and watch for this.

Neuropraxia may occur from simple stretch injury, tethering over a pin, or entrapment in soft tissue, particularly the peroneal nerve. *Immediately* stop lengthening in this scenario. It has been shown that immediate decompression of the affected nerve as soon as the injury is recognized improves recovery.[13] Do not hesitate to slow the rate of lengthening if there are soft tissue problems or poor distraction callus. Speed up lengthening if there is concern over premature consolidation of callus.

THE GURU SAYS...

Limb lengthening surgeons are "bone farmers." To cultivate the growth of healthy new bone, the biological and mechanical environments surrounding the regenerate bone need persistent vigilance and occasional manipulation. Remember, regenerate bone should be visible on the radiograph by the third week. The goal is to create a smooth column of regenerate bone that is visible stretching from one bone end to the other. Do not continue lengthening when there is no visible bone at the distraction site "black hole" on the radiograph.

CHRISTOPHER IOBST

THE GURU SAYS...

The increased soft tissue movement that occurs around periarticular half pins and wires is thought to contribute to the development of pin site infections. Try to limit the movement by keeping a dressing on these pin sites to stabilize the skin at all times.

CHRISTOPHER IOBST

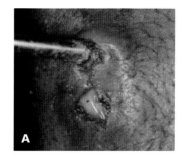

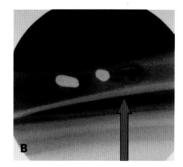

Figure 28-18 A: Pin tract infection with erythema, swelling and purulence noted at pin site. **B:** X-ray after removal of this pin demonstrates osseous changes consistent with osteomyelitis (arrow).

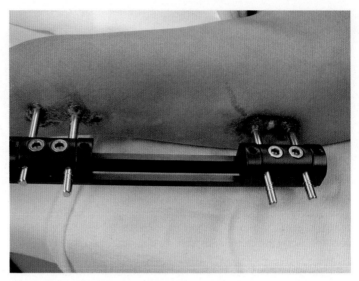

Figure 28-19 Pin sites may show local drainage and inflammatory tissue with the possibility of infection. Consider antibiotics and irrigation with whirlpool, Jacuzzi, etc.

It is better to remove the fixator 1 month too late than 1 day too early. Fracture or bending of the regenerate after removal of the device is reported as high as 10% to 15% in some series (Fig. 28-20). One method of helping to avoid this complication is to lengthen through the metaphysis when possible, as the bending strength of bone is related to the fourth power of the radius of the bone. There is unfortunately no infallible method of predicting when the device can be safely removed, though many have been studied. One criterion is that radiographs should show cortical bone and the beginning of a medullary canal of the regenerate in two planes. **ORTHOPAEDICS 101: When transitioning out of external fixation for fracture or limb lengthening, remove the device from**

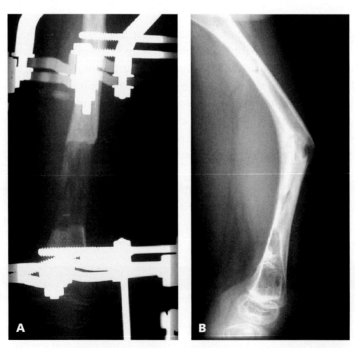

Figure 28-20 Fracture through the area of regenerate bone in a femoral lengthening and subsequent deformity.

the half pins or the spanning struts from the rings in the clinic and plan for operative half pin or ring removal a week later. **If the patient breaks the callus during that week, the device can be reapplied. (Because of the soft tissue tension from the lengthening, many of these fractures shorten and may be difficult to reduce.)** Avoid forceful manipulation of a stiff knee while the patient is under anesthesia, as this may cause significant injury to the cartilage or lead to iatrogenic physeal fracture. Following removal of the external fixator, stay out of trouble by recognizing (and sharing with the parents) that the remaining bone is weak and at risk for fracture (Fig. 28-21; see Fig. 28-18). As fracture through callus or pin-site is most likely following device removal, consider protection of the lengthened bone with a brace and/or crutches.

If the patient complains over the phone to your assistant that the device is becoming harder to turn, think:

- End of device limit for distraction
- Premature bone consolidation
- Turning the device wrong way
- Device malfunction

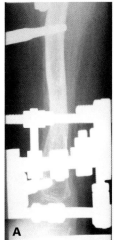
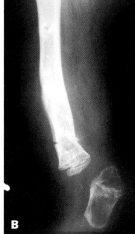
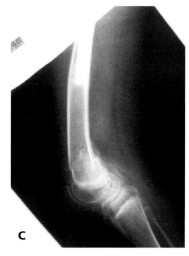

Figure 28-21 A, B: Fracture through a pin hole following device removal. **C:** Following removal of the external fixator, a distal femoral metaphyseal fracture occurred through the osteopenic bone. This is the same child seen in Figure 28-14.

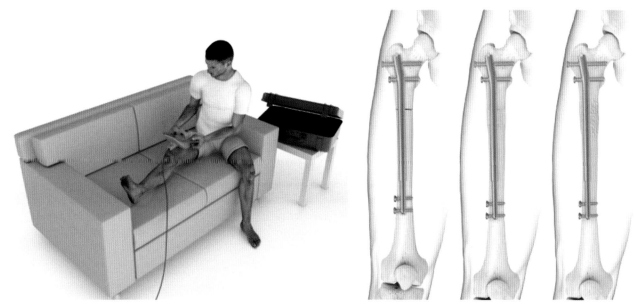

Figure 28-22 The Precice Nail (NuVasive, San Diego, CA) is lengthened using an external magnet. The patient distracts his leg three times a day for 0.33 mm. (We usually recommend 0.25 mm three or four times per day.) (Used with the permission of the University of Wisconsin Division of Pediatric Orthopaedics.)

Common Problems With Intramedullary Lengthenings

For decades, surgeons and engineers have labored to avoid the complications and problems created by transfixing wires and half pins from external fixation. Intramedullary devices have been developed in the past that require ratcheting of the limb or the use of external batteries. Current new technology uses magnetically driven intramedullary devices to lengthen long bones (Fig. 28-22). This technology is similar to that used in patients requiring growing rods in early onset scoliosis. Intramedullary nails have revolutionized limb lengthening in children, yet important pitfalls exist:

- Soft tissue contractures can still occur with intramedullary devices, and vigilance is still required to detect and treat joint contractures.
- This device is not used much in tibias of children with open growth plates. Magnetic lengthening plates may someday fill this niche.

- The diameter of the femur must be able to be reamed to at least 10 mm to accept the smallest device. (Don't forget to vent the femur as mentioned above for closed shortening.)

- When using the device in the femur of growing patients, the nail needs to go into the tip of the trochanter. **ORTHOPAEDICS 101: Whether nailing an immature femur for trauma or for limb lengthening, never use a piriformis fossa in order to avoid iatrogenic avascular necrosis (AVN).**
- It can be difficult to pass the straight portion of the rod down the tip of the trochanter without producing varus at the site of a proximal osteotomy. Blocking screws can help with this.

- The processes of lengthening and consolidation of limb lengthening still exist even though the device is hidden. Children must remain on protected weight bearing until sufficient callus is noted radiographically.

THE GURU SAYS...

To be safe, maintain touch-down weight bearing during the distraction phase and the first month of the consolidation phase when using internal lengthening nails. Then weight bearing status can be progressively advanced on a monthly basis according to the maturation of the regenerate bone.

If weight bearing is an issue, the lengthening nail can be exchanged for a trauma nail at any point once the distraction phase is completed. Weight bearing can then be advanced more aggressively with a trauma nail in place.

CHRISTOPHER IOBST

- The rod needs to be removed after a year.

THE GURU SAYS...

Because it is anticipated that the nail will be removed 9 to 12 months after insertion, you can make the removal process easier by leaving the interlocking pegs slightly proud during insertion and avoiding placement of an end cap.

CHRISTOPHER IOBST

Staying Out of Trouble With Leg Length Discrepancy

- Limb lengths must be verified by imaging and physical examination, as both methods are subject to error.
- Adequate preparation of parental and patient expectations is essential.
- Do not be greedy in lengthening; consider the middle way of combined contralateral epiphysiodesis and lengthening.
- Assess family and patient for coping abilities—get a psychologist involved before surgery if in doubt.
- Double-check radiographic measurements and calculations of final LLD before surgery—there is a high error rate in predicting final LLD.
- During lengthening focus on the soft tissues, alignment, and adjacent joints, not just radiographs of miraculous new bone.
- Golden rule: As in other aspects of life, function is more important than length.

SOURCES OF WISDOM

1. Hellsing AL. Leg length inequality: a prospective study of young men during their military service. *Ups J Med Sci.* 1988;93(3):245-253.
2. Song KM, Halliday SE, Little DG. The effect of limb-length discrepancy on gait. *J Bone Joint Surg Am.* 1997;79(11):1690-1698.
3. Ireland J, Kessel L. Hip adduction/abduction deformity and apparent leg-length inequality. *Clin Orthop Relat Res.* 1980;(153):156-157.
4. Kemnitz S, Moens P, Fabry G. Percutaneous epiphysiodesis for leg length discrepancy. *J Pediatr Orthop B.* 2003;12(1):69-71.

5. Blair VP III, Walker SJ, Sheridan JJ, et al. Epiphysiodesis: a problem of timing. *J Pediatr Orthop.* 1982;2(3):281-284.

6. Cundy P, Paterson D, Morris L, et al. Skeletal age estimation in leg length discrepancy. *J Pediatr Orthop.* 1988;8(5):513-515.

7. Moseley CF. A straight-line graph for leg-length discrepancies. *J Bone Joint Surg Am.* 1977;59(2):174-179.

8. Paley D, Bhave A, Herzenberg JE, et al. Multiplier method for predicting limb-length discrepancy. *J Bone Joint Surg Am.* 2000;82-A(10):1432-1446.

9. Sabharwal S, Paley D, Bhave A, Herzenberg JE. Growth patterns after lengthening of congenitally short lower limbs in young children. *J Pediatr Orthop.* 2000;20(2):137-145.

10. Surdam JW, Morris CD, DeWeese JD, et al. Leg length inequality and epiphysiodesis: review of 96 cases. *J Pediatr Orthop.* 2003;23(3):381-384.

11. McCarthy JJ, Burke T, McCarthy MC. Need for concomitant proximal fibular epiphysiodesis when performing a proximal tibial epiphysiodesis. *J Pediatr Orthop.* 2003;23(1):52-54.

12. Birch JG, Walsh SJ, Small JM, et al. Syme amputation for the treatment of fibular deficiency. An evaluation of long-term physical and psychological functional status. *J Bone Joint Surg Am.* 1999;81(11):1511-1518.

13. Nogueira MP, Paley D, Bhave A, et al. Nerve lesions associated with limb-lengthening. *J Bone Joint Surg Am.* 2003;85A(8):1502-1510.

14. Gordon JE, Kelly-Hahn J, Carpenter CJ, et al. Pin site care during external fixation in children: results of a nihilistic approach. *J Pediatr Orthop.* 2000;20(2):163-165.

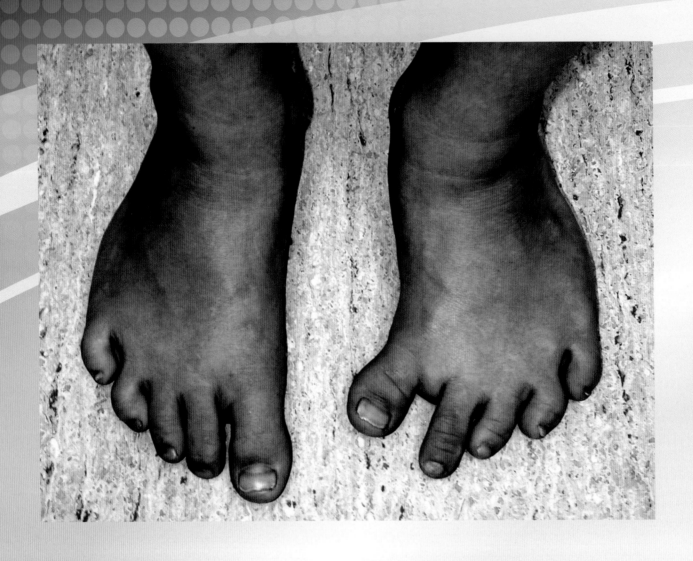

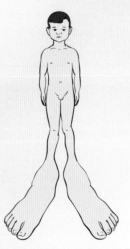

How some parents seem to see their children. (Adapted from Wenger DR, Rang M, eds. *The Art and Practice of Children's Orthopaedics.* New York, NY: Raven Press; 1993.)

Chapter 29

Foot Problems

KENNETH J. NOONAN, MD, MHCDS and VINCENT S. MOSCA, MD

Guru: Todd A. Milbrandt, MD

Clubfoot

While an entire book can be written on clubfoot, we will just stick to a limited number of pitfalls. Clubfoot is frequently part of an underlying syndrome, thus a complete history and physical examination is warranted to uncover other abnormalities. Clubfoot is also associated with tarsal coalition tibia and fibular hemimelia.[1] There is no indication for pelvis radiographs, as there is no known association between clubfoot and developmental dysplasia of the hip (DDH).[2] Regardless, all children being evaluated for musculoskeletal problems should have a careful hip examination; parents love it when you "check under the hood." Imaging of hips should be based purely on risk factors or findings suggestive of DDH.

All clubfeet will benefit from initial treatment with the Ponseti method, a series of manipulations and cast applications, which, when combined with a heel cord tenotomy, provides initial correction of the idiopathic clubfoot in up to 95% of patients.[3] Even children with syndromic clubfeet (who have a higher rate of residual deformity) will have some improvement in their deformity. Some practitioners have very good success with the Ponseti method in these feet, and they cite the need to go slow in these stiff feet and the need for many more casts than is usual in idiopathic clubfeet. In our opinion, the main pitfalls in use of the Ponseti method result from deviation from the prescribed technique as described by the originator.[4]

Ponseti Method

Pitfalls in Manipulation

▶ Hyperpronation of the first ray. The foot should be initially supinated. The foot should remain supinated throughout the casting procedure; as increased correction is obtained, the supination naturally decreases to a more normal alignment.
▶ Attempting to place the foot in a dorsiflexed position prior to correcting the hindfoot. This will block the eversion and abduction of the calcaneus underneath the talus, subsequently preventing full correction of the clubfoot. One should maintain the foot in equinus during the sessions of manipulation and casting.
▶ Errantly positioning pressure over the calcaneal cuboid joint.[5] This will block the reduction of the calcaneus underneath the talus and prevent subtalar correction. Fulcrum of pressure should be positioned over the head of the talus.

Pitfalls in Casting

▶ Casting children who are agitated. Babies are comforted with bottle-feeding during the casting procedure.[6] Low lighting in a private room (rather than in a large cast room) is also soothing.
▶ Failure to use long leg casts. Long leg cast application is always used and is integral to the success of the method. The cast must be applied in two sections. The short leg section is applied and carefully molded around the foot before extending the cast above the knee. Trying to focus simultaneously on the foot mold while keeping the knee in a fixed position risks poor foot pressure application as well as bunching up of the cast padding in the popliteal fossa.
▶ Pressure sores from the manipulation and casting in patients with spina bifida or arthrogryposis (Fig. 29-1)
▶ Placing too much or too little padding around the foot and ankle. Two or three layers of cotton roll are sufficient before application of the plaster cast
▶ Attempting to cast the foot in correction beyond that obtained by manipulation
▶ Pressure in the popliteal fossa from the proximal trim line of the short leg cast when converting to the long leg cast
▶ Overtrimming. When trimming the cast down, don't expose too much of the dorsal aspect of the foot proximal to the metatarsophalangeal joints, as this will often lead to a tourniquet effect and swelling of the toes

(Continued)

Pitfalls in Heel Cord Tenotomy

- ▶ Performing tenotomy before the heel is in valgus and foot abduction of greater than 60° is noted. This will block the eversion of the calcaneus in the subtalar joint and lead to midfoot breech and a rocker bottom deformity. *If you are a newbie, do these in the OR until comfortable.*

- ▶ Holding the ankle in excessive forced dorsiflexion prior to tenotomy will result in difficulty in palpation of the Achilles tendon.

- ▶ Injecting large amounts of lidocaine around the tendon will make palpation difficult. We put lidocaine cream on first. Do the procedures and then inject marcaine or lidocaine after tenotomy. Wait 15 minutes before applying the cast.

- ▶ Performing a tenotomy at the cutaneous heel crease (Fig. 29-2, dashed arrow) can be difficult and potentially detrimental, as you will be too distal and potentially into the substance of the Achilles tendon insertion on the calcaneus. Tenotomy needs to be approximately 1 centimeter proximal to the distal heel crease (Fig. 29-2, solid arrow).

- ▶ Incomplete tenotomy should be suspected when there is no palpable "pop" and an immediate increase in dorsiflexion of approximately 15° to 30°. The tendon should be revisited with the knife to complete the transection.

- ▶ Transection of local venous structures, and possibly the peroneal artery, has been noted.[7] When excessive bleeding occurs, simple pressure on the heel cord for an additional 3 to 4 minutes before placing in a long leg cast is usually all that is necessary.

Pitfalls in Abduction Bracing

- ▶ Noncompliant use of the abduction orthosis.[3,8] Successful use of an orthosis is associated with prevention of deformity recurrence.

- ▶ Errors in fitting of the abduction orthosis include deviation from the shoulder width positioning of the shoes and standard external rotation of the feet of 50° to 70°.

- ▶ Pressure sores can result from poor fit of the shoes. For the first week the skin should be checked at each diaper change to detect and treat potential blisters or other pressure phenomena.

Some clubfeet can develop a "complex clubfoot" pattern during the Ponseti method. When wondering if the foot you're treating is developing this pattern, think reflex sympathetic dystrophy. Besides retraction of the great toe and full plantar crease as described by Ponseti; if the foot is red, very swollen, and the child absolutely hates to have the foot touched (reflex sympathetic dystrophy–like symptoms) you are likely dealing with a complex

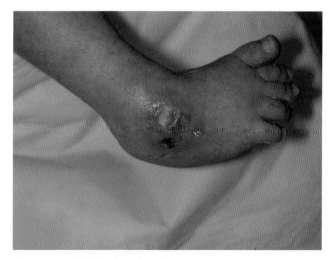

Figure 29-1 This 9-month-old girl with arthrogryposis has developed a pressure sore over her talus head from a Ponseti cast. **KEY POINT: In stiff feet go slow; in** *all* **feet don't cast the foot beyond what is obtained during manipulation.** (Used with the permission of the University of Wisconsin Division of Pediatric Orthopaedics.)

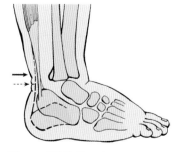

Figure 29-2 Tenotomy locations.

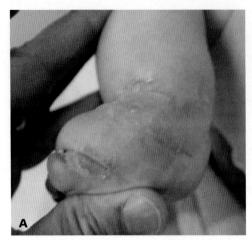 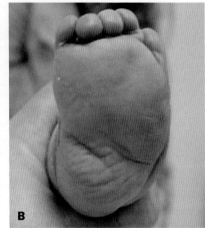

Figure 29-3 A: A complex clubfoot is diagnosed when the foot becomes swollen and red and is very irritated. **B:** The great toe is retracted and a full plantar crease is seen. (Used with the permission of the University of Wisconsin Division of Pediatric Orthopaedics.)

clubfoot pattern (Fig. 29-3). In these cases, the best thing to do is to *stop treatment*. Give the child a few weeks' break and start again; albeit more slowly. **ORTHOPAEDICS 101: Don't apply the cast beyond the degree obtained with manipulation.**

With the Ponseti method, over 98% of clubfeet will have good initial correction and will not need extensive posterior medial release. Over time, recurrent or residual deformity in clubfeet can be present in up to a third of patients. Repeat serial casting should be performed for these feet. If full deformity correction cannot be obtained, an ala carte approach to surgical correction is taken in these feet. For instance, posterior contracture can be managed with a repeat tenotomy, open Achilles lengthening, or even posterior release of the ankle joint. Dynamic forefoot supination is best managed with an anterior tibialis transfer to the lateral cuneiform.

During clubfoot surgery for residual or recurrent deformity, preservation of vascular supply should be the number one priority. Absence or a substantial reduction in the size and flow of the anterior tibial artery occurs in approximately 90% of limbs with clubfoot. Preservation of the posterior tibial artery should be a surgeon's number one priority. One should consider not fully exsanguinating the foot prior to tourniquet inflation in order to visualize the posterior tibial neurovascular bundle. Although uncommon, the posterior tibial artery may be absent in a clubfoot.[9] If the posterior tibial vascular bundle cannot be located at the time of surgery, even after the tourniquet is taken down, a hypertrophied peroneal vascular bundle may be present and should be carefully protected.

Metatarsus Adductus

It is hard to get in trouble with this condition as long as you make the right diagnosis and don't treat it. First, make certain there is normal ankle dorsiflexion; if not, it is *not* metatarsus adductus (MTA) and may be a clubfoot. Look at the hindfoot; if there is significant valgus, think of a skewfoot (Fig. 29-4). It may be difficult to differentiate between MTA and skewfoot with radiographs in infants as the navicular is not yet ossified (Fig. 29-5). MTA may also be confused with a metatarsal longitudinal epiphyseal bracket (Fig. 29-6).

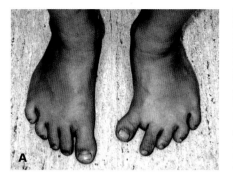 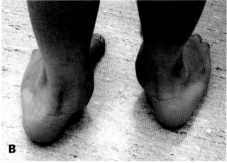

Figure 29-4 This child has bilateral foot deformities. **A:** Viewed from the top, he has bilateral metatarsus adductus in which the left is worse than the right. **B:** From behind, the child has severe hindfoot valgus. This child must have a skewfoot or variant as children with metatarsus adductus have a normal hindfoot.

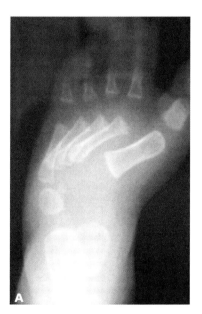 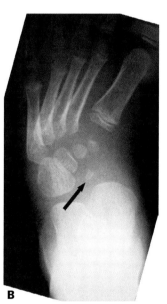

Figure 29-5 Serial radiographs of the less involved right foot from Figure 29-4 confirm that this is a classic skewfoot. The initial radiographs at presentation (**A**) are inconclusive and could be metatarsus adductus or skew foot. **B:** With time and further development, it becomes clear the navicular is laterally displaced (arrow) on the head of the talus and the forefoot is adducted on the midfoot. In combination with hind foot valgus, this is considered a skewfoot.

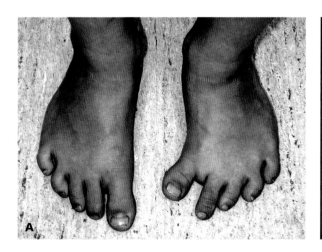 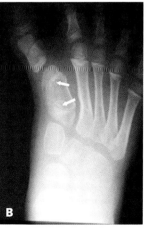

Figure 29-6 A. The presenting picture demonstrates that the left foot has severe asymmetric metatarsus adductus of the first ray. **B:** Radiograph of the left foot reveals the child has a bracket epiphysis (arrows) of the first ray. Most practitioners would recommend resection of the medial aspect of the growth plate.

In the extraordinarily unlikely event that surgery is needed for MTA, do not do a capsular release as this leads to poor results. We recommend an osteotomy of the medial cuneiform, rather than the first metatarsal, both to avoid the proximal physis of the first metatarsal, and for better correction. Lateral osteotomies may be of the second to fifth metatarsals or the cuboid.

Positional Calcaneovalgus

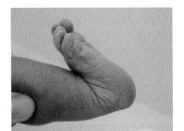

Figure 29-7 Calcaneal valgus in a newborn. It is not unusual for the dorsum of the foot to be touching the leg anterior to the tibia.

This is a very common deformity in newborns. Although the appearance of the foot may be striking and can be confused with congenital vertical talus, spontaneous correction is the rule (Fig. 29-7). Having the parents perform stretching exercises may help the babies a little, but it can help the parents *a lot* and will keep the grandparents happy that something is being done. "Apparent calcaneal valgus feet" may in fact be posterior medial bowing of the tibia, which usually corrects spontaneously but may result in a 3- to 6-cm leg length discrepancy at maturity.

Congenital Vertical Talus

Congenital vertical talus (CVT) is an uncommon foot deformity in young infants and may not be quite as obvious as some other foot deformities. CVT is characterized by a flat everted foot, which, in some respects, has the opposite appearance of a clubfoot, in which the foot is in cavus and inversion. Both deformities have Achilles tendon contractures. In the clubfoot, the equinus deformity is obvious. In CVT, the ankle doesn't appear to be in equinus because of the dorsiflexion contracture of the anterior/dorsal structures. This results in a midfoot breech with a rocker bottom and plantar prominence of the talar head (makes foot look flat). To stay out of trouble, the provider has to do three things:

1. Confirm the diagnosis of CVT in contradistinction to an oblique talus, positional calcaneovalgus, posteromedial bowing of the tibia, or is just a really flat foot (Fig. 29-8).
2. Determine whether the child with CVT has one of the associated diagnoses that are present in 50% of patients. (Consider genetics and neurology consults.)
3. Treat the CVT foot with Dobbs method of correction.

By definition, CVT is a fixed dorsal dislocation of the navicular on the head of the talus. As the navicular is not ossified until about 3 years of age, and cannot be seen on plain radiographs, we rely on the relationship of the axis of the talus and the first metatarsal. The diagnosis is confirmed on the plantar flexed lateral radiograph by observing that the axis of the talus passes plantar to that of the first metatarsal (Fig. 29-8B and C). Avoid the pitfall of believing that if the two axes become parallel,

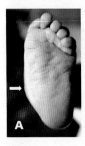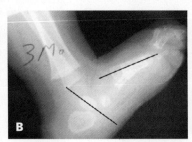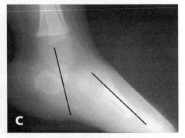

Figure 29-8 Three-month-old with vertical talus. **A:** Rocker bottom medial prominence characteristic of vertical talus. **B:** Lateral radiograph of foot is nondiagnostic. Although the axis of the talus is plantar to that of the first metatarsal, this radiograph is consistent with an oblique talus as well as vertical talus. **C:** Lateral radiograph in forced plantar-flexion confirms the diagnosis of vertical talus as the axis of the talus and first metatarsal still do not line up and the talus remains quite vertical relative to the first metatarsal.

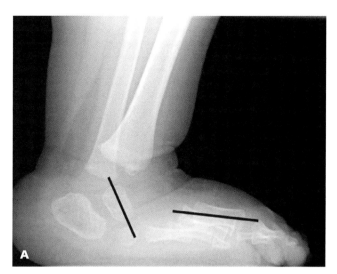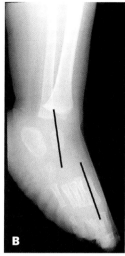

Figure 29-9 Example of a child with vertical talus (**A**) in which the axes of the talus and first metatarsal become nearly parallel in plantar flexion (**B**), but the axis of the first metatarsal is translated dorsal to that of the talus. Recall that the definition of a vertical talus is a fixed, dorsal dislocation of the navicular relative to the talus to help understand why this radiograph is consistent with a vertical talus.

there is no vertical talus. Dorsal translation of the first metatarsal axis in relation to that of the talus indicates dorsal dislocation at the talonavicular joint (Fig. 29-9). The axis of the talus remains vertically aligned with the axis of the tibia on the dorsiflexion lateral radiograph. An oblique talus is on the spectrum between flat foot and CVT; consider it a CVT without a lot of anterior contracture and without dislocation of the navicular. It is characterized by incomplete dorsiflexion of the talus in the ankle mortice, as seen on the dorsiflexion lateral view (normal is 90°) (Fig. 29-10A). There is fair alignment of the talus and first metatarsal on the plantar flexion lateral radiograph (Fig. 29-10B). The exact definition of an oblique talus is debated, but stretching and heel cord tenotomy may be effective.

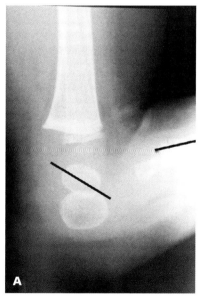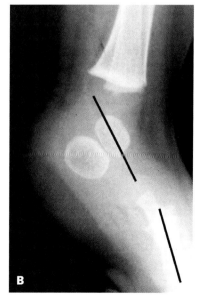

Figure 29-10 A: Child with an oblique talus. Note that this radiograph shows a quite similar relationship between the talus and first metatarsal as that seen in Figure 29-9. **B:** With plantar flexion, the axis of the talus and first metatarsal significantly change their relationship.

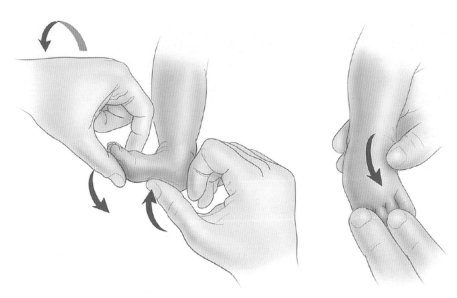

Figure 29-11 Dobbs method of manipulation in congenital vertical talus. The thumb of one hand is placed on the head of the talus for counterpressure while the other hand gently stretches the foot into plantar flexion and inversion. The heel should not be touched, so as to allow the calcaneus to slide from a valgus to a varus position under the talus. (From Dobbs MB, Purcell DB, Nunley R, Morcuende JA. Early results of a new method of treatment for idiopathic congenital vertical talus: surgical technique. *J Bone Joint Surg Am*. 2007;89(suppl 2, Pt 1):111-121.)

> **THE GURU SAYS...**
>
> During the pinning of the talonavicular joint in the operating room, at times it is necessary to open the joint to ensure reduction. Also it is important to pin the talonavicular joint before performing the Achilles tenotomy. This allows for the foot to be a lever for dorsiflexion. Burying the pin can extend the time that it is in place (up to 8 weeks casting).
>
> TODD A. MILBRANDT

Clubfeet and CVT are different in shape, and patients with CVT are also more likely to have an associated condition; yet historically, they both share a similar evolution toward nonoperative treatment. In the past, the CVT foot was treated with extensive surgical release just as clubfeet were treated with wide posterior medial release. Ponseti developed his nonoperative method of treatment for clubfoot, and it is no small coincidence that one of his protégés, Dr. Matt Dobbs, developed a similar approach for CVT. With his method, the foot is manipulated by plantar flexing and inverting the forefoot against plantar-medial pressure on the head of the talus (Fig. 29-11). Serial manipulations and long leg cast applications are carried out just as with clubfoot management. Once the anterior tibialis and long toe extensors have stretched and the talonavicular joint is aligned, the child goes to the operating room for talonavicular joint pinning and Achilles tenotomy (Fig. 29-12).

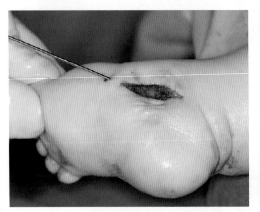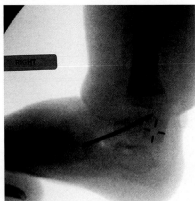

Figure 29-12 After ensuring the talonavicular joint is reduced and pinned, the Achilles tendon is lengthened. (From Dobbs MB, Purcell DB, Nunley R, Morcuende JA. Early results of a new method of treatment for idiopathic congenital vertical talus: surgical technique. *J Bone Joint Surg Am*. 2007;89(suppl 2, Pt 1):111-121.)

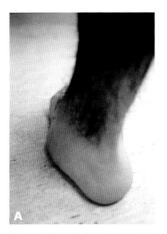
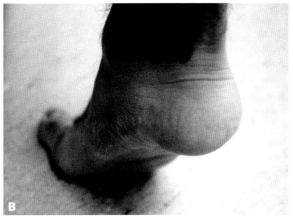

Figure 29-13 **A:** In normal weight-bearing position, this patient has a very flat foot. **B:** When standing on his toes, the arch is visible. This dynamic change with foot position defines a flexible flatfoot.

Flatfoot

Flatfoot is the normal and expected foot shape in infants. Its appearance is due in part to excessive subcutaneous fat, but also due to true valgus alignment of the bones and joints. As part of development, the longitudinal arch of the foot becomes more pronounced and the fat disappears. Flatfoot is present in 23% of adults and is usually asymptomatic.[10] The key to staying out of trouble with this condition is in recognizing that the flatfoot is one of several normal foot shapes seen in children and adults (Fig. 29-13). A predictor for symptoms and the possible need for treatment is to verify whether the hindfoot motion is rigid; stiff flatfeet tend to be more symptomatic than flexible feet. Causes of rigid flatfoot include tarsal coalition, vertical talus, neuromuscular condition, inflammatory arthritis, infection, and connective tissue disorders such as arthrogryposis (Fig. 29-14).

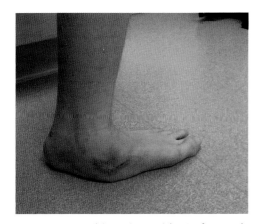
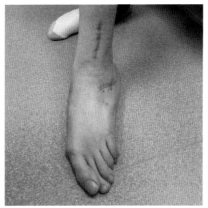

Figure 29-14 This patient with Marfan syndrome underwent lateral column lengthening with medial talonavicular plication and posterior tibialis advancement for painful flatfoot. This stunning failure in surgical execution is likely due to his intrinsic connective tissue disorder. The patient may have done better with a limited talonavicular fusion instead of medial plication. (Used with the permission of the University of Wisconsin Division of Pediatric Orthopaedics.)

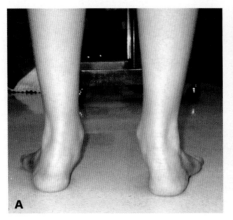 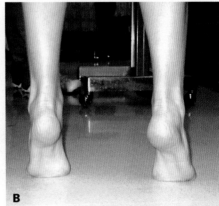

Figure 29-15 A: Patient with flatfeet and hindfoot valgus. **B:** When standing on the toes, the hindfoot goes into varus, proving the hindfoot is mobile, and the arch elevates, thus confirming a flexible flatfoot.

Rigidity can be determined by observing the child rising up to stand on the toes, as the flexible hindfoot will move from a valgus to varus position (Fig. 29-15). Hindfoot mobility can also be assessed by cupping the heel in the examiner's hand and shifting from side to side (inverting and everting) (Fig. 29-16). Although most flexible flatfeet are asymptomatic, rigidity does not predict the need for treatment as we have seen *many* rigid flatfeet that are pain free. **ORTHOPAEDICS 101: Regardless of the "form" of the foot, it's the presence of altered function (pain, sores, and difficult shoe wear) that dictates treatment.**

Once an asymptomatic, flexible flatfoot has been diagnosed, share with the parents that this is not a problem, but a normal variation. It may be helpful to share with parents that studies of both military recruits and grocery store employees who are on their feet much of the day found that flexible flatfeet are not a source of disability in adults.[10,11] It has been shown that wearing corrective shoes or inserts does not influence the course of flexible flatfoot in children.[12] Furthermore, shoe modifications during childhood have been shown to be a negative experience and associated with lower self-esteem in adult life.[13] While not prescribing "something" may get you in trouble with the parents; above all, we must not do harm to the child. Podiatrists tend to recommend rigid orthotics, which can be painful particularly in those with an Achilles tendon contracture or rigid flatfeet. Children who have undergone "elective orthotic excision" with complete relief of patient pain and parental guilt are among our most grateful families.

Dr. Skaggs Adds

After asking thousands of families the same question over two decades, only one family in my career thus far answered "no." The question is, "Did the podiatrist recommend an orthotic?" I am curious to see how long insurance companies continue to pay for these in asymptomatic flatfeet.

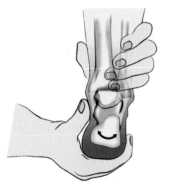

R.W.Williams

Figure 29-16 Hindfoot mobility can be assessed by cupping the heel and shifting it from side to side (inverting and everting).

Orthotics for Asymptomatic Flatfeet

Many children with *asymptomatic* flatfeet are seen by podiatrists, physical therapists, school teachers, physical education teachers, helicopter grandparents, and other experts in pediatric foot development (read: sarcasm) who recommend "special shoes" and orthotics. The family will have been exposed to several fallacies:
- Their child is doomed to a lifetime of painful crippling foot problems if this is not fixed with an $90 leather shoe that will need to be worn all the time and will have to be replaced every 6 months as they grow.
- Orthotic treatment will help the child develop an arch with growth as evidenced by the fact that when a child has an arch support in, they now have an arch. (The author is fond of explaining that shoe lifts may make him appear 6 feet tall, yet when he is barefoot he is still 5 feet 9 inches.)
- Having an arch will guarantee that their feet will be pain free for the remainder of their days as Olympic athletes.
- The pain that their child is having with their $400 new hard custom insert is good for them.

We should treat based on symptoms, and not on whether the flatfoot deformity is "flexible" or "rigid." For painful idiopathic flexible flatfoot deformities without Achilles tendon contractures, over-the-counter soft shoe inserts, available at many drug and sporting goods stores, will often relieve symptoms of diffuse foot aching. The over-the-counter orthotic is an economical start, but if it fails custom orthotics with modifications may be more effective. Often parents will arrive to clinic and say they failed "orthotic treatment from their podiatrist." It's important that families understand that all orthotics are not created equal. Similarly, all shoes are not the same. There are many types of shoes—running shoes, hiking boots, sandals, and stilettos—just because they are all shoes doesn't mean they're all equally comfortable. There is no evidence that one type of shoe over the other helps the foot develop in any way. We advise families to choose what is comfortable for the child, and easy on the pocketbook. We have found orthotics from podiatrists tend to be hard and painful; in contrast a soft accommodative over-the-counter insert may do the trick.

Painful flexible flatfeet may be associated with an accessory navicular and/or tight heel cord. An easily overlooked part of flatfoot assessment is contracture of the Achilles tendon. This can be evaluated by passively dorsiflexing the ankle with the knee in full extension and while inverting the hindfoot and holding the subtalar joint in neutral to slight varus. If, when tested in this manner, at least 10° of ankle dorsiflexion is not possible, the child may complain of pain under the medial midfoot. A painful flatfoot with a tight Achilles tendon will warrant treatment. This starts with twice-daily Achilles tendon stretching while maintaining neutral alignment of the subtalar joint and knee extension.

Consider surgery for flatfeet only as the last resort. Several core principles include:

1. It is essential that foot radiographs are taken with the child bearing weight (Fig. 29-17), and be aware that many of the radiographs patients bring with them will not be.

2. Long-term studies demonstrate that fusions within the foot lead to degenerative changes at adjacent joints. Fusions, and in particular triple arthrodesis,

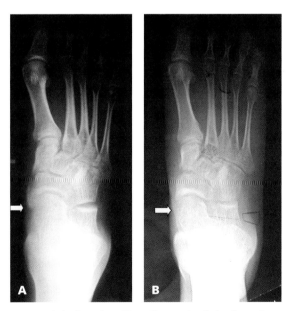

Figure 29-17 A: Non–weight-bearing AP radiograph of the foot demonstrates reasonable alignment of the talonavicular joint (arrow). **B:** Weight-bearing view of the same child's foot taken moments later demonstrates medial subluxation of the talar head relative to the navicular (arrow).

should be avoided if possible, and used only as a last resort.[14-16] Extra-articular osteotomies and soft tissue plications and lengthenings should adequately manage the majority of painful flatfoot deformities in children. The calcaneal lengthening osteotomy, with associated procedures, has been reported to achieve good pain relief and restored function while preserving subtalar motion.[17] One should consider selective fusions (talonavicular) in those patients with connective tissue and spastic disorders (see Fig. 29-14).

3. Subtalar arthroereisis with synthetic or metal implants has been used frequently by podiatrists. We have seen disasters, primarily related to the creation or enhancement of pain. We recommend staying away from these implants until they have been shown to be equal in safety and efficacy to the calcaneal lengthening osteotomy.

4. Keep in mind that compensatory forefoot supination has developed in flatfeet to balance out the extreme hindfoot valgus. Thus, surgery to correct the hind foot, such as a calcaneal lengthening or slide, may uncover a supinated forefoot that needs to be treated concurrently with a midfoot osteotomy.

Surgical options for the painful flat foot without accessory navicular or tarsal coalition include calcaneal sliding osteotomies and calcaneal lengthening osteotomy.

Staying Out of Trouble With Calcaneal Lengthening Osteotomy

✳ With distraction of the calcaneal fragments, the cuboid may subluxate dorsally and result in incomplete deformity correction. This can be prevented by inserting a 2-mm smooth Steinmann pin in a retrograde direction from the dorsum of the forefoot, through the cuboid, and across the center of the calcaneocuboid joint (with the foot held in the flatfoot position) after creating the osteotomy but before distracting it. The wire is then advanced through the graft and into the posterior calcaneal fragment.

✳ The peroneus brevis must be lengthened and the aponeurosis of the abductor digiti minimi released in order to enable full and untethered distraction of the calcaneal fragments.

✳ The peroneus longus must not be lengthened, as this is a muscle that pronates the supinated forefoot.

✳ Plication of the redundant talonavicular joint capsule and the tibialis posterior tendon is recommended to create soft-tissue balance of the hindfoot.

✳ Be wary of wound complications over the sinus tarsi. This area has thin skin to begin with and you are stretching it over an allograft. Careful skin handling technique is recommended.

✳ If the calcaneal osteotomy doesn't open adequately, think of four things:
  ✳ Plantar periosteum or long plantar ligament, not the plantar fascia, is tethering. Cut with a scalpel or scissors.
  ✳ Dorsal talonavicular capsule is incompletely released.
  ✳ Medial or plantar calcaneal cortex is still intact. Plantar—easy to get into bone during subperiosteal elevation—consider using an osteotome with a joker elevator protecting the soft tissues.
  ✳ Steinmann pin joy sticks in the proximal and distal calcaneal fragments may be in the talus.

✳ Don't crush the calcaneus with the laminar spreader or the graft.

✳ A tendoachilles lengthening or a gastrocnemius recession will be needed in essentially all cases.

Tarsal Coalitions

Tarsal coalitions are a common cause of foot pain in older children and adolescents and also may be a cause for a history of frequent ankle sprains. The diagnosis of a tarsal coalition should be strongly suspected from the physical examination, based on decreased subtalar joint motion and inability to voluntarily or passively invert the hindfoot (see Fig. 29-16). Many children with a tarsal coalition present with rigid heel valgus and tightness of the peroneal tendons (Fig. 29-18).

Standard AP and lateral radiographs may not always clearly demonstrate tarsal coalitions, but they do provide lots of clues. Oblique views are usually diagnostic of a calcaneonavicular coalition (Fig. 29-19). A talocalcaneal coalition may be seen on a Harris view if you are lucky enough to get a perfect shot, but is most reliably seen on a CT scan. A series of 48 patients found the C-sign of Lateur on the lateral radiograph to be present in all patients with flatfeet, but present in only 40% of those with tarsal coalitions[18] (Fig. 29-20), *so an absence of the C-sign does not rule out a tarsal coalition.* A dorsal spur off the head of the talus is not a degenerative condition but a result of talonavicular capsule traction from excessive motion at this joint (Fig. 29-21). This sign is suggestive for a subtalar coalition and a CT scan should be considered. A CT scan should also be considered for all feet in which a calcaneonavicular coalition has been identified on plain radiographs because of the possibility of a coincidental talocalcaneal coalition in the same foot. A second coalition was identified in 20% of patients undergoing CT scans for tarsal coalition at the Texas Scottish Rite Hospital, though this population from a tertiary pediatric center may be skewed toward more severe cases.[19]

One common clinical scenario is the older child with lateral sinus tarsi pain and decreased hindfoot motion. If the plain X-rays and CT scan do not show any sign of a bony coalition, we routinely order an MRI looking for a thickened

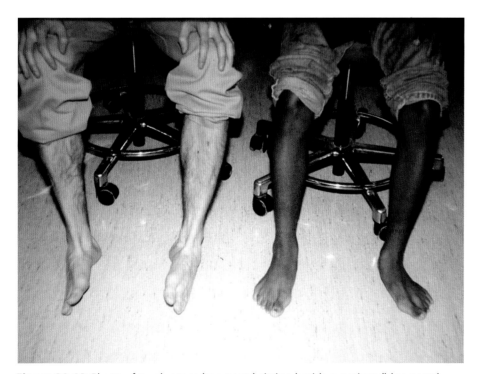

Figure 29-18 Photo of a volunteer (tan pants) sitting beside a patient (blue pants) with frequent recurrent ankle sprains. Both are trying to invert their feet, but the patient cannot do due to bilateral tarsal coalitions.

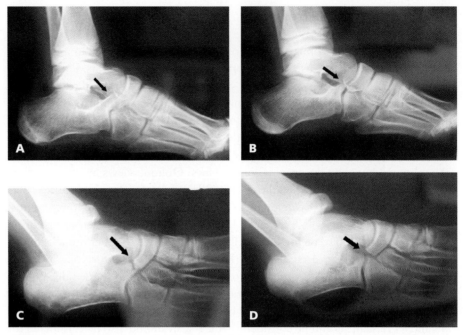

Figure 29-19 **A:** On a lateral radiograph of the foot, a calcaneonavicular coalition is difficult to identify conclusively. The arrow points to an elongated anterior process of the calcaneus ("anteater" sign), which is suggestive of a calcaneonavicular coalition. **B:** The contralateral normal foot for comparison. **C:** An oblique view clearly demonstrates the calcaneonavicular coalition or bar (arrow). **D:** The contralateral normal foot for comparison demonstrates no coalition (arrow).

fibrous calcaneal-navicular band. If there is T2 edema at the anterior process of the calcaneus or at the navicular (Fig. 29-22), one could hypothesize this to be the pain generator.

Most children and adults with tarsal coalitions are asymptomatic, so another pitfall is in treating something that doesn't need treatment. Pain onset is usually between ages 8 and 16 years in those who become symptomatic. The exact sites and sources of pain in tarsal coalitions are not well established. A few weeks of immobilization in a cast or walking boot may get a child through a symptomatic

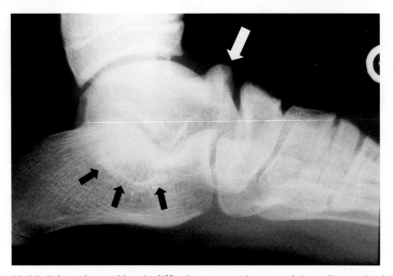

Figure 29-20 Talar calcaneal bar is difficult to appreciate on plain radiographs; however, talar beaking (white arrow) and the C-sign (black arrows) suggest this coalition may be present.

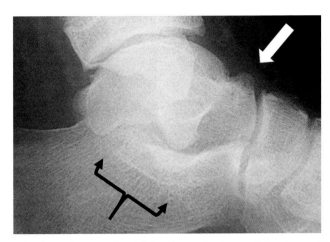

Figure 29-21 This lateral X-ray of a child with a subtalar coalition has a faint C-sign (bracket) and a traction spur off of the talus head (arrow). It is presumed that decreased subtalar motion leads to compensatory increases motion at the Chopart joints. (Used with the permission of the University of Wisconsin Division of Pediatric Orthopaedics.)

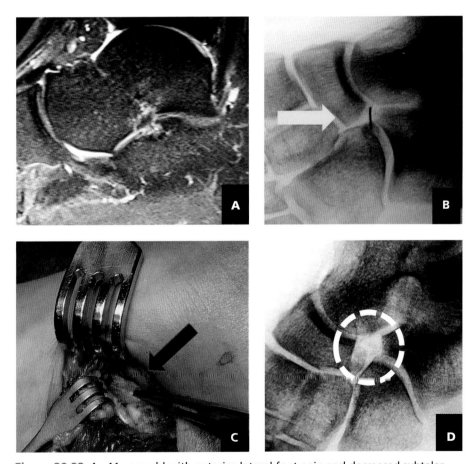

Figure 29-22 An 11-year-old with anterior lateral foot pain and decreased subtalar motion undergoes an MRI. **A:** MRI demonstrates a thickened band with questionable edema on T2 sequencing. **B:** An injection (arrow) of the calcaneal navicular articulation with marcaine relieved her pain. **C:** Surgical exposure demonstrates a thickened band (arrow). **D:** Intraoperative fluoroscopic image demonstrates complete resection (circle). (Used with the permission of the University of Wisconsin Division of Pediatric Orthopaedics.)

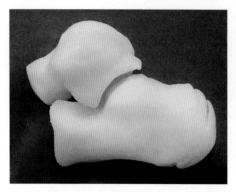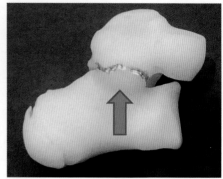

Figure 29-23 CT scan images of an older child with subtalar coalition can be used for 3D printing of the hindfoot, which can be used intraoperatively to help localize the coalition. The blue arrow demonstrates the coalition. (Used with the permission of the University of Wisconsin Division of Pediatric Orthopaedics.)

period, and save the child from surgery. Unfortunately, it is our experience that in most children who present with painful tarsal coalitions, pain will return after immobilization, and surgery is likely. In cases of fibrous calcaneal navicular coalitions, one could consider a diagnostic injection with Marcaine to confirm the cause of the pain.

The standard surgical treatment for coalition is resection of the bridging osteocartilaginous or fibrous tissue. The EDB tendon and muscle were once used as interposition material but have been abandoned by most surgeons due to their small volume, which does not fill the cavity, and the uncosmetic appearance that results over the resection site. Subtalar coalitions are particularly difficult to resect, as it can be difficult to find the proper extent and plane of bony coalition. Finding the joint anterior and posterior to the coalition can help. We have had 3D printed foot models available in the operating room to use for comparison (Fig. 29-23). Use of intraoperative CT can confirm that the resection is complete and in some centers this can be paired with intraoperative navigation (Fig. 29-24). Calcaneal navicular coalitions are slightly easier to resect, but try to avoid the pitfalls of injury to the talonavicular and calcaneal cuboid joint. In patients with very large coalitions, pain may actually be a result of hindfoot malalignment; some authors recommend calcaneal sliding or lengthening osteotomies in these cases.

At the time of surgery, be aware of how many coalitions exist in the foot and have a plan for your approach to each. Recurrent discomfort occurs at times due

THE GURU SAYS...

The most common coalition that is treated is the calcaneal navicular coalition. Resection of this coalition requires a large segment of bone to be removed. This can be a deep dark hole. The common mistake is to make an inadequate resection on the plantar surface of the coalition. This will lead to early recurrence and pain. Interposition material can be fat from the buttock, or the medial knee.

TODD A. MILBRANDT

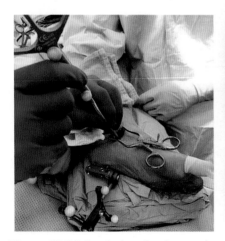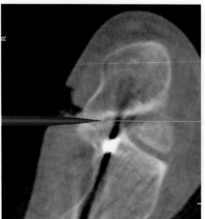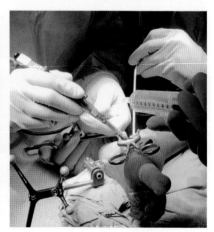

Figure 29-24 Surgical navigation can be used intraoperatively for removal of a subtalar coalition. (Used with the permission of the University of Wisconsin Division of Pediatric Orthopaedics.)

to inadequate resection, particularly of the talocalcaneal coalitions. Make certain that adequate bone is removed at the primary surgery so that normal cartilage and joint is seen at the periphery of the resection, and full inversion of the heel does not cause impingement at the region of resection. Last, but not least, as with any operation to treat pain in the feet, make the patient and family aware that pain relief cannot be guaranteed.

Cavus Foot Deformities

While flatfeet can be considered a normal foot variant, high arches are rarely present at birth. Progressive elevation of the arch or arches should cause one to wonder whether an underlying disorder is present. An underlying neuromuscular diagnosis is suspected until proven otherwise. It has been reported that two-thirds of patients with painful and progressive arch elevation have an underlying neurologic problem that turns out to be Charcot-Marie-Tooth about 50% of the time.[20] If there are bilateral cavus feet, think of neuromuscular disease. A unilateral cavus foot should elicit a Pavlovian response and cause one to reach for the spine MRI order form. These patients should have a total spinal cord MRI to rule out structural abnormalities. Note that progressive cavus deformities in CMT are never symmetric in onset. One foot always leads the other.

As a spine examination is not complete without inspection of the feet, examination of a child with a cavus foot is not complete without inspection of the spine. If the underlying neuromuscular problem is treatable such as a tethered cord, get on with it before treating the foot. Treatment for progressive cavus deformity with pain and instability is surgical. Make certain the parents understand that the foot deformity is not the problem, but is the result of the problem. It is possible that future surgery will be needed, as the underlying disease progresses in many cases.

Once an underlying diagnosis is made, the management of the flexible cavus foot in the young child can include orthotic treatment. Surgical treatment is *indicated* once the patient has pain under the metatarsal heads or along the lateral border of the foot, ankle instability exists, or there is stiff/rigid forefoot pronation or hindfoot varus. It is beyond the scope of this chapter to discuss the nuances of cavus foot reconstruction, as these are complicated procedures with multiple decision points. There are several surgical considerations: Which tissues need to be released and which tendons need to be transferred? Which bones need to be osteotomized? In bilateral cases should you do both feet at once? Do you perform the surgery in stages? What about clawed toes? The surgical options for the different deformities are shown in Table 29-1; what is chosen depends on the baseline disease, the age of the patient, the degree of the deformity, and the experience of the surgeon.

Accessory Bones

Accessory bones of the foot are often discovered on radiographs for minor trauma and are mistaken for fractures. Remember that more than 20% of children have at least one accessory bone that can be seen on radiographs.[21]

ACCESSORY NAVICULAR

Many think that nearly all children and adolescents who have a symptomatic accessory navicular become asymptomatic when they reach skeletal maturity, suggesting that surgery should be delayed and used only as a last resort. Use of a

TABLE 29-1 Surgical Options to Consider for Foot Problems

For cavus
Plantar fascia release
Peroneus longus to brevis transfer
First cuneiform osteotomy
First metatarsal osteotomy
Naviculectomy +/– cuboid osteotomy
Japas midfoot osteotomy

For varus
Posterior tibialis lengthening
Posterior tibialis transfer
Anterior tibialis transfer
Calcaneal osteotomy

For claw toes
EHL transfer to first metatarsal with:
  Extensor hallicus brevis to EHL transfer *or*
  Great toe IP arthrodesis
Long toe flexor release
DeVries resection arthroplasty of IP joint

EHL, extensor hallicus longus; IP, interphalangeal

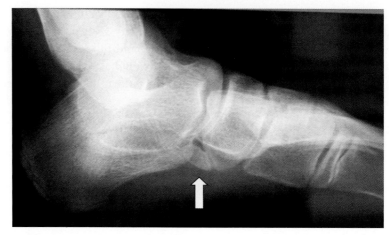

Figure 29-25 Accessory navicular (arrow).

medial longitudinal arch support may exacerbate the symptoms by adding more pressure to the region, whereas a UCBL (University of California Biomechanics Laboratory) shoe insert may unweight the painful area by bringing the heel into varus and elevating the arch of the foot. Surgical excision of the accessory navicular without rerouting of the posterior tibial tendon has been reported to have good results.[22] Any surgery in a painful weight-bearing region of the foot is prone to continued discomfort, however (Fig. 29-25). Stay out of trouble by using absorbable suture and avoid suture anchors, which can become prominent. *Keep it simple.* Results of excision in adolescent patients in whom the accessory navicular has just fused can be poor. Careful evaluation for other causes of foot pain is warranted.

OS TRIGONUM

Os trigonum is a normal variant present in 13% of children, where the flexor hallucis longus passes in the groove along the posterior talus. The trouble with this accessory bone is that it can fracture and cause pain or become symptomatic in ballet dancers and other athletes due to prolonged weight bearing in equinus. A fractured os trigonum may have a rough or sharp border along the talus, in contrast to an unfused os trigonum with a smooth border (Fig. 29-26). The difficulty

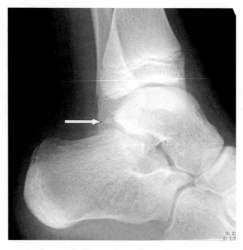

Figure 29-26 Os trigonum (arrow). Note that the edges are smooth, suggesting that this is not a fracture.

for practitioners is to determine whether the os trigonum is the pain generator. Pain in the posterior part of the ankle with extreme plantar flexion is a good clue. An MRI that reveals increase signal on T2 sequences is another predictor. Finally, a selective diagnostic injection under ultrasound with Marcaine at the site of edema is a good predictor of results from surgical excision. Very slick surgeons can remove these with an arthroscope, but we prefer a small open approach. Use of a fluoroscopy can help identify the level of the incision.

APOPHYSIS AT BASE OF FIFTH METATARSAL

Although not really an accessory bone, the apophysis at the base of the fifth metatarsal where the peroneus brevis attaches is often confused with a fracture by the unknowing (Fig. 29-27).

Köhler Disease

This condition is no trouble as long as you recognize it and do not confuse it with infection, fracture, or something more serious. Do not treat if there are no symptoms, but immobilization for a few weeks in a cast should help relieve discomfort. Multiple ossification centers of the navicular are a normal finding yet may be confused with Köhler disease (Fig. 29-28).

Bunions (Juvenile Hallux Valgus)

Many series report a higher recurrence rate following bunion surgery in adolescents than in adults. Stay out of trouble by delaying surgery until skeletal maturity, if possible. If surgery is needed, an opening-wedge osteotomy of the medial cuneiform is a particularly good choice if the metatarsal-cuneiform joint is medially deviated, the metatarsal (MT) growth plate is open, and the first metatarsal is shorter than the second. Assess the distal metatarsal articular angle (DMAA) and the congruity of the first metatarsal phalangeal (MTP) joint. Concurrently perform a medially based closing wedge osteotomy of the distal end of the first MT if the DMAA is high and the joint is congruous (Fig. 29-29). Do *not* release the soft tissues on the lateral aspect of the first MTP joint in this situation or risk avascular necrosis (AVN) of the MT head. If the DMAA is normal and the joint is laterally subluxated, release the lateral joint soft tissues and do not perform a distal metatarsal osteotomy.

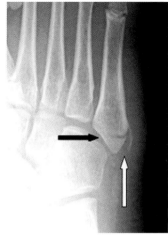

Figure 29-27 AP radiograph of a child's foot demonstrating the normal apophysis of the fifth metatarsal where the peroneus brevis tendon attaches (white arrow), which is more or less parallel to the long axis of the metatarsal. This normal apophysis is not to be confused with a fracture of the proximal fifth metatarsal (black arrow), which tends to occur perpendicular to the long axis of the metatarsal.

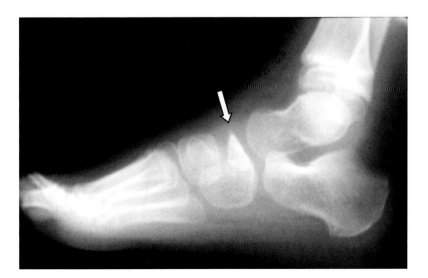

Figure 29-28 Lateral view of a child with foot pain demonstrates Köhler disease. Arrow points to collapsed, avascular navicular.

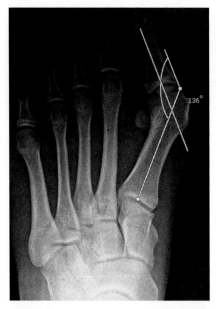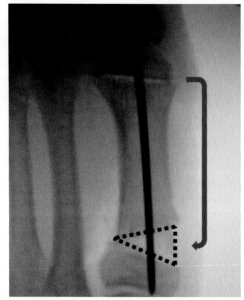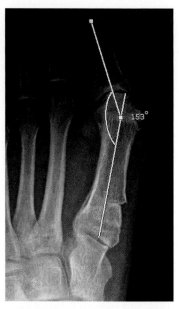

Figure 29-29 Adolescent bunion correction should be recommended with great restraint and with trepidation. It is best managed with bilevel osteotomy of the first metatarsal. (Used with the permission of the University of Wisconsin Division of Pediatric Orthopaedics.)

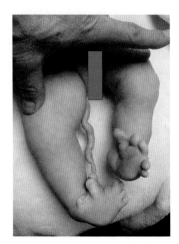

Figure 29-30 A 9-month-old girl with left tibial hemimelia and bilateral polydactyly. The extra toes are the least of her challenges. (Used with the permission of the University of Wisconsin Division of Pediatric Orthopaedics.)

Polydactyly

Polydactyly is common and usually an isolated finding, although it can be associated with Ellis-Van-Creveld syndrome, Down syndrome, and tibial hemimelia (Fig. 29-30). Thus, you should be on the lookout for underlying disorders when encountering polydactyly. Look carefully at the radiographic shadow of the first MT in cases of duplication of the hallux, because of the common association of longitudinal (Fig. 29-31) epiphyseal bracket. Without resection of the central portion of this abnormal C-shaped growth plate, the first MT will be short and result in long-term disability.

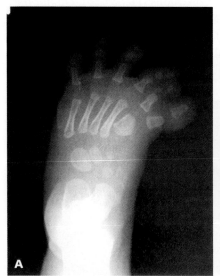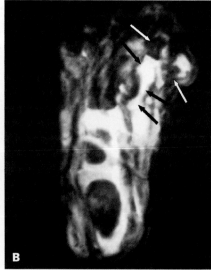

Figure 29-31 A: AP radiograph of a foot with preaxial duplication in a 1-month-old child. The abnormally shaped first MT is characteristic of a longitudinal epiphyseal bracket. **B:** An MRI at age 7 mo demonstrates the cartilage (black arrows) wrapping around the first MT, confirming the diagnosis of a longitudinal epiphyseal bracket. The proximal phalange of each of the two great toes is shown by white arrows.

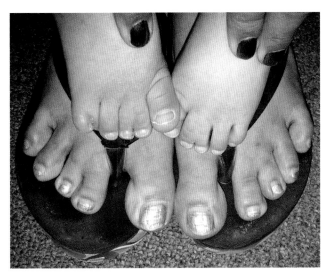

Figure 29-32 Mother and daughter with syndactyly between the second and third toes. Can't blame dad for this one. (Used with the permission of the University of Wisconsin Division of Pediatric Orthopaedics.)

In contrast, absent toes may signify an underlying longitudinal deficiency, most commonly fibular hemimelia, and may be associated with other conditions such as a leg length discrepancy, ball and socket ankle, or absent ACL.

Syndactyly

Syndactyly of the toes is rarely symptomatic and can be made much worse with surgery. Syndactyly between the second and third toes is extremely common, frequently bilateral, often hereditary (Fig. 29-32), and essentially never a cause of pain or disability. Make the parents take their shoes off, as they may have a very shallow syndactyly that they never noticed. Excessive scarring and unhappiness with cosmetic appearance are not uncommon following surgical separation. But don't worry, plastic surgeons don't read this book, so you may refer patients who demand surgery to them.

Congenital Curly Toes

Curly toes are a common concern for parents and they often ask why the second toe is overlapping the third and can the second toe be fixed? It usually takes a moment to educate the family that the cause of the deformity is a tight toe flexor to the third toe which gives the second toe room to wander laterally. One pitfall is failing to recognize that the long toe flexors to digits 4 and 5 may also be tight. Treatment is not needed unless there is pain, skin maceration, calluses, or difficulty with shoeing. If treatment is indicated, tenotomy of the long tendon of that toe is usually curative.

Congenital Overriding Fifth Toe

Overriding fifth toe is another lesser toe deformity that can be irritating in about 50% of patients. This is a not just a tight extensor tendon. It is a dorsomedial translation of the toe that would require long toe extensor lengthening, V-Y capsulotomy and pinning of the MTP joint once reduced. Although the Butler procedure has been shown to effectively correct the deformity, the procedure is associated with risk to the vascularity of the toe.

Staying Out of Trouble With Foot Problems

* Focus on function and not appearance. It's hard to make an asymptomatic patient better with surgery designed to make the foot look different.

* Perform fusions of the foot only as an absolute last resort.

* Foot deformities are often a reflection of underlying neuromuscular conditions, especially in cavus deformities.
    * For a cavus foot, look for an underlying neurologic condition.
    * For a vertical talus, look for an underlying neurologic condition or syndrome.

Run from surgical correction for the juvenile bunion, syndactyly, congenital overriding 5th toe.

* Flatfoot is a normal variant. An asymptomatic, isolated flatfoot does not require treatment.

* For the Ponseti clubfoot method, long leg casts are essential, and results are dependent on parental follow-through with bracing.

With the Ponseti Method make sure parents understand that their compliance for bracing is critical to maintain correction.

SOURCES OF WISDOM

1. Caskey PM, Lester EL. Association of fibular hemimelia and clubfoot. *J Pediatr Orthop.* 2002;22(4):522-525.
2. Westberry DE, Davids JR, Pugh LI. Clubfoot and developmental dysplasia of the hip: value of screening hip radiographs in children with clubfoot. *J Pediatr Orthop.* 2003;23(4):503-507.
3. Morcuende JA, Dolan LA, Dietz FR, et al. Radial reduction in the rate of extensive corrective surgery for clubfoot using the Ponseti method. *Pediatrics.* 2004;113(2):376-380.
4. Ponseti IV. *Congenital Clubfoot: Fundamentals of Treatment.* Oxford: Oxford University Press; 1996.
5. Kite JH. Principles involved in the treatment of congenital club-foot. *J Bone Joint Surg Am.* 1939;21:595-606.
6. Milbrandt T, Kryscio R, Muchow R, et al. Oral sucrose for pain relief during clubfoot casting: a double-blinded randomized controlled trial. *J Pediatr Orthop.* 2018;38(8):430-435.
7. Dobbs MB, Gordon JE, Walton T, et al. Bleeding complications following percutaneous tendoachilles tenotomy in the treatment of clubfoot deformity. *J Pediatr Orthop.* 2004;24(4):353-357.
8. Dobbs MB, Rudzki JR, Purcell DB, et al. Factors predictive of outcome after use of the Ponseti method for the treatment of idiopathic clubfeet. *J Bone Joint Surg Am.* 2004;86A(1):22-27.
9. Dobbs MB, Gordon JE, Schoenecker PL. Absent posterior tibial artery associated with idiopathic clubfoot: a report of two cases. *J Bone Joint Surg Am.* 2004;86(3):599-602.
10. Harris R, Beath T. *Army Foot Survey: An Investigation of Foot Ailments in Canadian Soldiers.* Ottawa, ON: National Research Council of Canada; 1947.
11. Hogan MT, Staheli LT. Arch height and lower limb pain: an adult civilian study. *Foot Ankle Int.* 2002;23(1):43-47.
12. Wenger DR, Mauldin D, Speck G, et al. Corrective shoes and inserts as treatment for flexible flatfoot in infants and children. *J Bone Joint Surg Am.* 1989;71(6):800-810.
13. Driano AN, Staheli LT. Psychosocial development and corrective shoewear use in childhood. *J Pediatr Orthop.* 1998;18(3):346-349.
14. Seymour N. The late results of naviculo-cuneiform fusion. *J Bone Joint Surg Br.* 1967;49(3):558-559.
15. Angus PD, Cowell HR. Triple arthrodesis: a critical long-term review. *J Bone Joint Surg Br.* 1986;68(2):260-265.
16. Tenuta J, Shelton YA, Miller F. Long-term follow-up of triple arthrodesis in patients with cerebral palsy. *J Pediatr Orthop.* 1993;13(6):713-716.
17. Mosca VS. Calcaneal lengthening for valgus deformity of the hindfoot: results in children who had severe, symptomatic flatfoot and skewfoot. *J Bone Joint Surg Am.* 1995;77(4):500-512.
18. Brown RR, Rosenberg ZS, Thornhill BA. The C sign: more specific for flatfoot deformity than subtalar coalition. *Skeletal Radiol.* 2001;30(2):84-87.
19. Clarke PM. Multiple tarsal coalitions in the same foot. *J Pediatr Orthop.* 1997;17(6):777-780.

20. Brewerton D, Sandifer P, Sweetnam DR. "Idiopathic" pes cavus: an investigation into its aetiology. *Br Med J.* 1963;2:659-661.
21. Shands A. The accessory bones of the foot. *South Med Surg.* 1931;9:326.
22. Bennett GL, Weiner DS, Leighley B. Surgical treatment of symptomatic accessory tarsal navicular. *J Pediatr Orthop.* 1990;10(4):445-449.

FOR FURTHER ENLIGHTENMENT

Katz DA, Albanese EL, Levinsohn EM, et al. Pulsed color-flow Doppler analysis of arterial deficiency in idiopathic clubfoot. *J Pediatr Orthop.* 2003;23(1):84-87.

Kuo KN, Jansen LD. Rotatory dorsal subluxation of the navicular: a complication of clubfoot surgery. *J Pediatr Orthop.* 1998;18(6):770-774.

Mosca VS. The cavus foot. *J Pediatr Orthop.* 2001;21(4):423-424.

Mosca VS. The child's foot: principles of management. *J Pediatr Orthop.* 1998;18(3):281-282.

Rogers JG, Geho WB. Fibrodysplasia ossificans progressiva: a survey of forty-two cases. *J Bone Joint Surg Am.* 1979;61(6A):909-914.

Spero CR, Simon GS, Tornetta P III. Clubfeet and tarsal coalition. *J Pediatr Orthop.* 1994;14(3):372-376.

Stevens PM, Otis S. Ankle valgus and clubfeet. *J Pediatr Orthop.* 1999;19(4):515-517.

Yang JS, Dobbs MB. Treatment of congenital vertical talus: comparison of minimally invasive and extensive soft-tissue release procedures at minimum five-year follow-up. *J Bone Joint Surg Am.* 2015;97(16):1354-1365.

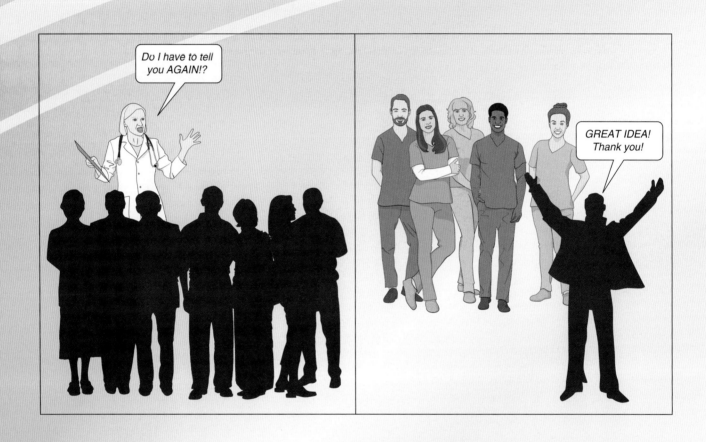

PRACTICE MANAGEMENT

Chapter 30

Leading Your Team

**DAVID L. SKAGGS, MD, MMM, JOHN M. (JACK) FLYNN, MD,
MININDER S. KOCHER, MD, MPH,
KENNETH J. NOONAN, MD, MHCDS, and
MICHAEL G. VITALE, MD, MPH**

Guru: Paul S. Viviano

Compared with the average person, you are probably already an expert in most of the topics of this book, except this one. This chapter may be one of the best opportunities to improve yourself and help your patients. Leading a team is a completely different skill than getting good grades, getting into medical school, or matching into a competitive residency. Self-discipline, intelligence, and drive got you this far, but those qualities alone will not result in optimal patient care. We have all seen extraordinarily talented surgeons get in their own way and fail. Many more surgeons fail, or get into trouble, because of interpersonal skills, not surgical skill or knowledge.

Surgeons freshly out of fellowship or residency have put in their 10 000 hours of medical training but have probably had very little training to lead a team. From their first day on the job, they are then expected to lead teams in the operating room, clinic, and office. A freshly minted surgeon tends to focus on being exceptional in the operating room and may fail to appreciate that their citizenship and the ability to work within a team will be the metric that their new colleagues and coworkers will use to judge them (Fig. 30-1). The stakes are high, and it is easy for a new surgeon to get a reputation as being a jerk. This chapter is aimed at the newly trained surgeon, but some pearls should be found by experienced leaders as well.

Words of Caution for the Truly New Attending

Building your team, like building your practice, takes time and effort. Avoid the pitfall of expecting your team to be like that of your fellowship director's right from the start. If you are lucky, a nurse or scrub technician who regularly works with your senior partner will volunteer for "junior duty" to take you under their wing. One should be extremely cognizant and appreciative of this gift and ask that person for feedback on how you and your team can improve. It is likely your team will likely include members who are less experienced or less motivated than the best teams. Your team will have no way of knowing your preferences unless you tell them. This is probably best done in writing so that they are both tangible and can be shared with others as there is often more turnover on less established teams. A weekly email to your team regarding your plan for the cases and your anticipated equipment needs is a good start. It is also a good opportunity to share successes such as a preop and postop radiograph of a case that went well. Assume good intentions from your team until proven otherwise.

Although we have arguably the best job on the planet, it can be quite stressful or frustrating at times. Even in your first year of practice when you are dealing with complications, it is unacceptable for you to take your stress out on the team. In order to avoid doing so you need to allow yourself time and opportunity to decompress. You don't want your entire team going on the emotional roller coaster that the first few years of practice often entail.

—*Dr. Lindsay Andras*
Attending Surgeon, Children's Hospital Los Angeles, 7 years into practice

---

Emotional intelligence (EQ) has been shown to be twice as important for effective leadership as IQ and technical skill combined. EQ comprises traits within the domains of self-awareness (e.g., self-confidence, emotional self-awareness), social awareness (e.g., empathy and organizational awareness), self-management (e.g., self-control, adaptability), and relationship management (e.g., influence, conflict management, teamwork, leadership).[1] The good news is that, unlike IQ, EQ can improve over one's life. In order to improve EQ, one has to *want* to improve it. One must have a genuine desire to be more empathetic to others, as well as more self-aware and open to change. While EQ may seem a little soft, it has been shown

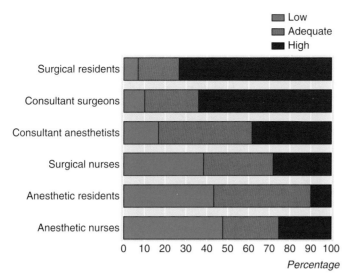

Figure 30-1 Surgeons in the operating room view the level of teamwork as much higher than nursing and anesthesia do. (Reproduced from Sexton JB, Thomas EJ, Helmreich RL. Error, stress, and teamwork in medicine and aviation: cross sectional surveys. *BMJ* 2000;320(7237):745-749; with permission from BMJ Publishing Group Ltd.)

that of the most predictive factors in success of any military unit is the emotional intelligence of the leader, and EQ is now a focus of leadership training in the military.

When Google sought to identify a common factor of their highest functioning teams, they concluded that psychological safety was the most important factor.[2] Harvard Business School professor Amy Edmondson defines psychological safety as a "shared belief held by members of a team that the team is safe for interpersonal risk-taking." Members of the team feel "a sense of confidence that the team will not embarrass, reject or punish someone for speaking up." As a leader you can help create that culture by showing your vulnerability, sharing mistakes you made, asking and listening to everyone's opinions, and not allowing some member of the team to talk over others. Realize that when someone makes a suggestion, they are taking a risk of being rejected or embarrassed. Thank team members for even bad ideas and they will remain engaged and helpful.

Steve Jobs, who everyone thought was the secret to Apple's success, said, "The secret to my success is that we've gone to exceptional lengths to hire the best people in the world." You should go to extraordinary lengths to identify, recruit, and retain the best people. Simultaneously, be mindful that a single toxic team member can bring down the entire team and must be removed. When leaders tolerate mediocrity, it erodes their credibility and brings down the entire team. When you have to have a tough conversation with a team member not meeting expectations, do not do so until you are free from anger, and feel you truly want to help the person perform better. **TEAM LEADING 101: Be hard on the situation, but empathetic toward the person**. And document, document, document. Tell the person you will send them an email documenting the conversation. Human Resources generally demands multiple written warnings before someone can be removed, and putting something in writing is taken more seriously by the offender.

People will come to you with conflicts and real or perceived injustices. Stay out of trouble by always hearing both sides of the story before offering an opinion or taking sides. When you hear from the first person, say something like, "Thank you for telling me this, I take this seriously and will look into it and get back to you." Often just letting someone "vent" is enough to diffuse the situation.

Dr. Skaggs Adds

When working with a new nurse or scrub technician in the operating room, you might want to consider saying something like, "I am someone's father and I care very deeply about the health and recovery of each and every child. Please help me take the best care of this patient and avoid mistakes. Speak up if there is something I should know." There have been many, many times when suggestions by scrub technicians, implant reps, nurses, residents, or fellows have resulted in better patient care than I would have done alone. A highly functional and high performing team is the differentiator clinically.

Dr. Vitale Adds

I enjoy recognizing that I am not the smartest person in the room. In fact, my job is really more like a coach—identifying talent and orchestrating the playbook. Diversification of talent has huge benefits.

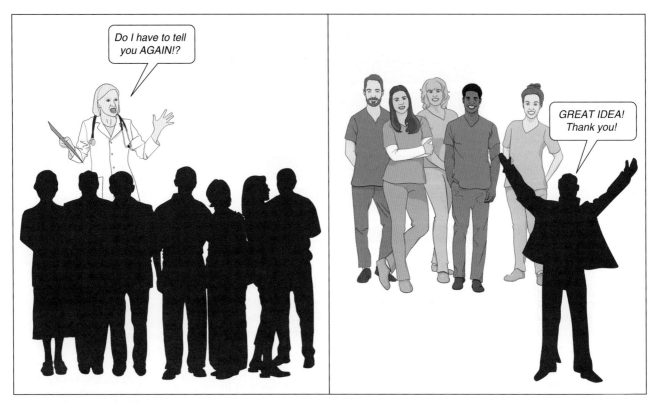

Figure 30-2 One of the best ways to stay out of trouble is to surround yourself with a great team of people with the shared mission of caring for children, pursuing excellence, and caring for each other.

> **THE GURU SAYS...**
>
> Leading with a sense of optimism and hope is one key consideration for your leadership profile. To be consistently optimistic and not negative or reactionary are among the hallmarks of an inspirational leader.
>
> PAUL S. VIVIANO

As a leader you have the opportunity and responsibility to create a culture of excellence, positivity, and accountability (Fig. 30-2). Of course, this starts with you as an example. Aim for the sweet spot where team members feel they are part of an elite team, and they *want* to work hard for pride, mission, and approval of other team members. Aim for a team that *wants* to come to work and enjoys returning to work after a vacation. Expressing a genuine interest in your team members' overall happiness and welfare, as well as lightness and humor, will help build the culture. Caring about your team members on both a personal level and professionally engenders loyalty and commitment.

Regularly praise team members, but remember to be most effective there should be an honest mix of positive and negative feedback. Gottam has shown that in marriages the "magic ratio" is 5 to 1.[3] This means that for every negative interaction during conflict, a stable and happy marriage has five (or more) positive interactions. Try to "catch them doing something right" as an effective way to give positive feedback and drive people to do their best. A good rule of thumb is to praise publicly and criticize privately.

> **Dr. Noonan Adds**
>
> After a particularly challenging case is managed well or the team performs above and beyond the call of duty, I will share a short email with the leadership of the OR. I express appreciation for the skills of the team, the efforts to perform at the highest level, and that I am honored to be a member of the team. Many times these emails are read in department meetings and provide a huge boost for morale.

A challenge for busy surgeons is to have enough time for one-on-one discussions with team members. Make yourself available; you may find it useful to walk through the office and clinic between surgeries. Ask people how things are going. People will tell you things when they see you in the hallway that they would not have otherwise told you if they had to make an appointment to see you. Knowing this "water cooler" information is invaluable. Ask a few trusted lieutenants to report to you if there is conflict or there are issues you should know about; early intervention can prevent major problems before they occur.

Daniel Pink tells us that what that high-functioning individuals are motivated by mission, mastery, and autonomy. We are lucky that our mission of helping children is clear, but it is often helpful to explicitly state this mission and keep the team focused and centered. Mastery of surgery and medicine is also an easy goal. So all we have to do as leaders, if Daniel Pink is correct, is get out of the way and allow our team members some autonomy. If you have hired the right people, they want to do great things.

> ### Two Pitfalls of Rookie Managers[4]
>
> 1. Worrying that if their team members do all the work, they get all the credit. Does anyone recognize the manager?
> 2. Hesitancy to let go and actually let others have real responsibility

Hospitals don't always subscribe to having specialized teams, as there are economies that the hospital benefits by having people that can cross cover on multiple services. That doesn't mean you cannot develop "your team." There are lots of informal opportunities to make people feel part of the team.

And, finally, some thoughts about dealing most effectively with the leaders above you. Perhaps approaching your leaders from a position of consciously shared mission and positivity is the best advice we can give. When your ability to care for patients is compromised by chronic issues that an institution does not seem to care about, we all feel frustrated and are tempted complain with justified indignation. A Dean of Faculty at a prestigious medical school recently noted that the angriest "problem" physicians were generally aggressive in advocating for and protecting their patients. Of course, approaching your superior with anger or confrontation can turn that relationship into an adversarial one, and you are less likely to effect change that can ultimately help your patients. The archetypal figure of a surgeon getting what they want by threats and demands should be historic and laughable. Such figures are polarizing and not effective members of present-day health care teams. Reflecting anger is never acceptable.

In general, health care executives and chairs genuinely want to provide the best care to patients and want to support doctors. If you can phrase your requests as opportunities to partner toward improving patient care or the work environment rather than complaints, you will likely have more impact. Try to feel that you are sitting on the same side of the table with them, working toward the same goal.

A basic principle for any negotiation is to understand the other person's needs. Often all you have to do is ask—there is a good chance your leaders see things you don't, and you may never know about if you don't ask them. Remember that orthopaedic leaders are more likely to be emotionally exhausted and unsatisfied with their positions than the surgeons under them. Approach them with empathy, and the favor may be returned.

While books are written on preparing yourself to be a good leader, one inarguable but often overlooked tool is getting enough sleep. This can be a real challenge for a busy surgeon. It has been shown that when bosses slept poorly, they were

Dr. Skaggs Adds

I love to say to a team member "Let's take a walk" as I leave clinic, go to the OR, or round on patients. Walking meetings are spontaneous, low stress, and the person you are with appreciates the one-on-one time in which you focus on them. Somehow people seem more open and willing to share when walking.

Dr. Vitale Adds

I will start my OR an hour late and have a breakfast meeting with the staff assigned to my room. They generally do not have time allocated to talk and plan away from their clinical responsibilities. This is a great opportunity to get people engaged without asking them to come in early or stay late. Consider some social events outside the hospital as a thank you for their effort.

Dr. Flynn Adds

It is very easy to develop blind spots as a leader that others are hesitant to point out to you. A 360° review can help you see them.[5] As you ascend as a leader, leadership is associated with "brain damage"[6] and lack of empathy. Beware of being "holier than thou"—getting more help than others in clinic, not taking call, getting a free pass and missing deadlines, harping on being on time when you're the one who's late, etc, etc, etc.

more likely to exhibit abusive behavior the next day, resulting in lower levels of engagement among subordinates.[7] Take comfort that as a leader you are sleeping for the welfare of others. Short naps can be like hitting a reset button for your mood.

Welcome leadership with open arms! It is one of the most enjoyable and deeply satisfying part of our profession. The effort you put into developing yourself as a leader and into leading your team will pay rich rewards throughout your career.

SOURCES OF WISDOM

1. Bradberry T, Greaves J. *Emotional Intelligence 2.0*. San Diego, CA: TalentSmart; 2009.
2. Duhigg C. What Google learned from its quest to build the perfect team. *NY Times*. February 25, 2016. Available at https://www.nytimes.com/2016/02/28/magazine/what-google-learned-from-its-quest-to-build-the-perfect-team.html.
3. Benson K. *The magic relationship ratio, according to science*. Gottam Institute; 2017. Available at https://www.gottman.com/blog/the-magic-relationship-ratio-according-science/.
4. HBR guide to coaching employees. *Harv Bus Rev*. 2014.
5. Nurudeen SM, Kwakye G, Berry WR, et al. Can 360-degree reviews help surgeons? Evaluation of multisource feedback for surgeons in a multi-institutional quality improvement project. *J Am Coll Surg*. 2015;221:837-844.
6. Useem J. Power causes brain damage. *Atlantic*. July/August 2017. Available at https://www.theatlantic.com/magazine/archive/2017/07/power-causes-brain-damage/528711/.
7. Barnes CM. Sleep well, lead better. *Harv Bus Rev*. September/October 2018. Available at https://hbr.org/2018/09/sleep-well-lead-better.

Index

Note: Page numbers followed by "f" indicate figures, "t" indicate tables and "b" indicate boxes.